The Founders of Operative Surgery

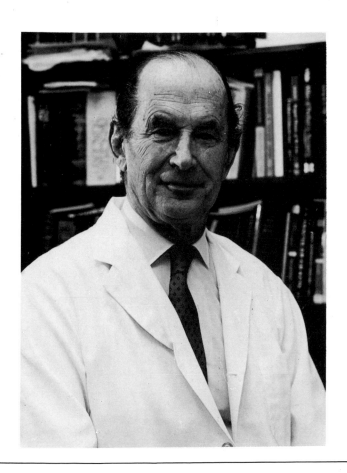

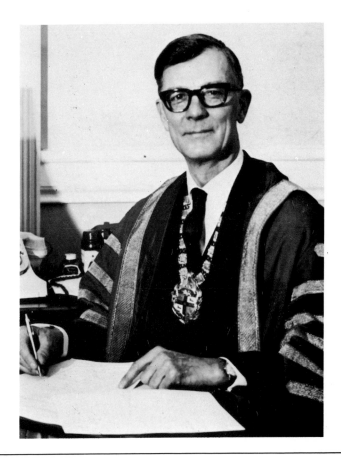

Charles Granville Rob MC, MChir, MD, FRCS, FACS
Professor of Surgery, Department of Surgery, Uniformed
Services University of the Health Sciences, F. Edward Hébert
School of Medicine, Bethesda, Maryland
Quondam: Professor of Surgery, St Mary's Hospital Medical
School, London 1950–1960;
Professor and Chairman, Department of Surgery, University of
Rochester, New York, 1960–1978;
Professor of Surgery, East Carolina University, 1978–1983

Lord Smith of Marlow KBE, MS, FRCS, Hon DSc
(Exeter and Leeds), Hon MD (Zurich), Hon FRACS,
Hon FRCS(Ed), Hon FACS, Hon FRCS(Can), Hon FRCSI,
Hon FCS(SA), Hon FDS
Honorary Consulting Surgeon, St George's Hospital, London
Quondam: Surgeon, St George's Hospital, London,
1946–1978;
President of the Royal College of Surgeons of England,
1973–1977

Rob & Smith's

Operative Surgery

Plastic Surgery

Fourth Edition

Rob & Smith's
Operative Surgery

General Editors

Hugh Dudley ChM, FRCS(Ed), FRACS, FRCS
Professor of Surgery, St Mary's Hospital, London, UK

David C. Carter MD, FRCS(Ed), FRCS(Glas)
St Mungo Professor of Surgery, University of Glasgow;
Honorary Consultant Surgeon, Royal Infirmary, Glasgow, UK

R. C. G. Russell MS, FRCS
Consultant Surgeon, Middlesex Hospital, St John's Hospital for Diseases of the Skin,
and Royal National Nose, Throat and Ear Hospital, London, UK

Rob & Smith's
Operative Surgery

Plastic Surgery

Fourth Edition

Edited by

T. L. Barclay ChM, FRCS, FRCS(Ed)
Formerly Consultant Plastic Surgeon, Bradford Royal Infirmary and St Luke's Hospital, Bradford, UK

and

Desmond A. Kernahan MD, FRCS(C), FACS
Chief, Division of Plastic Surgery, Children's Memorial Hospital, Chicago;
Professor of Surgery, North Western University Medical School, Chicago, Illinois, USA

Butterworths
London Boston Durban Singapore Sydney Toronto Wellington

© Butterworths 1986

First edition published in eight volumes 1956–1958
Second edition published in fourteen volumes 1968–1971
Third edition published in nineteen volumes 1976–1981
Fourth edition published 1983–

British Library Cataloguing in Publication Data

Rob, Charles
    Rob & Smith's operative surgery. – 4th ed.
    Plastic Surgery
    1. Surgery
    I. Title   II. Smith, Rodney Smith, *Baron*
    III. Barclay, T. L.   IV. Kernahan, Desmond A.
    V. Rob, Charles. Operative surgery
    617   RD31

    ISBN 0-407-00664-8

Library of Congress Cataloging in Publication Data
(Revised for volume 7)

Rob & Smith's operative surgery.

    Rev. ed. of: Operative surgery. 3rd ed. 1976–1981.
    Includes bibliographies and indexes.
    Contents; [1] Alimentary tract and abdominal wall.
1. General principles, oesophagus, stomach, duodenum,
small intestine, abdominal wall, hernia/edited by
Hugh Dudley – [2] Urology/edited by W. Scott
McDougal – [etc.] – [7] Plastic surgery/edited by
T. L. Barclay, Desmond A. Kernahan.
    1. Surgery, Operative–Collected works. I. Rob,
Charles. II. Smith of Marlow, Rodney Smith, Baron,
1914– . III. Dudley, Hugh A. F. (Hugh Arnold
Freeman) IV. Pories, Walter J. V. Carter, David C.
(David Craig) VI. Operative surgery. [DNLM: 1. Surgery,
Operative. WO 500 061 1982]
RD32.06   1983   617'.91   83-14465
ISBN 0-407-00651-6 (v. 1)

Photoset by Butterworths Litho Preparation Department
Printed by Blantyre Printing Ltd, London & Glasgow
Bound by Robert Hartnoll Ltd, Bodmin, Cornwall

Volumes and Editors

Alimentary Tract and Abdominal Wall

1 **General Principles · Oesophagus ·
   Stomach · Duodenum · Small Intestine ·
   Abdominal Wall · Hernia**

Hugh Dudley ChM, FRCS(Ed), FRACS, FRCS
Professor of Surgery, St Mary's Hospital, London, UK

2 **Liver · Portal Hypertension · Spleen ·
   Biliary Tract · Pancreas**

Hugh Dudley ChM, FRCS(Ed), FRACS, FRCS
Professor of Surgery, St Mary's Hospital, London, UK

3 **Colon, Rectum and Anus**

Ian P. Todd MS, MD(Tor), FRCS, DCH
Consulting Surgeon, St Bartholomew's Hospital, London;
Consultant Surgeon, St Mark's Hospital and
King Edward VII Hospital for Officers, London, UK

L. P. Fielding MB, FRCS
Chief of Surgery, St Mary's Hospital, Waterbury, Connecticut, USA;
Associate Professor of Surgery, Yale University, Connecticut, USA

Cardiac Surgery

Stuart W. Jamieson MB, FRCS, FACS
Professor and Head, Cardiothoracic Surgery,
University of Minnesota, Minneapolis, Minnesota, USA

Norman E. Shumway MD, PhD, FACS, FRCS
Professor and Chairman, Department of Cardiovascular Surgery,
Stanford University School of Medicine, California, USA

The Ear

John C. Ballantyne CBE, FRCS, HonFRCSI, DLO
Consultant Ear, Nose and Throat Surgeon,
Royal Free and King Edward VII Hospital for Officers, London, UK

Andrew Morrison FRCS
Senior Surgeon, Ear, Nose and Throat Department, The London Hospital, UK

General Principles, Breast and Extracranial Endocrines

Hugh Dudley ChM, FRCS(Ed), FRACS, FRCS
Professor of Surgery, St Mary's Hospital, London, UK

Walter J. Pories MD, FACS
Professor and Chairman, Department of Surgery, School of Medicine,
East Carolina University, Greenville, North Carolina, USA

Gynaecology and Obstetrics

J. M. Monaghan MB, FRCS(Ed), MRCOG
Consultant Surgeon, Regional Department of Gynaecological Oncology,
Queen Elizabeth Hospital, Gateshead, UK

The Hand

Rolfe Birch FRCS
Consultant Orthopaedic Surgeon, PNI Unit and Hand Clinic,
Royal National Orthopaedic Hospital, London and
St Mary's Hospital, London, UK

Donal Brooks MA, MB, FRCS, FRSCI
Consulting Orthopaedic Surgeon, University College Hospital
and Royal National Orthopaedic Hospital, London, UK;
Civilian Consultant in Hand Surgery to the Royal Navy and
Royal Air Force

Neurosurgery

Lindsay Symon TD, FRCS, FRCS(Ed)
Professor of Neurological Surgery, Institute of Neurology,
The National Hospital, Queen Square, London, UK

David G. T. Thomas MRCP, FRCSE
Senior Lecturer and Consultant Neurosurgeon,
Institute of Neurology, The National Hospital,
Queen Square, London, UK

Kemp Clarke MD
Professor and Chairman, Division of Neurological Surgery,
Southwestern Medical School, Dallas, Texas, USA

Nose and Throat

John C. Ballantyne CBE, FRCS, HonFRCSI, DLO
Consultant Ear, Nose and Throat Surgeon,
Royal Free and King Edward VII Hospital for Officers, London, UK

D. F. N. Harrison MD, MS, PhD, FRCS, FRACS
Professor of Laryngology and Otology,
Royal National Throat, Nose and Ear Hospital, London, UK

Ophthalmic Surgery

Thomas A. Rice MD
Assistant Clinical Professor of Ophthalmology,
Case Western Reserve University School of Medicine,
Cleveland, Ohio, USA;
formerly of the Wilmer Ophthalmological Institute

Ronald G. Michels MD
Professor of Ophthalmology, The Wilmer Ophthalmological Institute,
The Johns Hopkins University School of Medicine,
Maryland, USA

Walter W. J. Stark MD
Professor of Ophthalmology, The Wilmer Ophthalmological Institute,
The Johns Hopkins University School of Medicine,
Maryland, USA

Orthopaedics (in 2 volumes)

George Bentley ChM, FRCS
Professor of Orthopaedic Surgery, Institute of Orthopaedics,
Royal National Orthopaedic Hospital, London, UK

Paediatric Surgery

L. Spitz PhD, FRCS
Nuffield Professor of Paediatric Surgery and Honorary
Consultant Paediatric Surgeon, The Hospital for Sick Children,
Great Ormond Street, London, UK

H. Homewood Nixon MA, MB, BChir, FRCS, HonFAAP
Consultant Paediatric Surgeon, The Hospital for Sick Children,
Great Ormond Street, London and Paddington Green Children's
Hospital, St Mary's Hospital Group, London, UK

Plastic Surgery

T. L. Barclay ChM, FRCS, FRCS(Ed)
Formerly Consultant Plastic Surgeon, Bradford Royal Infirmary and
St Luke's Hospital, Bradford, West Yorkshire, UK

Desmond A. Kernahan MD, FRCS(C), FACS
Chief, Division of Plastic Surgery,
Children's Memorial Hospital, Chicago;
Professor of Surgery, North Western University
Medical School, Chicago, Illinois, USA

Thoracic Surgery

John W. Jackson MCh, FRCS
Formerly Consultant Thoracic Surgeon, Harefield Hospital, Middlesex, UK

D. K. C. Cooper PhD, FRCS, FACC
Associate Professor, Department of Cardiothoracic Surgery,
University of Cape Town Medical School and Groote Schuur Hospital, Cape
Town, South Africa

Trauma

John V. Robbs FRCS
Associate Professor of Surgery,
Department of Surgery, University of Natal, South Africa

Howard R. Champion FRCS
Chief, Trauma Service;
Director, Surgery Critical Care Services,
The Washington Hospital Center, Washington DC, USA

Donald Trunkey MD
Chairman, Department of Surgery, University of Portland, Portland, Oregon,
USA

Urology

W. Scott McDougal MD
Professor and Chairman, Department of Urology, Vanderbilt
University, Nashville, Tennessee, USA

Vascular Surgery

James A. DeWeese MD
Professor and Chairman, Division of Cardiothoracic Surgery,
University of Rochester Medical Center, Rochester, New York, USA

Contributors

Louis C. Argenta MD
Assistant Professor of Surgery, Section of Plastic and Reconstructive Surgery, University of Michigan Medical Center, Ann Arbor, Michigan, USA

Michael Awty MRCS, LRCP, FDS, RCS(Eng)
Consultant Oral and Maxillofacial Surgeon, Queen Victoria Hospital, East Grinstead, Sussex, UK

Bruce N. Bailey FRCS
Consultant Plastic Surgeon, Stoke Mandeville Hospital, Aylesbury, Buckinghamshire, UK

Vahram Y. Bakamjian MD
Chief Reconstructive Surgeon, Roswell Park Memorial Institute, New York, USA

T. L. Barclay ChM, FRCS, FRCS(Ed)
Formerly Consultant Plastic Surgeon, Bradford Royal Infirmary and St Luke's Hospital, Bradford, UK

Bruce S. Bauer MD, FACS, FAAP
Attending Plastic Surgeon, Division of Plastic Surgery, Children's Memorial Hospital, Chicago; Assistant Professor, Department of Surgery, Northwestern University Medical School, Chicago, Illinois, USA

D. C. Bodenham FRCS, FRCS(Ed)
Consultant Plastic Surgeon, Frenchay Hospital and United Bristol Hospitals, Bristol, UK

Nicholas M. Breach FRCS, FDS, RCS
Consultant Surgeon, Head and Neck Unit, The Royal Marsden Hospital, London, UK

I. W. Broomhead MA, MChir, FRCS
Consultant Plastic Surgeon, The Hospital for Sick Children and Guy's Hospital, London, UK

F. S. C. Browning FRCS
Consultant Plastic Surgeon, Leeds General Infirmary, Leeds, UK

Gary C. Burget MD, FACS
Plastic Surgeon, Chicago, Illinois, USA

Elethea H. Caldwell MD
Associate Professor of Plastic Surgery, University of Rochester School of Medicine and Dentistry, Rochester, New York, USA

James Calnan FRCP, FRCS
Professor of Plastic and Reconstructive Surgery, Royal Postgraduate Medical School, Hammersmith Hospital, London, UK

John R. Cobbett FRCS
Consultant Plastic Surgeon, The Queen Victoria Hospital, East Grinstead and Lewisham Hospital, London, UK

I. Kelman Cohen MD, FACS
Professor of Surgery, Division of Plastic and Reconstructive Surgery, Medical College of Virginia, Richmond, Virginia, USA

Bard Cosman MD
Formerly Professor of Clinical Surgery, Columbia University College of Physicians and Surgeons, New York, USA

R. L. G. Dawson FRCS
Formerly Plastic Surgeon, Mount Vernon Hospital, Northwood, Middlesex, and Royal Free Hospital, London, UK

Charles J. Devine Jr MD
Professor and Chairman, Department of Urology, Eastern Virginia Medical School, Norfolk, Virginia, USA

A. J. Evans FRCS
Consultant Plastic Surgeon, Westminster Hospital, London, Queen Mary's Hospital, Roehampton, and Croydon General Hospital, Croydon, UK

David M. Evans FRCS
Consultant Plastic Surgeon, Wexham Park Hospital, Slough and Ashford Hospital, Middlesex, UK

Gregory S. Georgiade MD
Assistant Professor, General and Plastic and Reconstructive Surgery, Duke University Medical Center, Durham, North Carolina, USA

Nicholas G. Georgiade MD, FACS
Chairman and Professor, Division of Plastic and Reconstructive Surgery, Duke University Medical Center, Durham, North Carolina, USA

Michael F. Green FRCS, FRCS(Ed)
Consultant Plastic Surgeon, Welsh Centre for Burns, Plastic and Reconstructive Surgery, St Lawrence Hospital, Chepstow, Wales, UK

Michael E. J. Hackett FRCS
Consultant Plastic Surgeon, The London Hospital, and St Andrew's Hospital, Billericay, UK

Kiyonori Harii MD
Associate Professor, Plastic Surgery, University of Tokyo Hospital, Tokyo, Japan

Ronald W. Hiles FRCS, FRCS(Ed)
Consultant Plastic Surgeon, Frenchay Hospital, Bristol, Avon, UK

Michael Hobsley TD, MA, MChir, PhD, FRCS
Professor of Surgery, Head of Department of Surgical Studies, Middlesex Hospital Medical School, and Consultant Surgeon, Middlesex and University College Hospitals, London, UK

Charles E. Horton MD
Professor and Chairman, Department of Plastic Surgery, Eastern Virginia Medical School, Norfolk, Virginia, USA

Norman C. Hughes OBE, FRCS, FRCSI
Consultant Plastic Surgeon, Royal Victoria Hospital, Belfast; Royal Belfast Hospital for Sick Children and The Ulster Hospital, Dundonald, Belfast, Northern Ireland

Norman E. Hugo MD
Professor of Surgery, College of Physicians and Surgeons, Columbia University; Chief, Plastic Surgery, Department of Surgery, Columbia-Presbyterian Medical Center, New York, USA

Ian T. Jackson MD, FRCS, FACS
Professor of Plastic Surgery, Head of Plastic Surgery, Mayo Foundation, Mayo Clinic, Rochester, Minnesota, USA

Percy H. Jayes FRCS
Formerly Consultant Plastic Surgeon, St Bartholomew's Hospital, London and Queen Victoria Hospital, East Grinstead, Sussex, UK

Bernard L. Kaye MD, DMD
Clinical Professor of Surgery (Plastic), University of Florida College of Medicine, Jacksonville, Florida, USA

Desmond A. Kernahan MD, FRCS(C), FACS
Chief, Division of Plastic Surgery, Children's Memorial Hospital, Chicago; Professor of Surgery, Northwestern University Medical School, Chicago, Illinois, USA

Christopher Khoo FRCS
Consultant Plastic Surgeon, Wexham Park Hospital, Slough, Berkshire, UK

Samuel E. Logan MD, PhD
Assistant Professor, Division of Plastic Surgery, Washington University School of Medicine, St Louis, Missouri, USA

Ian A. McGregor ChM, FRCS
Director, Plastic and Oral Surgery Unit, Canniesburn Hospital, Glasgow, UK

D. O. Maisels FRCS, FRCS(Ed)
Consultant Plastic Surgeon, Mersey Regional Health Authority; Clinical Lecturer in Plastic Surgery, University of Liverpool, Liverpool, UK

W. M. Manchester CBE, FRCS, FRACS, FACS
St Mark's Clinic, Auckland, New Zealand

Timothy A. Miller MD, FACS
Professor of Surgery, UCLA School of Medicine; Chief of Plastic Surgery, Wadsworth Veterans Hospital, Los Angeles, California, USA

H. Millesi MD
Head, Unit of Plastic and Reconstructive Surgery, I Chirurgische Universitatscklinik; Director, Ludwig Boltzmann Institute of Experimental Plastic Surgery, Vienna, Austria

John C. Mustardé FRCS, FRCS(Glas)
Consulting Plastic Surgeon, West of Scotland Regional Plastic Surgery Centre, Canniesburn Hospital, and Royal Hospital for Sick Children, Glasgow, Scotland, UK

John D. Noonan MD, FACS
Associate Professor, Division of Plastic Surgery, Albany Medical College, Albany, New York, USA

T. P. F. O'Connor FRCS, FRCSI
Consultant Plastic Surgeon, Southern Health Board, The Regional Hospital, Cork, Ireland

Kitaro Ohmori MD
Director, Department of Plastic and Reconstructive Surgery, Tokyo Metropolitan Police Hospital, Tokyo, Japan

John Q. Owsley Jr MD, FACS
Clinical Professor of Surgery, Department of Plastic Surgery, University of California Medical Center, San Francisco, California; Chairman, Department of Plastic Surgery, R. K. Davies Medical Center, San Francisco, California, USA

Carl G. Quillen MD
Clinical Assistant Professor of Plastic Surgery, College of Medicine and Dentistry, Newark, New Jersey, USA

Peter Randall MD, FACS
Professor of Plastic Surgery; Chief, Division of Plastic Surgery, Hospital of the University of Pennsylvania, Pennsylvania, USA

Paule Regnault MD, FRCS(C)
Former Professor, Agrégé de Clinique, Montreal University, Montreal, Canada

R. T. Routledge FRCS
Senior Consultant Plastic Surgeon, Frenchay Hospital, UK

Richard Carlton Schultz MD
Clinical Professor of Surgery and Chief, Division of Plastic Surgery, University of Illinois College of Medicine, Illinois, USA

David T. Sharpe MA, FRCS
Consultant Plastic Surgeon, St Luke's Hospital, Bradford, UK

J. Connell Shearin Jr MD
Associate Professor of Surgery, Division of Plastic Surgery, Bowman Gray School of Medicine, Winston Salem, North Carolina, USA

P. M. Stell ChM, FRCS
Professor of Otolaryngology, University of Liverpool, UK

G. Ian Taylor FRCS, FRACS
Consultant Plastic Surgeon, The Royal Melbourne Hospital; Senior Consultant Plastic Surgeon, Preston and Northcote Community Hospital; Associate Plastic Surgeon, The University of Melbourne, Australia

D. E. Tolhurst FRCS
Academisch Ziekenhuis Rotterdam, Rotterdam, The Netherlands

Luis O. Vasconez MD
Professor of Surgery and Chief, Division of Plastic Surgery, University of Alabama in Birmingham, Birmingham, Alabama, USA

Charles Viva FRCS, FRCS(Ed)
Senior Consultant Plastic Surgeon, North and South Teeside District, Hartlepool, South West Durham and General Hospital, Middlesbrough, UK

John Watson FRCS, FRCS(Ed)
Formerly Consultant Plastic Surgeon, The London Hospital; Queen Victoria Hospital, East Grinstead, Sussex, UK

G. Westbury FRCS, FRCP
Professor of Surgery, Institute of Cancer Research and Royal Marsden Hospital, London, UK

Contributing Medical Artists

John M. P. Booth

R. Callander

Michael Carroll MA
Medical Illustrator, 1228 East 54th Street, Chicago, Illinois 60615, USA

Angela Christie MMAA
11 West End, Pinner, Middlesex HA5 1BJ, UK

Peter Cox MMAA
2 Frome Villas, Frenchay, Bristol BS16 1TL, UK

Patrick Elliott
Medical Artist, 31 Moor Oaks Road, Broomhill, Sheffield S10 1BX, UK

K. Joy Graham FMAA, AIMBI
Senior Medical Artist, Queen Victoria Hospital, East Grinstead, Sussex RH19 3DZ, UK

Gwynne Gloege

Hooker Goodwin

Richard D. Howe
Medical Illustrator, 15 Robin Street, Rochester, NY 14613, USA

Barbara Hyams MA, AMI
Medical Illustrator, Poynings, Northchurch Common, Northchurch, Berkhamsted, Hertfordshire, UK

John W. Karapelou BS, AMI
Chief Medical Illustrator, College of Physicians and Surgeons, Columbia University, 630 West 168th Street, New York, NY 10032, USA

Y. Kitabatake

Robert N. Lane
Medical Illustrator, Studio 19a, Edith Grove, London SW10, UK

Denis C. Lee MA
Professor of Medical and Biological Illustration, University of Michigan Medical Center, Ann Arbor, Michigan, USA

Gillian Lee FMAA, AIMBI
Burnham, 15 Little Plucketts Way, Buckhurst Hill, Essex IG9 5QU, UK

Michael E. Leonard MA, AMI
Medical Illustrator, Division of Audiovisual Education, Duke University Medical Center, Durham, North Carolina 27710, USA

Patrick McDonnell AMI
50 rue Pernety, Atelier No 3, 75014 Paris, France

Helen McIlhenny
Medical Artist, Formerly of Department of Medical Illustration, Royal Victoria Hospital, Belfast, Ireland

Pam McMaghie

Douglas McManamny FRACS
Registrar, Department of Plastic Surgery, The Royal Melbourne Hospital, Melbourne, Australia

Robert L. Margulies MSc, AMI
Medical Illustrator, Duke University Medical Center, Durham, NC 27710, USA

Kevin Marks BA(Hons)
3 Hilltop Court, Grange Road, Upper Norwood, London SE19 3BQ, UK

A. Marrin

Sandra Neophytu MMAA
375 Canon Hill Lane, London SW20, UK

Gillian Oliver MMAA, AIMBI
71 Crawford Road, Hatfield, Hertfordshire AL10 0PF, UK

Ian Ramsden
Head, Department of Medical Illustration, Glasgow University, UK

Deborah K. Randall BA
Medical Illustrator, Children's Hospital of Philadelphia, Cleft Palate Clinic, Philadelphia, PA 19146, USA

William Schwarz

T. R. Tarrant
Moorfields Eye Hospital, High Holborn, London WC1V 7AN, UK

Contents

Preface

The fourth edition of the Plastic Surgery volume of the Operative Surgery series appears at a time when the practice of everyday plastic surgery is undergoing a marked change. Many of the older well-tried reconstructive procedures are being superseded by those involving flaps which have been designed with a better understanding of the blood supply of skin, fascia and muscle; the newer methods described in this volume have nevertheless been thoroughly worked up over the past few years, long enough for their reliability as well as their potential hazards and drawbacks to be evaluated.

There is no doubt that further refinements of these techniques are continually being made by thoughtful and ingenious plastic surgeons the world over, and the best of these, we hope, will be described in the next edition; how long it will be before a sufficient number of significant developments demand its production is anybody's guess. In the meantime we hope we have included most of the advances made in the seven years which have elapsed since the third edition was published, retaining the one volume format. At the same time we have tried to preserve, as did our predecessors, the emphasis on careful design and execution of operations without which plastic surgery loses its special standard of excellence and degenerates into second-rate patchwork.

We hope that the principles involved are sufficiently well described for the trainee plastic surgeon, or the surgeon in another specialty confronted with an unfamiliar reconstructive problem, to embark on a repair that will succeed. At the same time it should offer the trained plastic surgeon the experience of experts should he wish to refresh his memory of some of the procedures in common use in plastic surgery departments elsewhere.

T. L. Barclay
Desmond A. Kernahan

Illustrations by Helen McIlhenny

Basic techniques of excision and wound closure

Norman C. Hughes   OBE, FRCS, FRCSI
Consultant Plastic Surgeon, Royal Victoria Hospital, Belfast,
Royal Belfast Hospital for Sick Children and The Ulster Hospital, Dundonald, Belfast, Northern Ireland

PRIMARY WOUND CLOSURE

Preoperative

The objectives in primary wound closure are to achieve rapid healing with minimal scar formation. All possible precautions must be taken in order to prevent infection as this will interfere with healing of the wound more than any other single factor. Age and ethnic group have their effect in determining the structure and appearance of the scar and, in addition, each patient has his individual response to trauma. Local factors include the depth, situation and alignment of the wound, and the amount of tissue loss or death caused by the injury. By using a meticulous technique which places viable tissues in accurate apposition and avoids any additional trauma to the tissues, a surgeon can ensure that the ultimate scarring represents an irreducible minimum.

Indications

Wounds that are suitable for primary closure fall into one of two groups: those caused by sharp instruments where there is minimal trauma to the edges of the wound; and injuries which have involved some degree of crushing of the tissues, provided the wound edges can be sutured with acceptable tension following removal of devitalized tissue. If this condition cannot be met, and especially if further swelling of the tissues is anticipated, primary suture is not indicated. In these circumstances it is often advantageous to close the wound with a split-skin graft which can subsequently be excised. This achieves primary wound closure and avoids the dangers of suture under excessive tension.

Primary wound suture should be carried out within 6–8 hours from the time of injury as a general rule, but in the case of tissues with an exceptionally good blood supply (such as the head and neck) this time limit can be extended safely to 24 hours.

Contraindications

Deeply penetrating wounds associated with heavy contamination and severe muscle damage are not suitable for primary closure. It is not possible to guarantee the removal of all foreign and devitalized material and the risks of serious infection, possibly with anaerobic organisms, are very high. High velocity bullet wounds fall into this category because the deceleration which occurs as the missile traverses the tissues results in a massive release of energy, transient cavitation and widespread damage to deep structures.

When doubt exists it is better to limit initial surgery to the removal of foreign bodies and tissue which is certainly non-viable. Adequate drainage should be provided and further debridement may be carried out over the next few days as indicated by inspection of the wound. If no non-viable tissue remains the wound can safely be sutured after several days. If closure with sutures is not possible a split-skin graft will eliminate infection and accelerate healing.

Preoperative management

A careful clinical examination may indicate damage to deeper structures. This is particularly important in the upper limb where a small skin wound may overlie serious damage to nerves and tendons. However, a complete diagnosis can often only be made at formal surgical exploration, and this should be carried out if any doubt exists about the integrity of deep structures.

There may have been a considerable loss of blood especially from wounds of the head and neck commonly encountered in road traffic accidents. In such cases blood transfusions should of course be arranged.

Careful documentation of injuries should be made, and clinical photographs are helpful in this context.

Anaesthesia

Suitable operating conditions may, in different circumstances, be provided by general, regional block or local infiltration anaesthesia. Factors influencing the choice include the extent and distribution of the injuries and the age and temperament of the patient. Even quite minor injuries in young children are best dealt with under general anaesthesia.

Where there are injuries to the face the anaesthetic should be administered by an orotracheal or nasotracheal tube, the choice depending on the exact distribution of the wounds. Brachial block anaesthesia is a good alternative to general anaesthesia for wounds of the forearm and hand, particularly if the patient's condition is poor or if he has eaten recently.

1a–d

Instruments

The instruments required are contained in the basic plastic surgery set and will reflect the individual preference of the surgeon. It is important to maintain the instruments in good condition. Fine scissors, skin hooks, dissecting forceps and needle holders are easily damaged by inappropriate use. They are designed to deal with delicate tissues and light needles and suture material and should only be used for these purposes.

The Barron scalpel handle is octagonal in shape and is much better suited to finger tip control than the traditional flat handle. Disposable blades of sizes 10, 11 and 15 will meet most requirements.

The author uses the Gillies needle holder or the small Foster needle holder for the insertion of fine sutures. These instruments are also used in tying the knot in the suture material. The needle holder is used in conjunction with Adson's dissecting forceps.

Suture materials

Cutting needles are used for most purposes. The slim blade type of needle has a flat segment which is gripped by the needle holder. This eliminates the irritating needle flick which is so liable to occur with the conventional needle of a triangular cross-section.

A wide range of suitable suture material is available premounted on eyeless needles.

Preparation

After he has scrubbed up and put on his gown and gloves the surgeon should put on a further pair of gloves whilst cleansing the patient's skin with an antiseptic solution

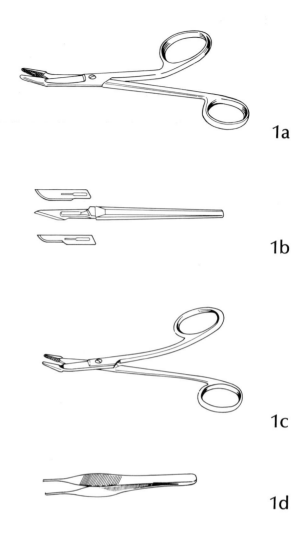

1a

1b

1c

1d

such as Cetrimide or chlorhexidine. The outer pair of gloves can then be discarded and the skin preparation completed using forceps. Hair may with advantage be shaved around wounds within the scalp but it is better to avoid cutting the hair immediately above the forehead as adequate regrowth is very slow. The eyebrows should never be shaved as the hairs provide a valuable guide to accurate wound suture.

Towels are applied to expose the full extent of the wound and also a skin graft donor site, should this be required.

The height of the operating table should be adjusted so that the surgeon can work in a comfortable position with his elbows at his sides and his forearms flexed to about 90°. This position permits a full range of wrist and hand movements, while relaxation of the shoulder girdle muscles minimizes fatigue and tremor. These considerations are of equal importance whether the surgeon is standing or sitting.

The operation

2

Detailed cleansing and inspection of the wound

The wound should be thoroughly cleansed with normal saline solution and all foreign bodies removed. This can be a tedious procedure where there is much ingrained gravel or dust, but unless it is carried out in a meticulous fashion the end result will be an ugly tattooed scar. Such disfigurement may be difficult to eradicate at a later stage, and in the case of widespread, deeply abraded areas satisfactory revision of the pigmented scar may be impossible.

In road traffic accidents multiple cubes of windscreen glass are often driven into the deeper layers of the tissue and must be identified and removed.

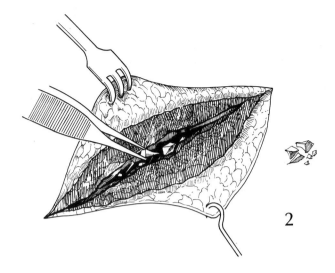

2

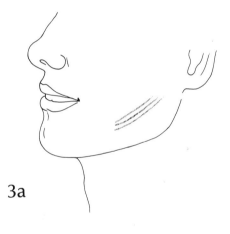

3a

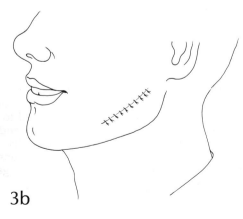

3b

3a & b

Debridement

Debridement is not usually required for clean cut wounds such as those caused by glass or sharp implements. In the case of untidy wounds all devitalized tissue and small skin tags should be excised.

Where there are multiple parallel wounds in close proximity, and provided the tissue can be spared, excision of the intervening skin bridges simplifies closure and results in a single linear scar.

Haematoma formation is a major cause of infection and wound breakdown. Meticulous haemostasis is of the utmost importance. Large blood vessels should be ligated, and it will be found that small bleeding points can be controlled rapidly using bipolar coagulation. This allows accurate haemostasis with a minimum of tissue necrosis. If complete haemostasis cannot be achieved for any reason drainage of the wound is mandatory.

4

Closure

General principles

Closure should be carried out in layers so that dead space is eliminated. Accurate repositioning of the wound edges is most important especially in the case of face injuries which often present as a very complex jig-saw. The eyebrows, eyelid margins, alar rims, columella and mucocutaneous junction of the lips are all well defined landmarks. When one of these is involved in the wound it should be accurately re-aligned at an early stage in the repair. In the case of the vermilion border of the lip it is very helpful to mark the exact position of the lip margin with ink as the red tissue will blanch under the pressure of the needle. Irregularities in the wound margin can often be matched with the other side of the wound and even wrinkle lines can provide pointers to the accurate repositioning of the tissues.

When there is a full-thickness laceration of the lip it is usually advisable to repair the mucous membrane first. An absorbable suture can be used with knots tied on the buccal surface. The muscle layer should then be repaired using an absorbable material preferably on a ⅝ circle needle. Particular attention should be paid to reconstituting the muscle at the lip margin or a notch deformity will result.

When a wound extends into the nostril it is essential to repair the mucosa first, working down to the alar margin, otherwise access will be impossible.

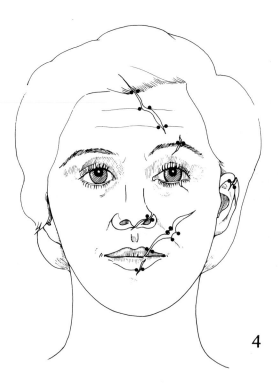

4

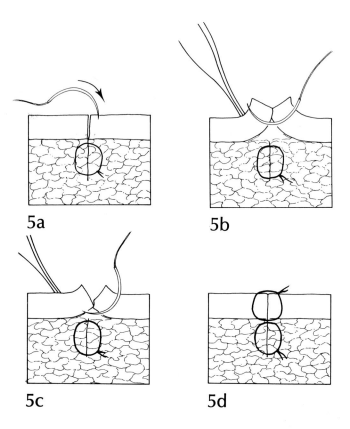

5a

5b

5c

5d

5a–d

Repair of the skin

The aim is accurate repositioning of the wound edges without the addition of further damage to the tissue. A fine curved cutting needle is used. With the forearm fully pronated the point of the needle is passed through the full-thickness of the dermis at right angles to the skin surface or even directed slightly away from the wound (a). As the forearm is supinated the curve of the needle causes the point to penetrate the dermis on the opposite side of the wound. Gentle pressure on the skin with closed Adson's forceps at a point just outside the arc of the needle will evert the skin as the needle point re-emerges (b). As an alternative technique, the skin edge can be held lightly with the Adson's forceps or with a skin hook, thus achieving eversion of the wound margin (c).

When the suture has been tied the knot should be brought to one side of the wound and the tension adjusted so that the skin edges are apposed without impairment of the blood supply (d). When sutures are tied too tightly tissue necrosis results and infection is more likely. The optimum distance between sutures will vary at different anatomical sites but on the face they should be 3–4 mm apart and placed about 2 mm from the wound edge.

In the case of scalp wounds it is advisable to use a strong needle and relatively heavy material. Closure can be carried out in a single layer or, if the galea aponeurotica is involved in the wound, it can be included in a vertical figure-of-8 suture.

6a–d

Use of adhesive skin closure strips

Small superficial wounds can sometimes be treated in a satisfactory manner by the application of sterile adhesive tapes (Steristrips), thus obviating the need for anaesthesia. Many of the finger tip injuries which occur so frequently in children can be managed by this technique. A series of adhesive tapes are applied across the end and down the sides of the finger so that the repositioned tip is held in correct position. As well as rendering anaesthesia unnecessary, the method avoids such additional trauma to the tissues as would result from the insertion of sutures.

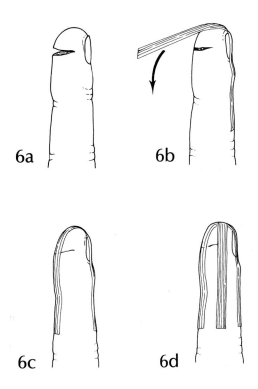

Postoperative care

Dressings

It is the author's practice to augment most suture lines with sterile adhesive tapes (Steristrips). These provide support for the wound, and as they are microporous maceration of the underlying skin is not a problem. Small wounds may require no further dressing but it is often found advantageous to appply a carefully controlled pressure dressing for the first 24–48 hours. Gauze swabs dampened with saline conform better and absorb ooze better than dry swabs. Gauze is covered with wool or gauze and the dressing held in position with a crêpe bandage or Elastoplast strapping. In the case of limb injuries elevation is of great importance in the prevention of oedema.

Removal of sutures

Sutures should be removed as early as possible consistent with adequate healing. Many factors influence this, such as the local blood supply, the direction of the wound and its tension, and the age and general condition of the patient, so that rigid rules are not appropriate. Wounds on the face usually heal rapidly and alternate sutures can be removed in 2–3 days and the remainder 2 days later. Steristrips are either left in place or re-applied in order to support the wound for a week or two. In the case of injuries to the wrist and hand where deep structures have been repaired, provided fine suture material has been used to close the skin it may safely be left *in situ* for several weeks until the plaster splint has been removed. Wounds on the hands of children can be closed with fine absorbable suture material such as 6/0 chromic catgut which avoids the distress and trauma of attempts at suture removal.

Late treatment

About 3 weeks after the sutures have been removed a programme of grease massage of the scars can be instituted. This may aid the dispersal of oedema and induration. The patient should be instructed to carry out this massage using lanolin, olive oil or Nivea cream but it is important to stress that massage is the important ingredient and not the mere application of a greasy substance.

SCAR EXCISION

Preoperative

Introduction

The aim of scar revision is reduced disfigurement or improved function. Such surgery should, therefore, only be undertaken when there is a high likelihood of effecting a significant improvement in one or both of these defects. Among the factors which need to be considered are the nature of the preceding trauma, the age of the patient and the situation and line of the scar in relation to normal lines of tension. Injuries in children often result in hypertrophic scars and these mature much less quickly than in adult patients. There is considerable individual variation in response to trauma and valuable information can be obtained by an inspection of scars from previous trauma or surgery.

Indications

Scars which are likely to benefit from revisional surgery usually fall into one of the following categories.

1. Scars with contour defects (puckered, elevated or depressed scars, or those which are stepped with a disparity between the skin levels on each side of the scar);
2. Scars that are adherent to underlying structures;
3. Scars that are pigmented due to retained foreign material;
4. Scars that are causing distortion of important features such as the lips or eyelids.

Attempts to camouflage these types of scar with cosmetic preparations are unlikely to be successful.

Contraindications

It is important to resist the temptation to revise scars which have only recently healed. They should be left for up to 12 months to allow natural resolution to occur. In many cases the degree of spontaneous improvement will make surgery unnecessary. In the others surgery will be technically easier and the chances of improvement much greater.

Certain anatomical regions so commonly produce hypertrophic scar as a response to injury or surgery that scar revision is not generally advisable. These sites include the deltoid and presternal areas. Repeated injections into the scar of small doses of triamcinalone often produce improvement and are preferable to excisional surgery.

Scars over the extensor aspects of the major joints, particularly the knee and elbow, always stretch. This is likely to recur following revision.

Anaesthesia

Local anaesthesia is satisfactory in many cases, and a solution containing a low concentration of adrenaline will reduce bleeding and facilitate the surgery. It is important to draw the plan of surgery before infiltrating the local anaesthetic as the volume of fluid will cause significant distortion of soft tissues. General anaesthesia is preferred when the patient is young or apprehensive, or when a major scar revision is to be undertaken.

The operations

7a–f

Total scar excision

A line is drawn with methylene blue to enclose the scar and 1–2 mm of adjacent skin. An incision is made through this line at right angles to the skin. Initially this incision is made through only part of the thickness of the dermis and is then continued through its full thickness. Accurate incision at the extremities of the scar is facilitated by the use of a No. 11 blade. A full-thickness excision of the scar is then completed. The wound edges should be slightly undermined just beneath the dermis thus making it easier to evert the skin edges when the wound is subsequently sutured. Fine absorbable suture material is used to bring together the deeper layers of the wound and placed so that the knots will be buried. The suture material is cut flush with the knot. Skin edges should now be almost in apposition and accurate closure is completed with fine nylon sutures.

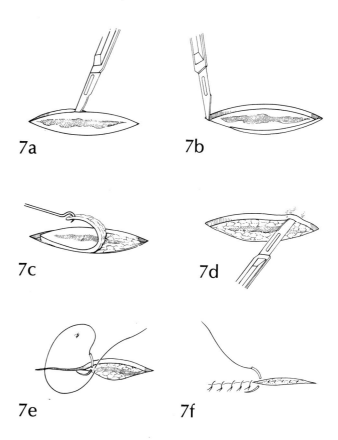

7a

7b

7c

7d

7e

7f

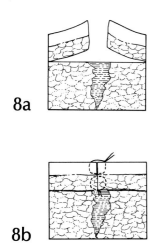

8a

8b

8a & b

Partial-thickness scar excision

Depressed scars can often be improved by this variation in technique. A deep portion of the scar is left *in situ*. Adjacent skin and subcutaneous tissues are mobilized and sutured in layers over the residual scar tissue. This increases the bulk of tissue in the region and helps to correct the depression.

9a–d

Serial excision of scars

Some scars are so wide that total excision would result in a wound which could not be closed with sutures. In many cases it it possible to remove a portion of the scar as a first stage followed by further excisions at intervals of about 6 months until the whole scar or a substantial portion of it has been excised. This technique is particularly valuable in reducing or eliminating areas of alopecia on the scalp due to scar tissue or split-skin grafting. An incision is made around one margin of the scar. The normal tissues adjacent to the scar are then widely undermined and advanced over the scarred area in order to assess the maximum possible excision that can be carried out with direct wound closure. After an interval the procedure is repeated on the opposite side of the scar.

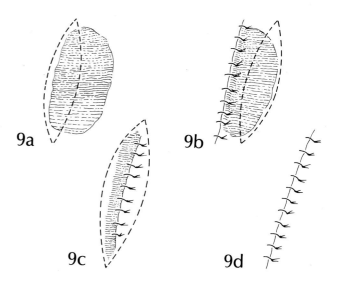

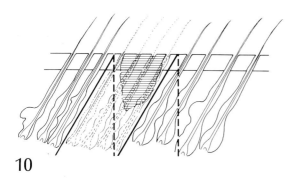

10

Scars in hair-bearing areas

When scars are to be revised in the scalp or eyebrows it is important to make the incisions parallel to the direction of the hair follicles. This minimizes damage to the hair follicles and prevents the development of a further broad hairless scar.

11a–h

Trapdoor and U-shaped scars

Trapdoor scars result from the elevation and subsequent replacement of small skin flaps. Contraction of the disc of scar underlying the flap leads to elevation of the overlying skin. This produces a conspicuous contour defect which is best treated by excising the area as an ellipse and suturing the defect as a straight line.

Contraction at the periphery of a U-shaped scar leads to bunching of the tissues contained within it. If sufficient tissue is available the best method of treatment is excision of the whole area and wound closure as in a trapdoor scar. If this is impossible only a segment of the scar should be excised at one time either as a simple ellipse with direct closure or by breaking the line of the scar by inserting several Z-plasties or by a W-plasty excision.

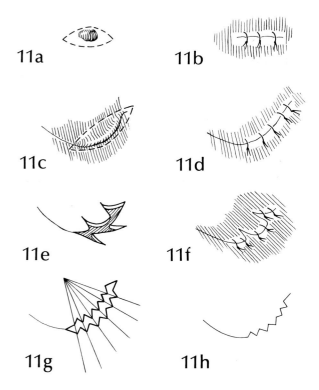

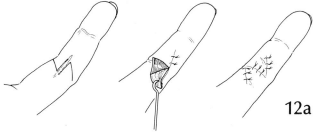

12a

12a–d

The place of Z-plasty in scar excision

The Z-plasty is a simple procedure involving the transposition of two triangular flaps. Tissue is advanced into the central portion of the Z, thus increasing its length and at the same time the common limb of the Z is altered in direction. The first effect is utilized in scars that cross concavities producing a tight web of tissue, or in scars that cross convex surfaces resulting in indentations (e.g. the lower border of the mandible). The second effect is particularly useful when treating scars which traverse the natural crease lines on the face. In such a situation the common limb of the Z can be repositioned in a favourable line. By this means a straight scar may be broken up into a number of smaller components, some of which are hidden in crease lines and, although the eventual scar is longer than the original, the overall effect is much less noticeable to the observer. Transposition of the flaps may also be used to reposition structures which have been misplaced in the original wound repair.

Technique

A plan is carefully marked out so that the common limb of the Z lies along the line of the scar to be excised and the ends of the other limbs lie in the line of a normal skin crease. All limbs of the Z should be of equal length. The 60° angle of the standard Z-plasty may need to be modified to place the limbs in the optimum direction. It should be noted that as the angle is reduced from 60° the lengthening effect is correspondingly reduced. After the scar has been excised the flaps are raised, transposed and sutured in their new position.

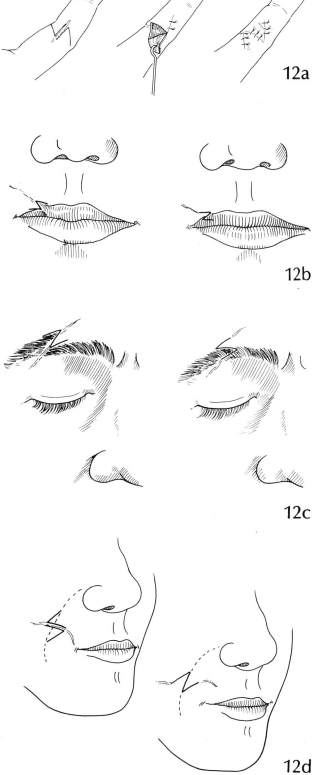

12b

12c

12d

13a & b

The place of the W-plasty in scar revision

Like the Z-plasty, the W-plasty may be used to break up the line of a scar on the face. Unlike the Z-plasty there is no increase in length between the ends of the scar. It may be used in situations where an increase in length would be a disadvantage. Like the Z-plasty, tissue is advanced from the side into the scar and both methods are dependent on a relative surplus of tissue at right angles to the scar. They should not be used where there is an increase in tension in this plane or where advancement of tissue would lead to distortion of an important structure such as the lip margin.

Technique

The scar is excised together with multiple 5 mm triangles of skin on either side and small isosceles triangles at each end. The triangles are planned so that they will interdigitate when the wound is sutured.

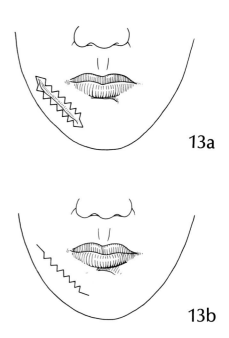

13a

13b

EXCISION OF TUMOURS WITH DIRECT CLOSURE OF DEFECT

Introduction

Many small lesions are suitable for excision and direct closure. They fall into three categories.

1. *Benign*, e.g. cutaneous papillomas, sebaceous cysts, dermoid cysts. Removal may be for cosmetic reasons or designed to prevent the occurrence of episodes of infection.
2. *Potentially malignant*, e.g. junctional cell naevi in sites liable to irritation, sebaceous naevi, senile keratoses. Excision is highly desirable in order to eliminate the risk of malignant change developing later.
3. *Malignant*, e.g. basal cell carcinomas, squamous carcinomas. Here the prime objective is complete removal of the tumour and the extent of the excision necessary to achieve this must never be compromised by consideration as to closure of the resulting defect. Experience is necessary to assess how much surrounding normal tissue should be removed. This varies with the type and nature of the lesion, but with a basal cell

growth 5–10 mm clearance all round is usually adequate while with a squamous cell carcinoma this margin should be increased to 10–15 mm.

If there is any doubt about the completeness of excision the application of a split-skin graft is preferable to direct closure or a flap repair, as it will permit the detection of any recurrence at an early stage. In the absence of recurrence it is a simple matter to excise the graft and carry out a definitive repair at a later date.

Pathological examination

All specimens, other than those benign lesions where the diagnosis is not in doubt, should be sent for histopathological examination. Preoperative biopsy is not advised; with small tumours the best biopsy is an excisional one.

The operations

14

Lines of election for scars

The most favourable lines for scars follow the skin wrinkles which form at right angles to the general direction of contracture of the underlying muscles.

As many of the lesions suitable for excision and direct closure occur on the face it is essential to appreciate these skin lines which are produced by the muscles of expression. They are not well marked in the young but become obvious in later life as the skin loses its elasticity. Favourable lines for facial scars are shown

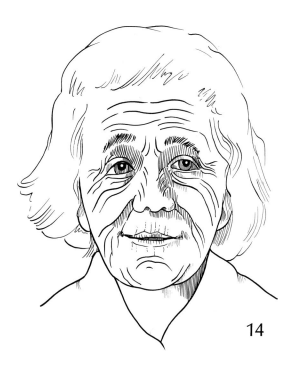

14

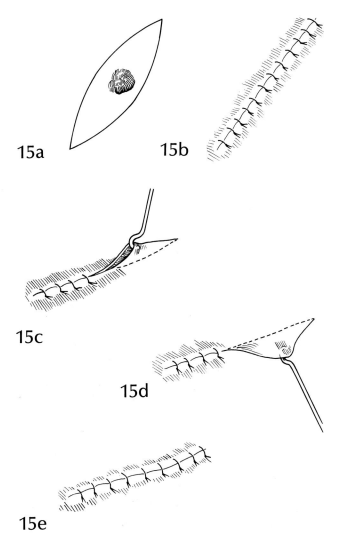

15a   15b

15c

15d

15e

15a–e

Simple elliptical excision

The ellipse is drawn around the part to be removed with its long axis ideally following a wrinkle line. The tissue within the ellipse, which includes the lesion together with the necessary margin of normal skin, is then excised and the wound edges are undermined sufficiently to permit closure in layers without undue tension on the suture line. Should 'dog ears' appear at the ends of the wound they are removed as shown. A skin hook is inserted in the end of the incision and the redundant tissue is elevated and incised around its base on one side. The resulting skin flap is then carried across the wound and the excess is removed.

16a & b

Excision using a lazy S 'ellipse'

With larger lesions more skin can be conserved to close the defect by off-setting the ends of the 'ellipse'. This method does not give a straight line closure, but in certain sites this is an advantage.

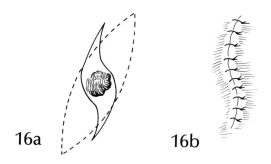

16a   16b

17a, b & c

Circular excision and closure with subcutaneous pedicle flaps

This technique also makes use of skin which would be discarded in a simple elliptical excision. After excising the lesion triangular subcutaneous pedicle flaps are advanced in V–Y fashion to close the defect.

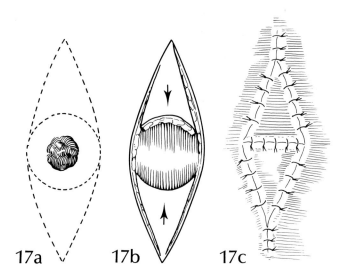

17a   17b   17c

18a   18b

18c   18d

18e   18f

Wedge excision and direct closure

Full-thickness wedge excision with closure in layers is particularly suitable for lesions on or near the free margins of the lips or eyelids. Up to a third of either lip or up to a quarter of either eyelid can be removed and the defect repaired by direct closure.

Technique

18a–f

Lip The tissue to be removed is outlined and the mucocutaneous junction is defined with tattoo marks. The lip is compressed on each side to limit blood loss and the incisions are made through the skin only using a No. 15 blade and then removal is completed with a No. 11 blade passed through the full-thickness of the lip. The muscle layer is defined by undermining the skin and mucous membrane and the defect is closed in three layers, the tattoo marks being used to achieve accurate re-alignment of the mucocutaneous junction.

A W excision instead of a V may be used for central lesions of the lower lip.

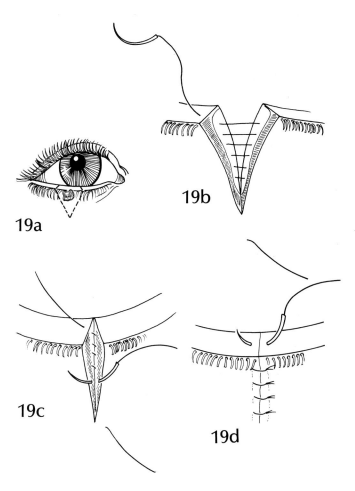

19a

19b

19c

19d

19a–d

Eyelid   The wedge to be removed is first marked on the skin and then excised. A continuous pull-out suture of 6/0 nylon is used to bring together the conjunctiva and tarsal plate from each side of the defect. The orbicularis muscle is sutured with 6/0 catgut and the skin is closed with interrupted sutures of fine nylon. A fine silk suture is used to approximate accurately the lid margin.

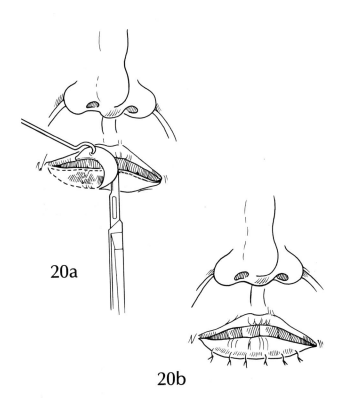

20a

20b

20a & b

Lip shave

This procedure is valuable for premalignant change extending along the red margin of the lip and can be combined with a wedge excision if required. The involved strip of mucosa is excised and the resulting defect repaired by advancement of the lining mucous membrane, only minimal undermining being required.

Further reading

Grabb, W. C, Smith, J. W. eds. Plastic surgery, a concise guide to clinical practice, 2nd edn. Boston: Little, Brown & Co., 1973

Converse, J. M. Kazanjian and Converse's surgical treatment of facial injuries, 3rd edn. Baltimore: Williams & Wilkins, 1974

McGregor, Ian A. ed. Fundamental Techniques of Plastic Surgery and their surgical applications, 6th edn. Edinburgh and London: Churchill Livingstone, 1975

Restoration of skin cover: the use of free grafts

Michael E. J. Hackett FRCS
Consultant Plastic Surgeon, The London Hospital and St Andrew's Hospital, Billericay, UK

Introduction

When an area of the body is partially or totally denuded of skin the following untoward events can occur.

1. Invasion by bacteria.
2. Loss of fluid, protein and energy.
3. Damage to important underlying structures such as nerves, vessels, tendons.
4. Pain.
5. Ugly scarring.

It would seem obvious that the sooner the defect is closed the better. In small lesions which will heal spontaneously the application of sterile dressings is adequate; in the case of full-thickness defects, apposition of the edges with sutures solves the problem. Larger defects are best closed permanently with the patient's own skin or temporarily with tissue resembling the patient's skin. This grafting procedure is often delayed unnecessarily because of the lack of available expertise, and what was previously a comparatively easy problem becomes much more difficult. Since grafting is such a simple procedure all that is needed is a little confidence and knowledge, and many defects can be closed early before the unpleasant events occur.

This chapter aims to enable a surgeon with no previous experience to perform some form of grafting whenever it is necessary.

General principles

Contraindications to skin grafting

Cross infection especially with streptococcus Grafting is carried out after control of the infection, which is usually best done by the application of local bactericidal agents, with or without systemic antibiotics.

Cortical bone denuded of periosteum; tendon denuded of paratenon; cartilage denuded of perichondrium If the areas are small (about 0.5 cm or less) a skin graft will occasionally bridge the gap, especially in children. Larger areas will require flap closure.

Heavily contaminated or irradiated areas If dirt or devitalized tissue can be effectively removed early, the area will often take a graft.

Factors contributing to the failure of grafts

Movement Grafts initially are sustained by plasmatic circulation which is rapidly replaced by ingrowth of host capillaries into the graft. Movement of a grafted area will break down these fragile connections and lead to graft loss. Therefore, complete immobilization of the grafted area will give the best chance of success.

Fluid collection beneath the graft This fluid may be blood or serum, both of which will inhibit the essential ingrowth of vessels into the graft.
   Absolute haemostasis must therefore be obtained prior to application of the graft, and even pressure must be applied over the graft to maintain complete apposition of the skin to the raw surface to prevent formation of seroma or haematoma. A haematoma will more effectively inhibit graft take than a seroma and should be evacuated as quickly as possible after formation.

Infection In clean surgical wounds this is rare, but in dirty wounds the streptococcus and pyocyaneus can destroy the graft even at a late stage. Testing of a contaminated raw area with a biological dressing prior to autografting will often prevent failure due to infection (*see below*).

Grafting on to unsuitable areas Irradiated tissue, bare bone, cartilage and tendons have already been mentioned. In traumatic wounds, fat which has been contused will also often have a poor take; if possible this should be removed as deep fascia and bare muscle take grafts readily, as do dermis and shaved scar tissue.

Varieties of tissue available to close raw areas effectively

Autograft This is the patient's own skin. If taken as a partial-thickness graft it can be stored under sterile conditions in a saline-soaked gauze for up to 3 weeks in a refrigerator at +4°C. Alternatively it can be taken as a full-thickness graft which includes all the layers of the skin.

Viable homograft This is partial-thickness skin taken from a fresh cadaver or a volunteer. It can be tissue typed, a good typing delaying the rejection of the tissue, and can be stored for 21 days in a refrigerator at +4°C or for a year in liquid nitrogen.

Viable xenograft This is available commercially and is usually partial-thickness porcine skin.

Freeze-dried homograft Taken from a cadaver within 3 days, this is reconstituted by soaking in saline. The freeze-drying process kills the tissue by removing the fluid component, but the architecture and most of its functions are retained.

Freeze-dried xenograft This is available commercially as lyophilized porcine skin.
   Freeze-dried homograft and xenograft are not true grafts, but biological dressings. However, they function similarly to grafts and are invaluable in this field.
   The easiest tissue to obtain and use is the commercially prepared xenograft. It can be shelf-stored for a year, is available in sheets of varying sizes enabling rapid and simple application even over large areas. Reconstitution in saline only takes a short time, so that one has virtually instant skin.

Autograft

This may be a partial-thickness (epidermis and a variable thickness of the dermis) or a full-thickness (all layers of skin) graft. In practice one uses a partial-thickness graft, a thick partial-thickness graft or a full-thickness graft. The thicker an autograft, the less it will contract, but the less chance it has of taking. Conversely, the thinner an autograft the better chance of success, but the greater the distortion as the graft contracts. Where contracture has to be avoided a thick partial-thickness graft is the best choice.

The treatment of the donor site differs with the depth. Partial-thickness donor sites will regenerate spontaneously, although a thick partial-thickness donor site may require grafting with a thin partial-thickness graft. The full-thickness donor site will require either grafting with partial-thickness skin or direct closure if this is possible.

Choice of depth of graft

Partial-thickness

1. Over a doubtful recipient area.
2. When contracture is not important, not possible or is desirable.
3. To obtain the maximum possibility of take.

Thick partial-thickness

1. Where contracture is to be avoided – flexion areas – especially in the fingers.
2. To fill a minimal concavity.

Full-thickness

1. To fill a full-thickness facial defect in order to achieve the best cosmetic effect.
2. To cover a defect on a flexor surface which has a good recipient bed.

The partial-thickness graft is by far the commonest type of graft used, and the method of obtaining it will be fully discussed in the following section.

Instruments

There are two types of instrument in common use: the free-hand knife and the dermatome. The free-hand knife has now been so modified that it is virtually fool-proof, and all that is needed to obtain a reasonable skin graft is a minimum of confidence and some simple instructions.

There are several types of knife but all have the same basic principle. The Watson knife is the most popular, but many people are deterred by the need to assemble and set this knife. This will therefore be discussed in some detail.

1, 2 & 3

Free-hand knife

Preparation of knife

The blades are disposable and are fitted as shown. To control the thickness of the graft to be taken, the calibration control is adjusted and the blade then locked by tightening the round nut at the opposite end of the knife. The usual calibration is 1.5 spaces to give a graft of about 0.3 mm (0.012 in). *N.B.* It is very important to check the gap between the blade and the knife by holding the knife up to the light before using it. If the knife has become misshapen during sterilization, the gap may be larger than intended or unequal.

This type of instrument has the following advantages.

1. It is not complicated and can be prepared and used quickly and simply.
2. It does not depend on the vagaries of motors or electrical supply.
3. It is inexpensive and therefore should be available in every theatre.
4. Given a reasonable donor site such as the thigh, a good graft can be taken without risk of failure, even when the surgeon is inexperienced.

A surgeon should become proficient at using this instrument early in his career. Wounds that require grafting are sometimes not treated, to the detriment of the patient, because of the surgeon's lack of confidence in his ability to take a graft. An expensive, complicated dermatome is quite unnecessary for obtaining good skin grafts.

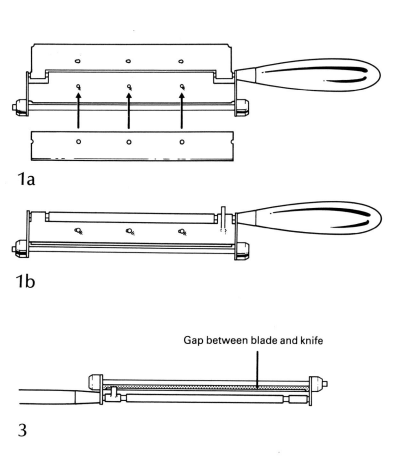

1a

1b

Gap between blade and knife

3

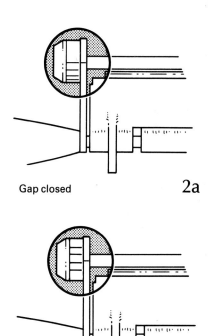

Gap closed   2a

Gap open 0.3 mm   2b

4

The De Silva knife

This is a useful instrument for taking small grafts in outpatient or casualty departments. It uses a standard sterilized razor blade as shown. The calibration setting is similar to the Watson knife, and it is used in the same way.

TECHNIQUE

Hairy donor areas are shaved preoperatively. The area of skin to be removed, the cutting edge of the knife, and the edge of one of the skin boards are all rubbed with a swab soaked in liquid paraffin. The ungreased skin board is placed at one end of the donor area, and pressure and traction are applied to make the skin tight. The assistant's other hand is used to broaden the donor site by pressing on the opposite side of the limb being 'cropped'.

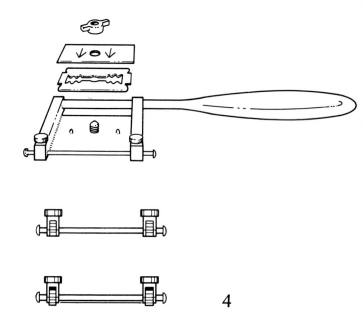

4

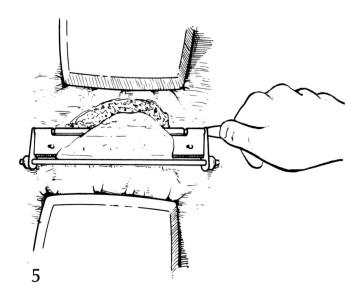

5

5

The greased board is placed 5 cm (2 in) in front of the ungreased board and countertraction and pressure are applied to make the skin tighter still. The knife is then applied to the skin in between the boards at an angle of about 30°. Side-to-side motions are made with the knife, about 13 mm (0.5 in) in each direction, minimal effort being made to advance it. The knife will move forward and the greased board should be moved at the same rate. It is important to note that if the knife has been set and fixed properly, it is virtually impossible to cut too deeply, so the procedure can be completed swiftly and with confidence, taking as long a strip of skin as is necessary. Continuous movement is essential and when sufficient skin is acquired the procedure is stopped by supinating the wrist while maintaining movement. This divides the skin cleanly.

The skin is then placed in a saline-soaked swab and stored carefully so that it is not inadvertently discarded. Warm compresses are applied to the donor site while further grafts are taken or until a dressing is applied.

6

Dermatomes

The electrically driven dermatome designed by Brown was the first mechanical instrument of this kind. There have been several modifications of this original idea and the instrument can now be run by electricity or compressed air.

When these instruments are available they may be used to take long sheets of skin of uniform depth with straight edges, not serrated edges as with hand knife grafts. Because of the straight margin of the cut a little more skin can be taken from a given area with slightly less blood loss. However, because of the more complex design and the dependency on some form of power, they are more likely to go wrong than the hand knife.

The blade fits on to a platform which moves mechanically from side to side, thus cutting the skin.

The blade is dropped on to two rivets and fixed by two screws on a securing plate. The depth of the graft is then determined by a calibration gauge which is set at 12 for a split-thickness graft.

The skin is prepared as above and the same procedure adopted as for a hand knife except that the steadying or non-greased board is not usually necessary and slightly more pressure is required to advance the knife. The dermatome can be used on any donor site and is usually slightly quicker than a hand knife. The big drawbacks with these instruments are their limited availability and a tendency to go wrong because of their complexity.

The Padgett and Reese dermatomes are useful in taking grafts from particular areas, such as the buttocks, but they necessitate the use of adhesive, are only kept in a few specialized theatres, and are expensive. They are probably best used in special circumstances by surgeons well versed in skin grafting. An excellent account of these instruments and their use can be found in Converse[1].

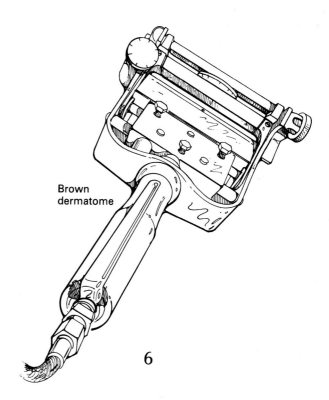

Brown dermatome

6

APPLICATION OF THE GRAFT

Poor application of the graft to the recipient site is a common cause of partial failure. The dermal side of the graft must be in contact with 100 per cent of the raw area and fixed there. If the recipient site is concave or flat the graft is just sewn securely into position. Sufficient sutures are required to ensure that there are no gaps at the graft edge where the graft is not in contact with the raw area. Complete haemostasis is desirable, but small residual haematomas will often be found under the graft after it has been sewn in. These are best flushed out with a chip syringe introduced under the graft. Persistent haematoma should be removed gently with non-toothed forceps. If firm pressure can then be applied over the graft for 5 minutes before the dressing is applied the incidence of haematoma is minimal.

In partial-thickness grafting the graft is best left exposed, if possible, and the area splinted. Otherwise, a firm dressing such as tulle gras, gauze and wool is applied. Two crêpe bandages are then applied – the first gently to maintain the graft in position, the second firmly to give pressure over the graft. Full-thickness grafts should be dressed and not left exposed.

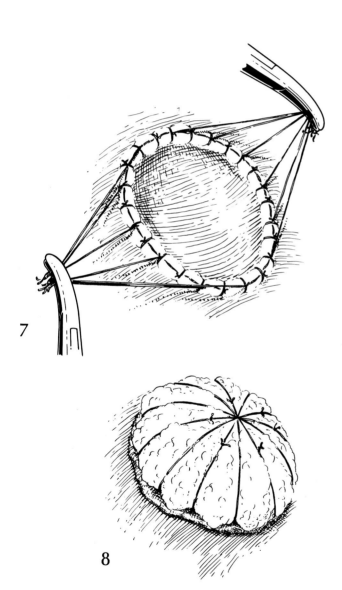

7

8

7 & 8

Should the recipient site be concave, the graft is held in place by a tie-over dressing. Here, alternate sutures are left long and a piece of non-adherent dressing is placed on the graft. Proflavine wool which has been lightly impregnated with paraffin is then tucked into the crevices around the edge of the graft and the centre is packed with the wool so that it is well above the level of the skin, allowing firm pressure to be applied when the long sutures are tied across. The object is to achieve contact between all areas of the graft and the recipient site. A strip of tulle gras is then applied around the dressing to protect any minimal raw areas. Full-thickness grafts are usually dressed in this way.

Partial-thickness grafts should be inspected daily if they are exposed but if dressed should be examined on the third day if applied to a suspect recipient site. If applied to a clean surgical wound they can be left without inspection for 5 days. When removing the dressings it is important to take great care not to disturb the graft. Two pairs of forceps should be used. One pair holds the graft *in situ* while the other pair eases off the dressing. If a tie-over dressing has been used the long sutures are first cut before the dressing is removed. Full-thickness grafts should be left undisturbed for a week or slightly longer, when the same care should be exercised.

Dressing the donor site

Warm compresses are applied to the donor site while further grafts are taken or until a dressing is applied. There are two common methods of dressing:

Mesh

The application of a greasy non-adherent mesh to the wound which is covered by a bulky absorptive dressing of gauze and wool. A double layer of this is advisable as leakage through the dressing can often lead to infection and is best avoided. Two crêpe bandages are then applied – one to keep the dressings in place and therefore applied comparatively gently, the second to provide pressure in an attempt to reduce exudation.

9

These dressings are best made before the patient is placed on the operating table. The tulle gras is laid on pieces of gauze of a suitable size to cover the donor site. Layers of wool are placed under the gauze to give an adequate thickness for absorption. Another piece of gauze is then placed on this wool so that the whole can be taken and applied directly. In the case of the thigh, two or three dressings may be needed if the whole thigh is to be stripped.

Preparation of dressings prior to the grafting can save up to half an hour of anaesthetic time for the patient. The exudation is reduced by rapid pressure application.

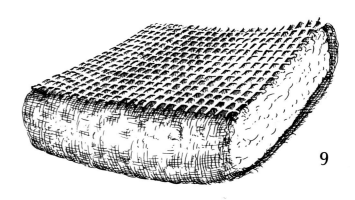

9

Artificial membrane

An artificial membrane, such as Opsite, applied to a donor site will often, though not always, relieve the pain associated with autografting. Apart from the humanitarian aspect this is an extremely important factor in that with little or no pain a patient with a donor site on his leg can be mobilized more quickly.

The skin around the donor site should be cleaned of all grease with ether or some solvent. It should be absolutely dry, which is sometimes difficult to attain if the oozing is profuse. The sheet of Opsite is held firmly by two assistants and a third removes the backing. The dressing is then applied to the skin at the side of the wound and lowered to cover the wound completely. Ideally cover should be completely watertight.

It is maintained that healing under this dressing may be quicker and the pain relief is often a definite advantage. In the author's experience the application of a bulky dressing in case of leakage is a wise precaution against infection. The dressings should be inspected daily to make sure they are firmly applied and have not leaked. It is important to impress on nursing staff that donor sites must not be taken down before 10 days at the earliest, unless infection is strongly suspected. The average healing time is 10 days, and in older patients it is often best to leave the dressing for several more days.

Full-thickness grafts

Full-thickness grafts include the epidermis and all levels of the dermis to the subcutaneous tissue. Such grafts are used, as already stated, in facial defects, usually following the removal of neoplastic lesions, or on a flexor surface with a good recipient bed. The donor sites for the face are postauricular, supraclavicular or nasolabial as these give the best colour match. The last can only be used in an older patient where the nasolabial fold is obvious. When this is so a graft 3–4 cm (7.5–10 inches) in diameter can be obtained and used anywhere on the face, but especially on the nose. The colour match is usually excellent and the donor site easy to manage and barely noticeable. For the hand or fingers the groin is often a good donor site or, alternatively, the thigh for larger grafts.

As stated previously, the advantages of these grafts are that they contract minimally and retain their characteris-tics well. The disadvantage is that the chances of take are smaller.

The graft can be taken in two ways:

1. The same as a partial-thickness graft, using a hand knife or dermatome, the only difference being that the setting is wider and the donor site must be closed with a partial-thickness graft. Taken this way with the correct setting, a minimal amount of unwanted subcutaneous tissue is adherent to the graft.
2. By cutting out a mapped-out area with a scalpel and then removing the adherent subcutaneous tissue. This is done by stretching the skin over the finger and gently cutting off the fat with a fine pair of curved scissors until the dermal surface is clean.

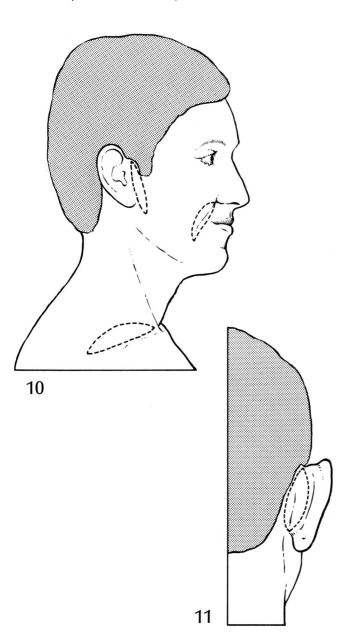

10

11

10 & 11

This second method is used especially when taking postauricular nasolabial or supraclavicular grafts. Full-thickness grafts must be designed to fit the defect they are to fill exactly, as overlap of skin minimizes the chance of take and gives a poor cosmetic result. A design of the defect must therefore first be taken on a piece of Jaconet, a sterile transparent material or even gauze. This is more easily done by placing the material over the defect after haemostasis has been obtained so that a slight blood-stained imprint is made. This can be cut out, placed back on the defect to check that it is a perfect fit and adjusted accordingly. The design is then placed over the donor site and outlined in ink. An incision is made around the design and an edge picked up with skin hooks.

Gentle dissection, including as little subcutaneous tissue as possible on the graft, is then performed. When the graft has been taken, it should be applied to the defect immediately and kept firmly in place by tie-over dressings. The donor site may be closed directly if small or with a split-thickness graft if larger. The dressings should be kept on full-thickness grafts for about a week and then the tie-over dressings carefully removed. It is seldom necessary to use large full-thickness grafts.

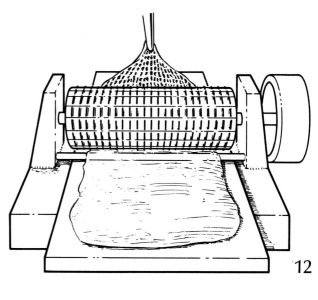

Mesh grafts

12 & 13

In cases where there is not sufficient autograft to allow complete cover of a raw area, such as in a large burn, the process enables the available skin to be expanded. The skin is perforated by passing it through a meshing machine and takes on a string-vest appearance. The gaps between the strands of skin can, by tension, be made as wide as required, but the most effective expansion is about 3:1, that is when applied the skin is made to cover 3 times its original area. Over a period of about 10 days the skin grows across the interstices of the mesh, and complete healing with the patient's own skin is obtained.

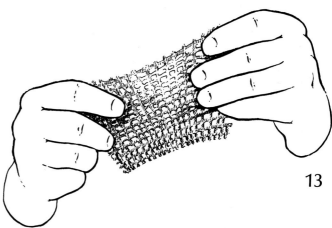

12

13

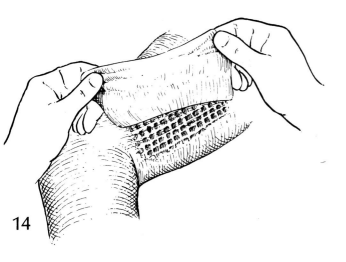

14

14

The best way to make sure that this occurs unimpeded is to cover the graft with a biological dressing. The raw interstices are then protected until they have healed over. The usual precaution against accumulation of fluid must be taken (see p.15).

Mesh grafting is unsatisfactory from a cosmetic standpoint in that the string-vest outline is obvious, and should therefore be avoided on the face. Because there is a tendency to contracture it should also not be used, if possible, over flexor areas, although this is not an absolute contraindication as the contracture can be minimized by adequate and prolonged splintage as described below.

Indications for mesh grafting

1. When there is a shortage of skin.
2. When cosmesis is not important.
3. In exudative areas such as varicose ulcers.
4. When a general anaesthetic is contraindicated, and the area required is larger than can be taken with infiltration of 30 ml of 1 per cent local anaesthetic.

Splintage

It is important to immobilize all grafts until they have become established, but in the case of flexor surfaces splinting is mandatory until the possibility of a flexion contracture has passed. The splint should be applied if possible immediately after surgery and be of such a form that it will not damage the graft by friction or pressure. The patient should only be allowed out of the splint for exercises and it must be firmly applied at night. This regimen may have to be followed for several months. The areas which appear to contract most quickly are the neck and the fingers, where correction can be most difficult. Absolute unnecessarily severe contractures are often seen because splintage was not applied very soon after grafting.

Delayed grafting

This is when the skin graft is taken, but applied at a later date.
   The advantages are:

1. Complete haemostasis.
2. Possible improvement of the recipient area.
3. Reduction in anaesthesia and theatre time.

The disadvantages are:

1. Possible increase of time in hospital.
2. Less secure fixation of the graft.
3. Possible discomfort for the patient.

   The recipient site can be covered either by saline soaks or biological dressing until the graft is applied. If it is infected the usual antibacterial preparations are used. When applied, the graft should be secured in place by Micropore or Steristrips to avoid hurting the patient by the use of sutures.
   The indications for this type of grafting are inability to obtain good haemostasis and a doubtful recipient bed.

General points

1. On areas thickly covered with granulation tissue, which is usually pale pink in colour when mature, the chance of take is improved by removing the granulations. This is best done with the edge of a ruler or some flat instrument.
2. If possible more skin than is necessary should be taken in order to be able to try again if the graft fails.
3. Skin should be stored in a refrigerator at $+4°C$ and not in the freezer compartment.
4. It is not necessary to spread skin on tulle gras before application. The less it is handled and allowed to come into contact with oily products the better.
5. When there is a contour defect intimate contact of graft to raw surface should be ensured. Nature tends to decrease the hollow with time.
6. When there is persistent oozing on the recipient site delayed grafting should be used or the graft should be inspected early to evacuate any haematoma.
7. When dealing with an infected area the skin should be taken first and the donor site closed before dealing with the recipient site to avoid the spread of infection.

Homograft and xenograft

The use of homograft or xenograft as viable tissue, or in the lyophilized form as a temporary substitute for a skin graft, is often valuable in providing adequate cover until permanent closure of a defect can be obtained. This is particularly so if important structures such as nerves, tendons or arteries are lying exposed in the wound.
   The following list shows the advantages of using these tissues.

1. Immediate availability of material for wound closure without disturbing the patient.
2. Diminution of fluid and protein loss.
3. Diminution of heat and energy loss.
4. Reduction in infection.
5. Reduction in pain.
6. Protection of vital structures.
7. Increase in mobility.
8. More economical use of autograft, by testing the recipient bed.
9. Psychological improvement.

   The freeze-dried tissue is dead and is therefore not a true graft but a biological dressing. It is minimally antigenic and is almost as effective as a true graft and will be considered as such.
   The commonest of these substances is freeze-dried porcine xenograft, which is available commercially. The tissue is soaked in saline for 30–45 minutes and can be applied to the raw area as long as the area is not grossly infected. The method of using homograft or xenograft in either form is virtually the same and will therefore be discussed as one entity assuming that the lyophilized tissue has been soaked in saline and reconstituted.
   Two kinds of defect will be considered: partial-thickness loss and full-thickness loss.

Partial-thickness loss

This occurs most commonly in thermal injury, but the depth may often be difficult to diagnose. The history and appearance will help. If there has been a scald or flash burn and the tissue is not leathery, has no coagulated vessels showing and is sensitive to pin-prick, the injury is probably partial-thickness. If in doubt it is worth while assuming a partial-thickness defect, especially in children.

The area involved should be cleaned, any blisters broken and removed and then the homograft or xenograft applied in as large sheets as possible, making sure there are no gaps and that the edges of the raw area are overlapped.

The object is to protect the lesion until the skin has generated. Therefore the dressing should, if possible, be left *in situ* until this occurs. Ideally, it should be left exposed but if this is not possible, as in a circumferential wound, then a firm dressing of tulle gras gauze and wool should be used to cover it. However, the wound should be inspected at least every 24 hours to make sure that there is no collection of fluid. Any fluid which has collected should be expressed, and if considerable the dressing should be removed, the raw surface cleaned with saline and a new graft applied. If there is no collection, the dressing should be left intact until it begins to peel off spontaneously. The peeled tissue should be cut off daily until the whole area is clean and healed. Meshed xenograft, which has the advantage of decreasing the accumulation of fluid, has recently been produced commercially.

It is important to appreciate that if this daily inspection is not carried out and fluid is allowed to accumulate, infection will occur and more harm will be done than if no treatment had been carried out.

Full-thickness defects

When applied to full-thickness defects the xenograft and homograft must be removed or changed in 4 days, otherwise copious bleeding will occur when they are stripped off with difficulty. The advantages of using this form of closure are that not only does it give instant protection and a 75 per cent functioning skin, but it also acts as a test of whether an autograft, if applied, would take. If the tissue becomes adherent it means almost certainly the autografting will succeed. This is particularly useful in traumatic wounds where treatment has been delayed or in chronic lesions such as varicose ulcers. Full-thickness burns must be excised first.

In a fresh, traumatic, full-thickness defect almost instant restoration of skin cover is possible, which is invaluable if vital structures have been exposed. If the area is dirty the usual cleaning should be performed and then the tissue applied. This enables more serious problems to be dealt with. The area can be left without change of tissue for up to 4 days, thus permitting eventual permanent closure of the defect under ideal conditions.

A good example is a patient who was involved in a motor-cycle accident. He had torn his femoral vessels and lost most of the skin and subcutaneous tissue from his groin. The vessels were repaired and it was then found that he had a reptured colon. The repaired vessels and skin defect were covered with lyophilized porcine skin and he then had surgery for his abdominal condition. Four days later, the xenograft having been untouched, flap closure of his groin was performed, his repaired vessels remaining clean and patent during this time.

In traumatic lesions where treatment has been delayed or in a chronic lesion, preparation with an antibacterial preparation such as Eusol may be necessary to cure gross infection. This should be applied 4 times a day for 48 hours. The xenograft or homograft is then applied and inspected daily, as previously mentioned – when the tissue becomes adherent, autografting is indicated.

If there is insufficient autograft to cover the full-thickness raw areas, for instance, in a large burn, xenograft or homograft can be used together with autograft to provide eventual complete cover.

The available autograft is cut into thin strips and alternated with 1.5 cm strips of xenograft or homograft – ideally viable and tissue-typed for a good match. As this is rejected, it is replaced with spreading autograft epithelium by 'creeping substitution'. Further surgery is, therefore, unnecessary. The size of the strips of the patient's own skin does not seem to influence the amount of outgrowth.

The mesh technique is a variation on this procedure as is the use of postage stamp grafts where inch square (2.5 cm^2) pieces of autograft are placed on a raw area with the idea of the pieces coalescing as they spread outwards. Postage stamp grafting is mainly used where the recipient bed is unfavourable and one expects less than a 100 per cent take. Pinch grafting where small pieces of combined partial and thick skin grafts are used is contraindicated.

The advent of freeze-dried biological dressings allows the adequate covering of raw areas quickly without a skin graft having to be taken. However, the wounds must be inspected daily to make sure that fluid is not accumulating, otherwise more harm than good may be done. In the treatment of partial-thickness defects it is often the only treatment required, but in larger full-thickness lesions it is only a method of providing temporary wound cover.

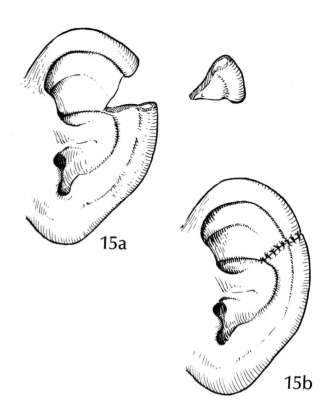

15a

15b

15 & 16

Composite grafts

This is a graft comprising not only skin but also usually subcutaneous tissue and cartilage. When part of the alar region of the nose is lost, the gap is often filled with such a composite graft from the ear. The size of the graft is limited and the centre should not be more than 1.5 cm from its ingrowing blood supply. When being transferred the tissue must be handled with great care and it is usually best left exposed postoperatively. The patient should be dissuaded from any activity for 1 week postoperatively as fluctuations in blood flow caused by movements of the head and trunk seem to inhibit take, as do sudden changes in temperature. The donor site can always be closed primarily.

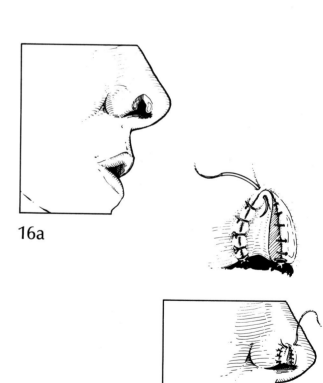

16a

16b

Hair-bearing grafts

17a & b

These are of two kinds: (a) full-thickness punch grafts 4–5 mm in diameter containing about 12–15 hair follicles or (b) strip grafts where lengths of full-thickness skin containing hair follicles are used. The donor sites are usually the temporal and occipital areas of the scalp where the hair is seldom lost – they retain this property when successfully transplanted.

In the punch variety, used mainly for the treatment of baldness, a slightly smaller recipient site is made with a 1 mm smaller punch, and the graft fitted in. It seldom requires fixation. A gap of 1 cm between grafts is left so the surgery must be repeated to fill these gaps. The donor sites usually heal spontaneously. Strip grafting is often used for replacement of lost eyebrows or to establish a hair-line. An incision is made and the tissue distracted to allow the graft to be inserted. Some fixation is required.

After the graft has taken, the hair eventually falls out and regrows in about 6 weeks, and the patient must be warned that this will happen.

It is important that the graft is orientated so that the hair grows in the direction required to give a natural effect.

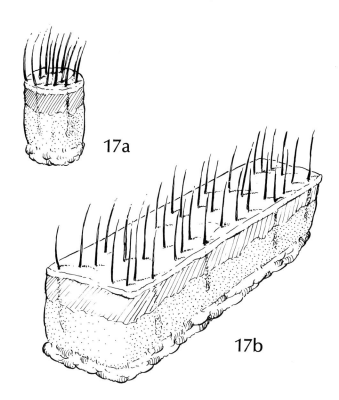

17a

17b

New concept in skin grafting in the use of cultured skin

This could be either cultured autograft, the patient's own skin or allograft from a different person. It takes three to four weeks for the skin to grow sufficiently to be of clinical use. The advantage of the allograft when cultured is that it seems to have lost the ability to cause rejection and can therefore be available when it is wanted. That is a bank can be built up and the wait of three to four weeks necessary when autograft is used, is eliminated. The skin comprises a layer of cultured keratinocytes 10–15 cells thick.

The results using cultured skin at present are considrably inferior to the use of routine skin grafts. In clinical situations varying from deep burns to excised tattoos, the take averages about 50%. However, the cosmetic results are probably superior and the need for painful, often difficult to obtain donor sites is eliminated. The logistic problems of this method are still considerable and only very specialised centres could provide the facility.

The routine use of cultured skin is not yet possible but the prospects for improvement in take and availability are good. Considerable further research is necessary and is being undertaken.

Reference

1. Converse, J., M. (ed.) Reconstructive plastic surgery: principles and procedures in correction, reconstruction and transplantation. Vol. 1, 2nd edn. pp. 27–30. Philadelphia: Saunders, 1977

Local skin flap repairs

F. S. C. Browning FRCS
Consultant Plastic Surgeon, Leeds General Infirmary, Leeds, UK

Introduction

The simplest repair of a skin defect is bilateral advancement produced by undermining the skin widely following elliptical excision of a lesion. When the defect is too large for this repair, then tissue must be brought in by using either a graft or a small local flap.

Flaps are the better form of repair in that they provide skin that gives a good match in colour, texture and contour and can provide hair growth. A small flap requires as much care in its planning and design as any large flap and successful repair calls for experience in its execution.

Many flaps are available but all have either advancement, transposition or rotation as their principal movement and it is sometimes safest to complete the excision before considering which flap is most suited to correcting the defect.

When designing a flap it must be remembered that the blood supply to the skin is being reduced by cutting along the three sides and subcutaneous plane of the flap. Thus on the limbs and trunk the ratio of flap length to flap width should not exceed 1:1.5, and it is as well to remember the Gillies definition that 'a flap is a partly attached piece of skin which is alive when you put it on and may die later'. On the face, which has a far richer blood supply, the ratio of length to breadth can be as great as 3:1.

When designing flaps on the face, care must be taken not to disturb important anatomical landmarks such as eyebrows, hairline and beardline, and on no account should eyebrows or frontal hairline be removed preoperatively.

Indications

Flaps must be used over bare bone and in the reconstruction of irradiated tissue. In areas of excision where two layers have been removed, for example the ala and eyelid, a flap must be used for reconstruction and covered with either a graft or a second flap.

Contraindications

Flaps should not be used if there is any doubt about the excision of a tumour being complete. It must be remembered that the malignancy, if it recurs, will extend into the deeper tissues before growing through the flap onto the surface. Therefore great care must be taken to ensure adequate clearance of the tumour when using this method of reconstruction.

When reconstructing infected areas, for example dog bites, it is better to achieve primary repair with a skin graft and then use what may be the only suitable flap for reconstruction once the area is clean and healed. Tissue where scars run across the base of the proposed flap cannot be used, as this reduces skin viability, nor can flaps be constructed from previous grafts.

Small flaps around the face can be used when performing repairs under local anaesthesia, but it must then be remembered to make allowances at the planning stage for the tissue oedema and swelling induced by injection of the anaesthetic.

Operative technique

As in all forms of plastic surgery, it is important to employ an atraumatic technique when raising the flaps, using hooks to handle the flap tissue and not forceps. It is best to incise round the flap, and to use a scalpel for the early dissection and blunt scissor dissection at the base of the flap to cause least disruption to the blood supply.

Attention to atraumatic technique throughout the operation will result in as little oedema as possible in the flap and thus cause less embarrassment to the circulation. Haemostasis is of prime importance and, in small flap surgery, bipolar coagulation will achieve this with minimal damage to the blood supply in the flap. Two-layer closure, using absorbable sutures in the deeper layer to take the tension, allows the use of a fine nylon suture for the final skin apposition. Barron's horizontal mattress sutures are ideal for suturing the flap, as they do not damage the subdermal plexus, thus ensuring a good blood supply to the wound edges and allowing primary wound healing.

Postoperatively the flap should be left exposed if possible and its colour observed. Oedema in the first 48 hours may impair circulation that appeared adequate at the time of surgery. Haematoma will reduce the flap blood supply and act as a good nidus for infection, which in turn will further impair the viability of the flap whose blood circulation has already been reduced. If the flap circulation becomes compromised, it is best to remove the sutures to relieve tension and to evacuate any haematoma. Once the oedema has settled, the flap can be resutured if necessary. It is better to allow the flap to survive by retraction and then resuture, than to persist with sutures under tension and lose the flap.

The operations

TRANSPOSITION FLAP

1

The excision margins are marked with Bonney's blue and a mapping pen.

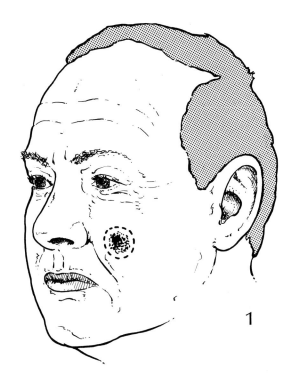

1

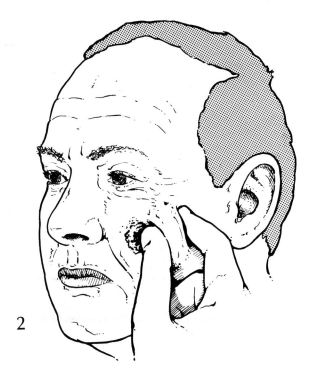

2

2

The skin next to the proposed defect is pinched to ensure that there is enough spare tissue for the planned flap. The flap is then outlined in ink, bearing in mind that any excess at its tip can be trimmed at the end of the procedure.

3

The length of the flap is checked to ensure that it can be transposed into the skin defect with little or no tension. When using such a flap on the skull it is important to remember that the bone is convex and that greater length will be required than when repairing a flap surface defect. The pivot point of the flap is at its base at the incision point furthest from the defect and the tightest line will be from the pivot point to the opposite lower corner of the flap.

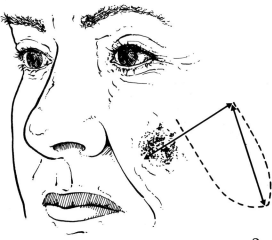

3

4

The skin is incised with a scalpel and dissection is continued through the subcutaneous fat, leaving the subdermal plexus intact.

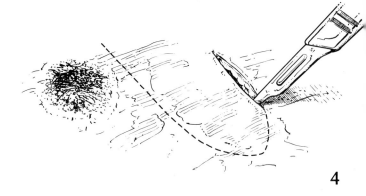

4

5

Holding the skin flap with a skin hook, blunt scissor dissection is then used in the base of the flap to maintain the integrity of the small blood vessels and ensure the best possible blood supply.

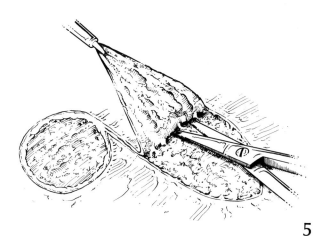

5

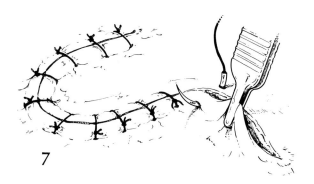

6

6 & 7

The edges of the recipient area are undermined by 2–3 mm but the hinge of the flap should be undermined widely to allow the skin to redistribute as widely as possible and so avoid a dog-ear (standing cone). If the dog-ear is still prominent at the end of the operation, it should be excised at a second stage, as any correction at the primary stage will reduce the base of the flap and lead to distal necrosis.

7

HALF-SIZED TRANSPOSITION FLAP

8

When using a transposition flap on the forehead the defect can be repaired by combining advancement of the edges with importation of a flap. It is possible to transpose a flap from the vertical plane which is only half the defect width.

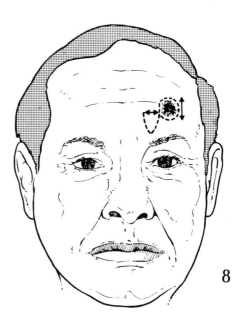

8

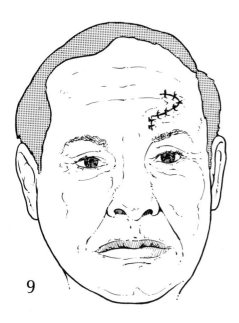

9

9

This will allow direct closure of the donor area with minimal tension and provide a repair without distortion of the hairline or eyebrow, which would result from direct closure of the defect.

BILOBED FLAP

10

In certain situations, for example on the nose, the donor defect resulting from a simple transposition flap cannot be closed directly. Esser in 1916 described a bilobed flap in which a second, smaller transposition flap is designed at right angles to the first transposition flap.

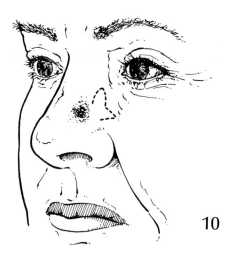

10

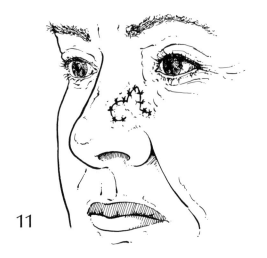

11

11

This is used to close the donor defect of the first transposition flap, and its own donor defect, being smaller, can then be closed directly.

LIMBERG FLAP

12

A Limberg flap is essentially a transposition flap which has been designed mathematically to close a rhomboid defect. The rhomboid must be an equilateral parallelogram with angles of 60° and 120°. The major advantage of creating a rhomboid defect and repairing it with a Limberg flap is that less tissue has to be excised than with straight elliptical excision. The sides of the defect and the short diagonal should all be the same length. To outline the flap the short diagonal (AD) should be extended by its own length; a line drawn parallel to the side of the rhomboid (EF) outlines the third side of the flap. As will be seen from this, there are four Limberg flaps available for any rhomboid defect. The orientation of the rhomboid is crucial in providing flap repair under minimal tension. The base of the triangle (DF) must be placed along the line of maximum extensibility (LME) which is at right angles to the relaxed skin tension line (RSTL). It is along this base line that maximum tension will result when closing the donor defect.

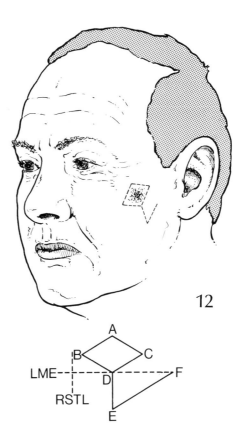

12

13

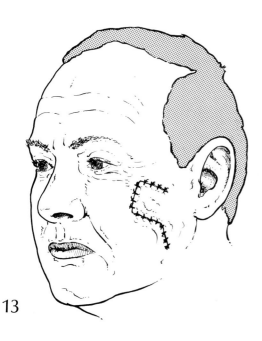

13

Limberg flaps are particularly useful for closing defects in the region of the nasolabial fold and temple, but great care must be taken when trying to close a defect over a convex surface, for example a frontal prominence. Multiple Limberg flaps can be used in closing larger skin defects.

DUFOURMENTAL FLAP

14

The Limberg flap can only be used in the repair of rhomboid defects where the acute angle is 60°. The Dufourmental flap can in theory be used for any rhomboid, but in practice it is useful only in rhomboids with an acute angle between 60° and 90°. If the angle is less than 60°, then direct closure is preferred. The Dufourmental flap is designed by extending side JK and axis GK of the rhomboid and bisecting the angle thus formed by a line (KL) which is the same length as the sides of the rhomboid. The third side of the flap (LM) is then drawn of equal length parallel to the long axis of the rhomboid defect.

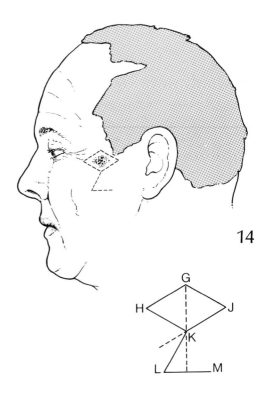

14

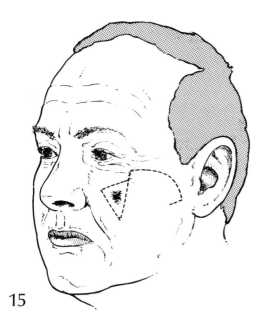

15

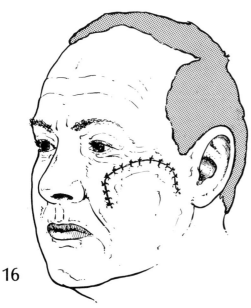

16

ROTATION FLAPS

15

Rotation flaps can be used to repair defects on the face. The defect is triangulated to form a segment of a circle and the flap is designed by extending the arc of the circle. The flap is then rotated in and the tension distributed over this long line. The pivot point of such a flap is not clear but it must be remembered that the larger the flap the less the tension resulting from the closure. Sometimes it is necessary to incorporate a back-cut in the design of the flap to reduce the tension.

16

This flap is often best used for the repair of defects in the region of the cheek and nasolabial fold in p-atients who have rounded cheeks and thus little excess tissue available for a transposition repair. The flap design can sometimes be improved by lengthening the advancing edge by 1 cm which reduces the tension on closure.

GLABELLAR FLAPS

17 & 18

When repairing a defect in the glabellar region, a flap can be used from the forehead based on one of the supraorbital vessels. This flap is almost triangular and is advanced downwards to close the defect, its own donor area being closed by direct suture, a V–Y advancement.

Dissection through the skin should be with a scalpel but that in the region of the base of the flap should be with scissors, deep to the muscle to avoid injury to the vascular pedicle.

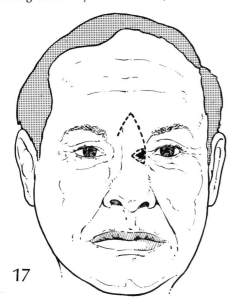

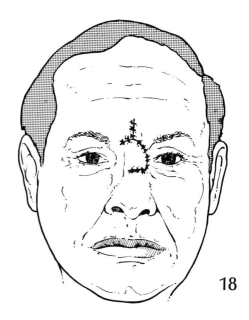

19 & 20

A similar technique can be used in repairing defects on the lower part of the nose. The whole of the skin on the dorsum of the nose can be raised as a flap, based on the opposite side of the nose, and advanced downwards.

However, when planning such a repair, the convexity of the bridge of the nose must be allowed for and often this flap advances less than would at first seem possible.

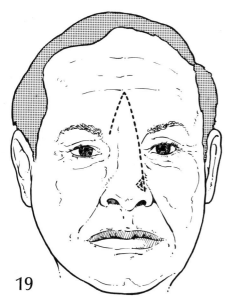

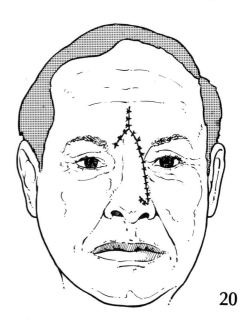

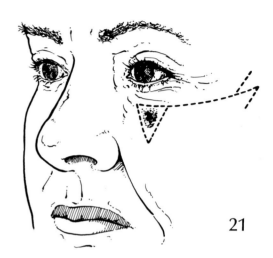

21

ADVANCEMENT WITH HALF Z-PLASTY (McGregor)

21 & 22

When correcting defects of the lower eyelid, an advancement flap can be used. It must be designed so that the lower lid is well supported and not dragged down to produce ectropion. The flap is designed with an upward curve out to the temple, where a back-cut is performed at 60° to allow advancement without tension. The triangular defect thus created is filled with a half Z-plasty from the upper margin of the incision.

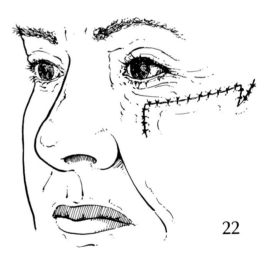

22

SUBCUTANEOUS PEDICLE FLAPS

In the small flaps described so far, the blood supply is based on the subdermal plexus, while the deep blood supply is divided. However, it is also possible to design flaps which will maintain integrity of the subcutaneous supply while the subdermal plexus is divided. Such flaps are used mainly to repair defects in the nasolabial fold.

23 & 24

The tissue to be excised is outlined as a square. The flap is then drawn as a triangle extending down the length of the nasolabial fold, with the upper limb made slightly longer than the lower. The skin is incised with a scalpel through to the subcutaneous fat. Dissection is then continued widely under the adjacent skin down through the fat to the muscle. Care must be taken not to separate the skin from the fat which is its only source of blood supply. The advancing edge of the triangular flap can be undermined slightly to allow closure without inversion.

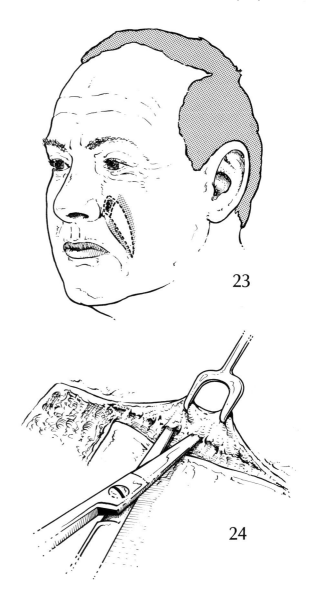

23

24

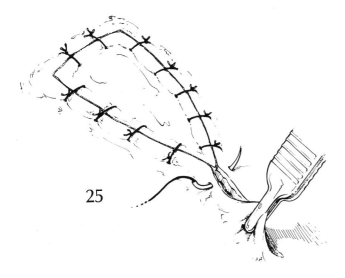

25

25

The donor area of the flap is closed by direct suture.

ISLAND FLAP FOR EAR DEFECTS

26a & b

Sometimes after excision of a neoplasm on the concha or helix, simple closure cannot be obtained (a). The defect can then be filled by a flap of postauricular skin (b).

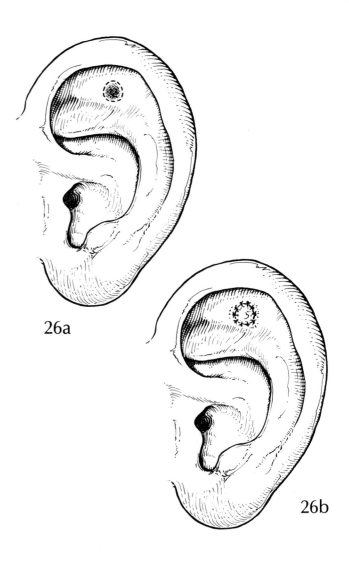

26a

26b

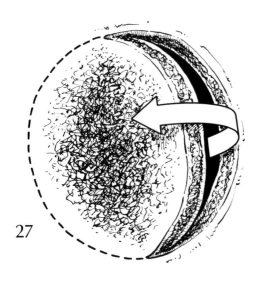

27

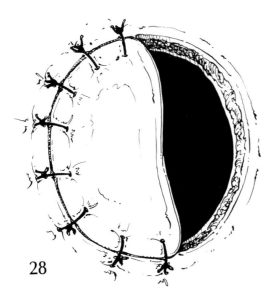

28

27 & 28

Following excision of the underlying cartilage, the skin at the posterior edge of the defect is incised through its full thickness and the incision carried round the upper and lower margins describing just over half a circle. This flap is then sutured to the anterior margin of the defect.

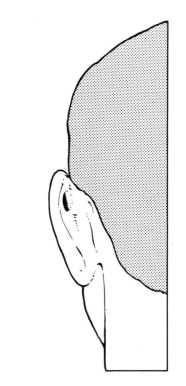

29–32

The skin on the anterior half of the back of the ear is now incised and dissected at the subdermal level, leaving a subcutaneous pedicle. This skin is now sutured to the posterior margin of the defect on the outer aspect of the ear. The donor defect in the postauricular region is closed by direct suture after excising excess tissue above and below as a triangle to produce an ellipse.

29

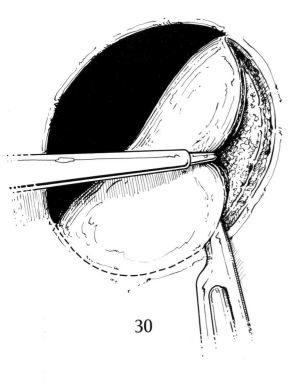

30

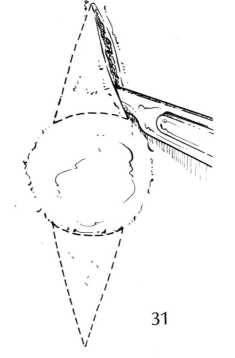

31

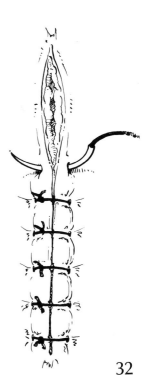

32

Further reading

Lister G.D., Gibson T. Closure of rhomboid skin defects: the flaps of Limberg and Dufourmental. British Journal of Plastic Surgery 1972; 25: 300–314

Borges A.F. Choosing the correct Limberg flap. Plastic and Reconstructive Surgery 1978; 62: 542–545

Herbert D.C., Harrison R.G. Nasolabial and subcutaneous pedicle flaps. British Journal of Plastic Surgery 1975; 28: 85–89

Masson J.K. A simple island flap for reconstruction of concha and helix defects. British Journal of Plastic Surgery 1972; 25: 399–403

Illustrations by Kevin Marks

Direct and indirect flaps

Charles Viva FRCS, FRCS(Ed)
Senior Consultant Plastic Surgeon, North and South Teeside District, Hartlepool and South West Durham, and General Hospital, Middlesbrough, UK

DIRECT FLAPS

A direct flap is raised at a site distant to a defect, developed as an open flap and transposed directly into the defect in one stage. A second operation is necessary to divide the pedicle of the flap when the blood supply from the periphery of the new site is assured.

Repair by direct flap should be considered when the defect is such that a local skin flap repair is impossible and the base of the defect is unsuitable for split skin grafting. The alternative is a free tissue transfer (see chapter on 'Restoration of skin cover: the use of free grafts', pp. 14–27). The method has the advantage of speed and simplicity in application, and is particularly useful for defects of the hands and fingers, the forearm and the lower leg. Successful repair depends on careful planning (which should always be done in reverse), taking into account the relationship of the recipient site to the donor site. Tension should be avoided, and where possible the flap should have an axial blood supply.

Pectoral and submammary flaps

1 & 2

Pectoral and submammary flaps may be used for circumferential defects of the thumb or fingers if the decision has been taken not to amputate the damaged digit.

A pattern is made of suitable size, taking into consideration the circumference and length of the defect.

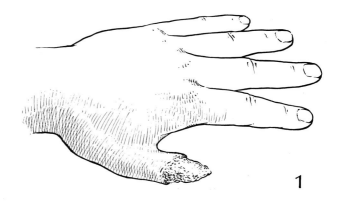

1

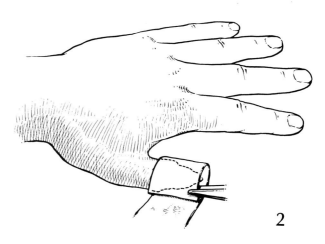

2

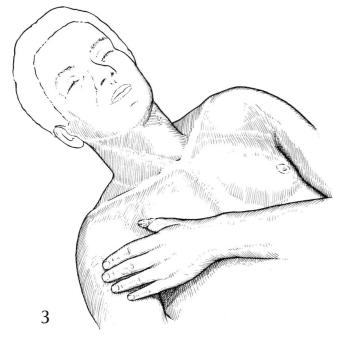

3

3 & 4

The thumb is placed at a convenient position on the chest wall, and the pattern is transferred to the chest wall.

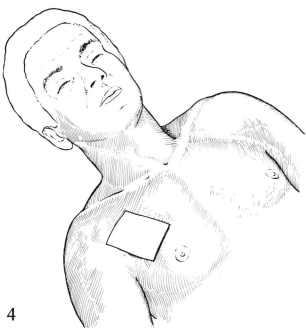

4

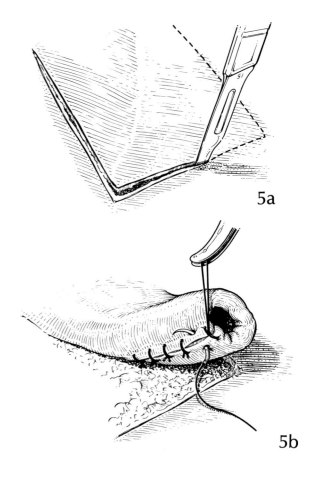

5a

5b

5a & b

The flap is then raised and tubed by suturing the sides together.

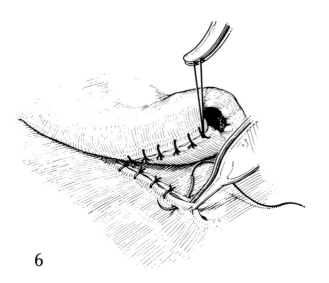

6

6

The secondary defect is repaired by direct suture (or skin graft).

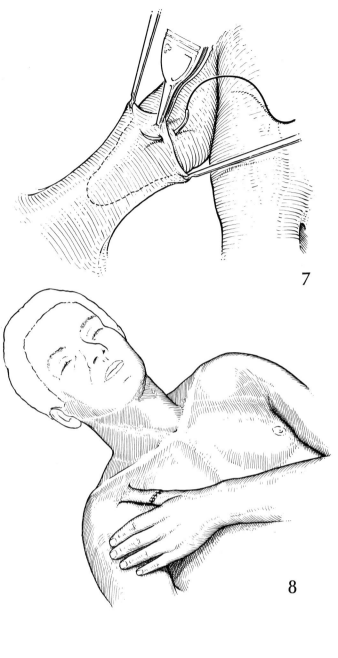

7

7 & 8

The stripped thumb is inserted into the tube and the end of the tube sutured to the margin of the defect. The seam of the tube should be aligned along the ulnar border of the thumb. The arm is immobilized on the trunk with Elastoplast.

8

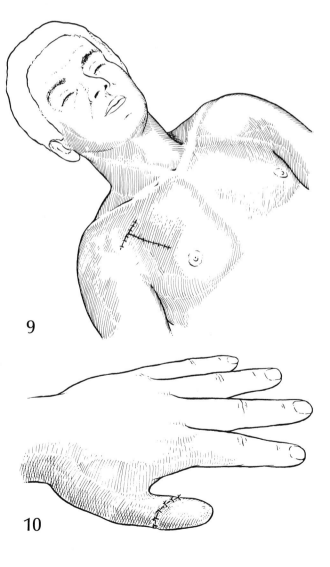

9

10

9 & 10

The pedicle is divided and inset after an interval of 3 weeks.

11

An alternative site for the tube is the inner side of the upper arm.

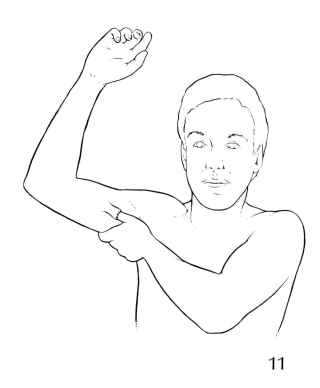

11

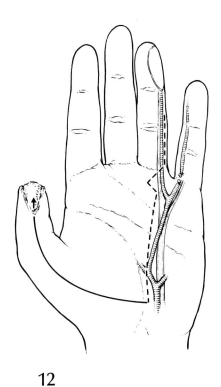

12

12

A neurovascular island flap is necessary to supply sensation to the anaesthetic flap reconstruction at a later date.

Flaps from the abdomen

Large defects on the hand or forearm are easily repaired by random direct flaps from the abdomen. Flaps may be raised on the upper, lower or lateral abdominal wall, depending on the ease of approximation of the defect to the trunk, and may be superiorly or inferiorly based. Defects on the distal forearm and hand are usually repaired by flaps raised on the contralateral abdominal wall, whereas those on the proximal forearm or upper arm require ipsilateral flaps.

13

The arm is placed on the abdomen to determine the most suitable site for the flap to be raised.

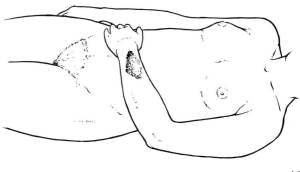

13

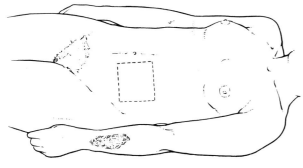

14

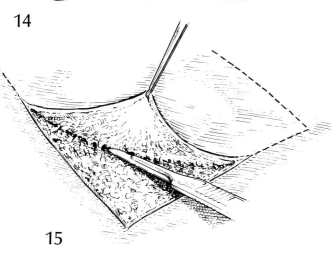

15

14 & 15

The flap is planned in reverse with a pattern. It is then raised with approximately 1 cm thickness of fat, taking care not to jeopardize the dermal and subdermal vascular plexus.

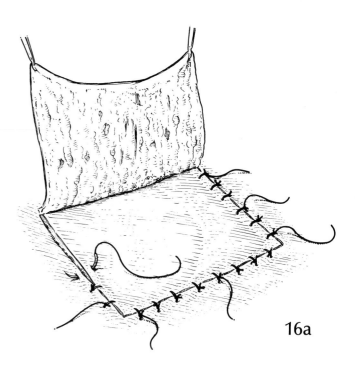

16a

16a & b

The secondary defect is closed by skin grafting (unless it is very small).

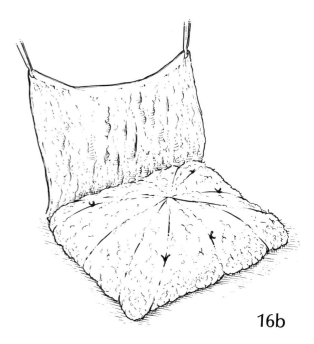

16b

17

The flap is sutured to the defect.

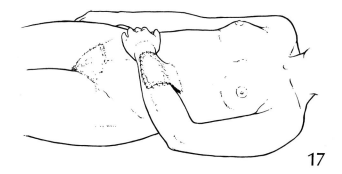

17

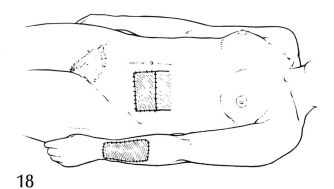

18

18

The pedicle is divided and inset after 3 weeks.

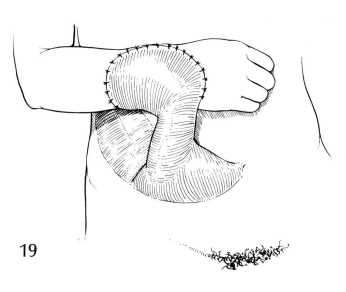

19

Groin flap

19

The groin flap is extremely useful, as it has an axial blood supply from the superficial external iliac artery and can be raised of a length-to-breadth ratio of 3:1 or 4:1 with safety. This allows some movement of uninjured digits to combat stasis oedema and resulting stiffness. The centre of the flap runs along the line of the inguinal ligament. The groin flap is a versatile flap which can be used for repair of defects of the thumb, finger or hand.

Direct flaps from the upper limb

The simplest of these is the cross-finger flap, which is useful to cover small defects on the volar aspect of a finger, when an adjacent finger is the donor site, or on the thumb, when the index, middle or ring finger can be used.

20a & b

The injured finger is placed touching the adjacent finger to determine the most suitable location for the flap, and the defect is outlined on a pattern.

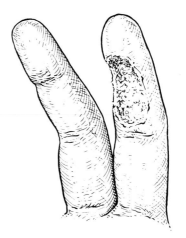

20a

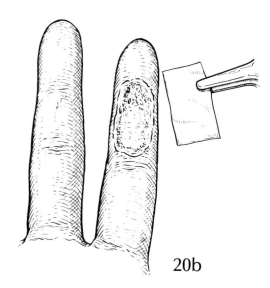

20b

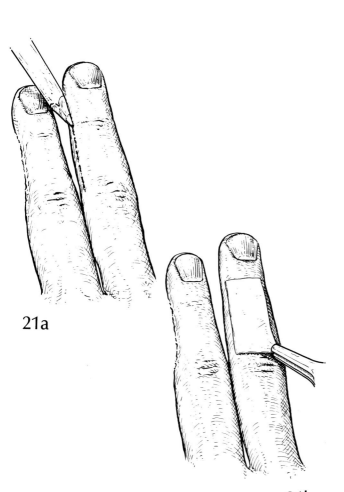

21a

21b

21a & b

The midaxial line is marked on the donor finger, and the pattern is placed on this finger with its edge at the midlateral line.

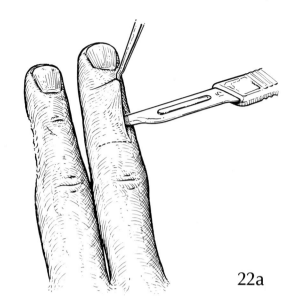

22a

22a, b & c

The flap is then raised, ligating the dorsal veins, and developed in the loose areolar tissue overlying the extensor tendon. The secondary defect is repaired by a partial thickness skin graft, and the flap is sutured into place. The pedicle is divided and inset 2 weeks later.

For larger defects, where insufficient donor skin is available on a finger, cross-forearm or cross-arm flaps can be used in a similar manner.

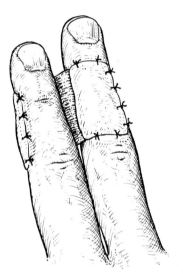

22b

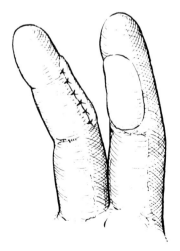

22c

Direct flaps in the lower limb

The well-known cross-leg flap is still in common use to provide full thickness cover over a fractured tibia. Many fractures which appeared to be heading towards non-union have been induced to unite without recourse to bone grafting merely by the provision of sound skin cover. Where a soft tissue defect on the lower leg is too large for repair by fasciocutaneous flap (*see* chapter on 'Fasciocutaneous flaps', pp. 56–58), and unsuitable for a free flap because of vascular damage or lack or suitable facilities, a cross-leg flap should always be considered.

23

The area to be covered is mapped out with a pattern.

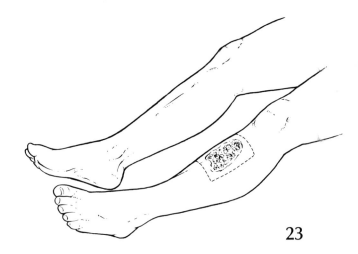

23

24

The limbs are positioned to find the least uncomfortable position for the patient, bearing in mind that the position has to be maintained for 3 weeks.

24

25

The pattern of the defect is placed on the recipient leg with the pedicle of the pattern corresponding to the pedicle of the proposed flap and then relaid on the donor leg to test the feasibility of the flap. If found to be unsuitable, the procedure is repeated until a satisfactory flap can be found. Meticulous planning is absolutely essential for the satisfactory outcome of a cross-leg flap repair, which is time-consuming and trying both for the surgeon and the patient.

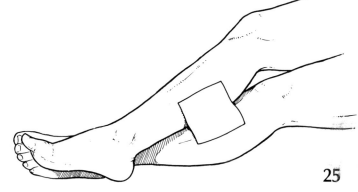

25

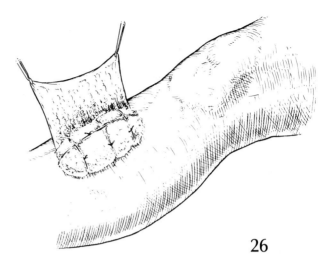

26

26

A generous flap is raised at the level of the deep fascia and a split thickness skin graft applied to the secondary defect.

27

The flap is placed over the defect, and the edges of the defect are excised to fit the flap, which is then sutured into place. The limb is immobilized in plaster of Paris, with Elastoplast, or by Vacupac, as appropriate.

The pedicle of the flap is divided after 3 weeks. It is often advisable to let the divided edge of the flap lie unsutured for 4–5 days before finally insetting it into the fourth side of the defect, as this helps to prevent marginal loss of tissue at the divided edge.

27

Cross-thigh flap

If the patient has good mobility of the knee joint, it may be possible to carry out a cross-thigh flap repair and thus avoid unsightly scarring on the calf. Planning has to be even more meticulous, and the method is usually unsuitable except in children.

Indirect flap

Flaps which need to be transported via an intermediary inset to their destination are called indirect flaps. The tubed pedicle is the classical example, and this can be used where a local or direct flap is impossible and a large amount of good quality skin is required, e.g. for defects on the scalp exposing bone and for neck contractures.

28

Tube pedicles can be raised on most areas of the body, but only the usual and most useful sites are illustrated here.

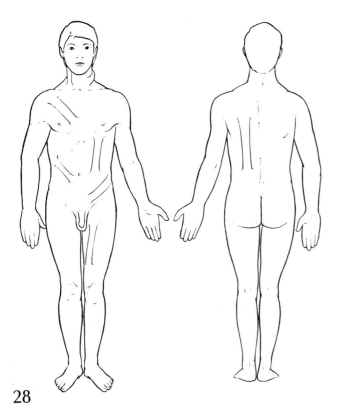

28

29

The lines of incision are marked. No absolute rules for dimensions exist, but in general a length-to-breadth ratio of 2.5:1 is satisfactory.

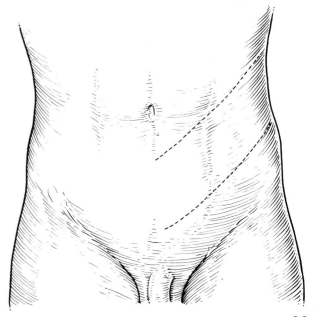

29

30

The lines are incised, and the strip of skin is developed in the plane of the loose areolar tissue just superficial to the fascia or scarpa.

31

The flap is handled with great care, using sutures or skin hooks along the margins.

32

The flap is tubed by placing a suture 3–4 cm from each end and using the sutures as retractors. The edges of the intervening portion of the tube are then carefully approximated with a continuous suture.

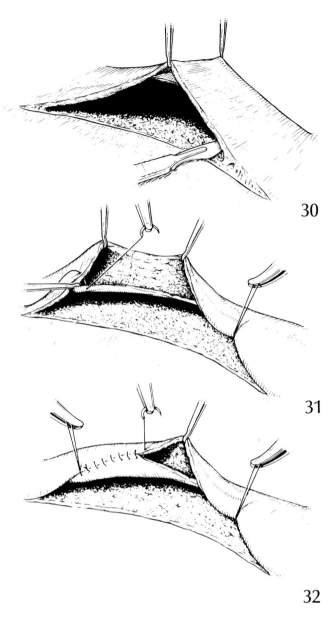

30

31

32

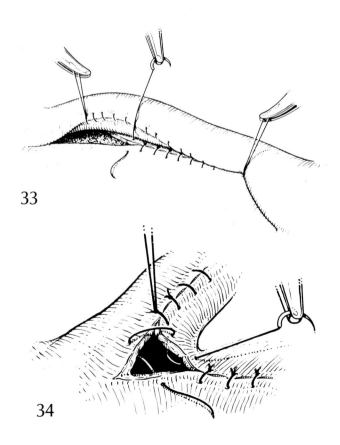

33

34

33

Next, the secondary defect is closed by undermining and approximation, or by skin grafting.

34

Care is taken to close the corners so that no defect remains. The tube cannot be transported with safety if any infected raw area remains. Dry gauze is placed under the tube pedicle to separate the suture line from the one which closes the secondary defect.

After an interval of 3 weeks, one end of the pedicle can be divided and attached to the intermediate carrier (usually the wrist).

Technique of intermediate attachment

35

The divided end of the tube is placed on the side of the wrist and the outline marked.

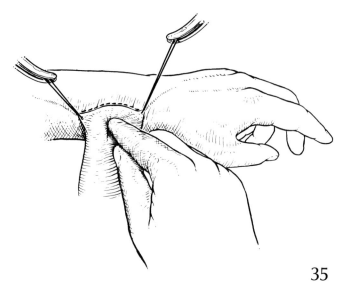

35

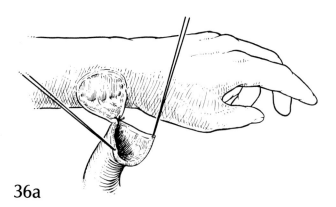

36a

36a & b

A flap of skin is then raised on the wrist like the leaf of a book (the return flap) and sutured to the edge of the inferior half of the cut end of the tube pedicle.

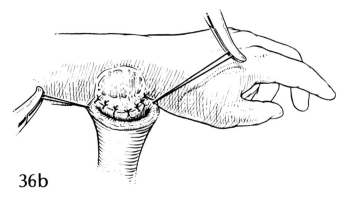

36b

37

The upper half is sutured to the half circle cut edge on the wrist.

Immobilization need not be complete, and Elastoplast will provide sufficient support and restraint.

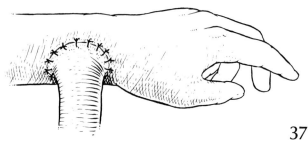

37

Transfer of the tube pedicle

After 3 weeks the second end of the tube is divided. This is attached to one edge of the defect, with only a small part of the return flap being used to obtain good closure along the seam; the remainder is discarded. The more of the tube that can be inset at this stage, the safer the final stage of detachment from the wrist and insetting, which is carried out after a further 3 weeks.

An alternative to the tube pedicle is the 'marsupial' flap described by Cuthbert[1], which allows a very broad piece of skin to be transported. The wrist attachment is achieved after the infolding of one-third of the flap has healed *in situ* on the abdomen.

In practice, where facilities for and expertise in microvascular surgery exist, the tube pedicle and marsupial flap methods of repair have been almost entirely superseded. However, the method still has applications, particularly in children and in the release of burns contractures, and is reliable and rewarding if carried out with proper attention to detail.

References

1. Cuthbert, J. B. The 'marsupial' skin flap. British Journal of Plastic Surgery 1949; 2: 125–131

Fasciocutaneous flaps

D. E. Tolhurst FRCS
Academisch Ziekenhuis Rotterdam, Rotterdam, The Netherlands

Introduction

It is only during the last 15 years that some significant advances have been made in the search for reliable flaps for the closure of complicated skin defects. Following Ger's demonstration of the value of muscle flaps[1], increasing experience with these flaps coupled with renewed interest in the exact anatomy of arteries supplying muscles led to the realization that many muscles will support an area of overlying skin whose boundaries can even be extended beyond those of the muscle itself. So was born the myocutaneous flap championed by McCraw[2].

In the late 1960s McGregor and Morgan[3] proposed a new classification of skin flaps; the well known delto-pectoral and groin flaps fell into the category of flaps with a system of axial vessels whilst all others, whose blood supply was not known to follow such a pattern, were termed random flaps. A vigorous search for axial pattern flaps ensued until attention began to be focused on myocutaneous flaps.

At the height of their popularity in 1980 Pontén[4] hit upon the idea of including the deep fascia with the overlying fat and skin in flaps on the lower leg. Such was their reliability that these fasciocutaneous flaps could be designed with a base to length ratio of 1:3, or more, on the lower leg. Tolhurst et al.[5,6] confirmed the safety of these flaps in the lower leg and applied the principle with success in other areas of the body such as the thigh, trunk and axilla.

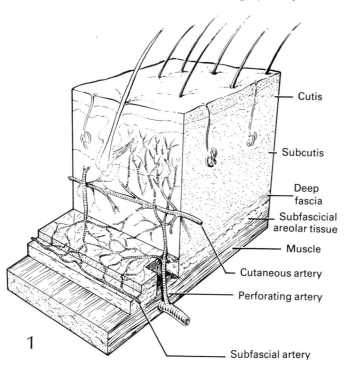

Cutis

Subcutis

Deep fascia

Subfascicial areolar tissue

Muscle

Cutaneous artery

Perforating artery

Subfascial artery

1

1

Although more detailed work is needed to clarify the precise role of the deep fascia as a vascular support to the overlying skin, Schäfer[7] has demonstrated three different arterial systems which are together responsible for the rich collateral circulation as well as the good perfusion of the deep fascia.

Wherever there is a layer of deep fascia in the body it is possible to raise a fasciocutaneous flap, and it is felt that random pattern flaps are even safer if they are raised together with the underlying deep fascia. Fasciocutaneous flaps have undoubtedly proved of the greatest use for the immediate closure of skin defects exposing bone or tendons in the lower leg. The technique of raising a fasciocutaneous flap, which combines the advantages of simplicity, lack of heavy bleeding, absence of secondary morbidity and impairment of function, with ease of dissection and transposition, will be demonstrated in the lower leg.

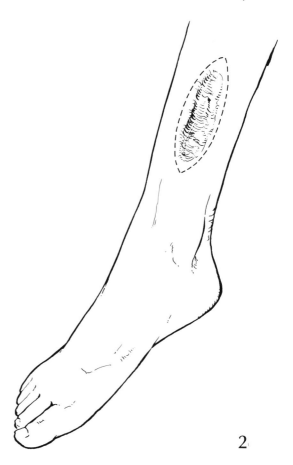

2

Technique

2

The margins of the wound to be closed are excised, and the defect is measured.

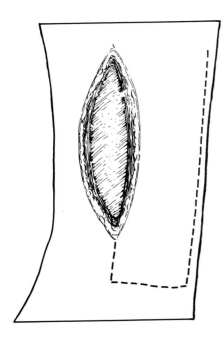

3

3

A flap is then outlined on the medial or lateral side of the defect, depending upon the availability of skin. The distal part of the flap should if possible exceed the length of the defect by a few centimetres in order to ensure that the defect can be comfortably covered after transposition of the flap. The base should be situated superiorly, and the length can be at least 3 times the breadth of the flap.

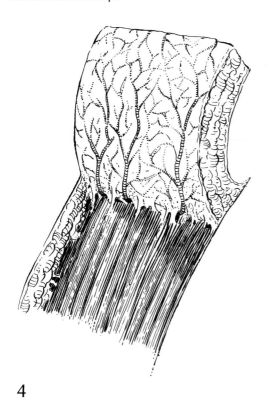

4

4

Cutting the flap is straightforward: the skin and fat are incised to deep fascia and the incision extended through the deep fascia. Starting distally the whole flap including the deep fascia is raised from the muscle. As the flap is raised a delicate plexus of vessels lying in a layer of loose areolar tissue on the deep surface of the fascia becomes visible. These vessels should be included with the fascia and, where encountered, perforating vessels are clamped and divided. As a rule there is very little bleeding from both surfaces.

If the flap is large and bulky it is sometimes helpful to tack the edges of the deep fascia to the subdermal tissue with a few Dexon sutures.

5

The flap is now transposed to cover the defect and the skin is sutured. An occasional suture between the bed of the defect and the deep fascia to help eliminate dead space does no harm. On the lower leg the donor defect is closed with a simple split skin graft, but on the trunk it is often possible to close the donor site by direct suture after wide undermining if the flap has been transposed through 90°.

A tie-over dressing is applied to the skin graft, the flap covered with a simple dressing and the leg encased in cotton wool and a firm bandage.

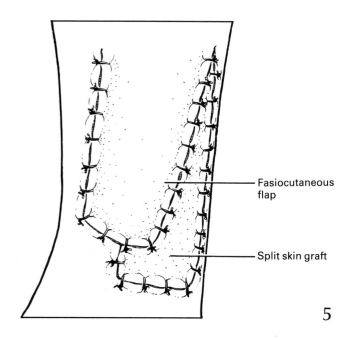

Fasiocutaneous flap

Split skin graft

5

References

1. Ger, R. The operative treatment of the advanced stasis ulcer: a preliminary communication. American Journal of Surgery 1966; 111: 659–663

2. McCraw, J. B., Dibbell, D. G. Experimental definition of independent myocutaneous vascular territories. Plastic and Reconstructive Surgery 1977; 60: 212–220

3. McGregor, I. A., Morgan, G. Axial and random pattern flaps. British Journal of Plastic Surgery 1973; 26: 202–213

4. Pontén, B. The fasciocutaneous flap: its use in soft tissue defects of the lower leg. British Journal of Plastic Surgery 1981; 34: 215–220

5. Tolhurst, D. E., Haeseker, B., Zeeman, R. J. Fasciocutaneous flaps. Chirurgia Plastica. 1982; 7: 11–21

6. Tolhurst, D. E., Haeseker, B. Fasciocutaneous flaps in the axillary region. British Journal of Plastic Surgery 1982; 35: 430–435

7. Schäfer, K. Das subcutane Gefäßsystem (untere Extremität): Mikropäparatorische Untersuchunger. Gegenbaurs Morphologisches Jahrbuch (Leipzig) 1975; 121: 492–514

Muscle, musculocutaneous and fasciocutaneous flaps

Luis O. Vasconez MD
Professor of Surgery and Chief, Division of Plastic Surgery, University of Alabama in Birmingham, USA

Samuel E. Logan MD, PhD
Assistant Professor, Division of Plastic Surgery, Washington University School of Medicine, St Louis, Missouri, USA

Introduction

1

Precise understanding of muscular blood supply has allowed the development of numerous *muscle and musculocutaneous flaps*. Because these are arterialized flaps, transfer can be made in a single stage. The key anatomical feature of a musculocutaneous flap is that the skin overlying the muscle is supplied from perforating musculocutaneous vessels. It is therefore possible to take an entire unit of muscle with overlying skin and expect it to survive so long as there is a dominant vascular pedicle. This concept has been extremely helpful in the design of flaps for the reconstruction of defects throughout the body. Experimental and clinical work has shown that muscle, because of its rich vascularity, encourages healing of chronically infected wounds that have been resistant to other modes of treatment.

Recent appreciation of skin territories supplied by fascial arteries and fasciocutaneous peforators has led to the concept of the *fasciocutaneous flap*. Although much more investigation is required, a number of clinically useful fasciocutaneous flaps have been developed.

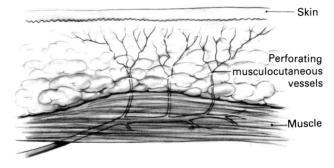

Skin

Perforating musculocutaneous vessels

Muscle

1

Choice of flaps

Several general considerations play a part in the selection of a suitable muscle or musculocutaneous flap to cover a particular defect.

1. The muscle should be adjacent to the surgical or traumatic defect, and should be expendable and of sufficient size to cover the defect. A muscle may be expendable because it is no longer needed, as with the gluteus muscle in non-ambulatory patients, or if there are synergistic muscles to compensate for its loss. Function can be preserved by splitting a muscle and using only a portion of it for transposition. Because the insertion of the muscle is divided, the transposed portion will lose its function and atrophy to approximately 50 per cent of its bulk. Although in theory the muscle can be returned to its original location and regain its function, this option has been used rarely, if at all.
2. The muscle should have a major vascular pedicle that nourishes the entire flap. Most musculocutaneous units have a major (dominant) vascular pedicle proximally and minor ones located distally. Certain muscles, such as the sartorius, have a segmental blood supply, with each segmental vessel supplying a small independent territory, which makes flap design more complex and less useful. Others, such as the latissimus dorsi musculocutaneous unit, have not only a major vascular pedicle entering at the proximal end but also multiple large perforators in the paravertebral area at the distal end, with multiple interconnections between these two systems. Consequently, in this particular unit, a distally based flap can be designed if some of the paravertebral perforators are preserved as the proximal thoracodorsal vascular bundle is divided.

   Some flaps, such as the tensor fasciae latae and inferior gluteal thigh, have associated sensory nerves that can be preserved, allowing the possibility of sensory units. Nevertheless, their application as sensory units needs further evaluation.
3. A defect in the donor area cannot be avoided. If, however, the musculocutaneous unit is used in an aesthetic reconstruction, such as the breast, a secondary defect of any proportion is undesirable.

The following muscle and musculocutaneous flaps have proved clinically useful:

1. Latissimus dorsi
2. Rectus abdominis
3. Pectoralis major
4. Trapezius (vertically designed)
5. Gluteus maximus
6. Rectus femoris
7. Tensor fasciae latae
8. Gastrocnemius
9. Soleus
10. Gracilis

Useful fasciocutaneous flaps have been obtained from the following sites:

1. Anterior thigh
2. Posterior inferior gluteal thigh
3. Gastrocnemius (posterior calf)
4. Parascapular

MUSCLE AND MUSCULOCUTANEOUS FLAPS

Latissimus dorsi

2

The major arterial supply of the latissimus dorsi muscle comes from the subscapular artery through the thoraco-dorsal artery and enters the muscle near its insertion into the humerus, where it divides into two main branches. A portion of the muscle with overlying skin can be elevated on either of these two main branches, allowing use of only half the muscle. The main pedicle will support the entire muscle and overlying skin. Similarly, the musculo-cutaneous unit can be based distally, preserving the large perforating vessels along the paravertebral area. This reversed latissimus unit, with its potentially wide axis of rotation, may be transposed to cover defects along the thoracolumbar area.

This flap is exceptionally safe and has been most useful for breast reconstruction after radical mastectomy. It is also the most popular free-flap donor site because of its long, reliable vascular pedicle, ease of dissection and acceptable donor defect.

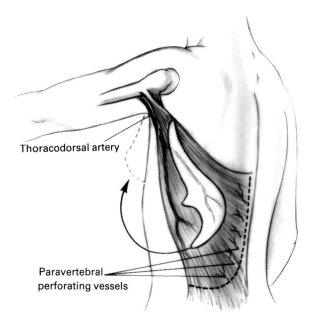

Thoracodorsal artery

Paravertebral perforating vessels

2

BREAST RECONSTRUCTION WITH LATISSIMUS DORSI

3

After radical or modified radical mastectomy, the latissimus dorsi can provide bulk to compensate for the missing or atrophic pectoralis major muscle, recreate the anterior axillary fold and provide excellent coverage for the silicone breast prosthesis. For successful transfer the latissimus dorsi must not have been devascularized or denervated during the mastectomy. The amount of muscle to be transferred is determined by the size and contour of the anterior defect to be reconstructed, and the skin island is designed and positioned so as to provide the optimum breast contour (*see Illustration 2*). Donor defects of up to 8 × 15 cm can be closed primarily; a larger defect requires a skin graft.

With the patient in the lateral position, the skin island (*see Illustration 2*) is incised down to the latissimus muscle and left attached to the underlying muscle. The surrounding skin flaps are elevated above the tip of the scapula superiorly but not quite reaching the iliac spine or middle of the back inferiorly and laterally. The skin island and latissimus muscle are elevated, leaving the underlying serratus in place. Dissection begins at the superior border of the latissimus just above the tip of the scapula (to avoid the scarring from the mastectomy along the anterior border of the latissimus) and proceeds inferomedially and inferolaterally. The flap is freed completely toward the axilla, allowing it to swing as a pendulum, and the vascular pedicle containing the thoracodorsal artery is identified and preserved. The flap is passed anteriorly through a tunnel high in the axilla, and the back incision is closed over a suction drain. The patient is then placed in the supine position and redraped, and the flap is inset in a previously marked line corresponding to the inframammary line and often disregarding the previous scar. If the pectoralis muscle is absent or atrophic, muscle is advanced into the infraclavicular hollow to offer potential correction.

A small opening in the incision is left laterally for submuscular placement of the silastic prosthesis. If possible, the final positioning and sizing should be done with the patient in a sitting position.

The commonest complication (occurring in up to 50 per cent of patients) is seroma at the donor site. Partial skin island loss occurs in less than 2 per cent of cases, and muscle loss is exceedingly rare, making this a very safe procedure. The colour discrepancy between the skin from the back and the adjacent anterior chest skin is most bothersome to the patient if the skin island is placed too high in the chest. Projection and a certain amount of ptosis are essential if one is to match the opposite breast.

Our own experience (Replogle and Vasconez, unpublished observations) indicates that in order to obtain projection the skin island must be placed vertically to increase the distance between the midsternal and mid-axillary line. For ptosis, the vertical distance has to be increased from the midclavicular line to the inframammary line. Different designs of skin islands, particularly of the lazy S or sickle variety, combine a vertical and a transverse component which are placed along the inframammary and anterior axillary lines respectively.

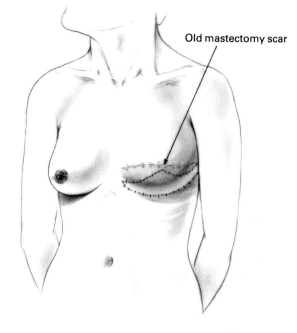

Old mastectomy scar

3

REVERSED LATISSIMUS DORSI FOR COVERAGE OF DEFECTS IN THE THORACOLUMBAR SPINE

This technique provides coverage for post-radiation wounds, post-surgery (laminectomy) wounds, and open wounds in the lumbar spine. It is also useful for closure of large meningomyelocele defects in children.

4 & 5

A transverse flap is outlined on the back, extending from the midback to the midaxillary line. This can then be rotated 90° and converted to an island with which to cover the defect in the lumbar region. Note the two rows of perforators located approximately 5 cm from the midline.

The flap is circumscribed down to and including the latissimus dorsi muscle. Elevation begins anteriorly, but care should be taken not to include the serratus anterior, which is identified by the different direction of its fibres. The dissection proceeds sharply up to the midback, encountering only an occasional perforator from the intercostal branches. At this point the dissection is continued with considerable care until at least one of the paravertebral perforators is identified. The superior and inferior incisions may be safely extended to the midline, but without undermining at this level. If a dog ear is not acceptable, or if one needs more length to cover the defect, the flap may be circumscribed as an island. The secondary defect can be closed primarily.

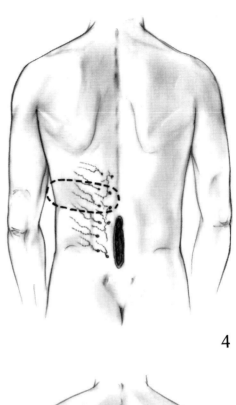

4

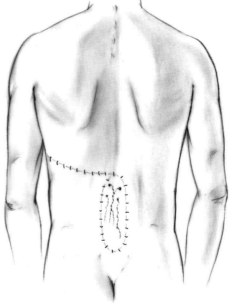

5

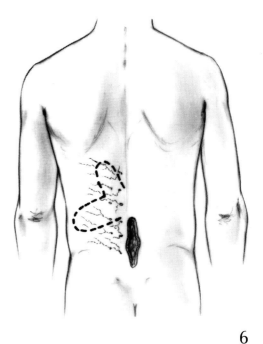

6

6 & 7

A bilobe design to facilitate closure of the secondary defect can also be used.

Several precautions are necessary when using the reversed latissimus flap. In patients with post-irradiation or open post-laminectomy wounds the perforators may have been damaged or divided. Similarly, there may be severe induration surrounding the wound, making design of an adjacent flap most troublesome. Whenever feasible, tissue should be taken from a non-irradiated area.

If there is a dural leak it is important that this is sealed with muscle; depending on the location of the defect, available possibilities include the latissimus (thoracolumbar), the trapezius (cervical wounds) and the gluteus (low lumbar).

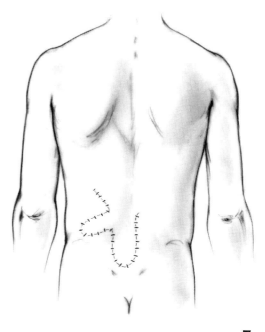

7

Rectus abdominis

The paired rectus abdominis muscles are important in flexing the vertebral column and tightening the abdominal wall. By increasing intra-abdominal pressure, they play a significant role in maintaining proper posture (particularly of the lumbar spine), in the prevention of back pain, and as an aid in defaecation and urination. Because of its exciting use in breast reconstruction, considerable interest in its anatomy and function has recently been generated.

8

The rectus abdominis receives its blood supply from two sources: (1) from the epigastric arcade that is composed of the superior and inferior epigastric vessels and (2) segmentally from the intercostal vessels. The rectus abdominis muscle will survive in its entirety with only one artery: the superior or inferior epigastric. This is an interesting physiological finding because in anatomical and post-mortem dye injection studies it is difficult to demonstrate continuity of the superior or inferior epigastric arcade throughout the muscle. The innervation is segmental and enters the muscle laterally. The epigastric arcade sends a row of perforators through the fascia which are of paramount importance in supplying the overlying skin. These anatomical facts play an important role in the design of safe musculocutaneous flaps, several of which are described below.

The rectus abdominis muscle, occasionally combined with the pectoralis muscle, has also been useful in the coverage of lower median sternotomy defects (*see Illustrations 25 and 26*).

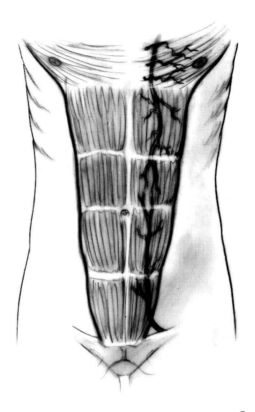

8

LOWER RECTUS ABDOMINIS

9 & 10

The larger vascular pedicle of the rectus abdominis is the inferior epigastric artery. The entire muscle could be dissected safely from its origin on the costal margin down to its insertion in the pelvis. As the muscle is freed, dividing the intercostal vessels as well as the superior epigastric artery, the arc of rotation of the inferiorly based muscle will demonstrate a tremendous reach. It has been used successfully for coverage of defects in the groin as well as for above-the-knee amputation stumps, and may also reach the lumbar area. This unit should be kept in mind, particularly when all the more conventional flaps have failed.

A variety of superior transverse skin islands can be designed on the inferiorly based rectus abdominis, providing a versatile musculocutaneous unit. Because of its wide arc of rotation the flap will cover defects in the trunk, pelvis and upper thigh. The 'flag flap of De la Plaza' is a variation with the skin island designed in the submammary area (De la Plaza, personal communication). Adequate mobilization allows direct closure by a reverse abdominoplasty and placement of the scar in the inframammary line.

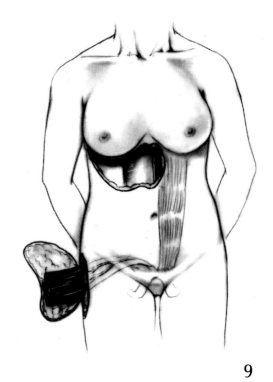

9

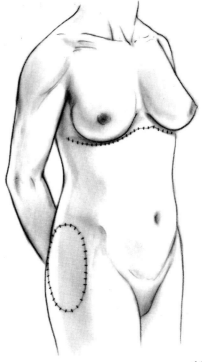

10

UPPER RECTUS ABDOMINIS FOR BREAST RECONSTRUCTION

This method has the advantage of using skin from the contralateral submammary area, similar in colour and texture, and transposing it to the mastectomy site, where there is a shortage of skin. It balances the torso of the patient and produces an acceptable scar that usually falls in the submammary area.

11, 12 & 13

A medially truncated ellipse is outlined on the contralateral submammary fold. The superior border is convex and extends above the inframammary line. The flap can safely extend to the anterior axillary line. It is elevated from lateral to medial until the lateral edge of the rectus muscle is encountered. The dissection proceeds by making the medial incision and opening the anterior rectus sheath (saving the linea alba) to expose the rectus abdominis muscle. A segment of muscle approximately 2 cm longer than the width of skin is included with the flap. It is important to suture ligate the superior epigastric vessels to avoid postoperative haematoma. The entire unit is transposed to the contralateral chest. Because the vascular pedicle is relatively short, and it is difficult and time-consuming to lengthen it, subperichondral resection of a portion of the seventh costal cartilage is most helpful in preserving and lengthening the underlying epigastric vessel. The flap should reach the contralateral anterior axillary line for a satisfactory reconstruction. A silastic implant may be inserted at the same time, but in this case the vascular pedicle should be freed even more to avoid excessive traction on the pedicle. In about 50 per cent of reconstructions there is no need for a silastic implant.

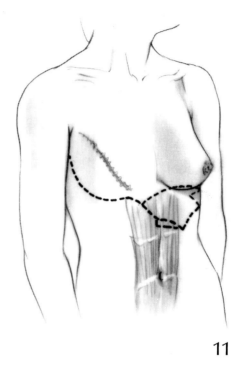

11

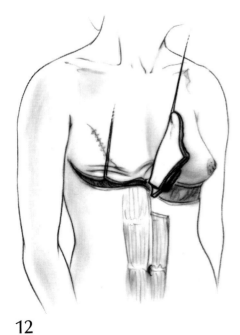

12

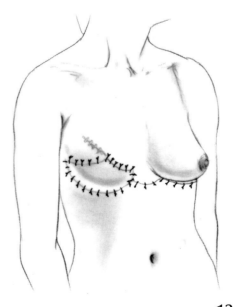

13

BREAST RECONSTRUCTION WITH A LOWER TRANSVERSE RECTUS ABDOMINIS FLAP

This most imaginative method of breast reconstruction, introduced by Hartrampf et al.[1], uses the skin of the infraumbilical area based on the rectus abdominis muscle.

14–17

The contralateral rectus abdominis is preferred, although the ipsilateral rectus can also be used. An ellipse of skin at the infraumbilical area is outlined, and four zones (1–4) of decreasing vascularity are envisioned. Dissection begins laterally at zone 4 and continues into zone 2, including skin and subcutaneous tissue but not the fascia. The perforating vessels that are divided between haemoclips in zone 2 are noted; these serve as a guide for their preservation in zone 1. After completing the superior incision the abdominal wall is elevated to the costal margin. A wide strip of anterior fascia is included with the underlying rectus muscle by making an incision just lateral to the midline and just medial to the lateral edge of the rectus fascia. The muscle is freed from the posterior sheath, and the intercostal vessels and nerves are divided. Only at the intersectiones tendineae is it necessary to use sharp dissection.

The anterior rectus fascia is carefully elevated with the flap in zone 1 to preserve the musculocutaneous perforators and to prevent their inadvertent disruption by traction or shearing. Some anterior rectus fascia should be left below the semilunar line to allow secure closure and avoid a postoperative hernia.

The chest incision is reopened on the mastectomy side and connected to the abdominal dissection through a subcutaneous tunnel. The muscle is divided at the semilunar line approximately 10 cm above the pubis, the inferior epigastric vessels are ligated, and the flap is transposed to the chest through a high subcutaneous tunnel. The lower aspect of the new incision is placed approximately 2–3 cm above the existing inframammary line. The reconstructed inframammary line will shift inferiorly postoperatively because of the abdominoplasty closure, the pull of the rectus muscle, and gravity.

Passage of the flap to the contralateral side should be high to avoid a bulge over the costal margin. Division of the origin of the rectus muscle at the costal margin further minimizes this bulge and lessens tension on the flap. This manoeuvre is done with relative safety because the superior epigastric vessels are well protected. The flap is inserted by placing the first suture correcting the midportion of the flap to correspond to the medial aspect of the inframammary line. Zone 2 of the flap forms the inframammary line and extends up towards the axilla. The most distal zone of the flap (zone 4) is discarded, while zone 3 is usually de-epithelialized and folded under to give projection and lateral fullness to the breast.

Because most of the mastectomy scars are quite high, the skin below the mastectomy scar should be excised to just above the inframammary line and the entire breast reconstructed with the infraumbilical skin.

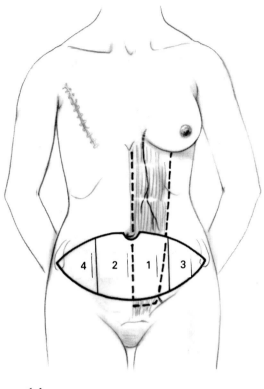

14

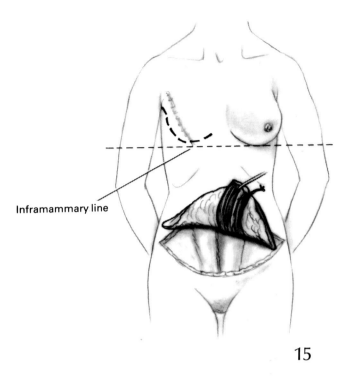

Inframammary line

15

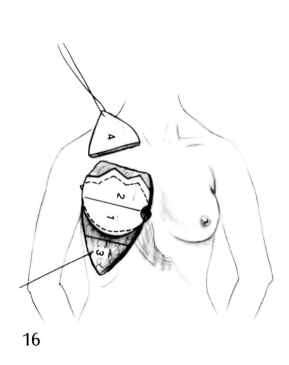

16

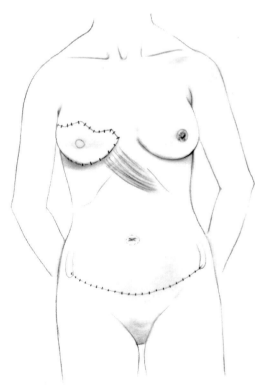

17

Pectoralis major

18

The major vascular pedicle to the pectoralis major muscle – the thoracoacromial artery, a branch of the axillary artery – is located just medial to the medial border of the pectoralis minor muscle. It is not necessary to include the entire pectoral muscle in elevating this unit so long as the vascular pedicle is preserved. The most useful skin is at the level of the costal margin, where the rectus fascia should be included, and a skin island can be designed as illustrated. Depending on the size of the skin island the donor defect can either be closed primarily or covered with a split thickness skin graft. If necessary, the skin over the sternum or the submammary area may also be included with an extended cutaneous territory. With its wide axis of rotation, this unit is most helpful in reconstructing defects of the head and neck.

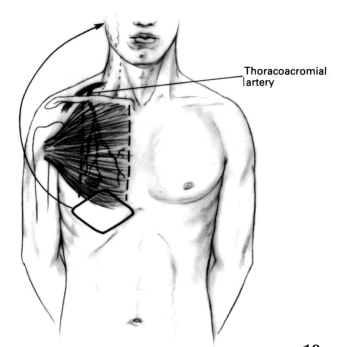

Thoracoacromial artery

18

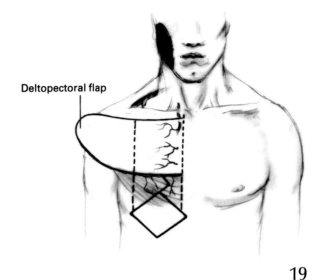

19

19, 20 & 21

Overlying the pectoralis major muscle is the skin territory
of the well-proven deltopectoral fasciocutaneous flap.
Because this flap receives its blood supply through
perforators from the internal mammary artery medially,
elevation of the deltopectoral flap does not interfere with
the simultaneous use of a pectoralis muscle or musculocutaneous flap. Combination of these two flaps provides a
versatile tool for reconstruction of full thickness cheek
defects and other defects requiring both coverage and
lining. For cheek reconstruction the pectoralis muscle
may be tunnelled subcutaneously as shown or constructed as a pedicle to be divided later. The deltopectoral
flap is later divided and returned to the chest wall.

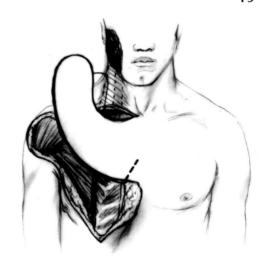

20

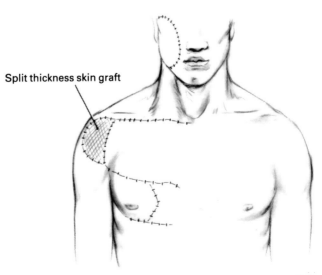

21

COVERAGE OF MEDIAN STERNOTOMY DEFECTS USING BILATERAL PECTORALIS MAJOR AND RECTUS ABDOMINIS MUSCLE

22

Open median sternotomy wounds, usually a result of complications after coronary arterial surgery, can be closed in a number of ways using the pectoralis major and the rectus abdominis muscles. The three options for closure are (1) advancement of both pectoralis muscles alone; (2) medial advancement of a composite of skin and muscle; and (3) a turnover flap of pectoralis muscle alone.

The pectoralis major muscles insert obliquely along the sixth rib and will not cover the lower mediastinum in larger defects. In such cases the rectus abdominis, superiorly based, is added.

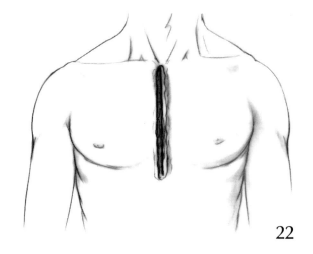

22

23

The wound and exposed edges of the sternum are debrided without entering the pleural cavities and resecting so far laterally that the internal mammary vessels or their perforators are divided. Following sternal debridement, the skin and muscle unit is freed bilaterally from the underlying chest wall as far laterally as possible, but preserving the pectoralis minor muscle as well as the major vascular pedicle to the pectoralis major. Incisions are made at the level of the anterior axillary fold, and the insertion of the pectoralis major muscle is divided bilaterally from the humerus.

Although advancement of the pectoralis muscle alone requires further dissection, since the muscle must also be freed from the overlying skin, the transposed muscle will stretch further and conform better to the defect, thus avoiding dead space in the mediastinal bed. For this reason we recommend this option whenever possible. On the other hand, medial advancement of skin and muscle as a unit is faster, relatively bloodless and likely to be just as successful. In both options the muscle is imbricated in the midline and will transpose over the mediastinal defect with little or no tension.

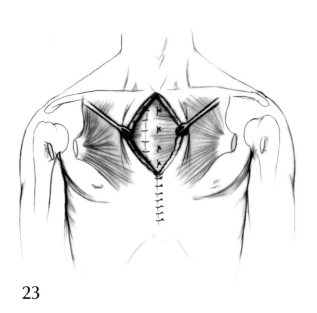

23

24

The third option is to reverse the pectoralis major by dividing its insertion from the humerus as well as its major thoracoacromial blood supply, turning it over like the page of a book and basing it on the perforators of the internal mammary artery. This will provide a considerable amount of muscle to fit into a large concave mediastinal defect.

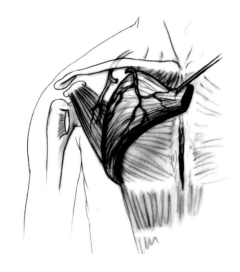

24

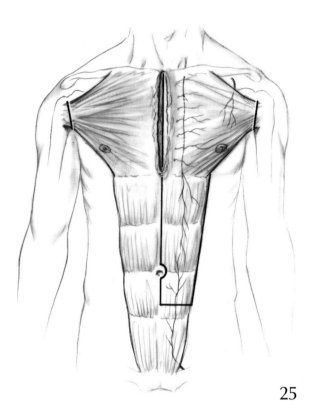

25 & 26

The pectoralis muscle will not cover the lowermost aspect of large mediastinal defects. In these cases the ipsilateral or contralateral rectus abdominis should be transposed. The mediastinal incision is extended inferiorly to below the umbilicus. The anterior rectus sheath is opened over the muscle, and the underlying rectus muscle is freed bluntly, except at the intersectiones tendineae, which requires sharp dissection. The amount of muscle needed to fill the defect is determined. Usually enough length can be obtained by dividing the muscle just below the umbilicus but above the semilunar line. If a wider arc of rotation is required, the muscle origin from the costal margin may be divided, converting the flap into an island. Care must be taken with the dissection near the xyphoid or along the seventh costal cartilage.

No attempt is made to reapproximate the sternum as clinical experience has shown that respiratory capacity is not impaired and assisted ventilation is not required.

25

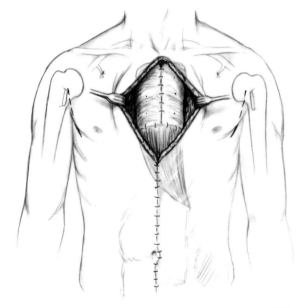

26

27

With proper mobilization, the wound is closed in layers, approximating the muscles, subcutaneous tissue and skin. If the rectus muscle is used the abdominal wound can be closed directly. The mediastinal wound may either be closed directly or the exposed muscle can be covered with a meshed split thickness skin graft.

Suction catheters, preferably silastic, are placed in the mediastinum but are removed after 48–72 hours to prevent any erosion of vital stuctures.

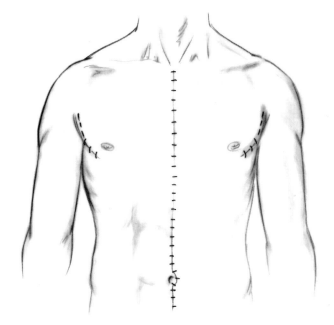

27

Precautions

1. Adequate debridement of the exposed sternum is essential.
2. If the pleural cavities are entered, chest tubes should be placed.
3. If the pectoralis muscles alone are used, there will be considerable potential dead space between muscle and overlying skin flaps, and this area should be suction drained.
4. Suction catheters in the mediastinum, even though they may be soft, should be removed as soon as possible (no later than 48–72 hours after insertion) to prevent erosion into the major vessels or trachea.

5. If the patient has had irradiation to the chest or a mastectomy, only the pectoralis major muscle from the contralateral side should be used, with the addition of the rectus abdominis. Omentum is safer than muscle in certain postradiation mediastinal wounds.
6. If the patient requires anticoagulants, heparin is preferred. Haematomas are common but are minimized by a combination of pressure dressings and suction catheters.

Trapezius

28

The major vascular supply of the trapezius is the transverse cervical artery, a branch of the subclavian artery, in the anterior neck. This vessel divides into a descending branch, the posterior scapular artery, and an ascending branch, the superficial cervical artery. The medial and inferior muscle fibres are expendable, and their use does not result in the shoulder-drooping deformity characteristic of the loss of the anterior muscle. For this reason vertically designed trapezius flaps have proved most useful and reliable.

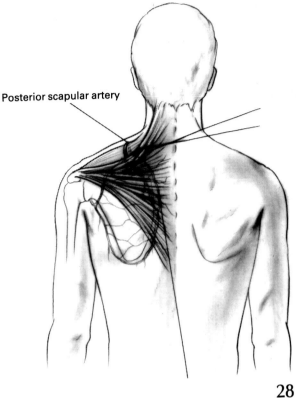

Posterior scapular artery

28

29

A portion of muscle can be used if the major arterial supply, the posterior scapular artery, is preserved. The usable skin territory of the musculocutaneous flap may safely extend up to 5 cm below the inferior border of the scapula, and the donor site can usually be closed primarily.

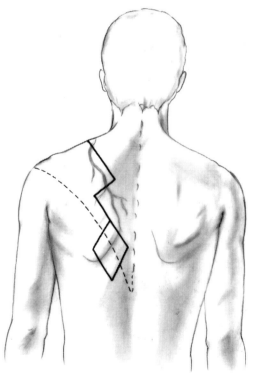

29

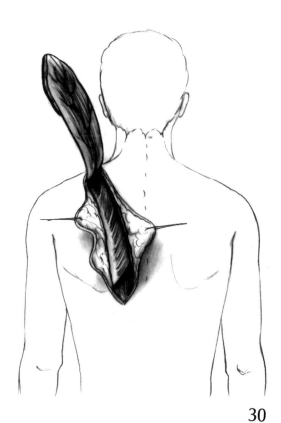

30

30 & 31

This muscle or musculocutaneous unit has a wide arc of rotation on its dominant pedicle at the base of the neck and is useful for reconstruction of defects in the head and neck, skull, shoulder and cervical spine.

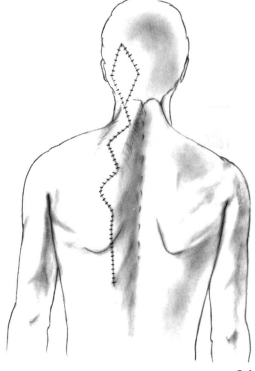

31

Gluteus maximus

32

The gluteus maximus is not an expendable muscle, except in paraplegics. In ambulatory patients it is essential for walking, and neither the inferior nor the superior position can be spared. Although the muscle is supplied by two discrete branches of the hypogastric artery – the superior and inferior gluteal arteries, both of which enter the muscle medially – the nerve supply accompanies the inferior gluteal artery. Division of the superior portion of the gluteus maximus would therefore of necessity denervate it. The gluteus maximus also receives its blood supply from the first branch of the profunda femoris that serves to form the cruciate anastomosis. The interconnections between this lateral blood supply and the superior and inferior gluteal arteries are multiple, and the muscle and overlying skin will survive on any of these three sources alone. The associated cutaneous territory includes the entire buttock area.

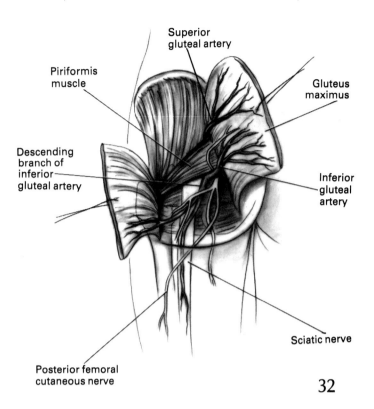

32

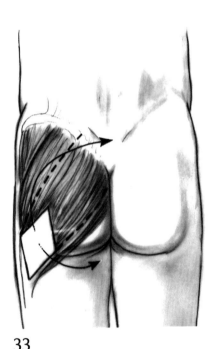

33

33

A variety of skin islands based on either the superior or the inferior gluteal arteries have been described. Although their vascular pedicle is relatively short and the arc of rotation limited, the sacrum can be reached with a superior island and the ischium with an inferior island. However, as indicated earlier, this technique is inappropriate for ambulatory patients, e.g. those with postradiation ulceration of the sacrum.

34 & 35

We favour the sliding gluteus maximus technique described by Ramirez, Orlander and Hurwitz[2], in which the muscle is freed bilaterally from its origin along the sacrum and from the gluteus medius, preserving the superior and inferior gluteal arteries as well as its nerve supply. Its inferior portion is freed along the sacrotuberous ligament, leaving it attached only by its insertion along the trochanter and the linea aspera of the femur. Once the muscle has been freed bilaterally, it will advance medially for at least 10 cm each side to allow coverage of the entire sacrum. The overlying skin will reach further with a V-Y advancement designed with its base along the sacrum and its sides along the superior and inferior border of the gluteus maximus, converging on its insertion in the greater trochanter. These skin incisions, together with moderate undermining, allow dissection of the muscle. Although difficult, the technique is worth while in ambulatory patients because of the preservation of function. The sliding gluteus maximus is the flap of choice for covering postradiation defects of the sacrum and for filling cavities in the sacral area after abdomino-perineal resections or colectomies for granulomatous colitis. It is superior to the commonly advocated gracilis flap, which is not sufficiently long or bulky to fill the cavities in the perineum.

The difficulties of dissection, particularly along the sacrotuberous ligament to free the muscle inferiorly, are due mainly to the anatomy of the area. The difference in texture, as well as a slight change in the direction of the fibres, facilitates recognition of the plane between the gluteus maximus and medius. The proximity to the sciatic nerve should be kept in mind. The dissection is bloody, particularly when freeing the insertion of the gluteus maximus from the sacrum and dividing the sacral vessels, which should be carefully controlled to avoid their retraction into the presacral space.

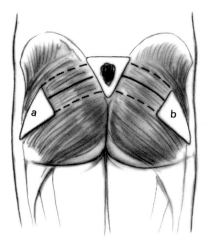

34

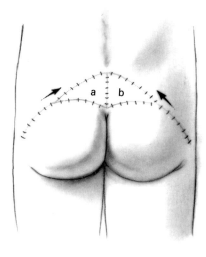

35

Rectus femoris

36

The rectus femoris muscle is part of the quadriceps group that flexes the thigh and extends the leg. This unit can be used to cover defects of the lower abdominal wall, perineum, trochanteric region and groin. The associated cutaneous territory on the anterior thigh between the sartorius and tensor fasciae latae can be elevated with the rectus femoris muscle or separately as a fasciocutaneous flap (see *Illustration 45*). In most cases the donor defect can be closed primarily. The lateral circumflex femoral artery, which enters the proximal muscle approximately 10 cm below the inguinal ligament, provides the vascular supply.

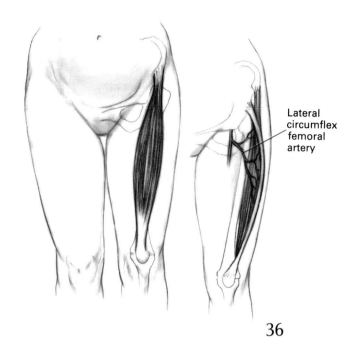

Lateral circumflex femoral artery

36

37

Tensor fasciae latae

37

The vascular supply of the tensor fasciae latae, the lateral circumflex branch of the profunda femoris, enters the muscle 8–10 cm below the anterior superior iliac spine. The muscle is proximal and relatively small. Distally, the flap is a skin–fascia unit, including the fascia lata. If necessary, a substantial territory on the anterolateral thigh can be elevated with the flap, and in most cases the donor defect can be closed primarily. The arc of rotation is almost 360°, and both anterior and posterior defects can be covered. This flap is most useful for covering trochanteric defects and may reach the ischium and sacrum. It has also proved to be an excellent alternative to the transposed sartorius muscle for covering the femoral vessels after a groin dissection. It is not recommended for reconstruction of postradiation wounds on the lower abdomen, particularly over the pubis, where the rectus femoris is the flap of choice.

The lateral cutaneous branch of T12 and the lateral femoral cutaneous nerve provide sensibility to the flaps.

Gastrocnemius

38a & b

The gastrocnemius and its associated skin territory on the posterior calf can be used as a muscle flap, a musculocutaneous flap or a fasciocutaneous unit. The sural branches from the popliteal artery supply the muscle with an independent vessel to both the medial and lateral muscular heads. In addition, a rich network of musculocutaneous perforators supplies the skin overlying the muscle. The skin territory of the musculocutaneous unit can be extended beyond the muscle itself for at least the same distance as the width of one of its heads. In fact, in the subfascial plexus, these musculocutaneous perforators are so richly interconnected with a direct axial branch off the popliteal artery that a sizeable fasciocutaneous flap is not only feasible but has also been shown to be reliable. This flap has the advantage of leaving the muscle intact.

For the muscle or musculocutaneous units, either the medial or lateral head can be used. If the soleus is intact, transposition of one of these heads results in only minimal functional deficit. Either head can be used for coverage of the knee or upper third of the leg. Because the medial head is somewhat longer and closer to the tibia, it is often chosen to cover tibial defects. Distal division of a portion of the tendinous attachment is necessary to allow rotation of either head. For the musculocutaneous unit or fasciocutaneous unit, the donor must be skin-grafted.

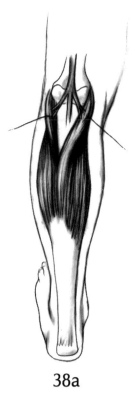

38a

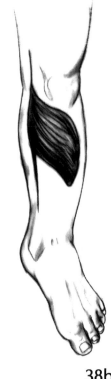

38b

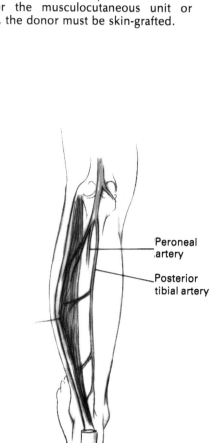

Peroneal artery

Posterior tibial artery

39a

39b

Soleus

39a & b

The soleus lies immediately beneath the gastrocnemius and is expendable in the ambulatory patient if the gastrocnemius is functional. The dominant vascular pedicle, a branch of the peroneal artery, enters the muscle 10–12 cm below the knee and can support the entire unit. There are also several minor distal pedicles (branches of the posterior tibial artery) whose division allows transposition of the muscular unit to cover defects in the midtibial region. Distally based flaps may be designed as indicated by the dashed lines if the nourishing vessels from the posterior tibial artery are preserved.

FASCIOCUTANEOUS FLAPS

Although musculocutaneous flaps have found wide acceptance in clinical practice, it has recently been shown that in a number of cases the underlying muscle need not be included for the skin and fascia to survive so long as there is a large proximal axial vessel or perforator. This has been beautifully demonstrated in the territory of the gastrocnemius by Pontén[3].

Gastrocnemius

40 & 41

The gastrocnemius musculocutaneous unit may be designed with the skin and fascia extending beyond the end of the muscle for at least 5–10 cm. At the proximal end of the muscle there are distinct, large perforators which form a wide anastomotic network on top of the fascia and supply the overlying skin. However, the main blood supply to this fasciocutaneous unit is a direct axial branch from the popliteal artery so that a skin and fascial flap can be raised over the gastrocnemius and transposed to cover defects on the proximal and medial third of the leg. There is no need to include the underlying muscle.

Indeed, there is now probably very little need for the classically designed gastrocnemius musculocutaneous unit, and either the muscle alone or the fasciocutaneous unit is used. The muscle alone is preferred for covering defects of the proximal third of the tibia or the knee joint. If additional length is needed, it may be converted to an island by dividing the muscle origin from the femoral condyles. In this way, a most unattractive defect in the back of the leg is avoided.

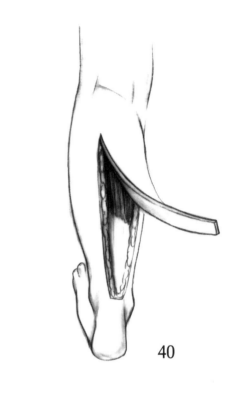

40

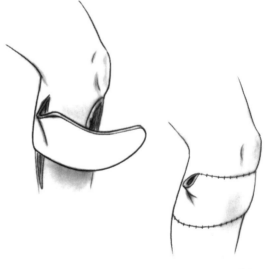

41

Thigh

42 & 43

Successful fasciocutaneous flaps have been raised any-where in the anterior thigh corresponding to the territory that has been outlined for the rectus femoris (*see Illustration 36*). The blood supply to this fasciocutaneous flap is dual, coming, perhaps, from a large perforator which leaves the muscle at the same level at which the major vascular pedicle enters it and from an inferiorly directed axial vessel from the cartwheel that exists at the femoral level. This cartwheel sends vessels laterally to correspond to the superficial circumflex iliac (the groin flap), superiorly to the superficial inferior epigastric (Shawn-Payne flap), and medially and inferiorly to conform to the unnamed fasciocutaneous flaps of the anterior thigh. If desired, the anterior thigh fascio-cutaneous flap may be used with the rectus femoris muscle, elevating each separately as illustrated.

In the medial thigh viable skin and fascial flaps can be raised over the territory corresponding to the gracilis, without including the muscle. This flap is expected to survive and is useful for covering defects in the ischium.

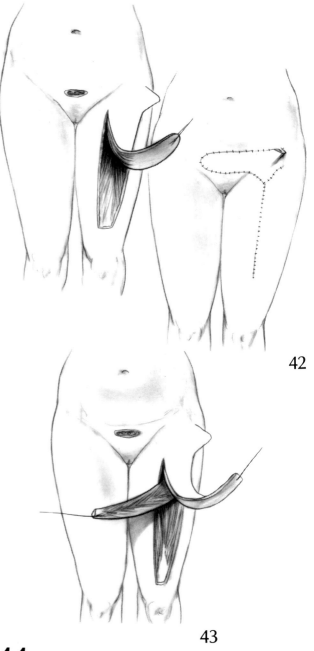

42

43

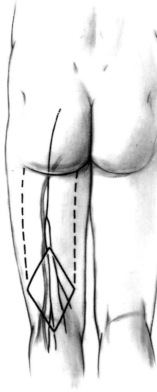

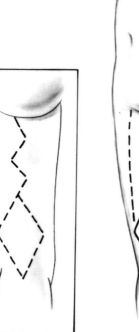

44

44

Inferior gluteal thigh flap

The inferior gluteal thigh flap, originally described by Hurwitz, Schwartz and Mathes[4], is a well-established and versatile fasciocutaneous flap, useful for covering ischial, trochanteric and pelvic defects. Its vascular supply comes from the descending branch of the inferior gluteal artery, and the posterior femoral cutaneous nerve provides sensibility to the flap. It may be designed either as a peninsula or as an island (*see inset*). The donor defect can often be closed primarily, but for wider flaps (more than 9–10 cm) a split thickness skin graft is usually required.

Parascapular flap

45a–b

This fasciocutaneous flap was first described and used by Tolhurst, Haescher and Zeeman[5] for the release of axillary contractures. The landmarks are as follows: the anterior border corresponds to the posterior axillary line; the width of the flap is approximately 7 cm; and its inferior border is at least 10 cm from the tip of the scapula.

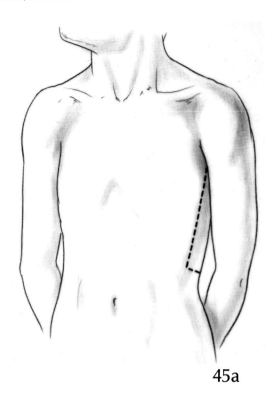

45a

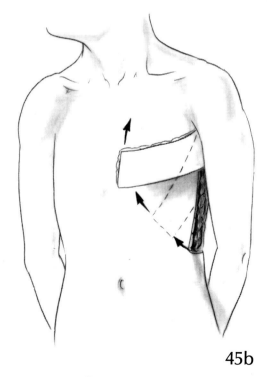

45b

45c–f

The flap is elevated with the deep fascia but sparing the latissimus dorsi. Three or four small perforators from the latissimus are divided. The flap is dissected superiorly to the triangular space formed by the teres major, the subscapularis and the large head of the triceps. This is the site where the vascular pedicle exits.

The blood supply is from an inferiorly directed branch of the circumflex scapular artery. The parent artery divides into two branches; one runs tranversely to supply the territory of the scapular flap, the other is an inferior branch that supplies the parascapular flap. The artery measures approximately 1 mm in diameter and is accompanied by two veins, each measuring 1.5 mm in diameter. The vascular pedicle penetrates the deep fascia and runs on top of it, forming an extensive fascial and subdermic plexus. The flap can be converted to an island so long as the deep fascia is spared and the vascular pedicle maintained.

This flap is most useful for covering defects in the axilla, the posterior arm and portions of the anterior thorax.

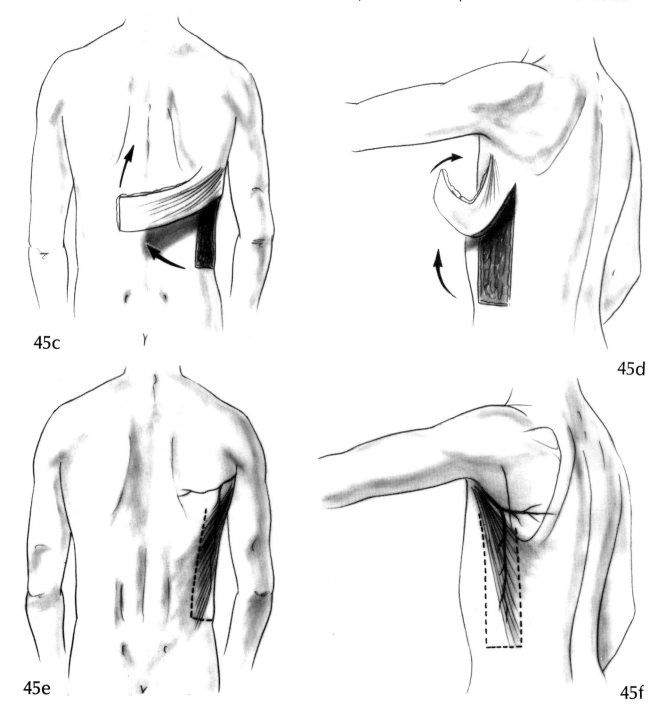

45c

45d

45e

45f

Other fasciocutaneous flaps

The tensor fasciae latae flap from the lateral thigh is also a type of fasciocutaneous flap. The muscle is relatively small, and there is a longitudinal vessel running on top of the fascia that nourishes the overlying skin.

Recently, a number of other fasciocutaneous flaps have all been described, corresponding to the territories of well-known musculocutaneous flaps. For example, in the region of the latissimus dorsi, fasciocutaneous flaps can be elevated to cover axillary defects. The reversed latissimus may be made into a fasciocutaneous flap – the muscle does not seem to be essential. The old thoraco-acromial flap, which was supplanted by the medially based deltopectoral flap, may also be raised safely without the muscle if care is taken to preserve the large perforator that exists at the same level at which the thoracoacromial vessel enters the pectoralis major muscle.

The deltopectoral flap is another important skin and fascial flap, as emphasized by Bakamjian (see chapter on 'Achievement of skin cover using the deltopectoral flap', pp. 128–133). This can also be made into a free flap based on the second perforator from the internal mammary artery.

Further experience and a better understanding of the vascular supply to muscle, fascia and skin are needed to allow more rational use of the different types of flaps, using muscle alone, muscle and skin, or skin and fascia as necessary.

Postoperative care: precautions and complications

In some cases, as with latissimus dorsi, vertical trapezius and tensor fasciae latae flaps, the donor defect can be closed primarily, but most defects require skin grafting when musculocutaneous or fasciocutaneous flaps have been used. The secondary defect is grafted immediately with a 1.5 × meshed graft. If muscle is transferred without skin it is covered with an unexpanded meshed graft.

Most postoperative problems result from either poor planning or technical error(s). Stretching of the muscle, musculocutaneous or fasciocutaneous unit reflects inadequate preoperative planning and can result in flap loss. Flap necrosis may be due to vascular injury during elevation of the flap or to kinking caused by trying to transpose the flap beyond its normal arc of rotation. Excessive pressure over the muscle, or tight tunnelling, is also detrimental.

Shearing forces that may disrupt the essential and delicate musculocutaneous perforators between muscle and overlying skin must be avoided. This can be accomplished by careful elevation, minimal flap manipulation, and suturing the dermis at the edge of the overlying skin island to the underlying muscle or fascia.

Loss of the functional donor muscle should be weighed against the anticipated gain from the procedure. Certain muscles, such as the gluteus maximus, which is necessary for climbing stairs, are indispensable in ambulatory patients. Loss of other units, for example of the tensor fasciae latae, medial gastrocnemius, latissimus dorsi and pectoralis major, tends to produce a relatively small functional deficit, although the secondary aesthetic defect may be considerable.

The flaps are initially bulky, but the muscle atrophies fairly quickly and will lose approximately 50 per cent of its bulk. Although the muscle may be divided or even returned to its original bed at a later date, the transfer is usually permanent.

Muscle and musculocutaneous flaps are especially useful for covering defects where local vascularity is inadequate and blood supply must be brought in from outside. They are the flaps of choice for replacement of radiation-damaged tissue. It has also been shown that well-vascularized muscle flaps are ideal for reconstructing defects in areas of potential or chronic infection.

If properly planned and executed, these units are remarkably safe, easy to manipulate and reliable.

References

1. Hartrampf, C. R., Scheflen, M., Black, P. W. Breast reconstruction with a transverse abdominal island flap. Plastic and Reconstructive Surgery 1982; 69: 216–225

2. Ramirez, O. M., Orlandor, J. C., Hurwitz, D. J. The sliding gluteus maximus myocutaneous flap: its relevance in ambulatory patients. Plastic and Reconstructive Surgery 1984; 74: 68–75

3. Pontén, B. The fasciocutaneous flap: its use in soft tissue defects of the lower leg. British Journal of Plastic Surgery 1981; 34: 215–220

4. Hurwitz, D. J., Swartz, W. M., Mathes, S. J. The gluteal thigh flap: a reliable sensate flap for the closure of buttock and perineal wounds. Plastic and Reconstructive Surgery 1981; 68: 521–532

5. Tolhurst, D. E., Haeseker, B., Zeeman, R. J. The development of the fasciocutaneous flap and its clinical applications. Plastic and Reconstructive Surgery 1983; 71: 597–606

Further reading

Ariyan, S. The pectoralis major myocutaneous flap. A versatile flap for reconstruction in the head and neck. Plastic and Reconstructive Surgery 1979; 63: 73–81

Bostwick, J. III, Nahai, F., Wallace, J. G., Vasconez, L. O. Sixty latissimus dorsi flaps. Plastic and Reconstructive Surgery 1979; 63: 31–41

Bostwick, J. III, Vasconez, L. O., Jurkiewicz, M. J. Breast reconstruction after a radical mastectomy. Plastic and Reconstructive Surgery 1978; 61: 682–693

Bunkis, J., Mulliken, J. B., Upton, T., Murray, J. E. The evolution of techniques for reconstruction of full-thickness cheek defects. Plastic and Reconstructive Surgery 1982; 70: 319–327

Haertsch, P. The surgical plane in the leg. British Journal of Plastic Surgery 1981; 34: 464–469

Jurkiewicz, M. J., Bostwick, J., Hester, R., Bishop, J. B., Cravet, J. Infected median sternotomy wound – successful treatment by muscle flaps. Annals of Surgery 1980; 191: 738–744

Mathes, S. J., Nahai, F. Clinical atlas of muscle and musculocutaneous flaps. St Louis: C. V. Mosby, 1979

Mathes, S. J., Nahai, F. Clinical application for muscle and musculocutaneous flaps. St Louis: C. V. Mosby, 1979

McCraw, J. B., Dibbell, D. G., Carraway, J. H. Clinical definition of independent myocutaneous vascular territories. Plastic and Reconstructive Surgery 1977; 60: 341–352

McCraw, J. B., Fishmann, J. M., Sharzer, L. A. The versatile gastrocnemius myocutaneous flap. Plastic and Reconstructive Surgery 1978; 62: 15–23

Nahai, F., Morales, L., Bone, D. K., Bostwick, J. Pectoralis major muscle turnover flaps for closure of the infected sternotomy wound with preservation of form and function. Plastic and Reconstructive Surgery 1982; 70: 471–474

Nahai, F., Silverton, J. S., Hill, H. G., Vasconez, L. O. The tensor fascia lata musculocutaneous flap. Annals of Plastic Surgery 1978; 1: 372–379

Orticochea, M. The musculocutaneous flap method: an immediate and heroic substitute for the method of delay. British Journal of Plastic Surgery 1972; 25: 106–110

Parry, S. W., Mathes, S. J. Bilateral gluteus maximus myocutaneous advancement flaps: sacral coverage for ambulatory patients. Annals of Plastic Surgery 1982; 8: 443–445

Vasconez, L. O., Bostwick, J. III, McCraw, J. Coverage of exposed bone by muscle transposition and skin grafting. Plastic and Reconstructive Surgery 1974; 53: 526–530

Vasconez, L. O., Psillakis, J., Johnson-Giebink, R. Breast reconstruction with contralateral rectus abdominis myocutaneous flap. Plastic and Reconstructive Surgery 1983; 71: 668–677

Vasconez, L. O., Schneider, W. J., Jurkiewicz, M. J. Pressure sores. Current Problems in Surgery 1977; 14: 1–62

Woods, J. E., Irons, G. B., Masson, J. K. Use of muscular, musculocutaneous and omental flaps to reconstruct difficult defects. Plastic and Reconstructive Surgery 1977; 59: 191–199

Illustrations by Y. Kitabatake

Restoration of skin cover by free flap transfer (microvascular technique)

Kitaro Ohmori MD
Director, Department of Plastic and Reconstructive Surgery, Tokyo Metropolitan Police Hospital, Tokyo, Japan

Kiyonori Harii MD
Associate Professor, Plastic Surgery, University of Tokyo Hospital, Tokyo, Japan

General considerations

Restoration of skin cover has been achieved chiefly by local flap, free skin grafting or distant flap techniques. Recently other techniques have been developed for this purpose, including free skin flap transfer with microvascular techniques.

1

In this operation a block of tissue nourished by an artery and a vein is raised in an island form, freed from its bed and directly transposed to the recipient defect. Transplantation of the freed tissue is accomplished by anastomoses of the prepared nourishing vessels of the recipient site to the pedicle vessels of the freed tissue, using an operating microscope. In this way the free tissue is well revascularized at the recipient site by means of microvascular surgery, and one-stage restoration of the skin cover can be achieved.

In order to perform this type of operation there are two important requirements: the technique of microsurgery, which is indispensable to free skin flap transfer, and knowledge of appropriate donor sites.

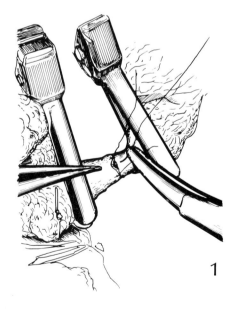

1

2

In planning a successful operation, selection of the recipient vessels is important as the free tissue must be revascularized by the blood flow in the recipient vessels. Based on this requirement the authors have used rather large vessels for the recipient arteries (*illustrated*). For the recipient vein(s), the venae comitantes of these arteries and/or cutaneous veins near the recipient site are selected and used.

Preoperative

Indications

Free flaps are used for the repair of any type of full-thickness skin loss when sufficient recipient vessels are available. It has been thought that free flap transfer is not indicated or is difficult when recipient vessels are not found near the recipient site. However this difficulty has been overcome by transferring recipient vessels with a long vascular cord from a distant place by using a free flap with a long vascular pedicle, or by filling the gap between the recipient and donor vessels by free omental transfer.

Of course, this free flap can be applied to poorly vascularized beds such as bare bone, exposed tendon and cartilage, and according to the authors' experience it can be applied to dirty infected wounds because the well revascularized flap may help to control the infection itself.

There are no age limitations, but most senile vessels offer some difficulty. However, it has been reported – and it is also the authors' experience – that this free flap can be transferred to unhealthy recipient vessels if great care is taken.

3

The maximum size of a free skin flap which is safe to transfer is not known, but a free groin flap of up to 20 cm² can be transferred in adults.

Contraindications

When a tissue defect can easily be treated by a local flap to restore skin cover, free flap transfer should not be used. In addition, since the free flap consists of normal skin with adipose tissue, it may be difficult to apply this technique to obese patients.

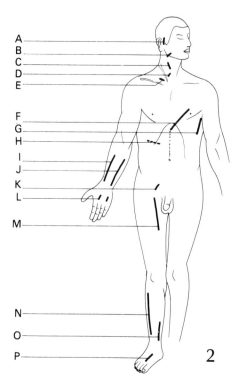

2

A = superficial temporal artery; B = facial artery; C = superior thyroid artery; D = inferior thyroid artery; E = transverse cervical artery; F = gastroepiploic artery; G = thoracodorsal artery; H = intercostal artery; I = radial artery; J = ulnar artery; K = epigastric vessels; L = common digital artery; M = profunda femoris artery; N = anterior tibial artery; O = posterior tibial artery; P = dorsalis pedis artery

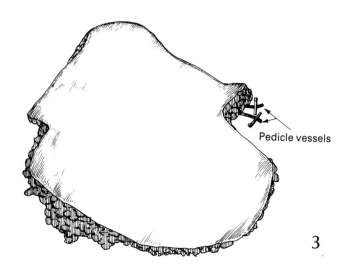

Pedicle vessels

3

4a & b

Selection of the donor flap

In planning the operation, one should be familiar with the specific nature of all kinds of donor flaps. In the authors' unit six kinds of free flaps have been used to restore skin cover.

For large-size skin restoration, the free groin flap (D) is the first choice while the free deltopectoral flap (B) has top quality skin and is applied to the reconstruction of the facial region. From the scalp and forehead region the free scalp flap and free forehead flap can be raised (A). The scalp flap, a hair-bearing free skin flap, is useful for reconstruction of hairy parts of the body. From the lateral thoracic region (C), three types of free flaps can be raised – one is only a skin flap, another is a musculocutaneous flap which is based on the latissimus dorsi muscle and the last is a flap with axillary hair. From the inside of the thigh a musculocutaneous flap based on the gracilis muscle can be raised (E). With this free flap, skin and muscle with motor function can be transferred in one stage. From the dorsal aspect of the foot, the dorsalis pedis flap (F) and first web space flap can be raised (G). The latter flap is used mainly as a free sensory flap for reconstruction of the hand.

For simple skin restoration it has been thought that the free groin flap is advantageous because the donor site is always covered by clothing.

In addition to the donor flaps mentioned above, various types of myocutaneous and other skin flaps, which are nourished by direct cutaneous arteries, have recently been successfully used as the source of donor flaps for microsurgical free flap transfer.

Of these donor flaps, the latissimus myocutaneous flap (H), the tensor fascia lata myocutaneous flap (I), or scapular flap (J) are employed for the restoration of skin defects by microsurgical free flap transfer. The advantages of these flaps are summarized as follows: (1) when the other donor areas have been damaged by the preceding trauma or previously used as donor sites these donor sites can be used as new donor sites; (2) when a myocutaneous flap is used as a donor flap the skin coverage as well as the muscle function can be restored in the recipient site, and (3) compared with the groin flap these flaps can have larger diameter vessels in the pedicle and this may facilitate anastomosis when the flap is transferred by means of microvascular surgery.

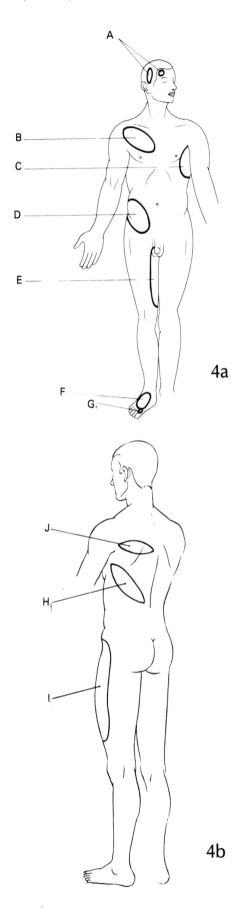

4a

4b

OUTLINE DESCRIPTION OF EACH FLAP

Free scalp and free forehead flaps

5

These free flaps are designed on the path of the superficial temporal vessels There are four types: totally hairy flaps (A); forehead skin flaps (B); and flaps including a part of the forehead skin (C); and the free temporo-occipital flap, which is an expanded totally hairy flap (D).

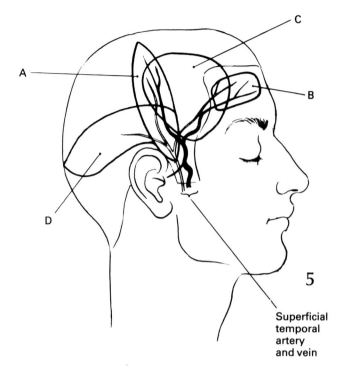

5

Superficial temporal artery and vein

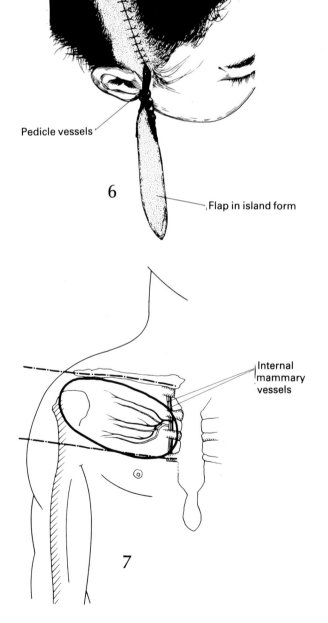

Pedicle vessels

6

Flap in island form

6

These flaps are raised in an island form after the vessels superficial temporal vessels have been found at the level of the tragus.

Free deltopectoral flap

7

This free flap is designed within the territory of the medially pedicled deltopectoral flap originally described by Bakamjian[1]. The base of the flap is located parasternally over the perforating branches of the internal mammary vessels; the upper border corresponds roughly to the clavicular line and the lower border is parallel to the upper border across the apex of the anterior axillary fold. The base of the free flap is designed over the second perforating branch.

In the authors' experience the second perforator of these internal mammary vessels is usually the most suitable for anastomosis, but when the third perforator is better this can be used.

Internal mammary vessels

7

8

The flap is raised from the lateral side inwards with dissection beneath the fascia of the pectoralis major. When the neurovascular bundle comes into view it is dissected within the pectoralis major muscle. Occasionally, however, the pedicle vessels do not form a complete neurovascular bundle at the level of the anterior surface of the pectoralis major muscle, so that great care is needed to find them.

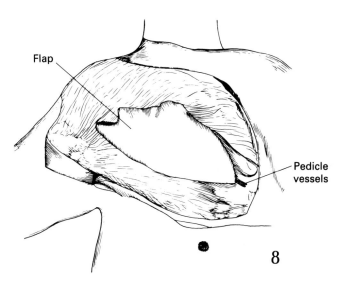

Free lateral thoracic flap

9

From the lateral thoracic and axillary region, free flaps are raised by using thoracodorsal, lateral thoracic and direct cutaneous vessels as the pedicle vessels. Direct cutaneous vessels nourish mainly the skin of the axilla and this type of free skin flap has been applied for reconstruction of the pubic hair. For simple skin restoration the thoracodorsal or lateral thoracic vessels are selectively used as the pedicle vessels of these free skin flaps, depending on the vascular pattern of the individual. When the free musculocutaneous compound flap includes the latissimus dorsi muscle, the thoracodorsal vessels and the motor nerve of this muscle are used for the vessels and motor nerve of the recipient site. In this case, one-stage reconstruction of the motor nerve and skin coverage can be achieved.

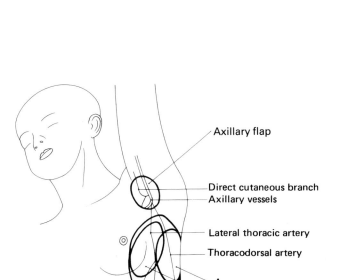

A = flap based on thoradordorsal artery; B = flap based on lateral thoracic artery; C = flap including whole system

10

On some special occasions, such as open skull defect, this free skin flap with ribs may be used for reconstruction.

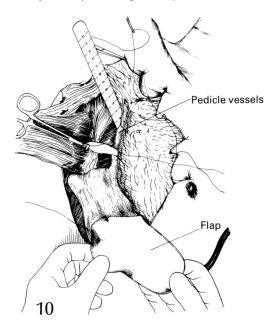

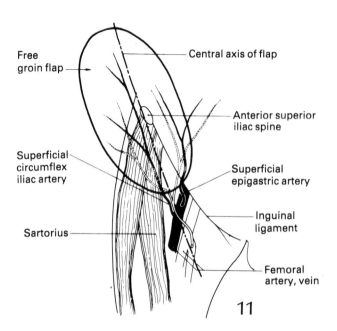

Free groin flap

Central axis of flap

Anterior superior iliac spine

Superficial circumflex iliac artery

Superficial epigastric artery

Inguinal ligament

Sartorius

Femoral artery, vein

11

Free groin flap

11 & 12

The central axis of this free groin flap is placed on the line connecting the anterosuperior iliac spine with a point 2.5 cm below the inguinal ligament on the femoral artery. The medial border of this design is located just above the femoral artery.

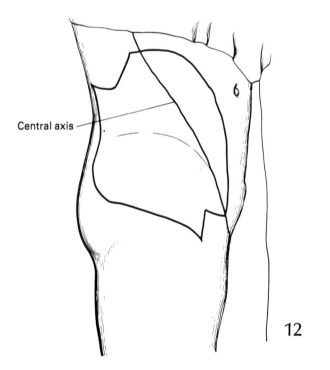

Central axis

12

13

The flap is raised from lateral to medial aspects, dissecting beneath the fascia of the sartorius muscle. When the dissection of the flap reaches the femoral artery and the pedicle arteries come into view, they should be dissected from their venae comitantes. The superficial drainage vein is found through the incision outlining the medial border of the flap.

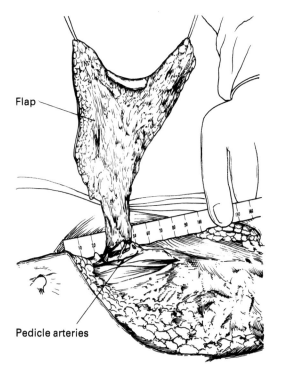

13

14

Application of a free groin flap presents problems not encountered with a pedicle groin flap. A free groin flap has to be raised in an island form by its pedicle vessels. (*Illustration 14* shows a close-up view of these pedicle vessels which are also shown in *Illustration 13*.) The vascular pedicle of the free groin flap has a more complex vascular pattern than that of other free skin flaps. It usually has two arteries and their venae comitantes and one superficial drainage vein, the superficial cutaneous vein (A), which runs directly into the great saphenous vein. The vessels to be anastomosed should be selected from these pedicle vessels because in the recipient site it is difficult to find vessels to match all the donor vessels and also because in free groin flap transfer it is not necessary to anastomose more than one artery and one vein.

The donor artery and vein to be anastomosed to the recipient vessels are selected as follows. When both the superficial epigastric artery and superficial circumflex iliac artery are found in the pedicle vessels, the larger is selected; when these have the same diameter it is preferable to select the superficial circumflex iliac artery. When a common trunk of the two arteries is found (B), there is no need for selection. If a good superficial drainage vein if found, it is better to select this vein for drainage but if the vena comitans (C) has a diameter large enough for anastomosis it will serve as a useful drainage vein.

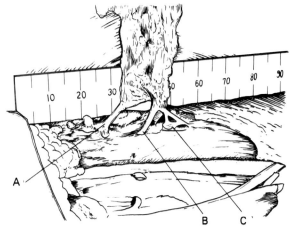

14

Free musculocutaneous compound flap

15

This island flap involves the gracilis muscle and the skin and adipose tissue above the muscle. The flap is raised in an island form by the nourishing vessels of the gracilis muscle, which enter the proximal one-third of the muscle belly. These nourishing vessels mostly emerge from the profunda femoris vessels.

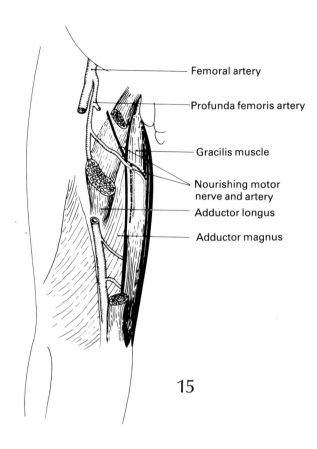

Femoral artery

Profunda femoris artery

Gracilis muscle

Nourishing motor nerve and artery

Adductor longus

Adductor magnus

15

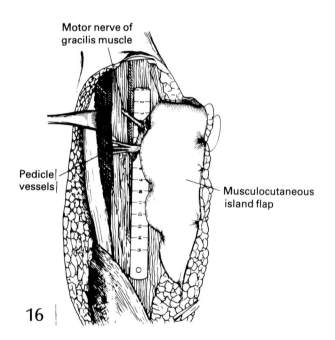

Motor nerve of gracilis muscle

Pedicle vessels

Musculocutaneous island flap

16

16

This flap can be used to reconstruct muscle function and provide skin coverage at the same time. When it is used for this purpose the motor nerve of the gracilis muscle, which is the anterior branch of the obturator nerve, should be anastomosed to the motor nerve in the recipient site when the flap is revascularized.

Free dorsalis pedis flap and free first web space flap

17 & 18

These free flaps are designed on the dorsal aspect of the foot.

The dorsalis pedis flap is centred over the pulsating path of the dorsalis pedis artery. When this flap is used as a free sensory flap the superficial peroneal nerve should be kept in the flap. Sensation of this free skin flap can be restored by anastomosis of this sensory nerve to the recipient site.

The pedicle vessels of this island flap are the dorsalis pedis artery and vein and the great and/or small saphenous vein(s), but the flap can be transferred as a free flap by anastomosing the dorsalis pedis artery and one of the venae comitantes of this artery.

The free first web space flap is raised in an island form on the dorsalis pedis vessels and the anterior tibial nerve, in the first web space of the foot.

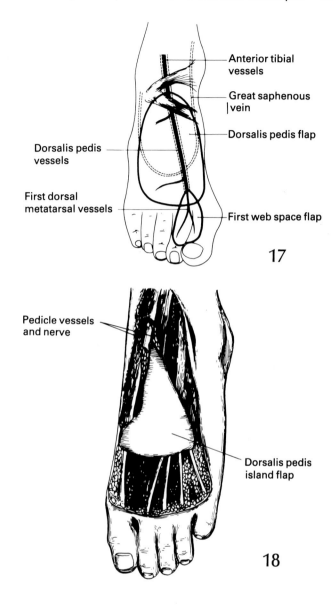

19

The free dorsalis pedis flap can be continuously raised with the first web space and/or the second toe and transferred as a free flap.

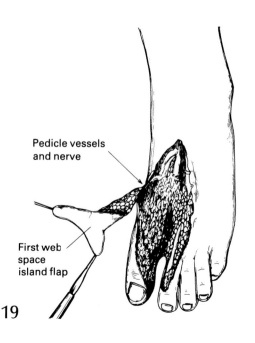

The operation

As an example, the operative steps are illustrated by a free groin flap transfer to the lower leg.

20

First, the nourishing vessels in the recipient site should be prepared for the tissue transfer, and then the recipient bed is prepared by excision of the scars or debridement. When the recipient vessels are located deeply, they should be brought closer to the surface to facilitate anastomoses.

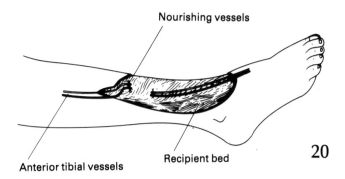

20

21

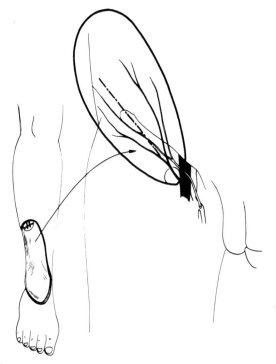

21

The accurate size and shape of the recipient site is traced on a sheet of paper and the locations of the recipient vessels are marked. The donor flap is designed by placing the marked positions of the recipient vessels over the nourishing vessels of the donor flap.

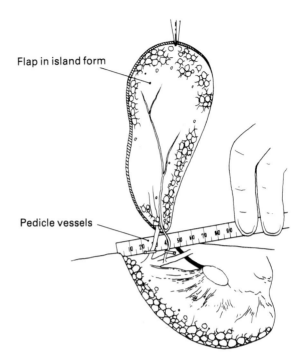

Flap in island form

Pedicle vessels

22

22

After the design of the flap is completed, the donor flap is raised in an island form on its pedicle vessels. The vessels to be anastomosed are selected and vascular clips are applied.

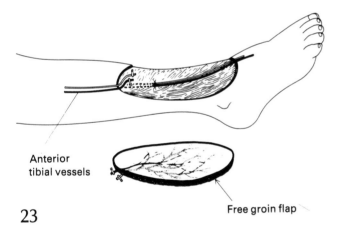

Anterior
tibial vessels

Free groin flap

23

23

The pedicle vessels of the donor island flap are then severed and the flap is transposed to the recipient site. The authors never irrigate the whole flap; only that part distal to the vascular clips is washed with heparinized saline solution.

A few stitches are applied to keep the free flap in position. At this stage the recipient and donor vessels should be placed near each other.

24

The operating microscope is brought into the micro-surgical operating field and then microvascular anastomoses are performed on the artery and vein.

After the anastomoses are accomplished the vascular clips are removed, and the circulation of the graft is checked. In most free flap transfers the transferred flap shows brisk dermal bleeding and a capillary flush is noticed soon after revascularization. In some cases revascularization takes more than a few minutes, but as long as the anastomosis is patent, circulation of the transferred flap becomes established within 15 minutes.

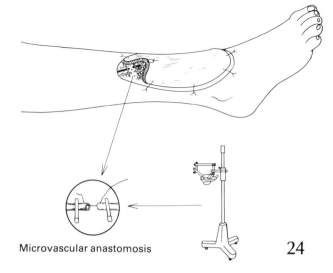
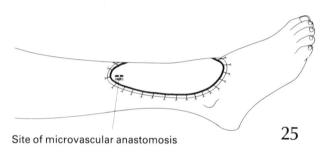

Microvascular anastomosis   **24**

25

The donor and recipient sites are closed after the circulation in the transferred flap is established.

Site of microvascular anastomosis   **25**

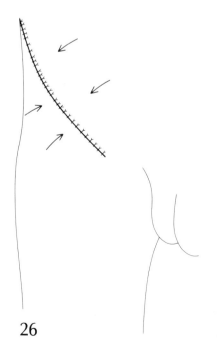

26

Closure of the donor defect can usually be achieved by direct approximation, but in some instances split skin grafting is required.

26

MICROVASCULAR TECHNIQUE

In free skin flap transfer the vessels to be anastomosed range from 0.8 to 4 mm in outside diameter. Therefore the microsurgical technique and implements should be set up to perform anastomoses of vessels of this size.

Implements

27

Operating microscope

Sophisticated operating microscopes with electrically controlled zoom optics and focus adjustment have increased the accuracy of free flap microsurgery. The Zeiss OPMi-6 type operating microscope as shown has been used in the authors' clinical cases. This microscope has a bright field of operative view, and its magnification and focus are controlled by foot pedals. A valuable feature is that the angle of the microscope can easily be adjusted to focus on any site in the operative field. Other types of Zeiss operating microscopes and other recently developed products by such manufacturers as Topcon are also very useful for this purpose.

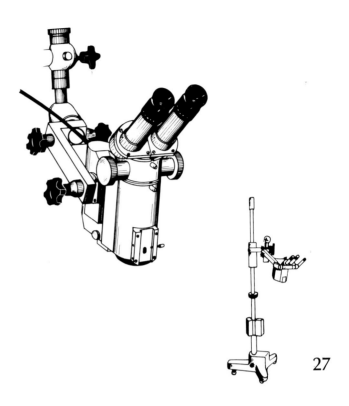

27

Micro-instruments

The following are essential for microvascular surgery.

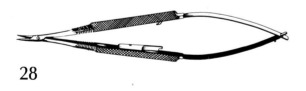

28

28

Spring-handled needle holder   Barraquer and Castroviejo type ophthalmic needle holders are available. The authors use a spring needle holder with lock or ratchet.

29

29

Spring-handled microscissors   Two types of microscissors are used. One has straight blades and the other curved. The straight-bladed scissors are used to cut the vessels and the curved ones to cut thread and connective tissues surrounding the vessels.

30

Microforceps Ordinary jeweller's forceps are employed. The authors use two pairs of No. 5 forceps for anastomoses of the vessels and two pairs of No. 2 forceps for dissection.

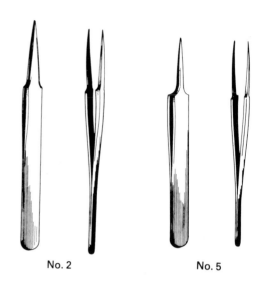

No. 2   No. 5   30

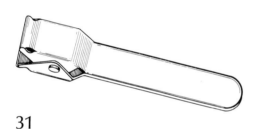

31

31

Microvascular clamps From among the various types of single and double clamps devised for microvascular anastomoses, the authors have selected the fine Heifetz's neurosurgical clips. The authors do not routinely use any of the double clamps devised by O'Brien, Ikuta, Acland, Kleinert or Tamai because even though double clamps faciliatate approximation of vascular stumps, the actual tension and torsion of the anastomosed vessels cannot be determined after the double clamps are applied.

32

Suture materials

Various suture materials are now commercially available from Ethicon, Davis and Geck, S & T, Microfine and Crown. The authors prefer to use the 10/0 monofilament nylon with a ⅜ circle tapered-point atraumatic needle less than 100 μm in calibre (such as Crown 10/0 DY and S & T 10V43).

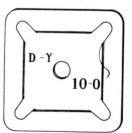

32

Surgeon's position and handling of tools

33

The surgeon must sit down on the surgical chair with his elbow and wrist placed on a stable table. Physiological tremor is an inevitable feature of muscle activity but factors that may aggravate tremor should be avoided. Steadier hand movement can be obtained by supporting the arm and instruments distally. In this respect, wrist support is more important than elbow support.

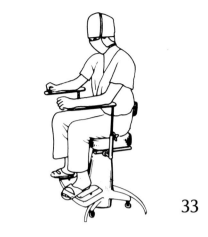

33

34

All instruments should be held by an external precision grip with the middle finger supporting the tip of the instrument. The spring-handle should be controlled by thumb movement. This grip permits easy finger movement, which facilitates rotation of the needle holder and makes anastomoses in deeper places possible. The internal precision grip may be used but the authors are not familiar with this.

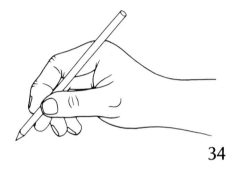

34

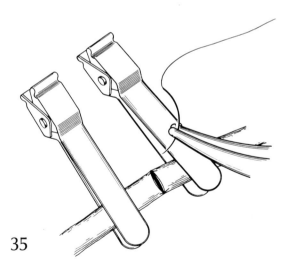

35

35

When the needle is to be held by a needle holder, it should not be held at the proximal end because this would make the needle easy to break and bend and would also make the needle tip unstable.

To ensure atraumatic vascular anastomoses the surgeon should hold the instrument gently and proceed as slowly as possible, and he should always watch the microsurgical operative field at a suitable magnification.

36

To obtain the best view of the vascular structure he should not hesitate to use a heparinized saline solution (20 i.u./ml saline) to wash out blood clots on the vascular stump. For this purpose the authors use a 10 ml syringe with a hypodermic needle with a bent tip.

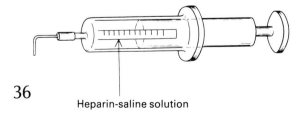

36

Heparin-saline solution

Selection of needle holder and management of suture material

In most cases the microsurgical plane is not horizontal and the surgeon cannot place his assistants in a good position. Therefore, the authors routinely have one surgeon perform microvascular anastomoses. In this case, one difficulty in suturing the small vessels under the operating microscope lies in controlling the barely visible suture materials. There are two types of needle holder used for this purpose, one with a ratchet and one without, and management of suture materials is closely related to the type chosen.

In using a needle holder without a ratchet, there are different ways to control the barely visible suture materials.

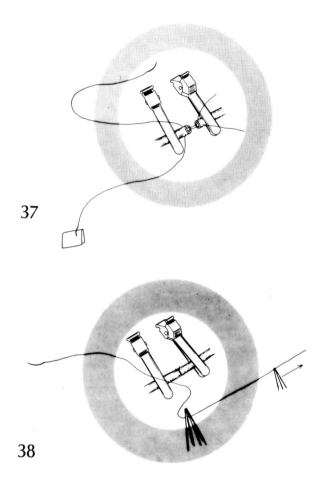

37

37

After the needle has been passed through the vascular wall it can be positioned by naked eye outside the field of microscope vision. Then, after the knot has been tied and the thread cut under the operating microscope, the needle is again picked up using the naked eye. Using this method the surgeon cannot continuously observe the working field of microscope vision unless he has an assistant. It is possible to select a particular spot inside the vision at the lowest magnification because the lowest magnification gives a wider vision, but the needle can be lost as a result of bleeding or swabbing of the operative field.

38

Another way of using the needle holder without a ratchet is to place the needle aside so as not to interfere with the anastomoses. The knot is then tied with microforceps and needle holder, and the thread is cut. The thread is then placed between the tips of the forceps held in one hand and pulled backward by the needle holder held in the other hand, so that the needle automatically comes back into the operative view of the microscope. This would be an ideal method when the needle is attached to the thread, but the small needle is temporarily lost from vision, which is undesirable, and also it is easy to break the junction of needle and thread. This technique, therefore, involves some risk.

38

39

Owing to the above requirements and considerations the authors have used needle holders with a ratchet. The needle can be held without locking the ratchet while it is being passed through the vascular wall. After it has passed through the walls of both vascular stumps, the needle is held by the needle holder and the thread is slowly pulled through until the end appears in the field of vision. The ratchet of the needle holder is then locked and the needle holder with needle is placed outside the field of the operating microscope. Tying of the thread is accomplished with two pairs of No. 5 forceps. In this way the needle and thread can be kept continuously in the same position without losing them in the complicated operative field. Many microsurgeons hesitate to use a needle holder with a ratchet because they are afraid of hand tremor when locking the ratchet. The authors, however, always use the ratchet outside the field of vision, thus avoiding hazardous tremor.

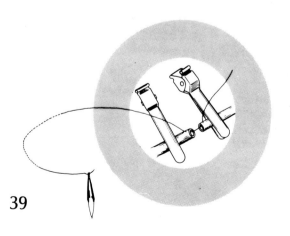

39

Suturing the vessels

40

Each bite should be of full thickness and equal to approximately twice the thickness of the vascular wall.

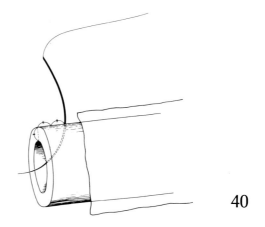

40

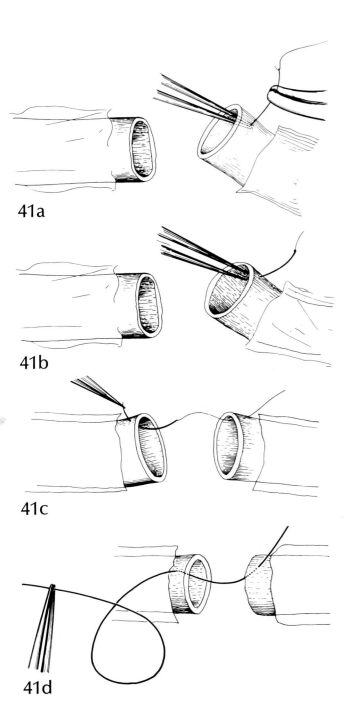

41a

41b

41c

41d

41a–d

The needle penetrates the vascular wall on the right segment when the surgeon is right-handed, while the No. 5 microforceps are applied as a counterpressor on the left segment. The needle then penetrates the left vascular wall from inside to outside while the surgeon watches the vascular lumen.

42a–e

The tip of the needle is picked up by No. 5 forceps in the left hand and gently withdrawn from the vascular wall. The needle is then held by a needle holder in the right hand and the thread is pulled gently until its end comes into the working field of the operating microscope. The needle is then retained in the needle holder with the ratchet locked. Tying is accomplished by two pairs of No. 5 forceps.

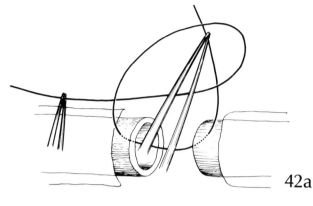

42a

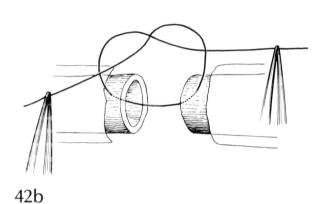

42b

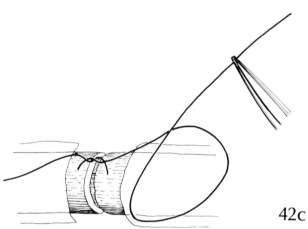

42c

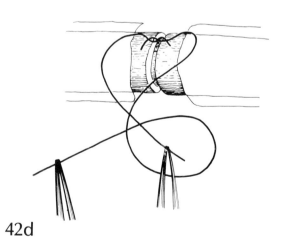

42d

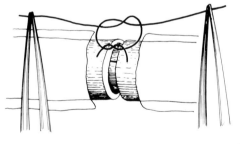

42e

Stitches

Stitches may be classified as key stitches or intermediate stitches. The key stitches are important in maintaining good balance between stitches on the two stumps, especially in cases involving different diameters. The intermediate stitches are applied to get a good approxima-

tion of the intima of the vessels to be anastomosed. With either type of stitch, one has to make sure of full-thickness bites in the vascular wall. The best way to ensure this is for the surgeon to watch the vascular lumen where the needle penetrates.

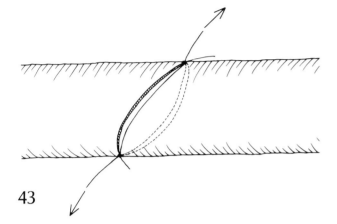

43

Key stitches

43

Placement of the key stitches is closely related to the number of stitches and is considered in two groups. In one, the key stitches are placed 180° apart.

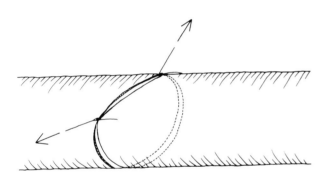

44

44

In the other they are placed in eccentric biangulation. This was described by Cobbett (1967). Eccentric biangulation allows the posterior edge to fall away from the needle point and avoids the error of pricking the opposite intima when the needle is passed through the anterior intima.

The first stitch is placed a little anterior to the furthest point but not at the centre of the anterior side. In this way the second stitch can be applied at a certain angle away from the first stitch, while watching the vascular lumen. These first and second stitches are the key stitches. The exact angle and the number of intermediate stitches to come in between these two stitches are decided by the total number of stitches to be used in the anastomoses. Thus, the first stitch is applied mainly to bring both segments together and the second stitch decides the total number and balance of stitches.

45

Intermediate stitches

When two intermediate stitches are required, the farther stitch should be performed first and left untied, then the nearer stitch is inserted and tied. In this way, when the needle penetrates the right segment, No. 5 forceps can be used as a counterpressor to ensure a full-thickness bite. When the needle penetrates the left segment, the vascular lumen can be observed by pulling the adventitia on the left segment, and a full-thickness bite can be achieved from inside to outside, while watching the vascular lumen. When three intermediate stitches are required the farthest one can be tied and the other two are applied just as described above.

The anterior wall of the vessel is repaired first, and after turning the vessels by rotation of the vascular clips the posterior vascular wall is repaired.

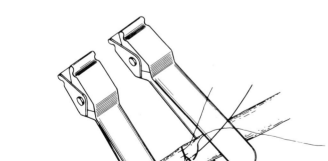

45

46

Patency test

The patency of an anastomosis is checked in the following way. A pair of microforceps is placed at a point immediately distal (downstream) to the anastomosis and closed; then another pair is used to squeeze the blood out of the downsteam segment and is placed at a point downstream from the first pair. Next, the first pair of forceps is released. If the anastomosis is patent the empty space will be quickly filled with blood flowing through the anastomosis.

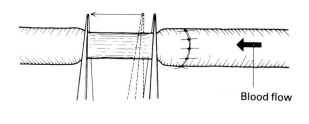

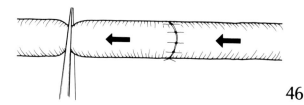

Blood flow

46

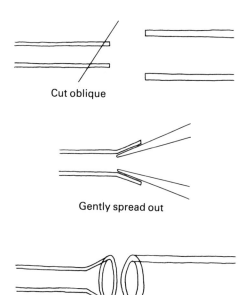

Cut oblique

Gently spread out

To match the larger circumference

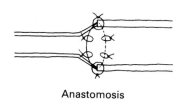

Anastomosis

47

47

Clinical free flap microsurgery

In free flap microvascular anastomoses the vessels to be anastomosed have different external diameters and wall thicknesses. The difference has been overcome by end-to-end anastomoses after obliquely cutting the smaller vessel and gently spreading it out to match the circumference of the larger one. The diameter of the vessels ranges from 1 mm to greater than 3 mm. Interrupted suture anastomosis is used with approximately 6–12 stitches; usually 7–10 stitches are required.

Anastomosis

Arterial anastomosis

48

The recipient and donor arteries are brought into the same operative field under the operating microscope without any tension or torsion. Both stumps are kept moist and should be irrigated with a heparinized saline solution to wash out the blood clots.

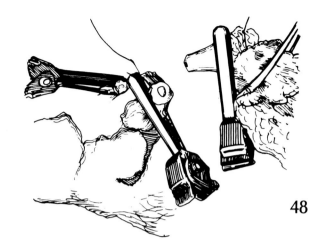

48

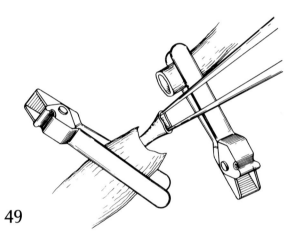

49

49

In many instances the stump is collapsed and No. 5 microforceps are gently inserted into the vascular lumen and gently spread out.

50

When the vascular stumps are washed and enlarged, the fibrous structure surrounding the arteries is loosened.

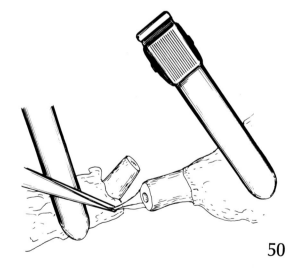

50

51

Usually, the fibrous strands drooping over the stump from the arterial wall are gently pulled away from the stump and, together with the adventitia extending over the stump, resected with microscissors.

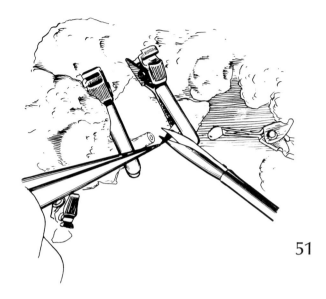

51

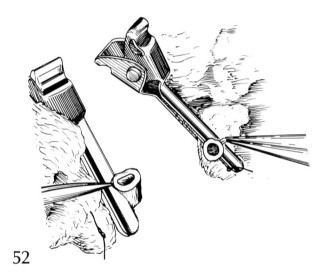

52

52

After this operative manoeuvre, both stumps are cleaned and prepared for anastomosis.

53

The first key stitch is applied on the anterior surface of the artery at a point slightly toward the surgeon from the farthest anterior end.

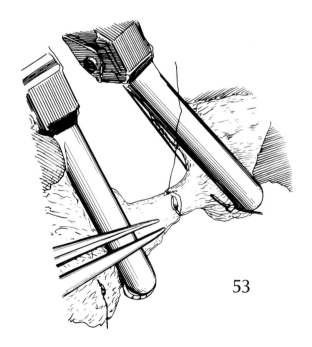

53

54

The second key stitch is placed approximately 150° from the first one, and an intermediate stitch is inserted between the two key stitches.

The number of intermediate stitches depends on the diameter and wall thickness of the arteries to be anastomosed. Approximately 8 stitches are required for repairing 1 mm arteries and 10 stitches for 1.5 mm arteries. Accurate apposition of each stitch and balance of the stitches may reduce the total number of stitches. In case of anastomosis between vessels of different diameters the total number of stitches is dependent on the smaller diameter.

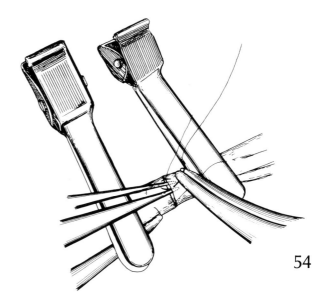

54

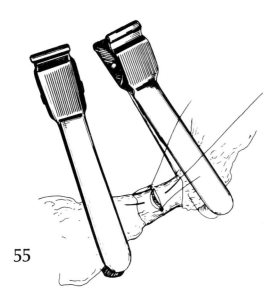

55

55

Each stitch should be a full-thickness bite of the vascular wall.

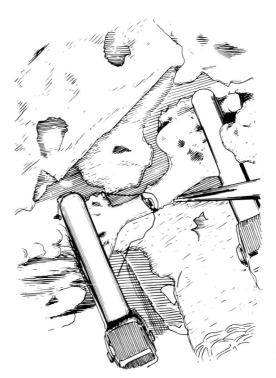

56

56

After repair of the anterior side of the vessel is completed, the vessel is rotated, ready for repair of the posterior side. At this stage, the intimal side of the vascular repair of the anterior vascular wall can be checked.

57

After vascular repair of the posterior side is accomplished in the same manner as on the anterior side, the vessel is rotated back to the original position.

Venous anastomosis

There are no great differences between arterial and venous anastomoses because most of the veins to be anastomosed in clinical cases have thick vascular walls. However, in some cases, the vascular wall of the vein is so thin that anastomosis is difficult. In this situation the veins on both sides flatten and it is difficult to estimate the angle from the centre of the vascular lumen, but it is easy to rotate the vessels, so that the key stitches can be applied 180° apart. The stitches are fewer than in arteries of the same diameter.

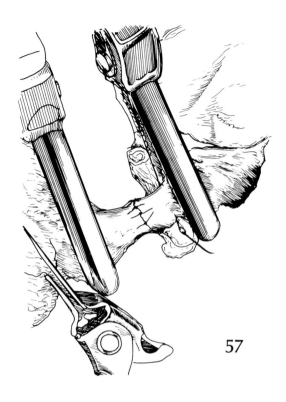

57

58

58

Removal of clips

Vascular clips are removed after the arterial and venous anastomoses have been made. The authors routinely remove the clips in the following order: first, the clip on the proximal side of the venous anastomosis; second, that on the distal side; third, that on the distal side of the arterial anastomosis; and finally the clip on the proximal side of the arterial anastomosis. If the anastomoses are satisfactory, the blood flow through the arterial anastomosis is vigorous and pulsation can be observed on the distal side. Venous backflow is noticed soon after the revascularization of the free tissue. Circulation of the flap can be established within 15 minutes.

Postoperative care

Postoperative care is easy in most cases. No anticoagulants are used during or after an operation as satisfactory anastomoses do not require them.

Comment

'Free skin flap transfer'[3] using microvascular surgery has been described based on the authors' own experience with more than 200 clinical cases. Success rate in this series was approximately 90 per cent. Development of the two elements – microvascular surgery and free skin flap transfer – made it possible to apply this operative procedure clinically.

Concerning the vascular basis of flaps, Milton[4] gives a good explanation of the island flap, which was employed between 60 and 80 years ago by Monks[5] and Esser[6]. Recently, McGregor and Jackson[7] and McGregor and Morgan[8] classified flaps into axial and random pattern flaps and their description of the groin flap pointed out the possibility of a free groin flap transfer. At the same time, the ideas of Daniel and Williams[9] on the vascularization of flaps and Taylor and Daniel's[10] descriptions of the vascular anatomy of various flaps well explain the basis on which various free skin flaps are commonly used today.

What has made free skin flap transfer possible is microvascular surgical technique. The history of vascular anastomoses dates back to Carrel[11], but Jacobson and Suarez[12] were the first to anastomose vessels of under 3 mm external diameter using an operating microscope. Later, improvement of technique, equipment and suture material by Buncke and Schulz[13] gave rise to the possibility of anastomosing vessels of about 1 mm external diameter. In 1967, Cobbett[2] devised the well-known eccentric bi-angulation method which, together with its modifications, is now applied clinically by many surgeons. Microsurgical techniques progressed along with thumb and digit replantations, starting with the first successful thumb replantation by Komatsu and Tamai[14] in 1968. In the early 1970s, the efforts of Acland[15] and other surgeons opened the way for clinical application of these techniques.

Later, following animal experiments by Goldwyn, Lamb and White[16], Krizek et al.,[17] Strauch and Murray[18] and other researchers, free skin flap transfer – a dream of reconstructive surgeons – reached a stage of maturity, with clinical successes being reported one after another by Harii and Ohmori[19–21], Daniel and Taylor[22], and O'Brien et al.[23] Thereafter, new free skin flaps have been applied clinically by numerous microsurgeons in different parts of the world. Articles written by the above-mentioned surgeons should be referred to by anyone who wishes to perform this type of operation.

References

1. Bakamjian, V. Y. A two stage method for pharyngoesophageal reconstruction with primary pectoral skin flap. Plastic and Reconstructive Surgery 1965; 36: 173–184

2. Cobbett, J. R. Microvascular surgery. Surgical Clinics of North America 1967; 47: 521–542

3. Harii, Ohmori, K. Free skin flap transfer. Clinics in Plastic Surgery 1976; 3: 111–127

4. Milton, S. H. Survival of experimental pedicle skin flaps. D. Phil. Oxford, 1967

5. Monks, G. H. The restoration of a lower eyelid by a new method. Boston Medical and Surgical Journal 1898; 139: 385

6. Esser, J. F. S. Island flaps. New York Medical Journal 1917; 106: 264–265

7. McGregor, I. A., Jackson, I. T. The groin flap. British Journal of Plastic Surgery 1972; 25: 3–16

8. McGregor, I. A., Morgan, G. Axial and random pattern flaps. British Journal of Plastic Surgery 1973; 26: 202–213

9. Daniel, R. K., Williams, H. B. The free transfer of skin flaps by microvascular anastomoses. An experimental study and reappraisal. Plastic and Reconstructive Surgery 1973; 52: 16–31

10. Taylor, G. I., Daniel, R. K. The anatomy of several free flap donor sites. Plastic and Reconstructive Surgery 1975; 56: 243–253

11. Carrel, A. La technique opératoire des anastomoses vasculaires et la transplantation des viscéres. Lyon Médicale 1902; 98: 859–864

12. Jacobson, J. H., Suarez, E. L. Microvascular surgery in anastomosis of small vessels. Surgical Forum 1960; 11: 243–245

13. Buncke, H. J., Jr., Schulz, W. P. Total ear reimplantation in the rabbit utilizing microminiature vascular anastomoses. British Journal of Plastic Surgery 1966; 19: 15–22

14. Komatsu, S., Tamai, S. Successful replantation of a completely cut-off thumb. Plastic and Reconstructive Surgery 1968; 42: 374–377

15. Acland, R. Thrombus formation in microvascular surgery: an experimental study of the effects of surgical trauma. Surgery 1973; 73: 766–771

16. Goldwyn, R. M., Lamb, D. L., White, W. L. An experimental study of large island flaps in dogs. Plastic and Reconstructive Surgery 1963; 31: 528–546

17. Krizek, T. J., Tani, T., Desprez, J. D., Kiehn, C. L. Experimental transplantation of composite grafts by microsurgical vascular anastomosis. Plastic and Reconstructive Surgery 1965; 36: 538–546

18. Strauch, B., Murray, D. E. Transfer of composite graft with immediate suture anastomosis of its vascular pedicle measuring less than 1 mm in external diameter using microsurgical techniques. Plastic and Reconstructive Surgery 1967; 40: 325–329

19. Harii, K., Ohmori, K., Ohmori, S. Successful clinical transfer of ten free flaps by microvascular anastomoses. Plastic and Reconstructive Surgery 1974; 53: 259–270

20. Harii, K., Ohmori, K., Ohmori, S. Hair transplantation with free scalp flaps. Plastic and Reconstructive Surgery 1974; 53: 410–413

21. Harii, K., Ohmori, K., Ohmori, S. Free deltopectoral skin flaps. British Journal of Plastic Surgery 1974; 27: 231–239

22. Daniel, R. K., Taylor, G. I. Distant transfer of an island flap by microvascular anastomoses. A clinical technique. Plastic and Reconstructive Surgery 1973; 52: 111–117

23. O'Brien, B. M., McLeod, A. M., Hayhurst, J. W., Morrison, W. A. Successful transfer of a large island flap from the groin to the foot by microvascular anastomoses. Plastic and Reconstructive Surgery 1973; 52: 271–278

Further reading

Baudet, J., Guimberteau, J. C., Nascimento, E. Successful clinical transfer of two free thoraco-dorsal axillary flaps. Plastic and Reconstructive Surgery 1976; 58: 680–688

Fujino, T., Harashina, T., Aoyagi, F. Reconstruction for aplasia of the breast and pectoral region by microvascular transfer of a free flap from the buttock. Plastic and Reconstructive Surgery 1975; 56: 178–181

Fujino, T., Harashina, T., Nakajima, T. Free skin flap from the retroauricular region to the nose. Plastic and Reconstructive Surgery 1976; 57: 338–341

Harii, K., Ohmori, K., Sekiguchi, J. The free musculocutaneous flap. Plastic and Reconstructive Surgery 1976; 57: 294–303

Harii, K., Ohmori, K., Torii, S., Murakimi, F., Kasai, Y., Skiguchi, J., Omori, S. Free groin flaps. British Journal of Plastic Surgery 1975; 28: 225–237

Ikuta, Y., Kubo, T., Tsurg, K. Free muscle transplantation by microsurgical technique to treat severe Volkmann's contracture. Plastic and Reconstructive Surgery 1976; 58: 407–411

Lendvay, P. G., Owen, E. R. Microvascular repair of completely severed digit. Fate of digital vessels after six months. Medical Journal of Australia 1970; 2: 818–820

McCraw, J. B., Furlow, L. T. The dorsalis pedis arterialized flap. A clinical study. Plastic and Reconstructive Surgery 1975; 55: 177–185

Ohmori, K. Free scalp flap. Plastic and Reconstructive Surgery 1980; 65: 42–49

Ohmori, K., Harii, K. Free groin flaps: their vascular basis. British Journal of Plastic Surgery 1975; 28: 238–246

Ohmori, K., Harii, K. Free dorsalis pedis sensory flap to the hand, with microvascular anastomoses. Plastic and Reconstructive Surgery 1976; 58: 546–554

Ohmori, K., Harii, K., Sekiguchi, J., Torii, S. The youngest free groin flap yet? British Journal Plastic Surgery 1977; 30: 273–276

Ohtsuka, H., Fujita, K., Shioya, N. Replantations and free flap transfers by microvascular surgery. Plastic and Reconstructive Surgery 1976; 58: 708–712

Orticochea, M. A method of total reconstruction of the penis. British Journal of Plastic Surgery 1976; 25: 347

Serafin, D., Georgiade, N. G., Peters, C. R. Microsurgical composite tissue transplantation. A method of immediate reconstruction of the head and neck. Clinics in Plastic Surgery 1976; 3: 447–457

Smith, J. W. Microsurgery: review of the literature and discussion of microtechniques. Plastic and Reconstructive Surgery 1966; 37: 227–245

Tamai, S., Horr, Y., Tatsumi, Y., Okuda, H. Hallux-to-thumb transfer with microsurgical technique: A case report in a 45-year-old woman. Journal of Hand Surgery 1977; 2: 152–155

Tissue expansion in reconstructive surgery

Louis C. Argenta MD
Assistant Professor, Surgery; Section of Plastic and Reconstructive Surgery, University of Michigan Medical Center, Ann Arbor, Michigan, USA

Introduction

Tissue expansion is a cosmetic refinement in reconstructive surgery that allows the surgeon to develop specific types of skin and subcutaneous tissue to correct specific defects. This process is effected by a silicone prosthesis which is placed beneath the appropriate skin and subcutaneous tissue and then is gradually expanded by intermittent percutaneous inflation. The overlying tissues become stretched, stimulating mitosis of the overlying skin to provide the required tissue. Skin expansion is an almost painless procedure that has been applied successfully to all areas of the body in patients of all ages.

The advantages of tissue expansion are as follows:

1. Minimal operative procedure with respect to risk, operative time, anaesthesia, and recovery.

2. There are no donor defects or new scars.
3. There is perfect colour and texture match to the recipient area.
4. The hairbearing and adnexal qualities of skin are preserved.
5. Sensation, if present, is preserved.
6. There is increased vascularity of expanded tissue to afford greater flap survival.

The disadvantages of tissue expansion are as follows:

1. Two operations are required, one to place the prosthesis, and one to remove it and mobilize tissue.
2. Multiple office visits are required for inflations.

113

EXPANSION PROSTHESIS

Multiple sizes and shapes of prostheses are available from various manufacturers. If custom prostheses are required they may be custom manufactured.

1

The prosthesis consists of a silicone bag (a) of various sizes and shapes. A separate, self-sealing inflation reservoir (b) is connected to the main reservoir by a silicone tube (c). Fluid is injected into the self-sealing inflation port, passes through the tubing, and into the main reservoir. Since there are no valves, fluid may be either injected or aspirated via the same port. Experimentally and clinically, the prosthesis has been hyper-inflated up to two times its recommended volume with minimal risk.

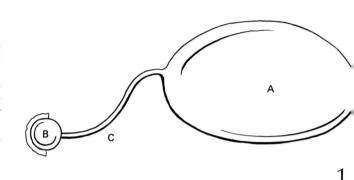

1

General principles of tissue expansion

The patient should be cooperative, motivated, fully informed and in reasonable health. The placement of the expansion prosthesis is individualized so that the tissue expanded is of the same colour, consistency, and hair bearing qualities as that of the skin to be replaced. Flaps should be planned as advancement or simple rotation flaps of the expanded tissue.

The prostheses are placed through previous scars, ideally in what will be the advancing edge of the flap. Careful dissection and haemostasis are mandatory. As large a prosthesis as will comfortably fit into the dissected space should be used. Excessively large, redundant prostheses may result in fold flaw erosion, while too small a prosthesis may not achieve the desired expansion. The inflation reservoir is placed as far from the prosthesis as necessary to avoid inadvertent puncture. Multiple prostheses around a defect are preferable to a single, larger implant. Only small amounts of saline are placed in the prosthesis initially – enough to minimize folding, but not enough to cause undue tension. Wounds are allowed to heal for at least two weeks before they are stressed with inflation.

There is a great variation in tissue tolerance to expansion. Each case is individualized. There should be no precise schedule for inflation or deadline for the second procedure. Saline is infused by percutaneous puncture of the inflation port with a 23 gauge needle, usually at weekly intervals. Enough saline is placed until the overlying skin becomes tense. Over-zealous inflation is avoided. During the process of expansion the overlying tissue becomes red; this rapidly subsides after removal of the prosthesis. Once complete expansion has been achieved the prosthesis is removed, and flaps can be advanced or rotated, incising as little of the capsular membrane as possible.

The operations

2

BREAST RECONSTRUCTION

Patients with qualitatively adequate, but quantitatively inadequate tissue after mastectomy, are candidates for reconstruction by tissue expansion. Excessive postradiation skin changes, skin grafts, or compromised skin are contraindications to this technique. A large, round prosthesis is placed through the initial mastectomy scar, and beneath the pectoralis major and superior portion of the serratus anterior muscles. The inflation reservoir is situated in the midaxillary line above the brassiere strap. Inflation is carried out at weekly or bi-weekly intervals until volume symmetry is obtained with the opposite side. The prosthesis is then over-inflated by 200 ml and allowed to remain in place for at least two months to develop ptosis. At a second operation a permanent prosthesis is placed. A nipple areolar reconstruction, if desired, can be accomplished simultaneously.

IMMEDIATE BREAST RECONSTRUCTION

Tissue expanders can be safely placed at the time of modified radical mastectomy in appropriately selected cases with low risk of recurrent disease. The prosthesis is placed beneath the pectoralis muscle, and the lateral defect closed with absorbable suture. No fluid is infused until complete healing of the usual thin flaps has taken place. At approximately one month the prosthesis is intermittently inflated until symmetry is achieved with the opposite side. A permanent prosthesis is placed after an over-expansion of 200 ml has been left in place 2–3 months. Expansion in the first three months after mastectomy is much more rapidly and easily carried out than delayed reconstruction.

3

CORRECTION OF CONGENITAL BREAST DEFORMITIES

Asymmetry secondary to unilateral hypoplasia may be corrected early in puberty as soon as it becomes significant. A prosthesis is introduced through a small transverse axillary incision, tunnelled down below the pectoralis muscle, and placed beneath the hypoplastic breast. The reservoir is positioned in the axilla with excessive redundancy of the connecting tubing so as to avoid tension when the arm is fully extended. Saline is infused at appropriate intervals so that the hypoplastic breast can be maintained at equal size to the normal developing breast. In Poland's syndrome a similar process is carried out in the subcutaneous space. At age 18, or when the opposite breast has ceased growing for two years, a permanent prosthesis is placed. If necessary the latissimus dorsi can be transferred at the time of permanent prosthesis placement to correct deficiencies in subcutaneous tissue and muscle.

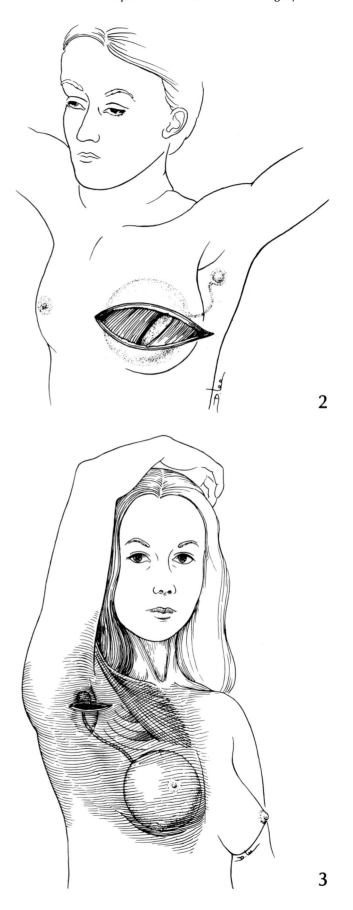

2

3

4

SCALP RECONSTRUCTION

Skin grafts, or lesions of the scalp, may be reconstructed with normal hair-bearing tissue by expanding adjacent scalp. Incisions are placed in what will be the advancing edge of the flap, usually at the junction of the lesion and the adjacent scalp. The prosthesis is placed beneath the galea with the reservoir situated low on the mastoid. After two weeks inflation is commenced. This may initially be quite difficult because of resistance of the galea. However, after one or two inflations this resistance is overcome and expansion proceeds rapidly at bi-weekly intervals. At a second procedure the expanders are removed and the scalp advanced. If insufficient expansion has been obtained the prosthesis may be left in place and re-expansion continued. Optimally, several expanders should be used around a specific defect to expedite the procedure.

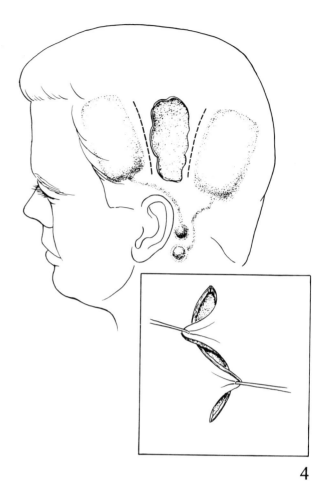

4

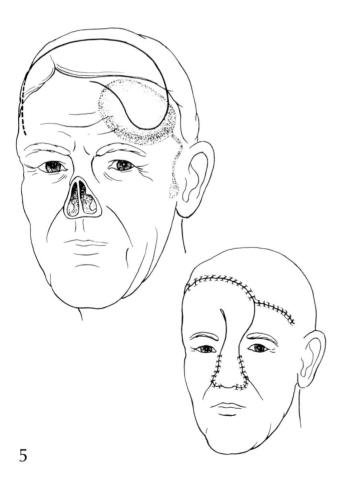

5

5

NASAL RECONSTRUCTION

Nasal reconstruction may be accomplished with forehead flaps without secondary skin grafting by first expanding the appropriate area of the forehead. This produces thin skin of the same consistency as the nose, which is especially useful for reconstruction of alar margins. The prosthesis is placed below the frontalis muscle with the reservoir anterior to the ear. Large, highly vascularized flaps can be obtained by this technique because of the increased vascularity occurring with tissue expansion. Defects can almost always be closed primarily.

An alternative procedure, not shown, combines the usual forehead turndown flap to reconstruct the nose with simultaneous placement of small expanders on either side of the defect created in the forehead. During the two weeks that the flap is allowed to mature on the nose the forehead is expanded, providing sufficient tissue for primary closure after division of the flap. It is imperative that adequate underlying support structures pre-exist or are reconstructed to avoid late irregularities and deformation.

6

DEFECTS OF THE TRUNK

Defects on the anterior or posterior chest or abdomen can be corrected by placement of multiple expanders around the defect. These are placed through incisions made along margins of the wound so that advancement flaps can be developed. Very large expanders can rapidly be inflated on the trunk with minimal resistance to cover large defects.

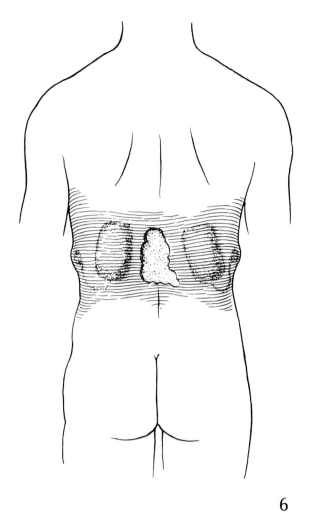

6

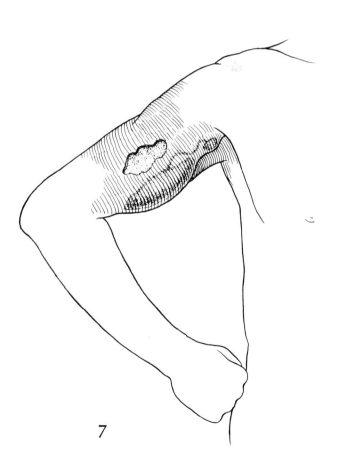

7

UPPER EXTREMITIES

Prostheses for reconstruction of defects of the arm should be placed axially around the specific defect. Inflation reservoirs should be placed within the same portion of the extremity and joints not traversed. The skin of the upper extremity tolerates expansion very rapidly and inflation can be carried out at weekly intervals. Advancement or simple rotation flaps are ideal. Care must be taken to protect tendons and cutaneous nerves during placement.

7

LOWER EXTREMITIES

8

Defects in the lower extremity are corrected by expansion of adjacent tissue above the fascial plane, preferably by multiple expanders. Care must be taken that the sum of the defect and the expanders do not occupy the entire circumference of the leg, otherwise distal lymphedema and infection may result.

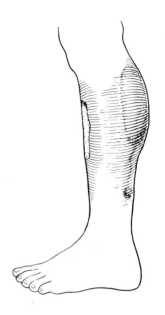

8

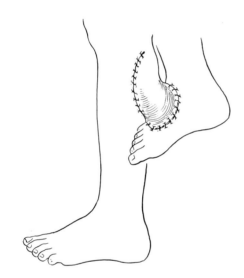

9

9

Advancement flaps

Expansion is ideally carried out with multiple expanders and simple advancement flaps. Such flaps can be used to cover contour defects as well as exposed bone after appropriate debridement.

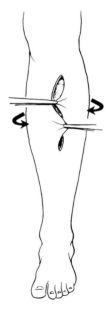

10

10

Cross leg flaps

As a primary step in cross leg flaps, large, well vascularized, dependable flaps can be developed on one leg prior to transfer to the opposite extremity. Because of the excess tissue generation, donor defects can usually be closed primarily.

Complications

Careful patient selection as with all procedures is mandatory. Perioperative antibiotics are employed, but not continued. Sterile technique during placement and inflation is mandatory, to avoid secondary contamination of the prosthesis. Expanders should not be used with haemangiomas, lymphangiomas, or adjacent to excessively contaminated wounds. Judicious inflation should be carried out to avoid necrosis of overlying tissue. If the overlying skin becomes blanched during inflation some fluid should be removed from the prosthesis. Once a prosthesis becomes exposed it should be removed if signs of infection develop. When exposure occurs near the termination of expansion additional expansion is usually well tolerated, and brief additional expansion can be carried out without excessive risk.

References

1. Argenta, L. C., Marks, M. W., Grabb, W. C. Selective use of serial expansion in breast reconstruction. Annals of Plastic Surgery 1983; 11: 188–195

2. Argenta, L. C., Watanabe, M. J., Grabb, W. C. The use of tissue expansion in head and neck reconstruction. Annals of Plastic Surgery 1983; 11: 31–37

3. Argenta, L. C., Watanabe, M. J., Grabb, W. C., Newmann, M. H. Soft tissue expanders in head and neck surgery. A new method of reconstruction. Plastic Surgery Forum 1981; Vol. IV

4. Austad, E. D., Pasyk, K. A., McClatchey, K. D., Cherry, G. W. Histomorphologic evaluation of guinea pig skin and soft tissue after controlled tissue expansion. Plastic Reconstructive Surgery 1982; 70: 705–710

5. Austad, E. D., Rose, G. L. A self-inflating tissue expander. Plastic and Reconstructive Surgery 1982; 70: 588–594

6. Radovan, C. Breast reconstruction after mastectomy using the temporary expander. Plastic and Reconstructive Surgery 1981; 69: 195–208

Illustrations by Ian Ramsden

The use of forehead flaps for lining

Ian A. McGregor   ChM, FRCS
Director, Plastic and Oral Surgery Unit, Canniesburn Hospital, Glasgow, UK

Introduction

In providing a replacement for buccal mucosa, forehead skin is used in the form of a temporal flap with its base extending from the lateral border of the eyebrow to the anterior border of the pinna at approximately the level of the zygomatic arch. Once raised, the flap is turned downwards and outwards, hinged on its base. The effect is to bring the flap into a position where it is lying against the skin of the cheek with its skin surface facing inwards, i.e. in the direction of the epithelial surface it is replacing. The proportion of the forehead skin used in the flap depends on the site and size of the defect it is to replace.

The method is used in two situations:

1. When the defect of the cheek is partial, involving part of its thickness up to, but not including, the skin; or
2. When the defect is of the full thickness of the cheek.

The operation

1

In the first situation a tunnel through the cheek is constructed, through which the flap is passed to bring its distal end inside the mouth where it can fill the defect.

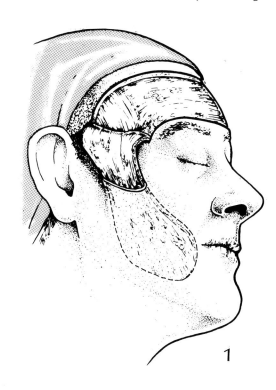

2

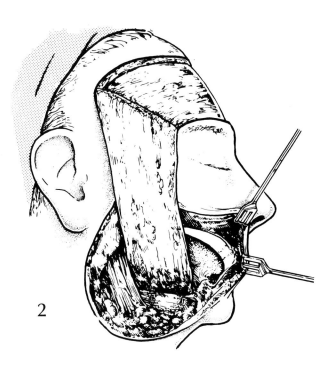

In the second a tunnel is less often needed. With the defect involving the full thickness of the cheek the turned-down flap straight away lies in a position which fills the mucosal defect. If the mucosal defect extends backwards in the mouth beyond the skin defect it may be necessary to use a tunnel to allow the flap to cover the entire intra-oral mucosal defect. This may happen if the intra-oral resection involves the mandible and postmolar triangle. In practice, the decision whether or not a tunnel is needed is usually clear cut.

3, 4 & 5

With the forehead skin reconstructing the mucosal element of the full thickness defect, a replacement for the skin element is also needed. This can most readily take the form of a deltopectoral flap, although alternative forms of skin cover, such as a local neck flap, are possible, if less satisfactory.

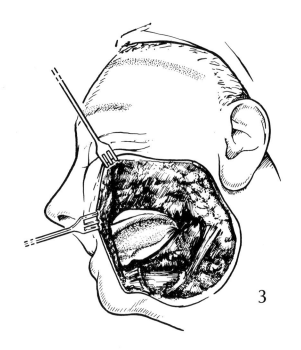

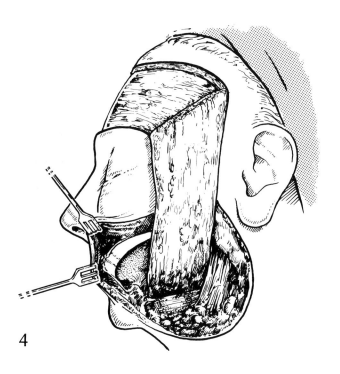

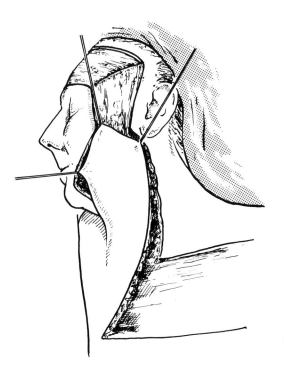

6 & 7

Site of the flap

The mucosal defect is usually, though not always, smaller than the area of skin available on the forehead and this gives the surgeon a choice of site. He can choose his site in such a way that it is symmetrical on the forehead and raise the flap on the temple only as far as is necessary to allow it to reach its destination without tension. Alternatively, he can raise the flap to the zygomatic arch and allow the forehead defect to select its own site, using reverse planning.

The ultimate cosmetic result is usually much the same whichever method of planning is used because the forehead defect is a partial one in nearly all instances.

The flap as so planned contains the anterior branch of the superficial temporal artery and the arteriovenous system of which this vessel is part allows it to sustain its highly advantageous length to breadth ratio.

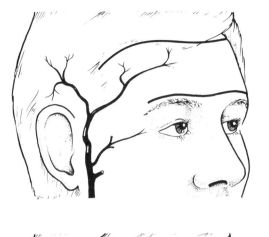

6

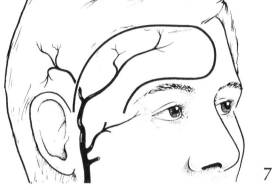

7

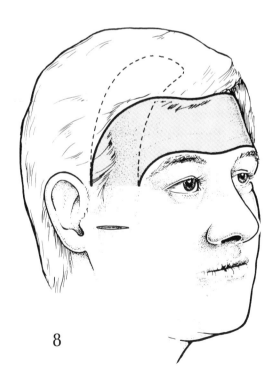

8

8

In the rare instance of a suitably bald patient an alternative, though basically similar, flap can be used, which uses the skin of the vertex as the donor site and the posterior branch of the superficial temporal vessels as its arteriovenous system. The flap, instead of curving forwards and upwards towards the forehead, passes directly upwards towards the vertex. The effect is to leave the secondary defect in a relatively unobtrusive area. A further consequence of using this flap is to leave the patient with a normally mobile forehead, an attribute which is lost with the standard forehead flap.

Dimensions of the flap

The length of the flap is determined in some degree by the length of the defect, but the selection of the site of the defect on the forehead also affects the length of the flap. This factor has already been discussed.

The breadth of the flap is usually made the width of the hairless forehead. The defects of cheek which are suitable for such a reconstruction have a breadth which would make use of the entire breadth of the hairless forehead necessary in the patient with a normal complement of hair.

9

Raising the flap

The flap is raised at the level of the pericranium. The frontalis muscle is raised with the flap to ensure that the flap contains its full quota of blood vessels. The temporal branch of the facial nerve is of necessity divided in the process. Beyond the temporal line the plane of elevation is immediately superficial to the temporal fascia.

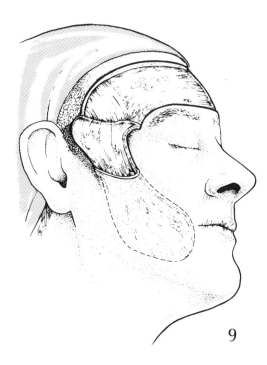

9

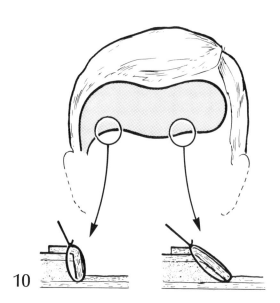

10

10

The split-skin graft used to cover the forehead defect is much thinner than the flap and as a result creates a hollow in the donor site. The hollow does become shallower with time but the immediate impact can be mitigated by bevelling the skin incision in the forehead. The effect of making the incision oblique rather than vertical is to produce an incline from the surrounding skin to the level of the graft and not an obvious step which would be the immediate result with a vertical incision.

Elevation of the flap is continued in the direction of the zygomatic arch as far as necessary, checking at intervals to see at which point in elevation the flap becomes capable of reaching its destination without tension. Elevation can be halted at this point.

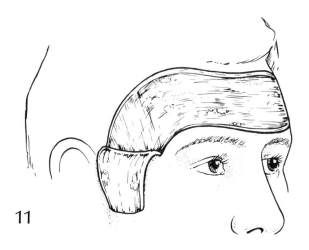

11

11

The secondary defect

The secondary defect is covered with a split-skin graft. This can be either *immediate* or *delayed*.

BOLUS GRAFTING

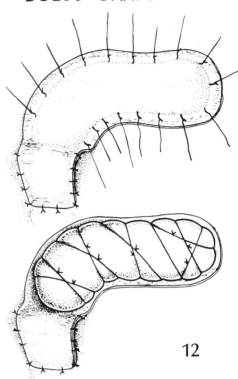

12

12

Immediate

Grafting is applied at the time of raising the flap, once haemostasis has been achieved, using a tie-over bolus of flavine wool followed by a crêpe bandage to provide overall cover.

DELAYED EXPOSED GRAFTING

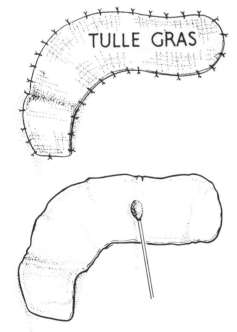

TULLE GRAS

13

13

Delayed grafting

Delayed grafting involves storing in the refrigerator until the defect is judged ready to receive it. In the interval between elevation of the flap and application of the graft steps must be taken to ensure that the pericranium is not allowed to become dry and mummified. This is most likely to happen immediately after the flap has been raised, under the heat of an operating room lamp. Drying can be prevented by covering the graft with an occlusive dressing. A convenient dressing is multilayer tulle gras, 0.5 cm thick, trimmed to fit the defect and loosely sutured to its margin.

This temporary dressing can be removed when the patient is back in bed. The raw surface is then dressed regularly until it is clean and free of all blood clot, on average for 3–5 days. The graft is then laid on the defect, overlapping its margins by 0.5 cm. Any air bubbles trapped underneath the graft are pressed out. No other protection of the graft is needed apart from reasonable patient care.

The proportion of the defect covered with the graft varies according to the taste of the surgeon. The entire defect can be grafted, including the forehead, temple and raw outer surface of the flap. If this is done, a considerable area of the graft has to be removed when the bridge segment of the flap is returned to the temple and forehead the second stage 3 weeks later. Alternatively, skin can be applied only to the area that the surgeon estimates will ultimately be covered with skin graft when the reconstruction is complete. The remaining raw surface, left ungrafted, is dressed until the bridge segment is returned.

14 & 15

Making the tunnel

When a tunnel is required it is important to use a technique which avoids damage to the facial nerve. This can be accomplished by using blunt dissection.

The skin is incised horizontally just in front of the ear, approximately 1.5 cm below the zygomatic arch, the length of the incision being two-thirds of the breadth of the flap. The incision is deepened to the level of the parotid gland, using the scalpel. With a hand inside the mouth to steady the tissues, McIndoe scissors with the points closed are thrust through the substance of the cheek in the direction of the defect. With the scissor tips in the mouth, the blades are opened and, held open, are withdrawn. The tunnel thus created is dilated with the gloved index finger until it is wide enough to accommodate the flap without constriction. This technique, although inelegant, is effective and has been found to avoid damage to the facial nerve.

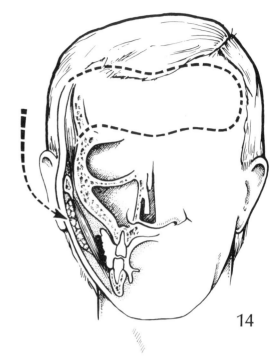

14

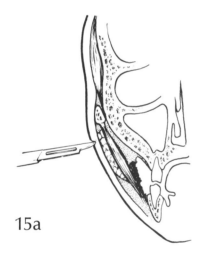

15a

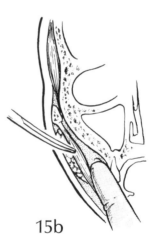

15b

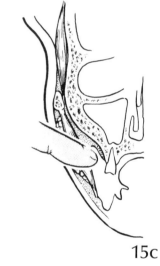

15c

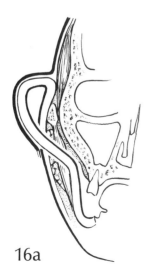

16a

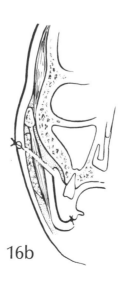

16b

16a & b

Transfer of the flap

The flap, turned down, is passed through the tunnel and its distal part is brought into an intra-oral position. The margin of the flap is sutured to the margin of the defect.

When a tunnel is not being used, the flap is merely turned down and laid into the defect, where again its margin is sutured to that of the defect.

In both instances, suture of the flap to the defect ends posteriorly where the flap passes from the distal inset segment on to the bridge segment or into the tunnel.

17 & 18

Return of the bridge segment

After 3 weeks the flap is ready to be divided along the line of the posterior margin of the defect.

If a tunnel has been used the flap is mobilized within it and after division the bridge segment is withdrawn and returned to the temple. If a tunnel has not been used, the bridge segment of the flap is merely turned upwards to its original site and insetting of the distal transferred segment inside the mouth is completed.

Any graft previously applied that prevents the bridge segment of the flap from being returned is, of course, excised. The bridge segment often tends to tube itself and this has to be undone by scoring and, if necessary, excising the scar tissue whose contraction has led the flap to become tubed.

If a tunnel has been used, steps should be taken to ensure that its opening into the mouth is not blocked by the posterior margin of the flap. To make certain that blocking does not occur, it is usual not to inset the flap posteriorly. The tunnel has to be left open to drain into the mouth as it heals.

The skin incision which marks the external opening of the tunnel is sutured after the edges have been mobilized.

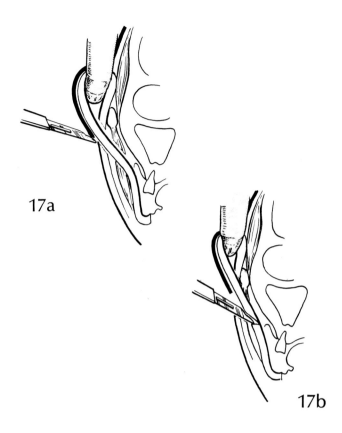

17a

17b

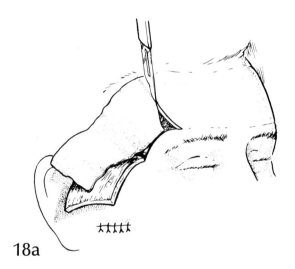

18a

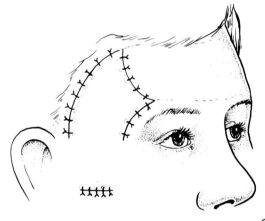

18b

Illustrations by Gillian Oliver

Achievement of skin cover using the deltopectoral flap

Vahram Y. Bakamjian MD
Chief Reconstructive Surgeon, Roswell Park Memorial Institute, New York, USA

The deltopectoral flap provides ample skin for immediate use on regions of the head and neck and is so versatile that the author now depends on it, almost to the exclusion of other flaps, in nearly all reconstructions following major resections for cancer[1-3]. In one move it can reach as high as the zygomatic arch and orbit on its own side. It is not hairy (or excessively so) over its deltoid part, which makes it suitable for lining the cavities of the mouth and pharynx. It has not usually been damaged by irradiation treatment for cancers of the head and neck, nor has it been compromised by incisions used to resect these tumours. It provides larger amounts of skin than either the forehead-temporal or the compound (myocutaneous) cervical flap, especially if one considers that twin flaps (one from each shoulder) are available to expand further the possibilities for reconstruction. And, last but not least, the donor area is hidden from view by clothing and is not objectionable to any significant degree, except rarely perhaps to young female patients.

Blood supply and flap design

1

Two axially vascular zones in the flap are connected to one another in series. The first receives intercostal perforating branches from the internal mammary artery that run horizontally outward to supply the breast and pectoral skin. The second receives one or two cutaneous branches from the thoracoacromial axis. These surface from muscle and pass into skin just medial to the deltopectoral groove and also spread outwards over the anterior aspect of the shoulder. Thus, blood flow in the raised flap, entering from the first into the second zone via dermal and subdermal anastomotic connections, can continue its axial flow without a reversal of current in the vasculature of the second zone. A random third zone may be added when more length or a greater area of skin is needed.

Two horizontal and nearly parallel lines, running outward from a parasternal base that spans the first four intercostal spaces, mark the borders of the pectoral portion. The first is at the level of the inferior border of the clavicle and the second at the level of the apex of the anterior axillary fold. Continuing from these two lines the outline of the deltoid portion ends with a curvilinear margin that extends to the anterolateral, lateral or posterolateral contour line of the shoulder, depending on the length required. When more skin is required in the reconstruction, downward extension over the anterolateral aspect of the upper arm may also be added in the shape of an L.

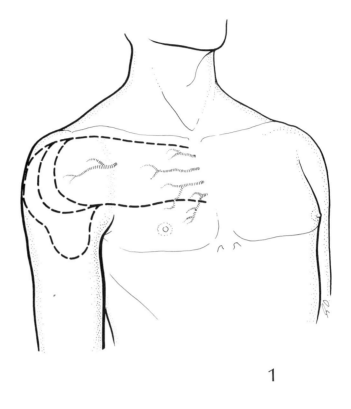

1

Flap elevation

2

Elevation begins at the tip and proceeds medially in the nearly bloodless plane beneath the deep fascia. Periodically it is stopped to test the reach of the flap to its intended destination. In this way it is often possible to stop short of the usual base of the flap, and sometimes to preserve the thoracoacromial cutaneous branch as additional guarantee for safety of the flap, such as when the emergence of that branch from muscle into skin is met at a point more medial and cephalad than usual.

2

Flap delay

Delay is not ordinarily required when using the standard flap, nor is it always necessary before using one of the extended forms of the flap, particularly in female patients in whom a rich blood supply from the internal mammary vessels to the breast can be expected. It should, however, be considered when poor circulation is suspected as, for example, in diabetes, arteriosclerosis and other infirmities associated with old age. Another indication may be that of a secondary reconstruction requiring a folding or prefabrication manoeuvre with an excessively long or large flap.

3

A simple and effective method of delay in a standard flap is to incise the total outline of the flap and to undermine the middle of the upper margin sufficiently to allow identification and division of the thoracoacromial vessel or vessels. This interrupts nearly all blood flow to and from the area of the flap except that entering and leaving its base. At the same time it avoids or minimizes the risks associated with haematoma, infection and fibrosis under the flap that are likely to result from a more extensive undermining.

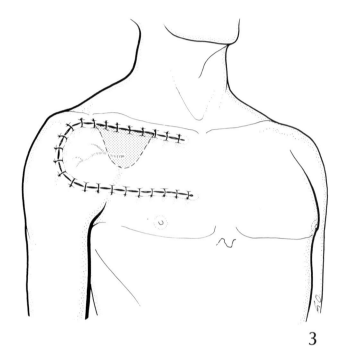

3

4

In order to produce a delay of equal effect on extended forms of the flap, the additional random zone at its periphery must also be undermined, interrupting the several small musculocutaneous branches that supply this area from the suprascapular and circumflex humeral vessels.

4

Applications

5 & 6

TRANSFER BY ROTATION

This allows the flap to cover easily one entire lateral side or the front of the neck. Any cervical skin that is infiltrated with cancer or damaged by irradiation can be sacrificed with impunity, therefore, and replaced, making resectable some advanced neck cancers that in the recent past would have been generally judged as inoperable.

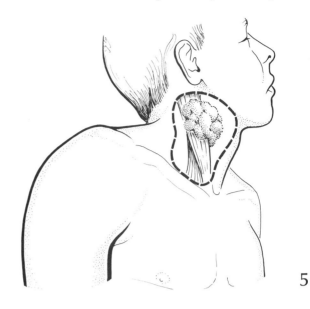

5

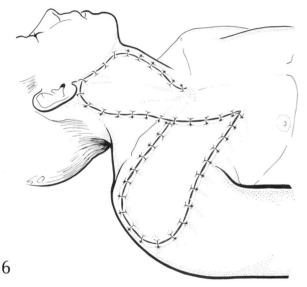

6

7 & 8

DE-EPITHELIZATION

By de-epithelizing the pedicle it can be passed subcutaneously. A trial pass is made under the intact bridge of cervical skin and the segment for de-epithelization is marked. The flap is then withdrawn and the epithelium is shaved off either free hand with the scalpel, or with a drum dermatome set to a thickness of 1/20 000 of an inch. (If properly removed, this skin can be grafted onto part of the donor wound.) This technique eliminates the need for later division of the pedicle, augments the contour of the dissected neck and reinforces the protection for vital structures exposed by the dissection.

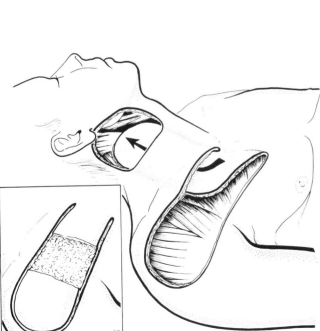

7

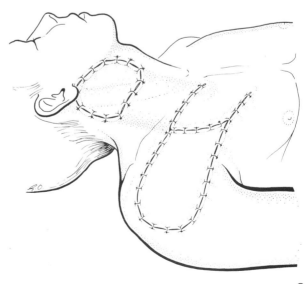

8

9–14

TUBING

This is the alternative method more commonly employed when applying the flap to high locations. It eliminates the raw surface from the bridge segment and spans the concavity of the neck thus reaching higher locations. Not having to conform to the neck concavity the intra-auricular, the auriculotemporal, lateral facial, orbitonasal and mentolabial regions fall within this range.

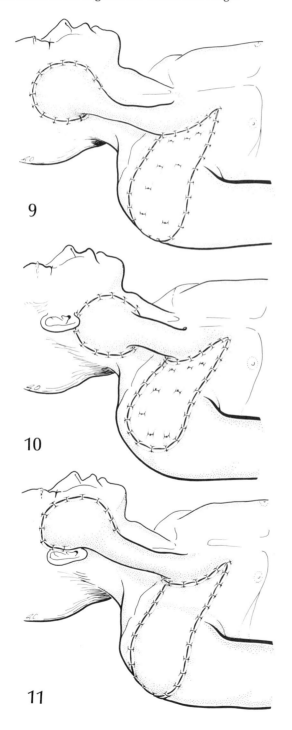

9

10

11

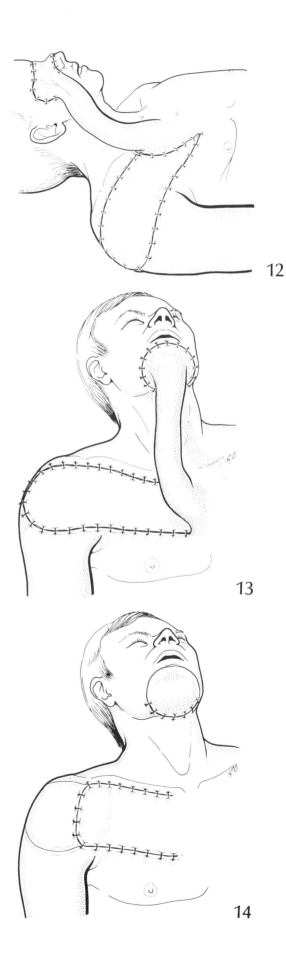

12

13

14

15 & 16

WALTZING

Instead of dividing and returning the tube pedicle to the chest wall, one can take advantage of the generous amount of skin available in the bridge segment and base of the flap and use it for any additional reconstruction required on the same or opposite side of the face. A delay of the base before waltzing may or may not be required, depending on the adequacy of the intial area of flap attachment. Illustrated is a case of multifocal cancer in facial skin severely damaged by irradiation; the method discussed was applied to cover both sides of the face.

Acknowledgement

The text for this chapter has been reproduced by kind permission of the publishers from: Barron, J. N. and Said, M. N. Operative Plastic and Reconstructive Surgery. Edinburgh: Churchill Livingstone, 1980.

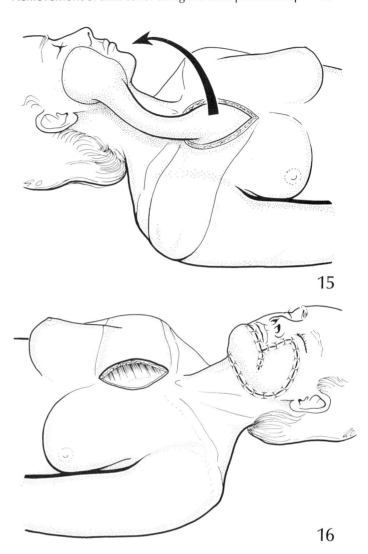

15

16

References

1. Bakamjian, V. Y. A two-stage method for pharyngoesophageal reconstruction with a primary pectoral skin flap. Plastic and Reconstructive Surgery 1965; 36: 173–184

2. Bakamjian, V. Y., Culf, N. K. and Bales, H. W. Versatility of deltopectoral flap in reconstruction following head and neck cancer surgery. In: Sanvenero-Roselli, G., Boggio-Rabutti G. (eds), Transactions of the Fourth International Congress of Plastic and Reconstructive Surgery, Rome, October, 1967, pp. 808–815. Amsterdam: Excerpta Medica, 1969

3. Bakamjian, V. Y., Long, M. and Rigg, B. Experience with the medially based deltopectoral flap in reconstructive surgery of the head and neck. British Journal of Plastic Surgery 1971; 24: 174–183

Illustrations by Kevin Marks

The pectoralis major myocutaneous flap

David T. Sharpe MA, FRCS
Consultant Plastic Surgeon, St Lukes Hospital, Bradford, UK

Introduction

The discovery of the pectoralis major flap represents a significant advance in reconstructive techniques for head and neck malignancy. The availability of a flap which can be raised immediately without recourse to previous delay has given the reconstructive surgeon greater versatility in the timing and performance of radical surgery.

The pectoralis major flap is a musculocutaneous flap. The skin relies for its survival on a long carrier pedicle of muscle, derived from the pectoralis major muscle, which carries its own blood supply. It is the length of this pedicle which gives the flap its wide range of uses. Providing the vessel remains intact the flap may be raised not only as a pedicle of skin and muscle but also as an island flap based only on the skeletonized muscle surrounding the vessel itself. The protection of this vessel therefore is paramount and accurate skin markings must be made to outline its course.

Preoperative

1

The pectoral branch of the acromiothoracic artery supplies the flap and is the main blood supply of the pectoralis major muscle. The thoracoacromial artery, a branch of the subclavian, passes under the clavicle obliquely, runs laterally under the fibres of the pectoralis major and then angles medially towards the xiphisternum. This constant vessel has as its surface markings a line drawn from a point just medial to the coracoid process obliquely to the xiphisternum[1]. It is the author's policy to map out the surface markings of the vessel using a dotted line before planning the skin flap itself. This planning can be carried out preoperatively. The pivot point of the flap is at the vascular hilum of the acromiothoracic vessels as they appear from under the clavicle and for all practical purposes corresponds to the coracoid process surface marking. The skin flap will extend below the nipple and will include all skin which overlies the pectoralis major flap directly. The skin flap can be further extended below the inferior margin of the pectoralis major muscle on to the anterior abdominal wall by up to 3 cm provided that the aponeurosis covering the anterior abdominal muscles remains attached to the pedicle[2]. This has the advantage that in fat women the inframammary skin may be used as an island, thus avoiding the use of fatty breast tissue.

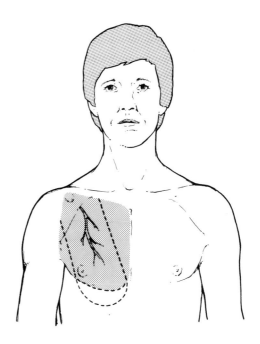

1

At this point it must be decided whether the deltopectoral flap on the ipsilateral side of the intended pectoralis major flap is to be preserved or not. A previously used deltopectoral flap is not a contraindication to using a pectoralis major flap. The underlying muscle will not have been disturbed and thus the vascular pedicle will have been protected. However the simplest method of raising the pectoralis major flap will involve cutting across the base of the potential deltopectoral flap. This can be avoided by raising the deltopectoral flap in its standard form thus revealing the underlying pectoralis major muscle. The flap may be replaced at the end of the procedure and preserved so that it may be used at a future time. This is a very important consideration as in many cases of head and neck malignancy the future use of further skin cover in the event of recurrence cannot be excluded[3].

At this stage of planning the flap, it is wise to consider whether the flap will be raised as a simple muscle and skin flap as in *Illustration 1*, or whether it will be raised as an island of skin based on the muscle and vascular pedicle only as in *Illustrations 2* and *3*.

The operation

The anaesthetized patient is placed in a position suitable for the excisional surgery. This will normally be supine or lateral. The preoperative planning markings are confirmed in ink. The skin flap or paddle is incised down to the fascia overlying the pectoralis major.

If the flap is to consist of an intact skin pedicle then this is incised by parallel incisions on each side of the surface markings of the vessel to the level of the clavicle (*see Illustration 1*). These incisions will later be developed directly through the pectoralis muscle itself until the underside of the fascia is reached.

2

If the flap is to be raised as an island sacrificing the deltopectoral flap then the incision extends upwards from the island of skin to the level of the clavicle along the surface markings of the vessel.

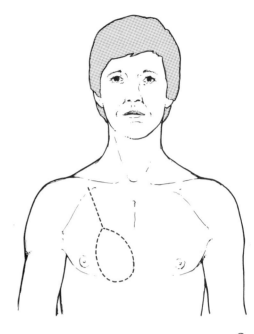

2

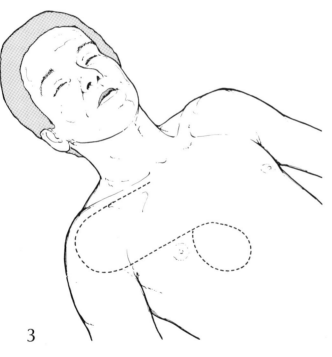

3

3 & 4

If, as is most commonly the case, the flap is to be raised as an island of skin with preservation of the deltopectoral flap then subsequent to the outlining of the island of skin a standard deltopectoral flap is raised. Particular care must be taken not to damage the perforating vessels passing through the origin of the pectoralis major muscle to supply the deltopectoral flap. In addition, the raised flap must be supported and covered with moist swabs to protect it.

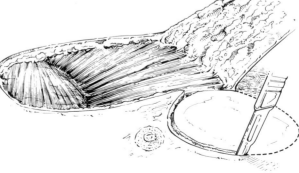

4

5

A strip of muscle containing the underlying feeding vessel is now raised. Using cutting diathermy, parallel incisions are made through the pectoralis major muscle at least 3 cm on each side of the original surface marking of the vessel. The lateral incision is made first and involves cutting the muscle almost at right angles.

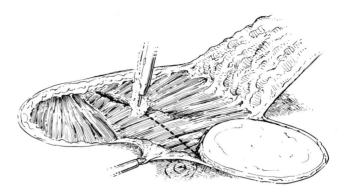

5

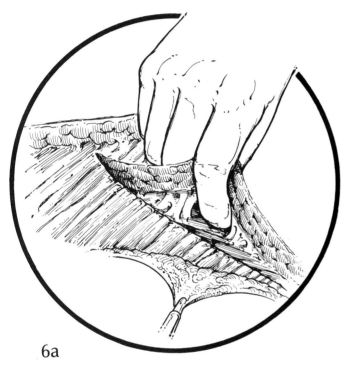

6a

6a & b

As soon as the underlying tissue plane of the pectoralis major muscle is encountered it is extended gently using the fingers and the underlying vessel is palpated. The medial incision can then be made.

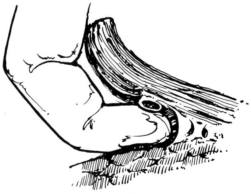

6b

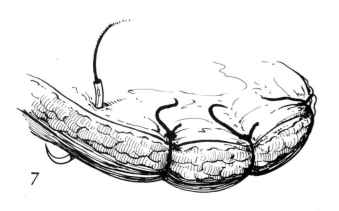

7

7

Before any attempt is made to raise the skin and muscle flap from the chest wall the attachment between the skin paddle and its underlying muscle must be reinforced by inserting several catgut sutures. If an extended paddle is required then the fascia continuing inferiorly beneath the pectoralis muscle is preserved along with the overlying skin.

8

The skin paddle is then raised, and with the underlying vessel in view the loose areolar tissue is dissected gently away along with the muscle pedicle. Other vessels will be encountered entering and supplying the muscle but it is only the thoracoacromial vessel which must be preserved to maintain viability. The flap may be raised right up to the hilum of the vascular pedicle beneath the clavicle, and the vascular pedicle itself may be skeletonized by excising all of the overlying muscle. However, it is preferable to maintain some of this muscle to act as a support. On a rare occasion the author has even removed the central section of the clavicle to gain an extra few centimetres of length, avoiding compression of the pedicle over the clavicle itself.

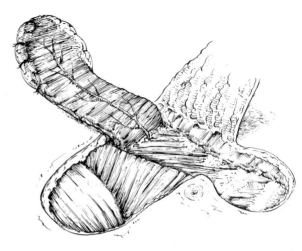

8

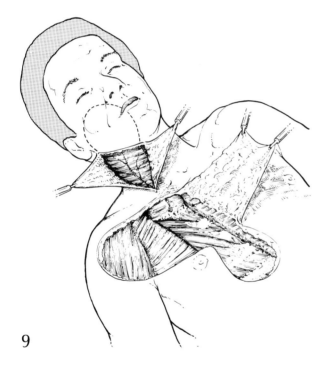

9

9

At this stage the pedicle and flap may be tunnelled into the neck under the intervening skin.

10

To ensure that the tunnel is sufficiently roomy it may even be better to incise and then resuture the skin bridge.

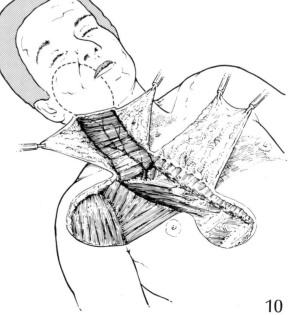

10

11

The skin paddle may be twisted through 180° if external skin cover is required or simply flip-flapped over for intraoral cover. An advantage of maintaining a wide muscular cuff to the vascular pedicle is that in block dissections of the neck the underlying great vessels will be protected.

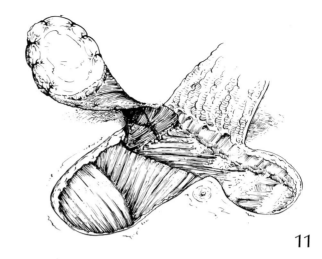

11

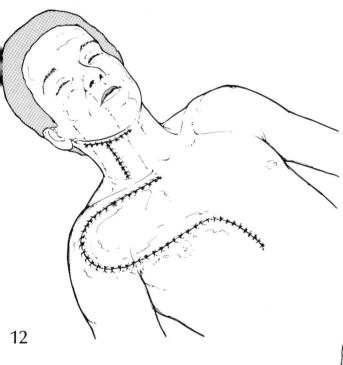

12

12

The donor site of the flap may be closed by undermining and direct suture.

13

Where direct suturing would result in distortion of the breast a split skin graft is preferred.

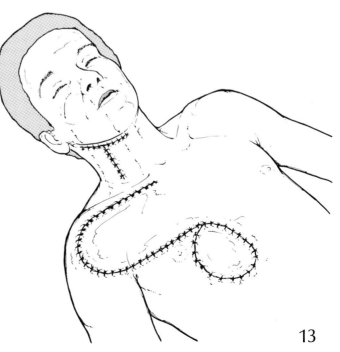

13

Assessment

In the author's experience the island pectoralis major flap described is very safe and reliable. However, there have been a number of occasions when the flap's viability has been in doubt either because poor technique has caused slight separation of the skin from the underlying muscle or because a large breast has forced the use of skin some distance from the underlying muscle. In these instances, intravenous fluorescein and ultraviolet light has proved to be an extremely reliable method of determining viability. Although survival of this flap with a negative fluorescein test has been reported, in the author's experience failure to fluoresce has always been followed by flap death provided that an adequate time (10 minutes) has elapsed from injection of the dye to examination under ultraviolet light. The knowledge that a flap is doomed means that another flap can be raised – either an ipsilateral deltopectoral flap or a controlateral flap. This approach has prevented potentially fatal intra-oral breakdown.

Before deciding whether to use the pectoralis major myocutaneous flap its advantages and disadvantages must be considered carefully.

Advantages

1. When used as an island flap a further staged procedure or separation may be avoided, and in many cases the patient is spared a temporary salivary fistula which may occur when a deltopectoral flap is used.
2. The flap avoids the previous delay which is sometimes needed when a long deltopectoral or forehead flap is required.
3. The donor defect may be disguised easily and may not be apparent in the dressed patient.

4. The carrier pedicle covers the major vessels following block dissection and also simulates the removed sternomastoid muscle.
5. The vascularized skin pedicle may aid healing in a previously irradiated area with a poor blood supply.
6. The increased blood supply provided by the pedicle may enhance the effectiveness of radiotherapy given following operation.

Disadvantages

1. The intra-oral use of this flap is inappropriate in a hairy-chested man.
2. The fat female breast may restrict the flap to a relatively small inframammary paddle, even when the breast has not overlain the flap. The author has lost one flap owing to an excessive amount of fat between the muscle and the skin. The fat resulted in too much traction on the small musculocutaneous vessels despite anchoring catgut sutures.
3. The carrier muscle, if too bulky, may obscure haematoma in block dissection of the neck. The muscle has on occasion produced a webbing effect in the neck and has to be divided at a later stage.

References

1. Ariyan, S. The pectoralis major myocutaneous flap. A versatile flap for reconstruction in the head and neck. Plastic and Reconstructive Surgery 1979; 62: 73–81

2. Magee, W. P., McCraw, J. B., Horton, C. E., McInnis, W. D. Pectoralis 'paddle' myocutaneous flaps. American Journal of Surgery 1980; 140: 507–513

3. McGregor, I. A. Fundamental techniques of plastic surgery, and their surgical applications. 7th edn. Edinburgh: Churchill Livingstone, 1980

Lattissimus dorsi myocutaneous flap for head and neck reconstruction

J. Connell Shearin, Jr. MD
Associate Professor of Surgery, Division of Plastic Surgery,
Bowman Gray School of Medicine, Winston Salem, North Carolina, USA

Carl G. Quillen MD
Assistant Professor of Plastic Surgery, College of Medicine and Dentistry, Newark, New Jersey, USA

Preoperative

Indications

The latissimus dorsi myocutaneous flap is an excellent source of tissue for any patient who needs tissue replacement in the head and neck area following major ablative cancer surgery or traumatic deformity.

Most regional flaps leave a deformity in the donor area of the head and neck region. The latissimus dorsi flap leaves no deformity in this area and also offers an excellent alternative tissue source when regional flaps are needed in addition or have been depleted.

The vascular supply to the flap is extremely constant and, since the flap is on its own artery and vein, it does not require a delay. A great mass of tissue can be transferred in the flap, enabling large defects to be filled in the head and neck areas. It also offers excellent protection against carotid blow-out in the irradiated neck.

Contraindications

The only limitations in the use of the flap would be in patients who have had irradiation to the axilla. Axillary dissection is not a contraindication to its use unless the subscapular artery and vein have been sacrificed during this dissection.

Preoperative preparation

The patient is given preoperative antibiotics and the axilla is scrubbed the night before surgery and again the morning of surgery. The area is shaved, with the preparation extending up onto the lateral chest and the arm and including the head and neck area involved in the reconstruction. A donor site for possible skin grafting is also prepared and draped.

1

Position of patient

Careful attention is given to placement and positioning of the patient on the operating table. Prevention of injury to the brachial plexus or its main branches as a result of stretching is a constant concern. The ulnar nerve at the elbow should be protected also. In simultaneous head and neck cancer surgery the arm can be elevated and the patient positioned either prior to the ablative surgery or after the head and neck procedure has been performed.

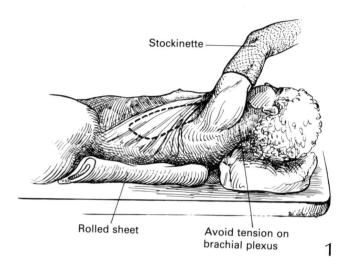

Stockinette

Rolled sheet   Avoid tension on brachial plexus

1

The operations

2

The incision

The flap is outlined in the dimensions needed from a minimum of 10 cm × 15 cm upward to 30 cm × 15–20 cm. The larger the flap, the greater will be the need for skin grafting the donor site. Most donor sites in the range of 10 cm × 20 cm can, however, be closed primarily, except in extremely thin individuals. The incision for the development of the flap follows the anterior curve of the upper part of the latissimus dorsi muscle. The flap should not overlap the muscle more than 2 cm anteriorly or posteriorly. The width of most flaps is smaller than the dimensions of the muscle body.

Exploration is first carried out through the subcutaneous tissue to the anterior border of the latissimus dorsi muscle using sharp dissection. Bleeding is controlled using electrocautery. An initial exploration is carried out in a filmy plane deep to the latissimus dorsi muscle to delineate the vascular pedicle of the muscle.

The latissimus dorsi myocutaneous flap is based on a dominant vascular pedicle from the thoracodorsal vessels which come off the axillary artery and vein. The vascular pedicle enters the proximal aspect of the latissimus dorsi muscle approximately 8–12 cm distal to the muscle's tendinous insertion into the humerus. The vascular pedicle continues in its branching down near the origin of the muscle from the iliac crest. The thoracodorsal nerve travels with the vascular pedicle.

Since the pedicle is the basis of the myocutaneous flap, it is imperative to ensure that it is intact before proceeding to incise the total flap. The flap pedicle is approximately 10–12 cm in length from the axillary vessel to its entrance into the latissimus dorsi muscle. It is the length of this pedicle that to some extent determines the overall length of the flap.

2

3

The outer perimeter of the flap is next incised and the incision is carried down to the latissimus dorsi muscle or 2 cm from its edge. Bleeding is controlled by electrocautery again. The tributary vessels arising from the subscapular pedicle to the serratus anterior and the pectoral muscles are easily divided and tied with 4/0 silk sutures. The circumflex scapular artery and vein (first branches off the subscapular trunk) may be divided if they appear to interfere with flow in the pedicle vessels when the flap is rotated. Usually the latter division of vessels is not necessary.

The muscle is next divided distally, parallel to but beneath the extent of the flap, using the electrocautery. Bleeding from the muscle is controlled by electrocautery or chromic catgut ties. The dissection then proceeds posteriorly in a similar fashion and the muscle is divided similarly. As the muscle is divided, it should be sewn to the subcutaneous tissue overlying it with 4/0 Dexon or 4/0 chromic sutures. This maintains stability between the tissue – that is, subcutaneous tissue – and skin and the muscle itself.

The final muscle division is done proximal to where the vascular pedicle enters the muscle. Frequently this is not necessary and the flap can be rotated without proximal muscle division. This division is done carefully and with the scalpel so as not to injure the vascular pedicle.

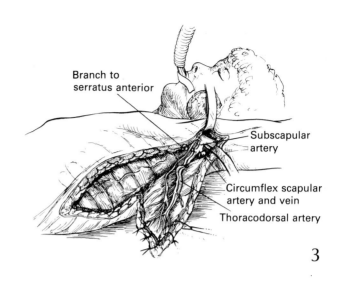

Branch to serratus anterior

Subscapular artery

Circumflex scapular artery and vein

Thoracodorsal artery

3

Bleeding is controlled by use of the cautery or with 4/0 Dexon or chromic ties. The thoracodorsal nerve is also divided at this time since intact innervation will cause undesirable movements of the face during rotational movements of the shoulder.

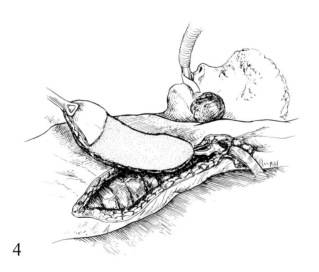

4

4

Before the flap is rotated, any de-epithelization (commonly needed so that the proximal portion of the flap can be placed beneath the neck skin) should be carried out using a sharp scalpel, with care being taken not to go deeper than the dermis. Split-thickness skin grafting can also be performed beneath the surface of the flap before it is rotated when grafting is needed in reconstruction of the head and neck.

5

Using blunt finger dissection, a tunnel is then created in the subcutaneous space superficial to the pectoralis muscle, extending superiorly into the base of the neck. The entire flap is passed through this tunnel by first passing two Kocher clamps parallel to each other, grasping the muscle and then rotating it and pulling the flap into position. Extreme care is taken not to twist the vascular pedicle. After the flap has been placed in position, it should be checked carefully to be sure that the capillary filling is adequate. The flap is sewn into position with horizontal mattress sutures into the dermis of the flap after being reinforced with subcutaneous sutures of 3/0 or 4/0 Dexon.

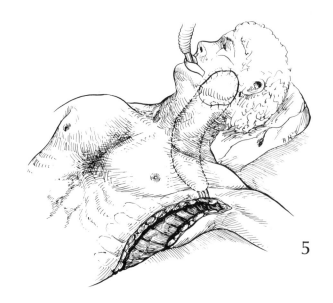

5

6

6

The donor site is then closed, usually under considerable tension but with few sequelae after the edges are undermined. Closure is effected with 2/0 or 0 Dexon and 5/0 nylon for the skin. If a large flap is used or the surgery is performed in a thin individual, the donor site may require split-thickness skin grafting for closure. A pliable suction catheter is left in place for 2–3 days in the donor site and drains are used as needed in the head and neck area.

Nasolabial flap reconstruction of intraoral defects

I. Kelman Cohen MD, FACS
Professor of Surgery, Division of Plastic and Reconstructive Surgery,
Medical College of Virginia, Richmond, Virginia, USA

Preoperative

Indications

After extirpation of intraoral neoplasm, inferiorly based nasolabial flaps are ideal to reconstruct modest to moderate size defects in the floor of the mouth. When based superiorly, they can reconstruct palatal or buccal defects and have even reached to cover nasal septal perforations. Even modest surgical defects remaining in the anterior floor of the mouth after tumour may lead to major functional defects. Simple closure may bind the lip and tongue, making denture-fitting and speech difficult. A tongue flap may result in a painful neuroma and decreased tongue mobility, and may cause drooling and poor articulation.

Contraindications

The author has never used these flaps for intraoral lining in infants or youths because he does not feel there is enough tissue laxity. The flap cannot be used if dentition impedes its passage. Absence of the anterior facial vessels or preoperative irradiation have not caused flap loss and are not contraindications.

Anaesthesia

Local or general anaesthesia may be used. If an orotracheal tube is used, it must be positioned so as not to interfere with flap passage.

The operation

1

Example of lesion

Resection of this midline ectopic salivary gland malignancy not involving bone is planned with bilateral supra-omohyoid neck dissections.

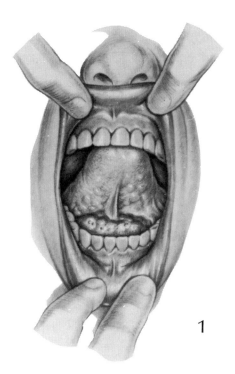

1

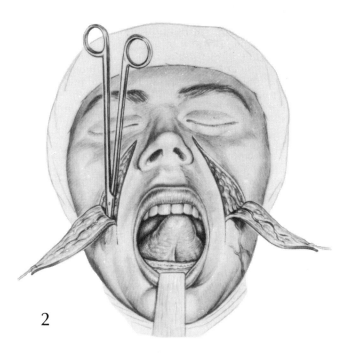

2

2

Flap elevation

Bilateral inferiorly based nasolabial flaps are outlined to cover the defect which has been created by wide excision of the tumour and a rim of adjacent mandible. Enough subcutaneous tissue is taken with the flap to assure adequate subdermal blood flow. Care is taken to avoid direct damage to the anterior facial artery or its branches within the flap. It is often necessary to undermine the flap base to achieve mobility for intraoral inset without tension.

3

De-epithelization

Alternatively, the base of the flap may be de-epithelized as shown on the left cheek (this is usually done free hand with a No. 15 blade) so that the skin wound can be closed primarily, avoiding a second procedure.

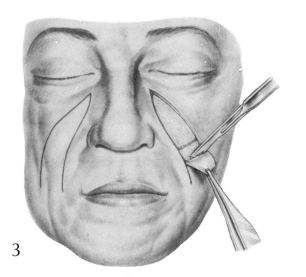

3

4

Flap placement

The tunnel from the cheek skin through the buccal mucosa is usually made by blunt scissor dissection and should be wide enough throughout to prevent constriction of the flap. One flap may suffice, but two can be used if needed. If the flap is simply raised without de-epithelization and passed transbuccally into the mouth as shown on the right cheek, secondary division at 3–6 weeks can be performed under local anaesthesia on an out-patient basis.

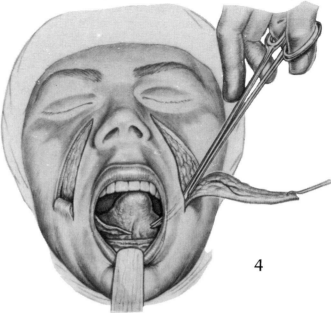

4

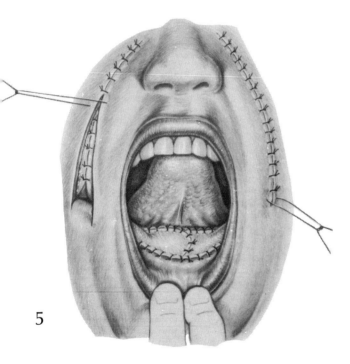

5

5

Wound closure

The flap closure will depend on the defect and position. In the case illustrated, two flaps have been used to cover the anterior floor of the mouth and rim of mandible. Thus, intraoral closure is obtained from flap to flap as well as to the anterior base of the tongue and mucosa of the labial sulcus. The tissue defect on the cheek is always closed primarily in two layers. Wide undermining is frequently needed. If the flap base has been de-epithelialized, total skin closure can be obtained; if not, one must be sure to leave the opening in skin at the base of the flap wide enough to prevent constriction of the pedicle.

6

Variation on flap

The flap may also be based superiorly and passed intraorally for reconstruction of buccal mucosal defects as well as defects of the hard palate.

Postoperative care

The flap must be protected from the teeth impinging on the base. A bite block may be necessary. Usual intraoral care is perfectly acceptable.

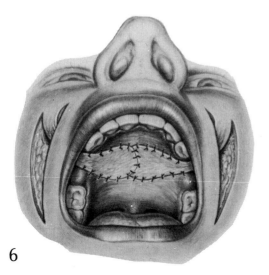

6

Illustrations by Robert N. Lane

Bone grafting in plastic and reconstructive surgery

W. M. Manchester CBE, FRCS, FRACS, FACS
St Mark's Clinic, Auckland, New Zealand

Introduction

It is still widely believed that free bone grafts die and merely act as a scaffolding for the ingrowth of new bone from the ends between which they are placed. It is well known that if a skin graft is placed on a haematoma, blood enters the vascular system of the graft and undergoes thrombosis; the graft becomes an infarct and dies. Because it is on the surface the fact that the graft becomes infarcted and is lost is obvious. If a skin graft is placed on a vascular bed without the intervention of blood, a connection is soon established between the vascular system of the graft and its bed, and the graft continues to live.

If the same technical standards are applied to free grafting of bone, particularly if it is largely of the more vascular cancellous variety, it seems almost certain that bone grafts will behave in much the same way as skin grafts do. This is borne out by clinical observation that if a bone graft has to be given more shape by one or more osteotomies, the osteotomies unite at the same rate as the ends of the graft that are in contact with normal bone, even when the graft is not in contact with any periosteum. This simply could not happen if the graft were dead. Other clinical evidence lends weight to this idea.

Of course, bone grafts are often placed in haematomas and then the earlier ideas might well apply, especially when the grafts are deeply buried and the necrosis is therefore aseptic. It is likely that this fact, and also the fact that, formerly, dense cortical tibial bone was used, gave rise to the original idea of the death of bone grafts.

Thus, provided that the technical standards are high enough, free grafting is still the ideal way to transfer bone from a donor to a recipient site and is likely to be used for many years to come. It is only fair to say that at present much work is being done on the transfer by microvascular anastomosis of compound flaps which may contain skin, bone and other tissues. Such flaps are available in the groin, where the ilium may be used as a source of bone complete with its skin cover. There is undoubtedly a great future for such flaps, for example in the immediate reconstruction of the mandible and floor of the mouth after resection of squamous cell carcinoma, particularly if the soft tissues have been damaged by radiotherapy. A compound flap is also available from the dorsum of the foot, where the skin and a metatarsal could be similarly used.

These methods are still in the developmental stage, and even after they are fully developed, there is no doubt that there will still be much scope for the free grafting of bone. Where there is adequate vascular soft tissue available it is still the method of choice.

The major sources of bone for grafting are: the ilium, the ribs and the tibia. In plastic and reconstructive surgery the main donor site is certainly the ilium as it provides a generous amount of cancellous bone, but it can also provide shims or plates of cortical bone, bicortical grafts mainly of cancellous bone and large masses of shaped bone such as are needed in hemimandibular reconstruction. It is readily accessible and the graft can be removed by another team of surgeons while the main operation is proceeding, for example in the head and neck region. The tibia is used when dense cortical bone is required. The ribs are used when long, narrow and flat pieces are needed. The ribs can then be split to open up more vascular spaces and also to make the bone go further.

Indications

Bone grafts are used in plastic and reconstructive surgery in the following circumstances.

1. In maxillofacial surgery.
   (a) For the treatment of ununited fractures of the mandible,
   (b) To speed union and fill gaps after mandibular and maxillary osteotomy.
   (c) To speed union, fill gaps and stabilize the facial and cranial bones after craniofacial and orbital surgery.
   (d) In the reconstruction of the hemimandible or any part of the mandible after resection of tumours.
   (e) In the reconstruction of the facial skeleton in facial microsomia.

2. In reconstructive rhinoplasty to provide a stable bridge.
3. In hand surgery to stabilize fractures and to provide a skeletal support for the reconstructed digits, combined usually with an island neurovascular pedicle flap or a free microneurovascular flap.
4. In cleft lip and palate surgery. Bone grafts are sometimes used to complete the alveolar arch either as a primary or as a secondary procedure. No agreement has been reached on the merit or otherwise of this procedure.

The most commonly used donor site is that of the ilium and only the method of obtaining bone from this area will be described here.

The operation

1

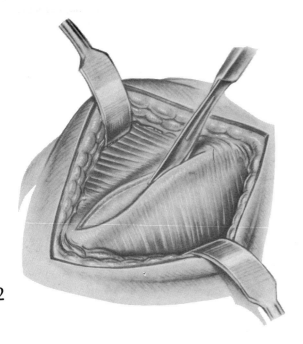

1

A hand on the lower abdomen, exercising firm pressure, displaces the skin medially. With the skin thus displaced, an incision marked out over the iliac crest ends up at a point below the crest, where it is likely to be less tender.

2

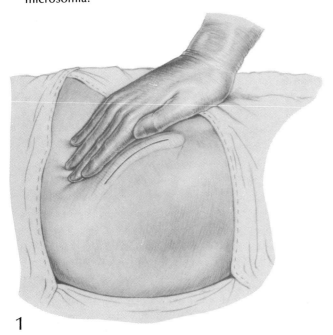

2

The incision is carried down to the iliac crest and then deliberately deepened in the space exactly between the origin of the abdominal musculature above and the origin of the gluteal muscles below.

3

It is carried right down to the bone and, taking great care to stay in the subperiosteal plane, the glutei are freed from the outer surface of the ilium. For most purposes it is better to leave the abdominal musculature attached to the iliac crest as the postoperative course is then much smoother. The iliac crest itself should be left intact.

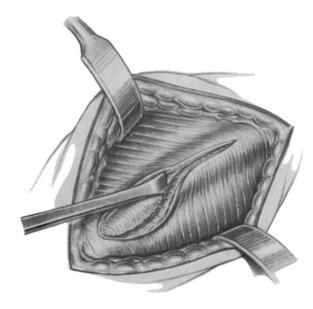

3

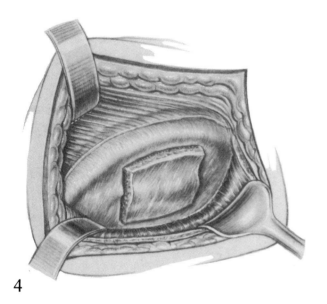

4

4

If a large block of bone is needed, it is removed from the region of the tuberosity where the bone is thickest. It is cut through the full thickness of the ilium by whatever means the surgeon prefers.

5

A bicortical piece of bone with a large thickness of cancellous bone is thus obtained. A piece of it can be suitably shaped for the required purpose.

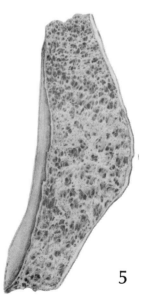

5

6

The outer and inner tables are removed from the block of cancellous bone which can then be cut with the scalpel to any shape and size required. Thin shims of cortical bone can be made from the inner table for subperiosteal grafting, for example in mandibular osteotomy. Alternatively, bicortical full-thickness blocks can be made.

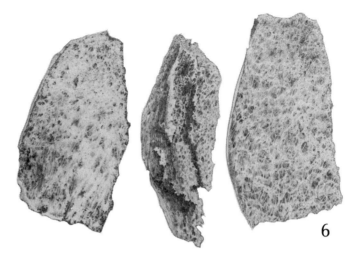

6

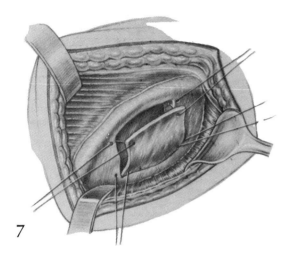

7

7

Often the outer table is not needed and it should be replaced, as X-rays taken years postoperatively show little regeneration.

8

A suction drain is then inserted in the wound and the aponeurotic layer closed with catgut stitches.

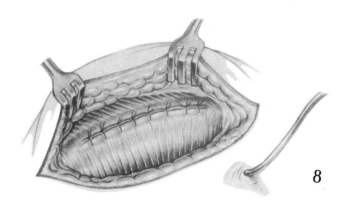

8

9

The skin is closed with a subcuticular stitch.

9

Immediate reconstruction of the hemimandible and temporomandibular joint

W. M. Manchester   CBE, FRCS, FRACS, FACS
St Mark's Clinic, Auckland, New Zealand

Preoperative

Indications

This method is indicated in any case where a tumour originating, say, in the region of the mandibular angle, extends upwards to the base of the condyle and forwards a variable distance into the body, and requires complete resection of the greater part of the hemimandible for its cure. Good examples are ameloblastoma, myxoma of the mandible and certain more aggressive tumours such as chondrosarcoma and osteogenic sarcoma. It has limited application even in the treatment of more malignant tumours such as certain carcinomas of the floor of the mouth.

The method of temporomandibular joint reconstruction depends on the fact that the temporomandibular joint has two synovial cavities, one above and one below the meniscus. The lower one is of course destroyed in the repair but the upper one is preserved. The remaining joint function is always good and is near-perfect in some cases.

Preoperative preparation

These tumours are commonest in early life and the best possible cosmetic and functional result should be aimed at. It is therefore important that the preoperative planning should make it possible to immobilize the graft in correct relation to the remaining part of the mandible and also to the upper jaw. This is in order that any remaining teeth on the lower jaw should occlude perfectly with the upper. In such young patients this is best achieved by the use of cast metal cap splints, a complete one for the upper jaw, and on the lower a splint only for those teeth that will remain after resection.

1

A removable fishplate enables these splints to be fixed in normal occlusal relationship. Details of the method of immobilization where one or other or both the jaws are edentulous have been described in the chapter on 'Fractures of the mandible', pp. 411–417.

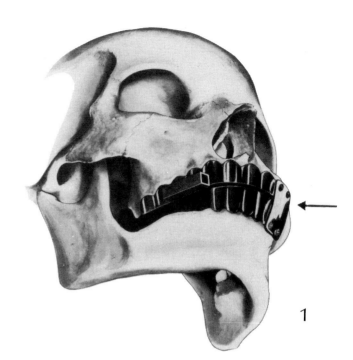

1

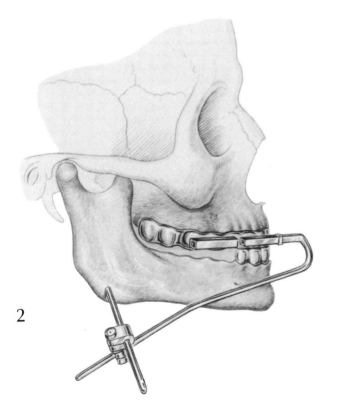

2

2

In addition it is necessary to provide on the upper splint a square tube which is soldered on to it on the same side as the tumour. A removable, adjustable caliper is made to fit into the square tube. The caliper is made in two pieces. The larger one, which fits into the square tube, is bent in such a way that it doubles back over the cheek to be positioned over the angle of the jaw. At this point a second smaller, straight rod is attached to the first with a universal joint which allows for adjustment. This caliper is designed to remove any guesswork from the positioning of the graft relative to the midline. Its use will become obvious later.

3

Before operation it is necessary also to prepare a pewter pattern of the required bone graft, using the normal side as a guide but with additional help from X-ray films. If necessary, it can be modified during the operation by reference to the excised piece of hemimandible.

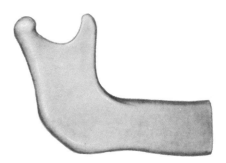

3

4

Position of patient

The position is determined by the fact that two operative areas must be prepared.

1. The patient has a low pillow or sandbag placed under the shoulders to give some extension of the neck, and the head is turned away from the side of the tumour.
2. Sandbags are placed above and below the ilium on the same side as the tumour so as to incline the pelvis towards the other side. Both legs are drawn over away from the side of the tumour. This presents the ilium to the operator in the best position for access to the donor site.

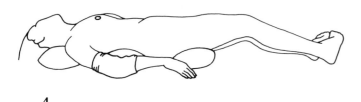

4

The operation

Exposure of the hemimandible

5

The incision extends from the point of the chin to a point well behind the anterior margin of the sternomastoid and comes well down into the neck in order to avoid the cervical branch of the facial nerve.

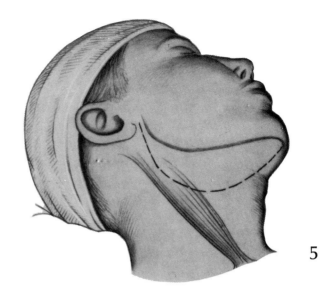

5

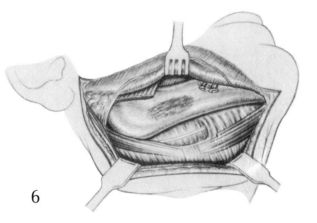

6

6

It is deepened through the platysma and the common facial vein is divided between ligatures. The facial artery is also divided between ligatures and the incision is carried down to the diseased half of the mandible. In the non-aggressive type of tumour the dissection then extends to expose the mandible subperiosteally for the most part so that the angle is clearly visible in the wound.

7

Immobilization of the mandible

The mandible is now immobilized to the maxilla by the application of the fishplate between the two splints. This ensures that the part of the mandible which will remain will be in normal occlusal relationship with the upper jaw.

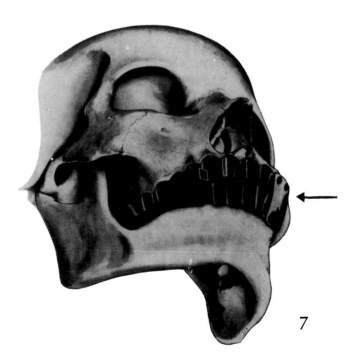

7

8

Determining the correct position of the angle

The adjustable caliper is inserted into the square tube on the side of the upper splint and, using the universal joint, the smaller rod is adjusted so that its free end just touches the exposed angle of the intact but diseased mandible. It is now indicating in space the exact position of the mandibular angle. The whole caliper is now removed and put to one side for later use.

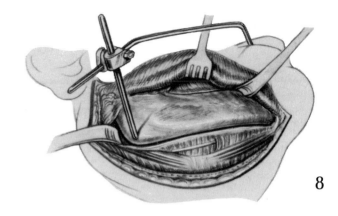

8

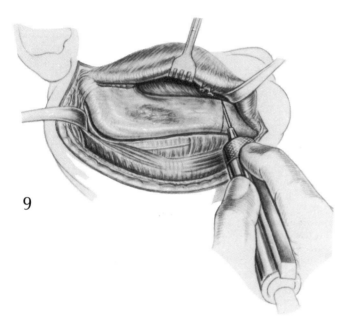

9

9

Removal of the diseased hemimandible.

The symphysis is then cleared subperiosteally and the point chosen for division. Using the Hall drill or any preferred type of saw, the mandible is cut through at this point. Starting in the symphyseal area and pulling it away from the midline, the excision of the diseased half of the mandible is completed subperiosteally for the most part, if the tumour is of the simple type, but taking with it a varying amount of soft tissue if it is more aggressive. Even in the simpler types it is usually necessary to sacrifice some of the lining of the mouth in the region of the alveolar ridge. It is possible by holding the hemimandible by its symphyseal end to clear the whole of the hemimandible under direct vision right up to the condylar process.

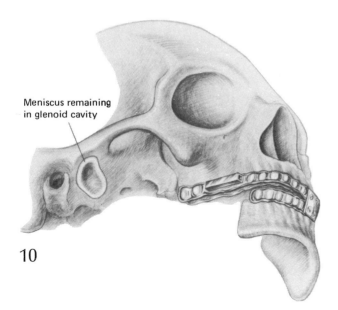

Meniscus remaining in glenoid cavity

10

10

Disarticulation of the temporomandibular joint

This is one of the most important parts of the procedure. The temporomandibular joint is disarticulated, but taking great care to do so in such a way as to leave the meniscus intact in the glenoid cavity. All bleeding must now be carefully controlled, and the use of diathermy is recommended.

11

Exposure of the ilium

The ilium on the same side as the tumour must be used as the curvature here is appropriate. The incision extends from the anterosuperior spine, well back along the line of the iliac crest but just below it, almost to the posterosuperior iliac spine. The incision is deepened and the muscles are elevated subperiosteally from the outer surface of practically the whole of the ilium.

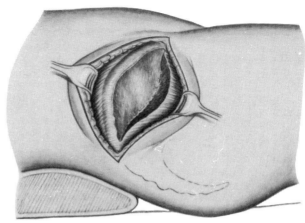

11

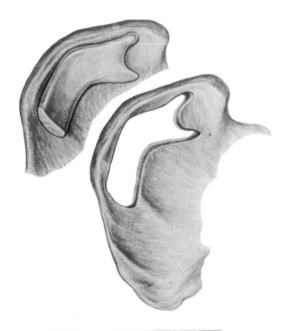

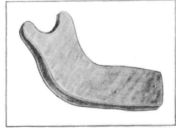

12

12

Removal and preparation of the bone graft

The previously prepared pewter pattern is then applied upside down to the outer surface of the ilium, but just below the level of the iliac crest which should be preserved intact in order not to interfere with the contour of this part of the body. The outline of the pattern is then chiselled into the outer surface of the ilium and the pewter pattern discarded. The piece of bone, now clearly outlined and in the shape of a hemimandible, is removed, including the full thickness of the ilium, either by using chisels or some preferred kind of bone saw. Further shaping is then carried out to make it into an exact replica of the normal hemimandible and also to remove some of the cortical bone to help in revascularization of the graft.

Closure of the iliac wound

The donor site is closed by a team of assistants to save time. Redivac suction drainage is used in order to prevent postoperative discomfort and complications.

13

The placing of the bone graft

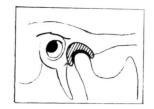

The condyle of the newly fashioned hemimandible is placed in the intact meniscus in the glenoid cavity and the symphyseal end is trimmed to fit exactly to the cut end of the remaining and immobilized hemimandible. The caliper is then re-inserted into the square tube on the upper splint and the bone graft adjusted so that its angle just touches the point of the caliper. In this way it is possible to be certain that it will occupy exactly the same relative position to the midline of the patient as did its predecessor. A single Kirschner wire is then inserted obliquely through the graft and into the symphyseal part of the remaining immobilized hemimandible to fix it in this position.

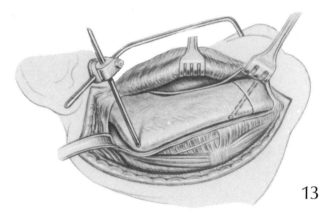

Bone grafting the symphyseal join

Pieces of cancellous bone of various shapes and sizes are available and these are packed in to fill any possible nooks and crannies around the line of union. A thin shim of cancellous bone overlaps the lingual and buccal sides of the line of junction. Redivac suction drains are introduced, one superficial to the bone graft and one deep to it, and the wound is closed carefully in layers to avoid any dead space.

13

14

Providing for greater curvature in larger grafts

When a complete hemimandible has to be reconstructed, sometimes the curvature of the ilium is insufficient. It can be increased by making a cut through the outer cortex and greenstick fracturing it. This opened-up cut can often be filled by a small wedge of bone.

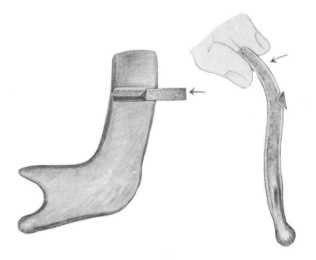

14

Postoperative care

Careful observation and supervision of the suction bottles is necessary in order to ensure that the vacuum is maintained, and these are removed only when the amount of exudate becomes less than, say, 10 ml/day. This applies equally to the donor site. The stitches are removed alternately on the fourth and fifth days in the case of the facial wound and on the 10th day in the case of the iliac wound. Four weeks after the operation the fishplate is removed and union is tested. It is usually found to be solidly united by this time. If it is not, the fishplate is left off but the splints are not yet removed. The patient is allowed to move the mandible gently but no great effort is made to increase the movement, which tends to increase spontaneously and will go on improving over a long period.

Illustrations by Gillian Oliver from originals by G. Ian Taylor and Douglas McManamny

Free composite bone flaps

G. Ian Taylor FRCS, FRACS
Consultant Plastic Surgeon, The Royal Melbourne Hospital;
Senior Consultant Plastic Surgeon, Preston and Northcote Community Hospital;
Associate Plastic Surgeon, The University of Melbourne, Australia

Introduction

The distant transfer of living bone and soft tissue by microvascular techniques now offers a reliable one-stage method of composite tissue repair in carefully selected patients. The method was first reported successfully in the experimental animal by Ostrup and Fredrickson[1] in 1974 and in man by Taylor, Miller and Ham[2] in 1975. The technique is usually considered by the author for those situations where the bone defect is large and where conventional bone grafting procedures have failed or are unavailable; where the alternative is a multiple staged procedure protracted over a long time interval; or where a superior result can be expected.

Donor sites

1

Basic research in fresh human cadaver dissections has uncovered many donor sites, some only recently reported. These include the fibula nourished by the peroneal or anterior tibial vessels; the iliac crest based on the deep circumflex iliac, the superficial circumflex iliac or the superior gluteal vessels; the rib based on the anterior or posterior intercostal vessels; the scapula designed on the circumflex scapular vessels; the humerus fed by the profunda brachii vessels; the radius and the ulna based on their correspondingly named vessels; and the metatarsal based on the dorsalis pedis stem.

Several of these composite bone flaps provide a short bone segment only and they are generally used where the prime concern is the soft tissue defect. However, the fibula and the iliac crest based on the deep circumflex iliac vessels each provide a large bone segment and can be combined with overlying skin. In our experience these two composite units have solved the majority of our clinical problems.

In general the fibula is best suited for the repair of a long bone and the iliac crest for a curved bone defect.

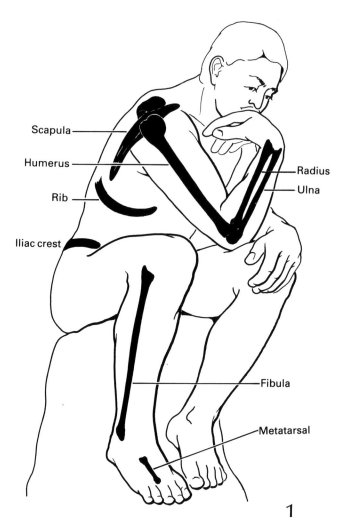

1

Indications

In most large centres throughout the world the success rate with these free vascularized composite bone flaps is over 90 per cent. Consequently they are being used in an expanding variety of clinical situations. Currently they are used primarily for the repair of large bone defects resulting from trauma or tumour ablation and after radical resection of congenital pseudoarthrosis of the tibia.

Mandibular defects

Much effort has focused on the reconstruction of this bone, and excellent results have been obtained with segments of radius[3] and metatarsal bone where a thin skin flap is required for intraoral lining and the bone defect is relatively small. The scapula[4] and rib[5] have also been used with good results.

2a–c

However, an exact replica of the hemimandible can be sculptured as a living graft from the iliac crest and this is ideal for large bone defects. Three different designs have been used.

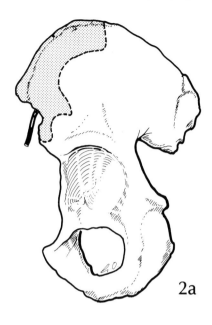

2a

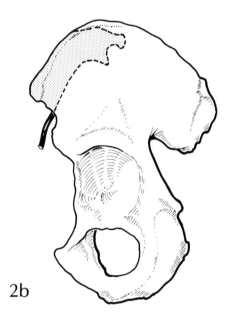

2b

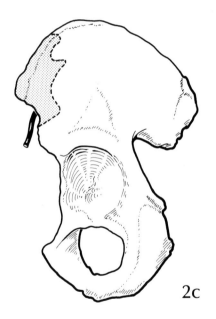

2c

3a–c

The curvature of the chin can be recreated with a wedge or step osteotomy of the iliac crest and in an adult the entire mandible can be reconstructed from one hip. In a child the iliac crest can be split, taking the graft from the inner cortex. This leaves the outer surface and hemiapophysis for normal hip development. The entire mandible can be reconstructed in a child but this requires grafts from both hips because of the relatively small size of the pelvis.

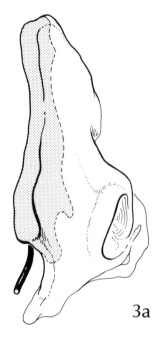

3a

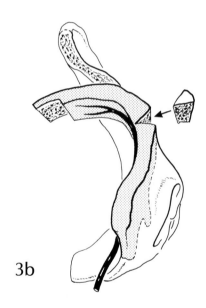

3b

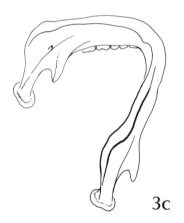

3c

Defects of upper and lower extremities

4

The fibula is ideally suited for the repair of a large defect in a long bone. It exactly matches the radius and the ulna, and fits snugly into the medullary cavity of the humerus, femur and tibia, serving as a 'biological Küntscher nail'. Its triangular cross-section and high proportion of cortical bone help to resist angular and rotational stress.

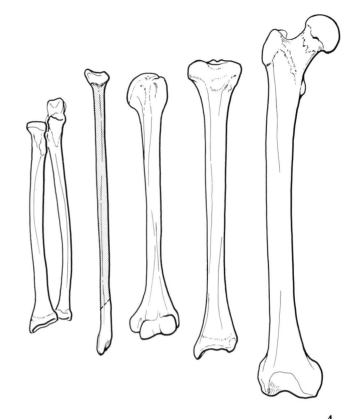

4

5

The curvature of the iliac crest conforms to defects of the pelvis, the longitudinal arches of the foot and the expanded bone architecture of the elbow, wrist, knee and ankle joints (*see below*).

In an adult a straight segment of bone of 6 to 8 cm in length can also be obtained from the anterior iliac crest. Beyond this the curvature presents a problem. However, the length of the graft can be extended to between 12 and 14 cm with a step or wedge osteotomy to straighten the bone. This provides a useful alternative graft for patients with bilateral leg injury or vascular anomaly which would preclude the use of the fibula. The blood supply from the deep circumflex iliac artery to the distal bone segment is preserved at the osteotomy site by careful subperiosteal stripping of the medial periosteum and the soft tissues attached to the iliac crest (*see below*).

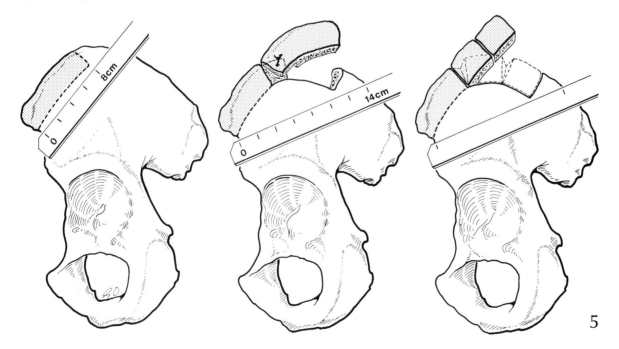

5

6

Defects of the tibia and associated soft tissues are very common, especially as the result of trauma. Where a free vascularized tissue transfer is indicated, the choice of flap depends on the size of the defect.

1. For tibial defects of less than 5–6 cm we use a free muscle or myocutaneous flap (most commonly the rectus abdominus or latissimus dorsi) combined with conventional free iliac bone grafts.
2. For bone defects of 5–8 cm a free vascularized iliac osteocutaneous flap based on the deep circumflex iliac artery is preferred.
3. For larger tibial defects a free vascularized fibular flap is ideal. If the soft tissue defect is large, this may require skin cover as the first stage. In some cases (and in expert hands) the two procedures can be combined.

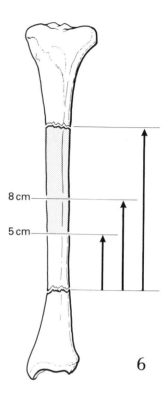

6

Preoperative

The recipe for success lies in careful preoperative planning.

1. Angiography should be performed several days before the transfer under regional or general anaesthesia to avoid arterial spasm. This is especially important in the lower limb in cases of trauma.
2. Bone replica models made of the donor and recipient bones have special application in reconstruction of the mandible.
3. Trial operations in cadavers are useful for identifying technical problems relating to the siting of the vascular anastomoses, the fixation of the bone graft and the orientation of the skin flap.
4. A pattern of the defect should be traced on clear X-ray film and transferred to the donor site (reverse planning). All incisions are marked the day before surgery.

The operations

THE FIBULA

Blood supply

7

The peroneal artery provides the dominant blood supply
to the shaft of the fibula. The endosteal (nutrient) supply is
represented by one or more branches entering the bone
just before its midpoint. While these enter the fibula, the
peroneal artery courses within or deep to the flexor
hallucis longus muscle. This muscle is the keystone to the
dissection of the bone flap.

The periosteal supply arises from the peroneal artery as
a series of arcades which encircle the fibula and
anastomose with similar branches of the anterior tibial
artery. The blood supply to the fibula is preserved by
including a sleeve of muscle around the bone. Only
1–2 mm of muscle is necessary on the anterior and
peroneal (lateral) surfaces of the fibula. However, on the
posterior surface this may be 1–2 cm thick, depending on
the proximity of the peroneal vessels to the fibula.

Provided the head of the fibula is left for knee stability
and the distal quarter of the bone for ankle stability,
between 22 and 26 cm of fibula are available for transfer in
an adult.

In addition to bone, the peroneal artery supplies muscle
and skin on the lateral side of the leg. Where bulk is
required the lateral half of the soleus may be included[6]
and covered with split skin. Similarly, a large segment of
the flexor hallucis longus muscle can be included for the
same purpose[7]. Fasciocutaneous perforators arise from
the peroneal artery in the middle and distal third of the
leg. They emerge in the intermuscular septum which
produces the groove between the soleus and the peroneal
muscles. Although a considerable area of skin is supplied,
we have included only a small skin island in some cases to
monitor the anastomoses.

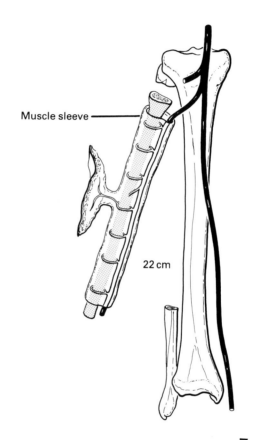

Muscle sleeve ——

22 cm

7

8 & 9

The anterior tibial artery supplies the head of the fibula, its growth plate and at least the proximal half of the shaft of the bone. The former supply arises from the beginning of the anterior tibial artery as a series of small ascending branches, and as twigs from its recurrent genicular branch. This is important for growth plate transfer (*see later*). The supply to the shaft is by a series of periosteal arcades which anastomose with those from the peroneal artery. Our injection studies of the anterior tibial artery reveal staining of the proximal two-thirds of the shaft, particularly within the medullary cavity.

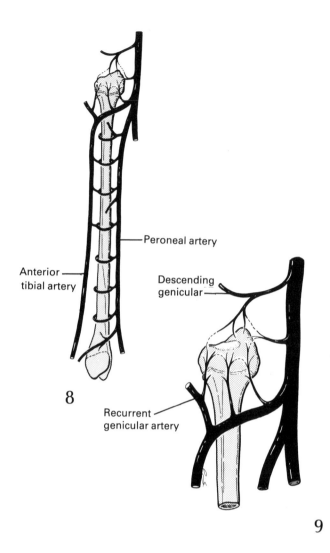

The incision

10

The dissection is performed under a tourniquet, using a lateral approach. The skin is incised in the groove between the peroneal and soleus muscles, and this incision is extended posteriorly at its upper end to identify and preserve the lateral popliteal nerve. The incision can include a skin island if desired, designed around one of the emerging fasciocutaneous perforators. The skin margins are elevated as flaps.

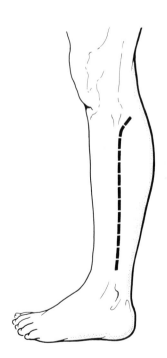

Dissection of bone flap

11

The peroneal and anterior tibial muscles are reflected with a scalpel, close to the periosteum. Care must be taken not to injure the anterior tibial vessels as they course close to the interosseous membrane. The flexor hallucis longus, sandwiched between the soleus muscle and the fibula in the distal two-thirds of the leg, is identified.

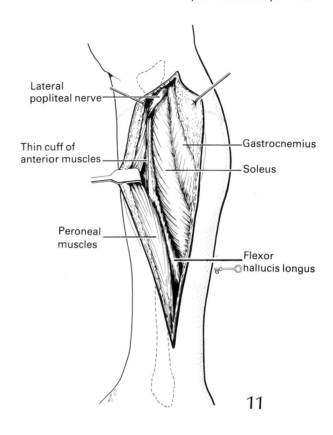

Lateral popliteal nerve

Thin cuff of anterior muscles

Peroneal muscles

Gastrocnemius

Soleus

Flexor hallucis longus

11

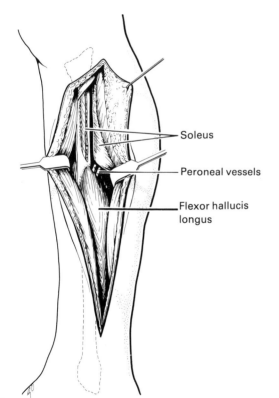

Soleus

Peroneal vessels

Flexor hallucis longus

12

12

An incision is made between these muscles, which are then separated by finger dissection. This reveals the peroneal vessels as they pass beneath the oblique upper border of the flexor hallucis longus. The soleus is then detached from the fibula. Care must be taken not to damage the short stout vascular pedicle which arises from the peroneal vessels and enters the soleus on the deep surface.

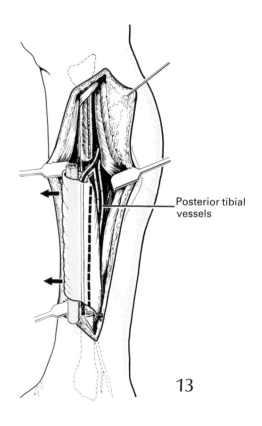

13

The fibula is divided at each end and the interosseous membrane is split longitudinally with scissors to facilitate further dissection. The peroneal vessels are identified distally, ligated and divided. Working from distal to proximal, the flexor hallucis longus and the tibialis posterior muscles are divided medial to the line of the peroneal vessels.

Posterior tibial vessels

13

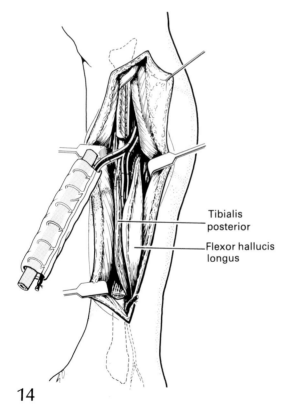

Tibialis posterior

Flexor hallucis longus

14

14

Finally the pedicle is dissected to its origin from the posterior tibial vessels. The tourniquet is released and the composite bone flap is left for 20 minutes to overcome any vessel spasm and to ensure vitality of all of its constituent parts.

Refinements

15

Although the peroneal artery and its two venae comitantes are of a large calibre, the pedicle is relatively short. This pedicle may be lengthened by suturing a vein graft loop (bearing in mind the direction of its valves) between the peroneal artery and one of its veins. This is done in comfort on a side table. The loop is then divided at the recipient site at the appropriate level. The technique is particularly useful in the reconstruction of the femur, as this bone is deeply buried in muscle and recipient vessels may be at a distance.

A musculoperiosteal flap is reflected from the fibula at each end and sutured at the recipient site to cover the bone graft junctions. Cancellous bone is also packed at each end beneath these flaps to hasten bone union.

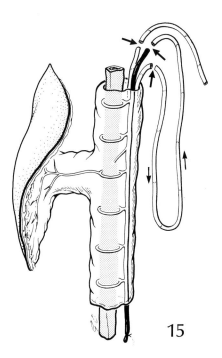

15

Clinical examples

Reconstruction of the ulna

16

This patient had an 8 cm traumatic defect of the ulna. The stumps of the ulna and its associated vessels were identified via a medially based volar flap and the bone and vessel ends were trimmed to healthy tissue.

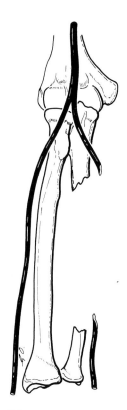

16

17

The flap was then isolated with a skin flap monitor in the donor leg and detached. (The skin flap has been omitted from this illustration for reasons of clarity.)

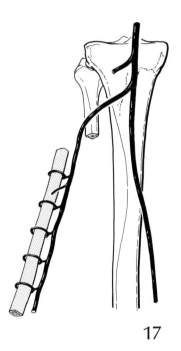

17

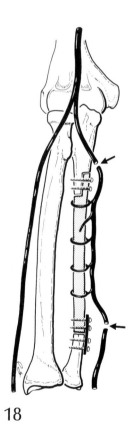

18

18

The fibula was fixed internally at the recipient site. (This may be done with small compression plates, or with screws after step-cutting the bone ends.) The peroneal artery was anastomosed to the ulnar artery at each end to reconstitute the damaged vessel. Proximal vein repairs only were performed in this patient.

The forearm and hand were immobilized in a plaster slab for one week. This was later converted to a full plaster cylinder. The bone ends were united at 8 weeks.

Reconstruction of the tibia

19

The stumps of the tibia are usually approached from behind or medially by reflecting the gastrocnemius and soleus muscles. Wherever possible the posterior tibial vessels are selected for the anastomosis, as they are of the largest calibre, most accessible, and in our experience least prone to spasm. In this patient with a traumatic defect of the tibia conventional transposition of the ipsilateral fibula had failed at the proximal end due to infection, resulting in a pseudoarthrosis (see *Illustration 21*).

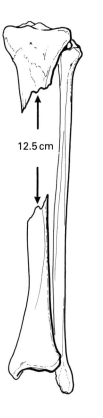

12.5 cm

19

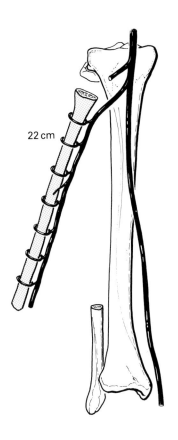

22 cm

20

The fibula from the donor leg was isolated simultaneously by a separate team. Periosteum was stripped from each end. In several similar cases it has been necessary to lengthen the vascular pedicle with a vein graft.

Although the traumatic defect was only 12.5 cm, the bone graft had to be longer (22 cm) as it was dowelled into each end of the tibia.

21

The bone graft was transferred and dowelled into the proximal tibial stump. A bone flap was elevated from the distal end of the tibia. The leg was distracted and the reverse end of the fibula slotted into the tibia. (An oblique cut of the fibula ensures that this end does not spring out of position.)

Rigid fixation is usually obtained with an external fixateur and compression of the bone graft. Whenever possible we avoid any form of internal fixation, especially screws placed through the fibula. The latter are potential sites for graft fracture.

Placing one of the external fixation screws through the tibia just beyond each end of the fibula will prevent 'telescoping' of the bone graft. The vessels are then joined by end-to-side anastomoses where possible.

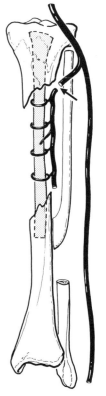

21

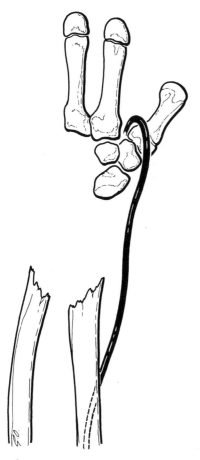

22

Epiphyseal transfer

22

This child lost the distal radius and ulna, together with a portion of the carpus, due to trauma. The distal stump of the radius, the carpus and the radial vessels were identified from the dorsal and radial aspects of the forearm. (The extensor tendons of the wrist have been omitted from this illustration for reasons of clarity.)

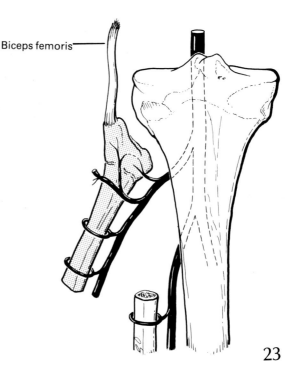

Biceps femoris

23

23

The proximal head and shaft of the fibula were isolated on the anterior tibial vessels. The composite bone flap included a longitudinal strip of attached biceps femoris tendon, as well as a thin cuff of anterior tibial and peroneal muscles. The shaft of the fibula was divided distally and the head of the fibula was disarticulated from the tibia. The anterior tibial vessels were divided at their origin and distally. The graft was carefully eased from beneath the lateral popliteal nerve and its muscular branches to the tibialis anterior. The remaining biceps tendon and its expansion to the deep fascia of the leg were stapled to the side of the tibia to ensure knee stability.

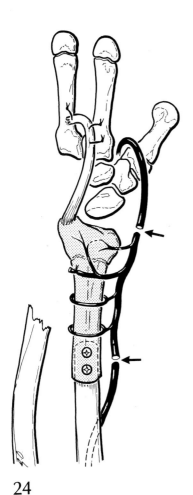

24

24

The composite bone flap was transferred and secured proximally to the radius with screws after step-cutting the bone ends. It was stabilized distally by passing the head of the fibula beneath the thumb extensors and long abductor tendons (omitted from diagram). The strip of biceps tendon attached to the head of the fibula was next woven through and around the insertion of the extensor carpi radialis longus and brevis tendons. The composite unit was revascularized by proximal and distal anastomoses to the radial vessels. Union of the fibula to the radius was evident at 6 weeks. At 1 year 14 mm of growth was evident, measured between the epiphyseal plate and a growth arrest line which had advanced along the fibular shaft.

THE ILIAC CREST

Blood supply

25

Although several vessels supply the iliac crest, we now prefer to design the graft on the deep circumflex iliac stem[8,9]. Its long pedicle (6–8 cm) and large calibre facilitates microvascular repairs. The deep circumflex iliac artery supplies the iliac crest and most of the wing of the ilium from its medial surface. A series of musculocutaneous branches are given off to supply the overlying skin of the iliac fossa. The artery usually terminates as the largest of these perforators, emerging 6–8 cm beyond the anterior superior iliac spine (ASIS). Parallel strips of the iliacus and abdominal wall muscles are included in the flap design to retain these periosteal and cutaneous branches.

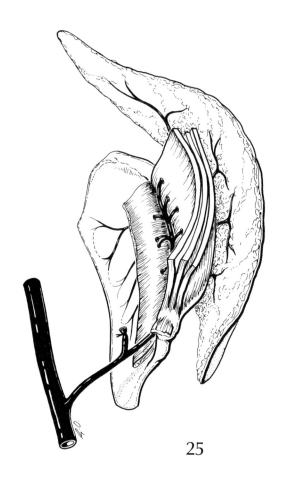

25

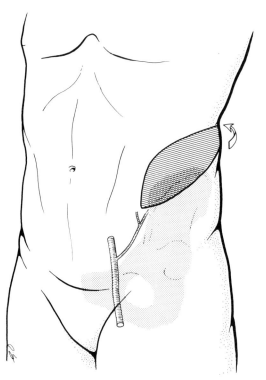

26

Dissection of the composite flap

26

The skin flap is designed two-thirds above and one-third below the anterior iliac crest. The anterior end of the flap should not extend further than 1–2 cm medial to the ASIS. If a large skin flap is required this should be extended posteriorly and upwards towards the inferior angle of the scapula.

27

An incision is made along the upper border of the iliac crest and carried forward above and parallel to the inguinal ligament. The skin flap is reflected downwards together with the loose areolar layer over the external oblique to within 1–2 cm of the iliac crest. At this stage the cutaneous perforators will be seen emerging through the muscle.

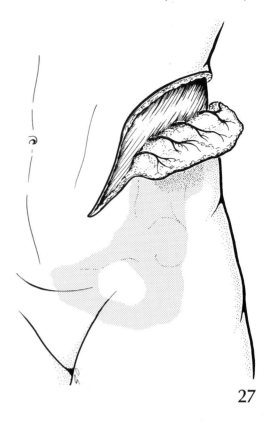

27

28

The external oblique is incised in the line of its fibres parallel to the anterior iliac crest, above the row of perforators. The incision is usually made 1–2 cm above the iliac crest and curved medially to lie just above the inguinal ligament. It is important to palpate the crest before making this incision as it is easily misplaced.

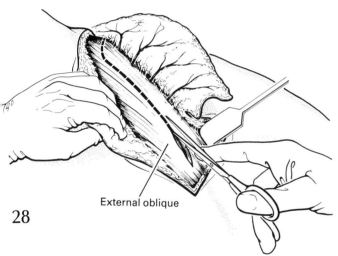

External oblique

28

29

The incision is deepened lateral to the anterior superior iliac spine, and the internal oblique, the transversus abdominis muscle and the transversalis fascia are then incised parallel to the anterior iliac crest and 1–2 cm from it. This usually exposes the ascending branch of the deep circumflex iliac artery, which is then ligated and divided. The index finger is inserted into the extraperitoneal space and passed medially behind the abdominal muscles and above the inguinal ligament. The deep circumflex iliac artery can be easily palpated and protected. The incision of the abdominal wall muscles is then carried through the inguinal canal to dissect the vascular pedicle. Here the deep circumflex iliac artery lies in a distinct fascial tunnel accompanied by its venae comitantes.

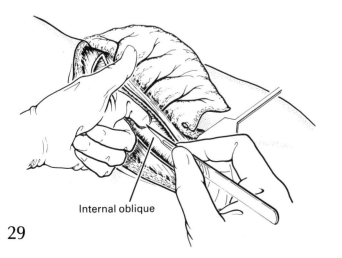

Internal oblique

29

30

The incision of the abdominal wall muscles is extended laterally above the iliac crest to its tuberosity. At this point the iliac crest curves away from the direction of the external oblique fibres. In order to avoid including too much muscle in the flap at this stage the incision is curved across the abdominal wall muscles and on to the iliac crest. If a long segment of iliac crest is required, only a narrow fringe of muscle is left attached to the bone beyond this point.

The groove formed by the union of the iliacus and transversalis fascia is identified in the iliac fossa. The deep circumflex iliac artery lies deep in this groove. The fibres of the iliacus are split 1 cm medial and parallel to this landmark and swept from the iliac fossa by blunt finger dissection.

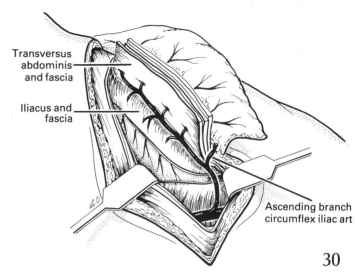

30

31

The lower border of the skin flap is incised next. The buttock and thigh muscles are then detached from the outer lip and surface of the ilium, and the inguinal ligament and other soft tissues from the ASIS.

The bone is sectioned, reflected medially on its vascular stalk and left for 20 minutes to overcome any vessel spasm. This is important, as the skin circulation especially may take several minutes to become re-established.

Particular care must be taken when repairing the donor site. In some cases holes drilled in the remaining wing of the ilium will help to secure the abdominal wall muscles, especially posteriorly.

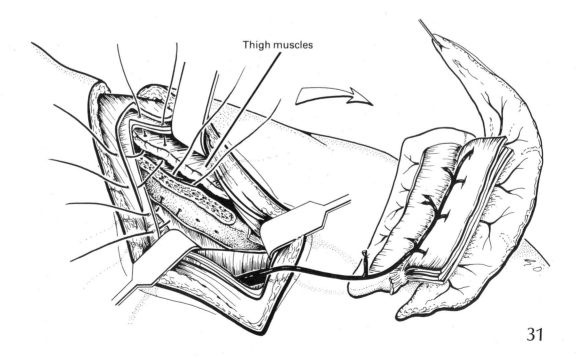

31

Clinical examples

Reconstruction of the mandible

Three methods of designing the hemimandible have been used (*see Illustration 2*). With the first and third designs the vascular pedicle will be sited at the angle of the new jaw. The second design will place the pedicle at the chin where it will reach recipient vessels on the contralateral side. The choice of design depends on the size of the bone defect and the availability of healthy recipient vessels (as determined by previous surgery or radiotherapy). The ipsilateral hip provides the largest graft and transfer of this bone flap will be described in a case of resection of recurrent tumour. Primary reconstruction is preferred whenever possible, and can be carried out before or after radiotherapy.

32

The tumour was excised by one surgical team. This included removal of a previous metal jaw prosthesis; the anterior half of the tongue and floor of the mouth; the entire remaining mandible except the right ramus; and skin from just below the lower lip to the level of the hyoid bone. A template was made of the required segment of mandible and skin and transferred to the ipsilateral hip.

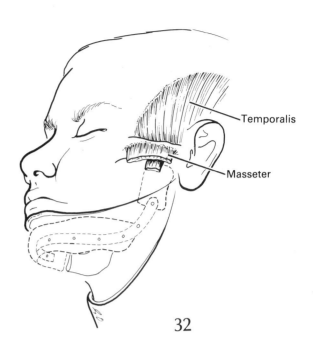

32

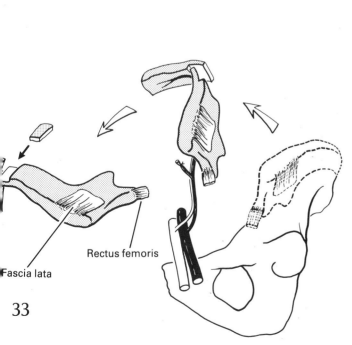

Fascia lata

Rectus femoris

33

33

The composite flap was isolated on its pedicle and included the entire iliac crest. It was planned so that the anterior inferior iliac spine became the head of the mandible; a segment of rectus femoris tendon provided capsular ligaments for the temporomandibular joint; the ASIS became the angle of the jaw; a flap of attached fascia lata could be used for re-attachment of the masseter muscle; a coronoid process could be sculptured from the ilium to re-attach the temporalis tendon; the parallel strips of attached abdominal wall muscle would repair the mylohyoid muscle in the floor of the mouth; and the skin of the iliac fossa would replace the chin and neck defect. In this case the oral mucosa could be closed directly.

An opening osteotomy of the iliac crest was made at the new chin site. This was performed from the outer cortex with a greenstick fracture of the inner surface. Care was taken to preserve intact the medial periosteum and the soft tissues attached to the rim of the iliac crest. A small keystone of bone was secured at the osteotomy site with wires. All of the manoeuvres were undertaken while the composite flap was still attached by its vascular pedicle in the groin. This shortens the ischaemic time after transfer.

34

The composite flap was transferred, fixed in position and revascularized by anastomosis to vessels in the neck. The bone was united at 6 weeks.

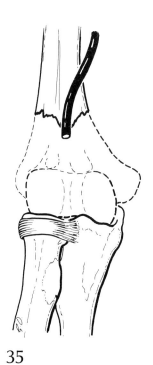

34

35

Reconstruction of the elbow

35

This defect of the lower end of the humerus was the result of a gun shot blast. Although the limb was flail, the forearm and hand retained remarkably good function. Reconstruction was carried out as a secondary procedure.

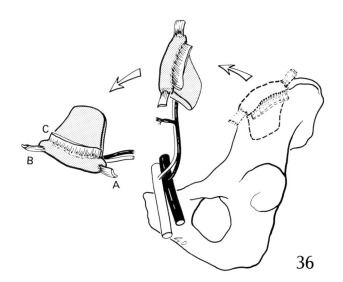

36

The deficient segment of humerus and associated soft tissues were designed from the iliac crest together with a flap of overlying skin (omitted from this illustration for reasons of clarity). The capsule and collateral ligaments of the elbow joint were designed from segments of the fascia lata and inguinal ligament and a stout flap of periosteum elevated from the iliac crest.

36

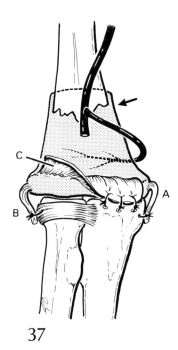

37

37

The composite bone flap was fixed at the elbow with a plate and screws and revascularized by anastomosis to the brachial vessels.

Reconstruction of the tibia

38, 39 & 40

A 6 cm traumatic defect of the distal tibia was repaired with a straight segment of the anterior iliac crest combined with a large skin flap.

The iliac bone was morticed into the tibial ends, taking care to align the graft within the line of weightbearing stress. The composite flap was revascularized by end-to-side anastomoses of the deep circumflex iliac artery to the posterior tibial vessels. The skin flap was sutured into the defect and an external fixateur provided rigid bone fixation.

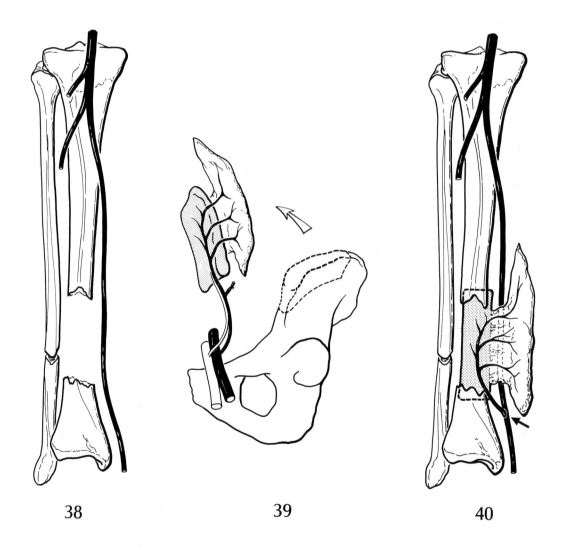

38   39   40

Results

We have used composite bone flaps in more than 60 cases, with a success rate of 93 per cent. Bone defects ranged from 6 to 20 cm. Stress fractures occurred in 6 of 28 grafts to the long bones of the lower extremity, and in each case the length of the graft exceeded 10 cm. However, callus was evident at the fracture site within 4 weeks, clearly demonstrating vascularity of the bone. Four of the six fractures united spontaneously, one resulted in a painless hypertrophic pseudoarthrosis and one required a supplementary operation.

The mandible was reconstructed with vascularized ilium in 20 patients. In four the intraoral suture line broke down, exposing a portion of the bone. In three of these patients an osteotomy had been performed at the chin point, and it was a portion of the distal bone segment which was bared. In each of these patients the wound healed spontaneously in 10 to 14 days by the process of granulation and epithelialization. The entire graft was exposed to saliva in the fourth patient. A successful secondary suture was performed on the seventh post-operative day. The outcome in these four patients provides strong support for the use of vascularized bone in difficult cases of jaw reconstruction, especially if the area has been or will be irradiated.

The rate of union at each end of the bone flap varies with the recipient bone. In the jaw it unites within 4 to 6 weeks; in the forearm union is evident between 8 and 12 weeks; and in the lower extremity between 4 and 6 months. Hypertrophy and remodelling of the bone were seen in all bone flaps subjected to weightbearing stress.

References

1. Ostrup, L. T., Fredrickson, J. M. Reconstruction of mandibular defects after radiation using a free living bone graft transferred by microvascular anastomose: an experimental study. Plastic and Reconstructive Surgery 1975; 55: 563–572

2. Taylor, G. I., Miller, G. D. H., Ham, F. J. The free vascularised bone graft: clinical extension of microvascular techniques. Plastic and Reconstructive Surgery 1975; 55: 533–544

3. Soutar, D. S., Scheker, L. R., Tanner, N. S. B., McGregor, I. A. The radial forearm flap: a versatile method for intra-oral reconstruction. British Journal of Plastic Surgery 1983; 36: 1–8

4. Toet, L., Bosse, J. P., Moufarrege, R., Papillon, J., Beauregard, G. The scapular crest pedicled bone graft. International Journal of Microsurgery 1981; 3: 257

5. Serafin, D., Riefkohl, R., Thomas, I., Georgiade, N. G. Vascularised rib-periosteal and osteocutaneous reconstruction of the maxilla and mandible: an assessment. Plastic and Reconstructive Surgery 1980; 66: 718–727

6. Baudet, J. Combined fibula and soleus muscle free flap transfer. International Journal of Microsurgery 1982; 4: 10

7. Taylor, G. I. The current status of free vascularised bone grafts. Clinics in Plastic Surgery 1983; 10: 185–209

8. Taylor, G. I., Townsend, P., Corlett, R. Superiority of the deep circumflex iliac vessels as the supply for free groin flaps. Plastic and Reconstructive Surgery 1979; 64: 595–604

9. Taylor G. I., Townsend, P., Corlett, R. Superiority of the deep circumflex iliac vessels as the supply for free groin flaps: clinical work. Plastic and Reconstructive Surgery 1979; 64: 745–759

Illustrations by Patrick McDonnell from originals by Deborah K. Randall

Triangular flap cleft lip repair

Peter Randall   MD, FACS
Professor of Plastic Surgery; Chief, Division of Plastic Surgery, Hospital of the University of Pennsylvania, Pennsylvania, USA

Introduction

Operations for repair of unilateral cleft lip should ideally be based on clearly defined landmarks, have a logical sequence, and produce a symmetrical lip in three dimensions, with near-normal dynamics for lip movement and facial expression. There is usually a deficiency of tissue along the cleft margins, including not only the lip but also the alveolus and the nostril tip, with a pulling of tissues toward the nasal spine medially and the piriform recess laterally. There is also distortion of the muscle orientation.

The aims of surgery are to reposition the displaced and atrophic alar cartilages and the displaced alar base; to reconstruct the nasal floor; to lengthen the medial side of the lip; to reorient the orbicularis oris muscle; to reposition the Cupid's bow and lip vermilion; and to reconstruct the buccal sulcus. These aims can be achieved in several different ways, the triangular flap operation being just one of many options.

Indications

1

I prefer to use the triangular flap repair for the more severe clefts, which usually are those with the Cupid's bow on the cleft side displaced upward 4 mm or more (in a 3-month-old child)[1], and the Millard rotation advancement technique for clefts with less distortion of the Cupid's bow[2].

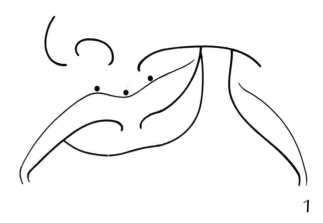

1

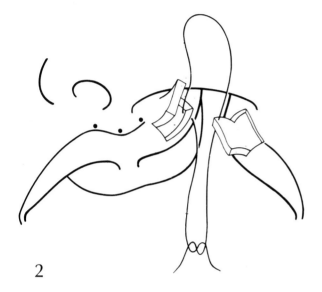

2

3

Overlapping flaps are raised using tissue at the cleft margin, which is usually discarded in the definitive repair.

Lip adhesion

2

If the cleft is very wide, so that closure would be under great tension, the wide complete cleft is first converted to an incomplete cleft with a 'lip adhesion' operation[3].

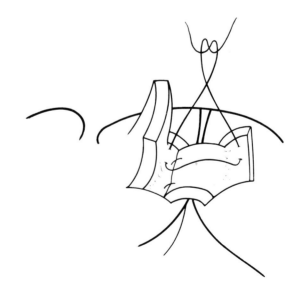

3

4

A relaxing incision is made laterally in the buccal sulcus, and the lip is undermined sufficiently to allow approximation of the cleft margins. The mucosal side is closed with 4/0 chromic catgut, and two or three similar catgut sutures are placed in the muscle. The skin side is closed with 6/0 nylon.

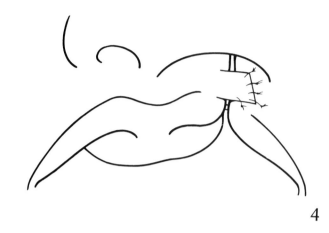

4

5

A tension suture is placed from the mucosal side using 2/0 or 3/0 nylon on a straight needle. This needle is passed all the way through the lip, exiting through the skin near the nasolabial fold. The needle is reinserted through the same hole, passed across within the lip through the repair, and out through the skin again near the nasolabial fold. The final pass goes back through the same hole in the skin and through the lip to the buccal mucosa. This stitch is left in 10 to 14 days. The definitive repair can be done after the lip has softened, which is usually between 3 and 6 months. The lip adhesion moulds the underlying bone, relieves the tension in the soft tissue and makes the key landmarks much easier to identify.

5

Preoperative

The child should be in good health and free from respiratory infections. If there is a cleft palate as well, there is usually some mucopurulent material in the nasopharynx. In itself, this is not a contraindication to surgery. A low haemoglobin in a child aged 1 to 2 months, however, is a contraindication to surgery. In a well-nourished infant surgery is usually undertaken at about 3 months of age.

Positioning

6

The most convenient position is to sit at the head of the operating table with an assistant to the right and the instrument nurse to the left. An instrument table is secured to the operating table so that it is within easy reach, above the patient's chest. General anaesthesia is used with a preformed orotracheal tube (Rae, NCC Division Mallinckott Inc.) taped to the midpoint of the chin. Intravenous fluids are given.

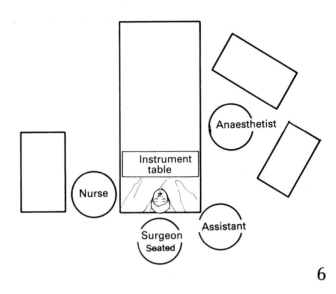

6

7

Exposure is improved by placing the footpad of the operating table under the infant's shoulders. After intubation the child is moved to the very end of the table and the headrest dropped slightly. The headpiece hinge is then located under the child's shoulders to allow adequate extension. If the child has a cleft palate the ears are checked by an otolaryngologist for fluid in the middle ear space. If present (in almost all patients) this tenaceous fluid should be removed by myringotomy and ventilating tubes placed in the myringotomy openings[4].

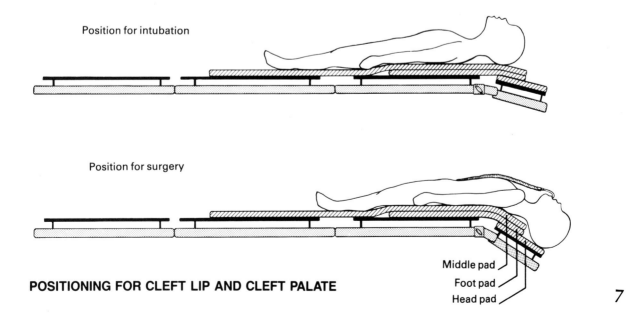

Position for intubation

Position for surgery

POSITIONING FOR CLEFT LIP AND CLEFT PALATE

Middle pad
Foot pad
Head pad

7

Markings

8

With the face aseptically prepared, and draped so that the entire face is exposed, the key landmarks are identified and marked. A 'nib' pen and methylene blue give particularly clear, fine points. The greatest difficulty in teaching inexperienced surgeons the lip markings is to ensure that they pick the key landmarks accurately.

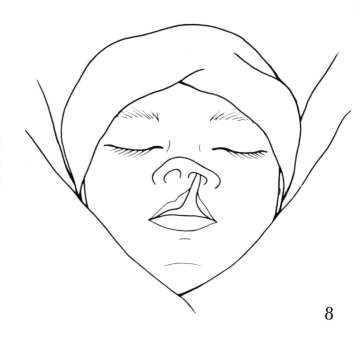

8

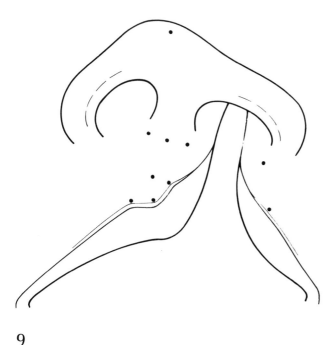

9

9

The 'white roll' at the junction of skin and vermilion is the key for the position of the lip incisions. The midline points at the skin/vermilion junction (the labial frenum helps with this location), the base of the columella and the tip of the nose (usually obtained by shifting these structures toward the midline), are marked first.

The peak of the Cupid's bow on the non-cleft side is marked next. Noting the 'white roll' at the skin/vermilion junction, the peak of the Cupid's bow is then marked on the cleft side (this is usually just where the skin/vermilion 'white roll' begins to disappear). The distance of these two points from the midline should be the same. The usual tendency is to try to save too much tissue on the cleft side, and this leads to asymmetries.

A mark is then made where the lip joins the base of the columella on each side. Another point is made laterally at the nostril base on the cleft side, so that when this point is approximated to the point at the base of the columella the ala on the cleft side will have the proper position and distance from the midline. Laterally, this point can be located slightly out on the lip so that in approximating this point to the columella base the ala will be turned inward.

10

Medially, the incision will extend from the base of the columella to the peak of the Cupid's bow and then at right angles into the midpoint of the philtrum. Laterally, a mark is placed on the skin/vermilion border, again where the 'white roll' and the vermilion have full thickness. (A common mistake made by surgeons in training is to try to save too much tissue and to move this point too far up into the cleft.) Measuring from the normal commisure to the peak of the Cupid's bow on the non-cleft side and using this to determine the lateral skin/vermilion point is frequently misleading because the tension on the cleft side differs from that on the normal side.

The distance on the medial side of the cleft from the base of the columella to the peak of the Cupid's bow is measured, and an equal distance is marked off on the lateral side from the point at the alar base, inscribing an arc close to the vermilion.

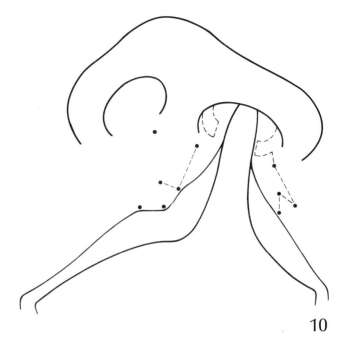

10

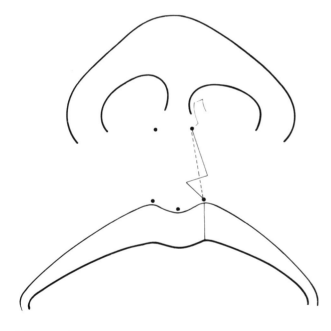

11

11

In looking at the completed lip repair it is clear that the distance from columella base to the peak of the Cupid's bow should be the same on each side. On the cleft side, this vertical line of measurement passes through the middle of the horizontal incision. The distance on the non-cleft side is easily measured, so that it is simply a matter of subtracting the vertical distance on the medial side of the cleft from the normal height on the non-cleft side to determine the width (diagonally) across the triangular flap[1]. The sum of these two measurements on the cleft side should equal the vertical height on the non-cleft side.

12

The triangular flap is sketched in on the lateral side and measured. If the flap is too small, the base is simply shifted along the arc to make it larger; if too large, it is shifted the other way. After the key points have been decided and before injecting vasoconstrictors, these points are tattooed in the skin with a nib pen or hypodermic needle and methylene blue.

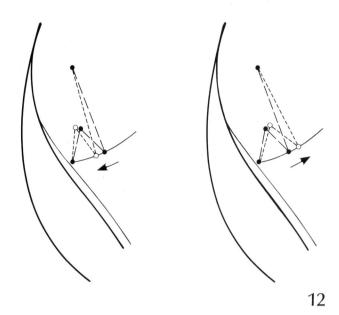

12

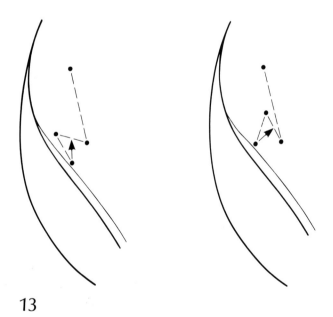

13

13

The most likely error and distortion seen as the child grows after the triangular flap operation is that the repaired side is too long. For this reason, I usually make the triangular flap no wider than 4 mm in a child aged 3 months, even though the calculations may call for a larger flap. Some surgeons always make the triangular flap 0.5–1.0 mm smaller than calculated. Should the lip eventually be too long, it can be shortened at a later stage by excising tissue either from the horizontal limb or in a horizontal incision just below the alar base and columella. If the horizontal limb of the triangular flap is used, the excision should be about twice as wide as one would want to elevate the vermilion border; if it is done at the alar base, it should be about three times as wide.

Occasionally, as described by Brauer and Wolfe[5], the vertical height of the unrepaired lateral side is far too long. In such a child, it is easy to excise a sizeable wedge of tissue at the level of the alar base at the time of the primary repair. The system of measurement would be the same as that described above. At the time of surgery, if more vertical height is needed, the incisions are simply advanced to make the flaps wider. Should the vertical height need to be reduced the flaps are separated as in a V–Y advancement to decrease the vertical distance. Thus, the design is flexible both at the time of the primary repair and at a secondary operation.

Vermilion

The incisions in the exposed vermilion are best made as straight lines paralleling the normal creases. This seems to give a better result than any type of interdigitating zigzag incision. Interestingly, the defects of a residual depression (whistling defect) and of redundancy of tissue in this area usually both call for the excision of more tissue. In the whistling deformity, the vermilion incision probably includes that portion of the vermilion where it turns up into the cleft, and this upward 'bend' is retained in the final result and must be excised.

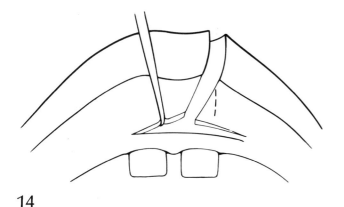

14

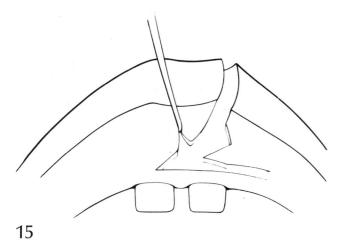

15

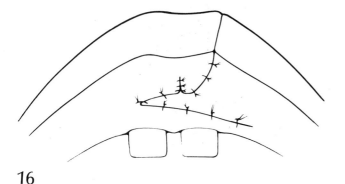

16

Buccal sulcus

14

There usually is a deficiency of tissue in the buccal mucosa in the midline and an excess laterally. The extreme of this midline deficiency is seen in the bilateral complete cleft where the sulcus may be missing completely.

15

In the unilateral incomplete cleft there may be no deficiency at all, and straight line closure of the mucosa is then possible.

If tissue is lacking centrally, a flap of mucosa is taken laterally and based superiorly. This flap includes underlying mucous glands and is switched across the midline adjacent to the buccal sulcus.

16

Often, the midline tubercle of the normal lip is also missing, and a slight protrusion can be produced centrally by closing the mucosa, as shown, with a slight advancement. In secondary repairs, this tubercle can be constructed with a simple V–Y advancement of buccal mucosa.

Muscle reorientation

17

One of the interesting recent developments in cleft lip repair is the technique of repositioning the orbicularis muscle, which can be badly malaligned. Fara[6] has shown that in stillborn children the fibres of the orbicularis oris muscle usually run parallel to the edge of the cleft. In severe clefts this means that instead of being in their usual horizontal position the fibres are vertical for much of their course, and at the alar base they are directed upward and laterally. If left in this position, contraction of the muscle, as when attempting to whistle, will produce an ugly distortion of the lip, with a marked 'orbicularis bulge' laterally. It is difficult to see how normal facial expression could be achieved without realigning the orbicularis muscle in a more horizontal direction[7].

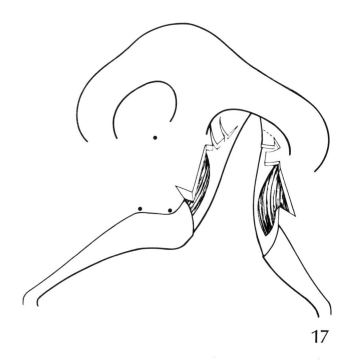

17

Kernahan et al.[8], and indeed Fara[6], have shown that in some patients the fibres do not lie parallel to each other in this vertical component, but are in complete disarray with no logical direction. Some surgeons prefer to excise this portion of the muscle and simply approximate those fibres which are further away from the cleft margin and more normally oriented.

Two methods of triangular flap repair will be described. It should be remembered that (a) in the normal uncleft lip the orbicularis fibres from each side interdigitate with each other, and that many of these fibres insert in the dermis just lateral to the philtrum columns. This produces the narrowing of the philtrum on pouting or whistling. (b) There are also very small slips of nasolabialis muscle which are vertical fibres located at the nostril base and which elevate the normal lip on smiling. Our crude attempts to reconstruct this delicate network of fibres and this interdigitating obviously fall far short of what is found in the normal lip.

Anaesthesia

The field is injected with lignocaine (lidocaine) 1 per cent with adrenaline (epinephrine) 1:100 000. A 2 or 3 ml syringe is used so that only very small quantities are injected and only a tiny amount in any one place. A 2½ inch (approx 6 cm) 25 gauge needle is used to minimize the number of skin punctures and to reduce further the amount injected. The field of injection includes nasolabial fold to nasolabial fold and to nasal tip. Careful studies have shown that adrenaline (epinephrine) in moderate doses is not a problem in children, even with halogen anaesthesia. So long as hypercarbia is avoided, quantities up to 10 μg/kg. can be used[9]. However, lignocaine (lidocaine) should not exceed 6 mg/kg, so that if more is needed it is better to mix the adrenaline (epinephrine) freshly in saline. It is best to wait for 7 minutes exactly after the last injection for maximum effect; during this time the markings can be checked again.

The operation

Skin, mucosa and muscle

18

The skin and mucosal incisions are made (haemostasis is achieved by a fine cautery at minimal intensity), and the lateral lip segment is then undermined in the subcutaneous layer directly on top of the muscle. The undermining is continued to the nasolabial fold superiorly and down to the skin vermilion border but not out to the lateral commissure. Similar undermining is carried out between muscle and mucosa close to the muscle, leaving the mucous glands intact. Medium-sized dissecting scissors, using mostly a spreading action, work well in this step. The medial skin and mucosa are undermined to a point about halfway between the philtrum on the normal side and the nasolabial fold. The mucosa is incised in the buccal sulcus laterally and medially (in minimal clefts this step can be omitted). In incomplete clefts the muscle across the line of the cleft is left intact so that after undermining it can be examined – with magnification, if necessary – to determine how much of the displaced muscle needs to be repositioned.

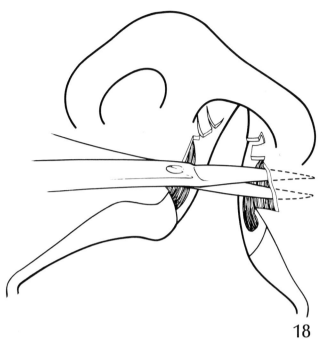

18

19

The muscle is then grasped with forceps at the alar base – a point which often appears to be almost tendinous – and a bold cut is made with scissors directly laterally above the forceps and to the nasolabial fold at the level of the alar base.

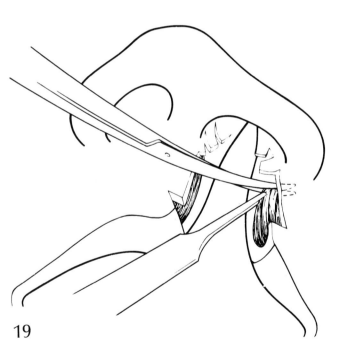

19

20

This cut is continued until the muscle can be brought down to the horizontal position. Occasionally, a bleeding vessel from a branch of the angular vessels is encountered at the limit of this incision; in a few cases this may require a suture tie of 5/0 chromic catgut.

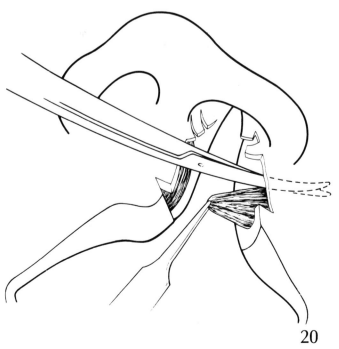

20

21

A similar incision is made on the medial side but the cut is not taken so far laterally. At about the position of the normal philtrum it is angled downward toward the free border of the lip and continued a short distance until the muscle can also be brought down into the horizontal position.

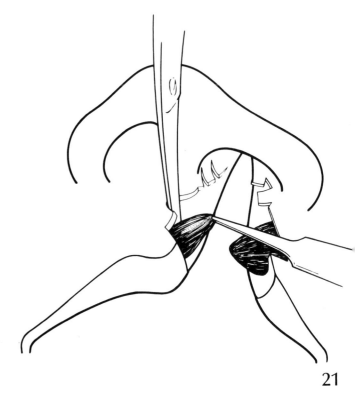

21

The nasal tip

22

After the lip has been dissected, the nasal tip dissection is done. This allows time for good haemostasis in the lip, as the added muscle dissection increases the likelihood of haematoma. If there is only minimal distortion of the nose, nothing is done to the alar cartilages. The alar base is simply rotated into a normal position. In a moderate to severe deformity the medial crus on the cleft side is dissected free using parallel incisions, one just inside the rim of the columella and the other in the membranous septum. The medial crura are separated and the medial crus on the cleft side is advanced toward the nasal tip into a slightly over-corrected position. The areolar tissue between the crura should be dissected off if the repositioned cartilage is to stay in position. The medial crus is secured with either a buried 5/0 chromic suture or several through-and-through sutures of the same material, or both. In an incomplete cleft these incisions are carried right across the nasal floor so that the nasal floor is rotated into the base of the columella behind the advanced medial crus, and the alar base is brought medially into a more normal position. Dissecting out a layer of dermis and subcutaneous tissue attached to the alar base, which can be sutured to the nasal spine, helps to maintain the alar base in its new position. This is the approach most frequently used by the author.

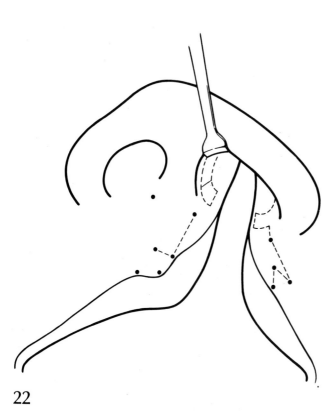

22

23 & 24

We used to dissect between skin and cartilage laterally so as to allow the ala to be rolled around – and many still prefer to do this step – but I think it can be omitted without any difficulty. Should the nostril rim still be pulled down, the usual problem is tightness laterally to the piriform recess.

A Z-plasty between the lateral alar crus and the anterior end of the inferior turbinate usually corrects this tightness.

Broadbent has stated that the problem with the unilateral cleft lip nose is not that the medial crus is pulled down but that the lateral crus is pulled laterally, and that this should be corrected by moving the lateral (rather than the medial) crus toward the alar dome.

His results support this point of view, and indeed it would seem that both problems exist if there is a deficiency of tissue both laterally and medially. The problem is how to correct both at the same time and still preserve an adequate blood supply to the alar cartilage and the vestibular skin. The consequence of too much scarring in the vestibule is vestibular stenosis, which is an extremely difficult complication to handle and which usually requires a full thickness skin graft.

In addition to these two defects, the alar cartilage in the unilateral cleft lip nose has often lost the overlap between the superior edge of the lateral crus and the inferior edge of the upper lateral cartilage. Occasionally this overlap can be re-established at the time of a tip rhinoplasty in an infant, but I usually prefer to approach this at an older age.

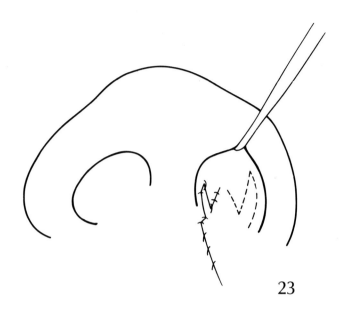

23

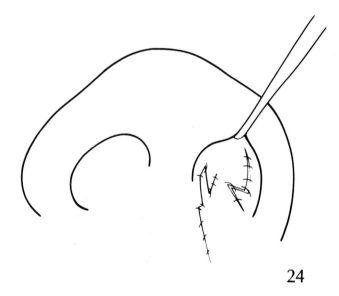

24

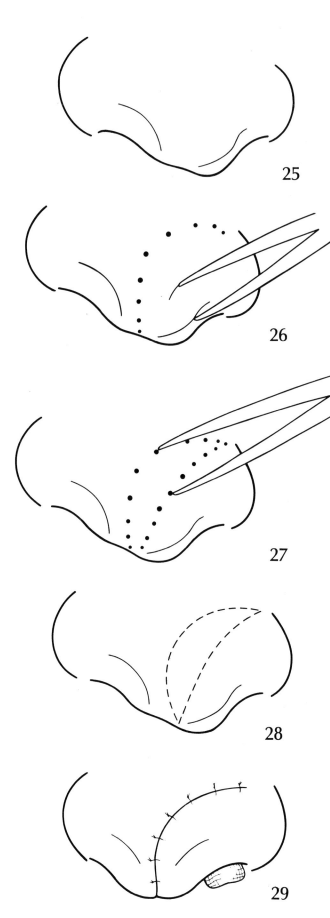

25–29

In the severely distorted cleft lip nose the rim incision does not allow sufficient correction, and if better correction is desired an external incision can be made in the nasal tip (although the author rarely uses this approach). This incision goes exactly up the midline of the columella, straight over the tip of the nose, and then curves around laterally at the inferior portion of the upper lateral cartilage. On the tip of the nose the incision has to be placed a little toward the non-cleft side, or it will not end up in the midline.

The incision can be used merely for access to the tip cartilages to achieve repositioning of these cartilages[10], or it can include excision of a crescent-shaped piece of nasal tip skin as it curves laterally, as suggested by Royster (unpublished observation). The width of this crescent is equal to the distance which the nostril margin has to be moved up.

These incisions usually heal surprisingly well in both white and black skin, particularly when made in infancy.

Closure of mucosa

Closure usually begins with the mucosa. A flap from the lateral side can be brought across the midline to reconstruct the buccal sulcus and a slight midline tubercle can be produced by advancing the midline mucosa as shown in *Illustrations 14–16*. 5/0 chromic catgut is used on the mucosa, 5/0 or 4/0 chromic catgut on the muscle and 6/0 nylon on the skin.

Closure of muscle

30

The muscle layer may be closed by overlapping the two flaps of muscles, placing the lateral flap medially between muscle and mucosa and using tacking sutures of 5/0 chromic catgut from the level of the vermilion up to the nasal spine. The medial flap is placed between muscle and skin at about the level of the skin/vermilion border. These muscle flaps are sutured muscle to muscle, except for one suture to the periosteal tissue at the nasal spine[7]. Initially, considerable overlap was used, but this seemed to produce an occasional tight lip and a drooping of the free border of the lip laterally so that now the overlap is done much more loosely, particularly at the inferior border.

Some surgeons prefer to divide the lateral muscle flap into two segments, suturing one up to the nasal spine and the other down in a more horizontal position[11]. It should be noted that if this step of dissecting out the oribicularis muscle is not carried out but the muscle is left intact with the overlying skin, as many prefer to do, some degree of reorientation is achieved by the rotation advancement, as this shifts the fibers inserting at the alar base over toward the nasal spine; however, this is not nearly as much as that achieved by bringing this point of muscle down to the level of the skin/vermilion junction. The triangular flap incision, if skin is left in continuity with the underlying muscle, will also reorient a very small amount of muscle, but only in the inferior portion of the lip.

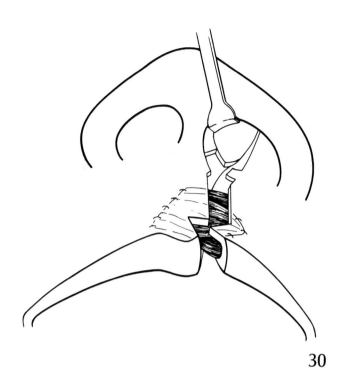

30

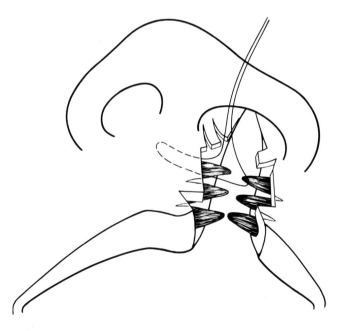

31

31

More recently we have attempted to interdigitate the muscle flaps by dividing the lateral and even the medial flap into three separate muscle bundles each. With one exception (*see below*), these are sutured to the dermis, an arrangement which is a little closer to the normal[12].

32 & 33

The superior lateral muscle bundle is sutured, not to dermis, but to the nasal spine. The superior medial bundle is next secured to dermis just below, not at, the alar base. This step brings the alar base around very nicely. The middle lateral bundle goes either to dermis just lateral to the normal philtral column or to dermis in the central part of the philtrum, producing a philtrum dimple. The middle medial muscle bundle is sutured to dermis lateral to the midpoint of the lateral skin incision, and the two inferior muscle bundles are loosely sutured to each other.

It is too early to tell whether this will be an improvement or not, but it is a crude imitation of the normal. Also, it completely omits the small vertical nasolabial fibres which elevate the central part of the lip on smiling and which are often absent or at least unrecognizable in infants with a cleft.

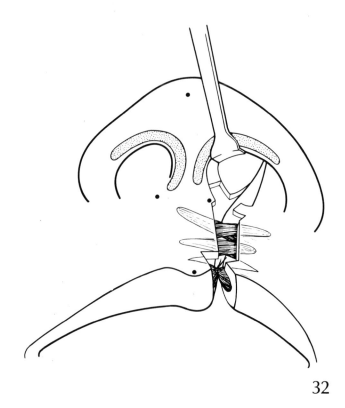

32

Closure of skin

A subcutaneous stitch of 5/0 chromic catgut is placed above and below the triangular flap and at the columellar base. Occasionally, one or more of these stitches can be omitted if the muscle closure relieves all tension on the skin. In some cases, a buried catgut stitch may be used in the vermilion. Key points are approximated with interrupted 6/0 nylon placed close to the skin margin. The intranasal incisions are then closed with tiny stitches of 5/0 chromic catgut. These sutures are tied with three knots and cut close to the knot so that they will fall out in a few days.

The free border of the lip is closed with 5/0 chromic catgut on the mucosal side and 6/0 nylon on the exposed vermilion. Lastly, a running suture of 6/0 nylon is used on the vertical skin incision and additional interrupted sutures, if needed, on the triangular flap.

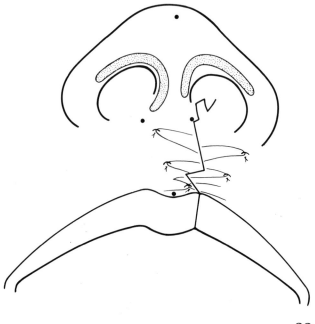

33

Postoperative care

34

The repaired nostril is packed with petrolatum gauze (for 24 hours). The lip is dressed with half-width Band-Aid® (Johnson and Johnson) which is changed after 2 and then every 6 hours. At each changing the incision is cleaned gently with soap and water. After 24 hours the Band-Aid is left off, but cleaning is continued. Antibiotic ointment is occasionally used on the suture line; systemic antibiotics are not used routinely. Elbow restraints are kept on constantly for about two weeks. Feeding with clear liquids is started as soon as the baby has recovered from anaesthesia and is increased to full liquid or semi-solid food within 24 to 48 hours. The use of a bottle with large holes in the nipple or a return to breast feeding is permitted after lip repair, as sucking puts little strain on the suture line. Sutures are removed after 4–6 days, preferably after a feed and occasionally under either sedation or light general anaesthesia.

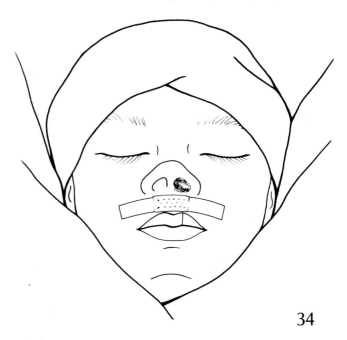

34

Complications

Wound breakdown rarely occurs. The most frequent causes are accidental bumping of the lip, wound infection or excess tension. If the lip is accidentally bumped or injured, causing a partial or complete dehiscence, immediate re-suture is usually successful although not as good as the original closure. In the case of dehiscence from infection or excess tension, re-suturing should not be attempted until the lip has become completely soft and pliable, which may take three to six months. Rarely a haematoma will need to be evacuated. Any additional scarring due to postoperative complications should not be revised surgically until the lip has become completely soft, which may take 12 to 24 months.

The best closure of any cleft is usually the first closure done in infancy, so great care must be taken to do it extremely well.

Acknowledgement

Illustrations 30–32 are reproduced with kind permission of the publishers of The Journal of Craniofacial Genetics and Developmental Biology.

References

1. Randall, P. A triangular flap operation for primary repair of unilateral clefts of the lip: the evolution of its surgery. Plastic and Reconstructive Surgery 1959; 23: 331–347

2. Millard, D. R. Cleft craft. Vol. 1. The unilateral deformity. Boston: Little, Brown and Co, 1976

3. Randall, P. A lip adhesion operation in cleft lip surgery. Plastic and Reconstructive Surgery 1965; 35: 371–376

4. Stool, S. E., Randall, P. Unexpected ear disease in infants with cleft palate. Cleft Palate Journal 1967; 4: 99–103

5. Brauer, R. O., Wolfe, L. E. Design for unilateral cleft lip repair to prevent a long lip. Plastic and Reconstructive Surgery 1978; 61: 190–197

6. Fara, M. Anatomy and arteriography of cleft lips in stillborn children. Plastic and Reconstructive Surgery 1968; 42: 29–36

7. Randall, P., Whitaker, L. A., LaRossa, D. D. The importance of muscle reconstruction in primary and secondary cleft lip repair. Plastic and Reconstructive Surgery 1974; 54: 316

8. Kernahan, D. A., Dado, D. V., Bauer, B. S. The anatomy of the orbicularis muscle in unilateral cleft lip: based on a three-dimensional histologic reconstruction. Plastic and Reconstructive Surgery 1984; 73: 875–881

9. Karl, H. W., Swedlow, D. N., Lee, K. W., Downes, J. J. Epinephrine–halothane interaction in children. Anesthesiology 1983; 58: 142–145

10. Berkeley, W. T. The cleft lip nose. Plastic and Reconstructive Surgery 1959; 23: 567–575

11. Kernahan, D. A., Bauer, B. S., Dado, D. V. Functional cleft lip repair: a sequential layered closure with orbicularis muscle realignment. In: Williams, B. H., ed. Transactions of the VIII International Congress of Plastic Surgery, p. 421. Montreal, 1983

12. Randall, P. Problems in cleft lip repair. Journal of Craniofacial Genetics and Developmental Biology 1985 (in press)

Illustrations by Kevin Marks

Rotation advancement repair of cleft lip

D. O. Maisels FRCS, FRCS(Ed)
Consultant Plastic Surgeon, Mersey Regional Health Authority;
Clinical Lecturer in Plastic Surgery, University of Liverpool, Liverpool, UK

Indications

This repair is indicated for a cleft of the lip of any degree of severity. One of the advantages of this operation is that it is based on the 'cut as you go' principle, so that complex preoperative measurements and markings are eliminated and each operation is tailored to the deformity in that particular case.

Preoperative considerations

Any associated malformations must be identified and treated appropriately. Genetic counselling should be offered to the parents. The infant must be thriving and taking feeds from a cup and spoon. The haemoglobin should be about 10 g/dl. The presence of upper respiratory infection must be excluded, as well as infection of the nose and throat with haemolytic streptococci.

Clefts of the primary palate only are best repaired when the infant is about 10 weeks old. For repairs of clefts of the primary and secondary palates presurgical orthodontic treatment should be completed. This calls for close cooperation with the orthodontist.

Anaesthesia

Oral endotracheal general anaesthesia with midline placement of the tube over the lower lip is most convenient.

Position of patient

The patient is placed supine on the special Frenchay cushion with the neck slightly extended.

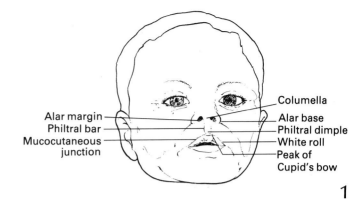

Alar margin
Philtral bar
Mucocutaneous junction
Columella
Alar base
Philtral dimple
White roll
Peak of Cupid's bow

1

The operation

1 & 2

The basic aim of the rotation advancement repair is repositioning of the displaced landmarks in their normal positions. It is therefore important to be familiar with these landmarks and anatomical features, and with the disposition of the fibres of the orbicularis oris sphincter in the normal lip.

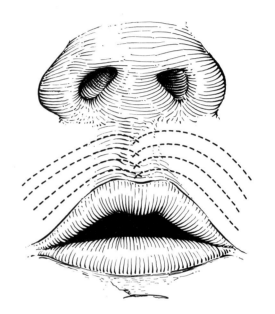

2

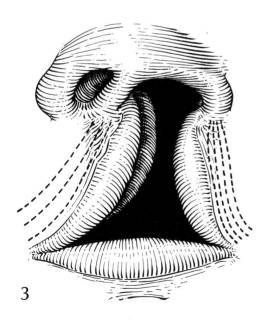

3

3

In the cleft lip the Cupid's bow is present but sloping up and towards the cleft side. The philtral bar is absent but both the dimple and the bar are present on the normal side. The premaxilla is displaced forward and slopes upwards parallel to the Cupid's bow. The vertical height of the lip and columella is reduced and the nostril margin is flattened and depressed. The alar base is displaced laterally and the muscle fibres are displaced as indicated by the dotted lines. It must be appreciated that in addition to the gap or failure of fusion there is a varying degree of absence of tissue.

4

The points of the Cupid's bow are tattooed with a needle dipped in Bonney's blue. It is also helpful to tattoo a series of dots along the mucocutaneous junctions on each side of the cleft, as these may be very difficult to recognize later on in the operation if the ink markings become obliterated. On the medial side a rotation flap is marked starting just over 1 mm above the peak of the Cupid's bow. The flap must not extend beyond the columella on the normal side, as this would lengthen the normal rather than the cleft side. If the lip is very short and more length is required, a back cut must be made at this point. This can be filled later by squaring the tip of the 'C' flap used to lengthen the columella (see *Illustration 10*) and/or the tip of the lateral advancement flap (see *Illustration 12*).

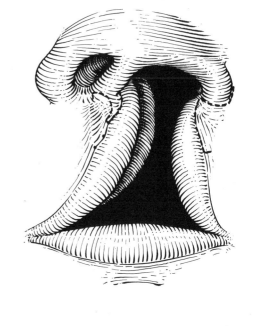

4

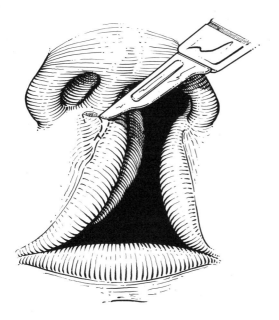

5

5

The incision through the skin is made with a No. 15 blade. A full-thickness incision is then made in this line with a No. 11 blade, angling the knife to preserve the muscle in the flap. The rotation incision is continued until the Cupid's bow lies horizontal.

6

The abnormal muscle attachments to the columella are freed and the skin and mucosa are then reflected to provide a good muscle flap. The 'white roll' which I prefer to fashion on the medial side and the 'C' flap consist of skin only.

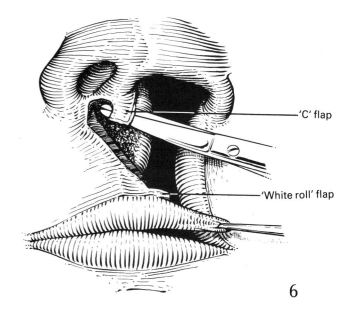

'C' flap

'White roll' flap

6

7 & 8

The incisions on the lateral side are made in a similar fashion, taking care that the incision along the mucocutaneous junction is long enough to match that on the medial side. This produces a triangular advancement flap which can be moved medially into the defect resulting from fashioning the rotation flap on the medial side. As this flap is advanced, it carries with it the alar base, thus correcting the alar flare. At the lateral or inferior end of the incision along the mucocutaneous junction a small recess is fashioned to accept the 'white roll' flap. This simulates the normal white roll and also breaks up the scar line where it crosses the mucocutaneous junction.

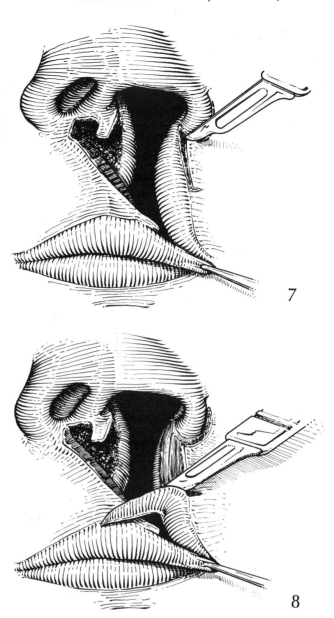

7

8

9

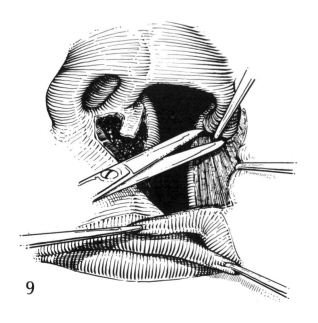

9

The skin must be reflected back from the muscle so that the muscle can be freed adequately from the alar base and a good muscle flap developed. If the anterior palate is to be repaired at the same operation, which is the usual practice in complete clefts of the lip and palate, this is now carried out.

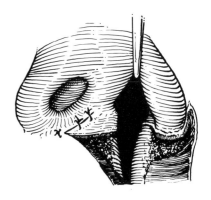

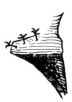

10

Suturing of the lip commences with the columellar lengthening. (It is helpful at this stage to have the assistant draw up the apex of the nostril with a skin hook.) Either 6/0 silk or 6/0 plain catgut is used for the skin. The latter usually obviates the need for formal suture removal or simplifies it to simple 'decapitation' of the outside portion of the stitch.

10

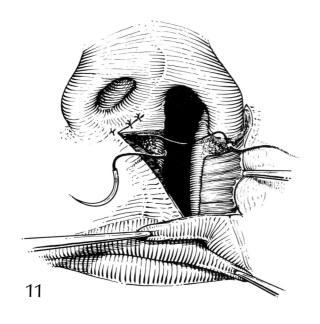

11

The alar base is advanced medially by a suture of 4/0 chromic catgut passed from the alar base to beneath the base of the columella. The muscle layer is then repaired with 4/0 chromic catgut.

11

12, 13 & 14

The vermilion flaps are cut square. Some surgeons advocate a Z-plasty here, but I have not found this necessary or helpful. It is, however, important to ensure that the mucosal edges are well freed so that there is no tendency to 'inroll' and produce a vermilion notch. Holding the mucosal sutures of 4/0 chromic catgut with an artery forceps aids eversion of the lip and simplifies closure of the mucosal layer, which is done last. Note that after completion of the repair the main scar lies in the line of the philtral bar, thus helping to conceal it.

Postoperative care

A Logan's bow helps to relieve strain on the suture line, especially when the baby cries. It also affords some protection against damage to the repair if the baby manages to roll on to his face. Arm splints may also be used to protect the repair from damage by the baby for a week or two.

A five-day course of penicillin is usually prescribed. Postoperative sedation is not required. On return to the ward, feeding is immediately commenced and this removes the need for other sedation. The wounds are, of course, kept clean and feeds are followed by a drink of clear fluid for the same purpose.

Further reading

Millard, D. R. Refinements in rotation-advancement cleft lip technique. Plastic and Reconstructive Surgery 1964; 33: 26–38

Millard, D. R. Cleft craft, Vol. 1. The unilateral deformity. Boston: Little, Brown and Co. 1976

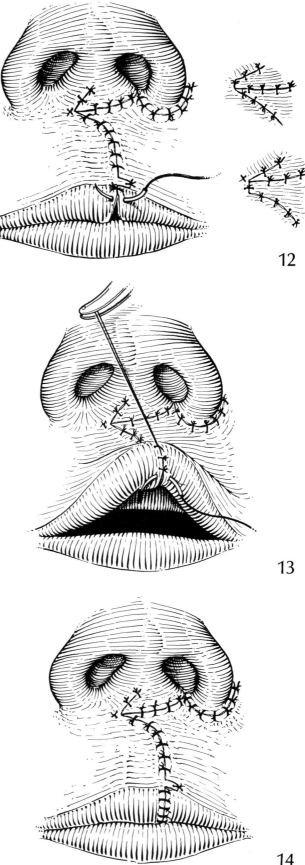

12

13

14

Cleft lip repair

Desmond A. Kernahan MD, FRCS(C), FACS
Chief, Division of Plastic Surgery, Children's Memorial Hospital, Chicago;
Professor of Surgery, Northwestern University Medical School, Chicago, Illinois, USA

PRIMARY REPAIR OF UNILATERAL CLEFT LIP

Preoperative

Indications

Presence of a congenital cleft of the lip, with or without cleft palate.

Preoperative considerations

1. The presence of associated malformation must be identified and treated appropriately.
2. Genetic counselling must be given to the parents.
3. The infant must be thriving and free from feeding problems.
4. Upper respiratory infection must be excluded.
5. Repair is generally performed at age 6–8 weeks.

Anaesthesia

Oral endotracheal general anaesthesia with a mid-line placement of the tube over the lower lip is most convenient. Local anaesthesia combined with basal sedation is an alternative.

Position of patient

Supine with head central on 'doughnut' and neck extended by rolled towels under shoulders.

The operation

1

Using a straight Keith needle (point dipped in methylene blue) the salient points in the architecture of the normal and cleft sides of the upper lip are tattooed. The following are observed: (1) length of lip on normal side (AB); (2) mid-points of Cupid's bow line and columella (C,C_1); (3) high point of Cupid's bow on cleft side (A_1); (4) site of the nasal threshold (B_1, B_2); (5) point at which white roll (junction of skin and vermilion) gives out on cleft side (A_2). AB–A_1 is the length by which the skin repair line on the cleft side must be elongated. Note the abnormal insertion of the bulging orbicularis oris muscle into the dermal skeleton on the lateral side of the cleft.

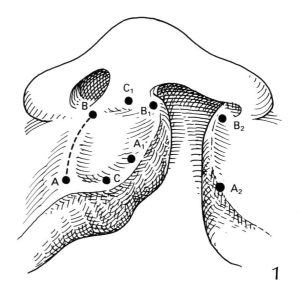

2

A thin strip of skin-mucosal junction on both sides of the cleft is pared and a mucosal flap is reflected on each side of the cleft.

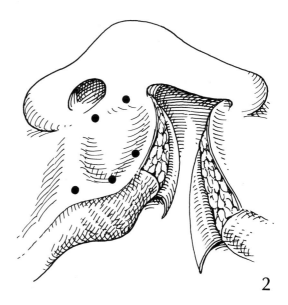

3

Subcutaneous undermining on the lateral side of the cleft frees the orbicularis muscle from its dermal attachment and from its attachment to the mucosa.

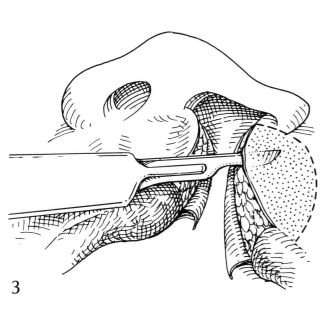

4

The tissue attachments of muscle around the alar base of the nose are divided.

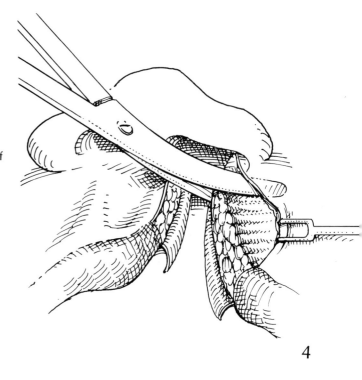

4

5

On the medial side of the cleft undermining creates a pocket beneath the nasal spine and the mid-line of the lip.

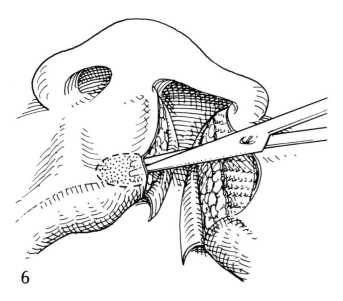

5

6

Undermining is used to create another pocket at the inferior lip border.

6

7

The muscle flap is split for 2–3 mm at the junction of its upper two-thirds and lower one-third.

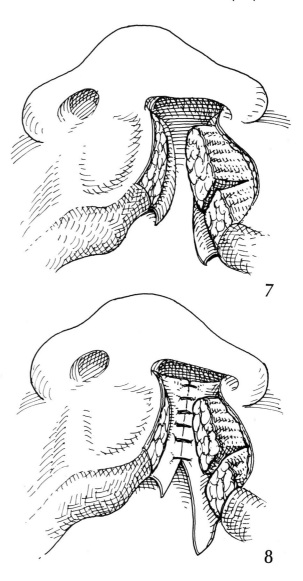

7

8

The upper portions of the mucosal flaps are trimmed and approximated.

8

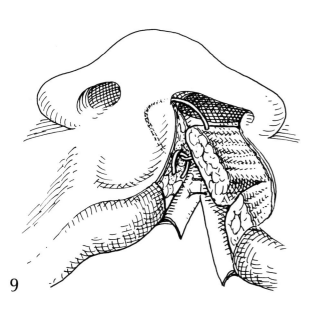

9

The upper part of the muscle flap is advanced and sutured with clear nylon into the pocket at the nasal spine.

9

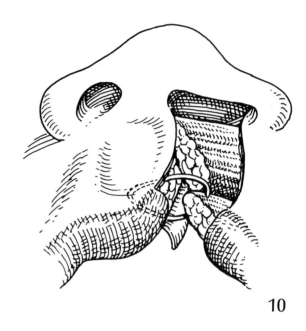

10

The lower part of the muscle flap is advanced and sutured with clear nylon into the pocket along the lip border.

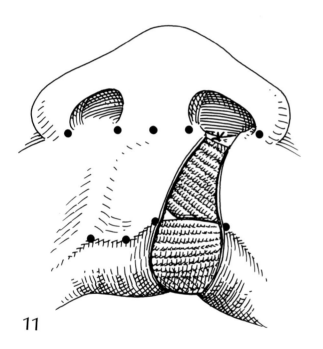

11

The muscle repair is shown completed, indicating how the line of muscle closure does not underlie the subsequent closure of the skin.

12a, b & c

Skin elongation is accomplished by Z-plasties, the first being placed under the nostril sill (12a). The flaps of this Z are transposed and sutured and if a balanced Cupid's bow line has not been achieved, a secondary smaller Z is planned just above the white roll of the lip to achieve a symmetrical repair (12b, c).

Postoperative care

The suture line is cleaned as needed with peroxide-soaked, cotton-tipped applicators. Topical antibiotic ointment is applied to prevent crusting. Elbow restraints are worn for 7–10 days to keep the baby's hands away from the mouth.

Intravenous feeding is maintained postoperatively until intake of oral clear fluids is established. Feeding of the infant's regular formula through a bulb syringe is commenced on the first postoperative day.

The sutures are removed 6–7 days postoperatively.

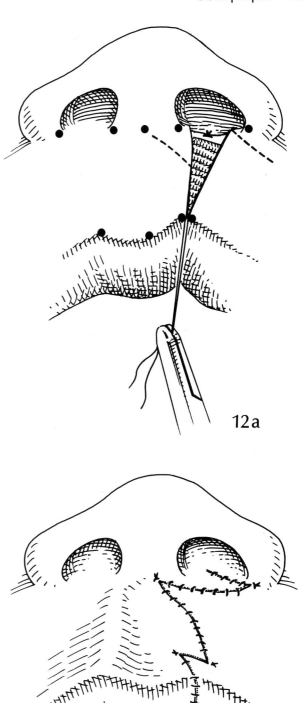

12a

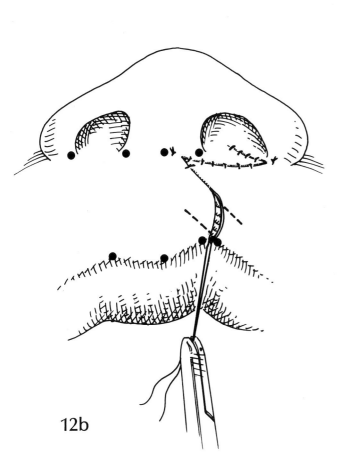

12b

12c

REPAIR OF BILATERAL CLEFT LIP

Introduction

The principal problem in repair of the bilateral cleft lip is the degree of protrusion of the premaxilla and prolabium relative to the lateral margin of the cleft.

If there is little or no protrusion, definitive repair of skin, mucosa and muscle may be carried out as a primary procedure. If the protrusion is up to 1.5 cm, adequate repair of the muscle layer is either extremely difficult or impossible and a lip adhesion which will mould the premaxilla back into the line of the dental arch should be performed as an initial step. In rare cases where the degree of projection of the premaxilla and prolabium is over 1.5 cm surgical recession of the premaxilla may be required before repair of the cleft can be achieved.

A well-repaired bilateral cleft lip should satisfy the following criteria. (1) The orbicularis oris should be in continuity across the centre of the upper lip. (2) The upper buccal sulcus should be deep and the prolabium not tethered to the underlying premaxilla. (3) A central notch at the lip border ('whistle deformity') should be avoided. (4) The prolabium should not be too wide. (5) The upper dental arch should be of good form and in correct relationship with the lower arch. (6) The lip should be symmetrical.

Repair of both sides of the bilateral cleft at one operation rather than repairing one side at a time helps to achieve these objectives.

The operation

13

Using a straight Keith needle the salient points in the architecture of the lip are tattooed. These are: (1) The point at which the white roll (skin–vermilion junction) gives out on the lateral side of the cleft (A, A_1). (2) The high point on the Cupid's bow line (B, B_1). (3) The centre of the prolabium (C). (4) The medial points of the nostril sills (D, D_1). (5) The base of the columella (E, E_1).

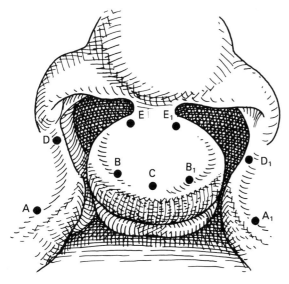

13

14

The lip is infiltrated with 0.5 per cent lignocaine (lidocaine) with 1:200 000 adrenaline (epinephrine) for haemostasis. The skin-mucosal junctions along both sides of the prolabium and along the lateral edges of the cleft are pared: mucosal flaps are then reflected.

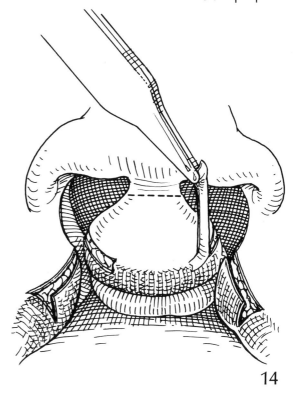

14

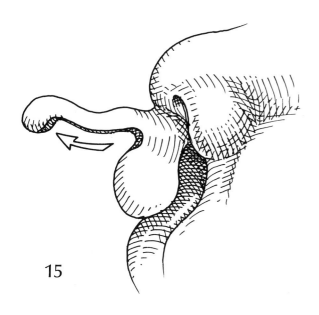

15

15

The mucosa of the prolabium is incised on its posterior aspect at its attachment to the premaxilla. It is undermined as a flap and elevated. The base of this flap lies between the points B and B_1. It will form the central tubercle of the reconstructed lip.

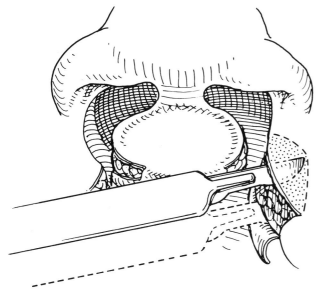

16

16

The orbicularis muscle is freed from its dermal and mucosal insertions.

17

The mucosal incision is extended laterally to allow mobilization of the mucosal flaps from the lateral sides of the cleft.

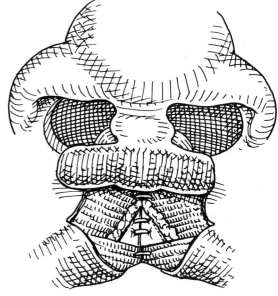

18

The lateral mucosal flaps are advanced and sutured in the midline to create a buccal sulcus. If the flaps fail to reach the midline they can be sutured to the upper edges of the mucosa which has been freed from the prolabium.

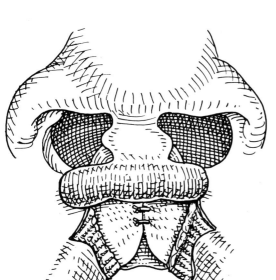
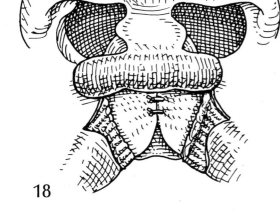

19

The muscle flaps are advanced and split at the junction of their middle and lower thirds as in unilateral lip repair. If the degree of premaxillary protrusion permits, they are sutured to each other in the midline. If this is not possible the muscle on either side is sutured to the soft tissue layer of the prolabium, resulting in a lip adhesion rather than a definitive repair.

20

The skin is now closed in a straight line, beginning above at the nasal floor.

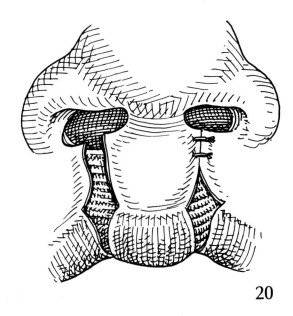

20

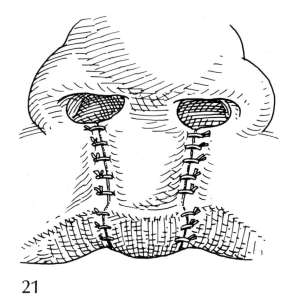

21

21

The mucosal flap from the prolabium is trimmed and inset to form the central tubercle of the repaired lip.

Postoperative care

As for unilateral cleft lip repair.

RECESSION OF PREMAXILLA IN BILATERAL CLEFT LIP

Preoperative

Indications

A premaxilla so protruberant (greater than 1.5 cm in front of the lateral elements of the cleft) that repair of the cleft is not feasible without risk of breakdown of the repair line due to tension.

Preoperative considerations

As for repair of cleft lip.

Anaesthesia

Oral endotracheal general anaesthesia with mid-line placement of the tube over the lower lip.

Position of patient

Supine with the head centrally placed on a 'doughnut' and the neck extended by rolled towels under the shoulders.

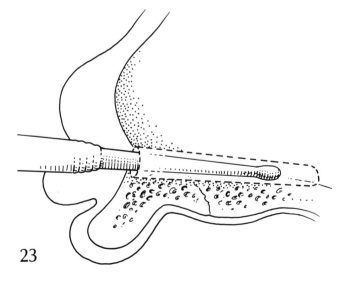

The operation

22

A small vertical incision is made on either side of the columella at the junction of the membranous and cartilaginous septum.

23

The lower free border of the cartilaginous septum is exposed and the mucosa over the septum elevated on either side to a point behind the prevomerine suture. The cartilaginous septum is lifted carefully out of the vomerine groove.

24

An incision is made intra-orally over the free inferior border of the vomer and the mucosa is elevated on either side of the vomer over an area appropriate to the required extent of recession of the premaxilla.

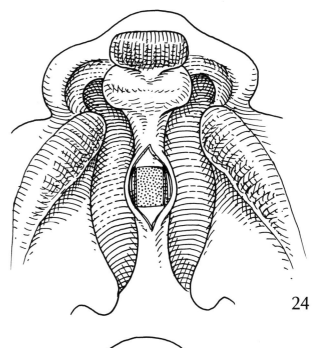

24

25

Bone is removed from the vomer with a fine curved rongeur. The amount of bone removed depends upon the degree of recession of the premaxilla required to bring the prolabium into line with the lateral sides of the cleft and permit surgical repair.

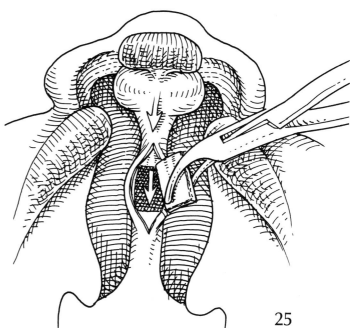

25

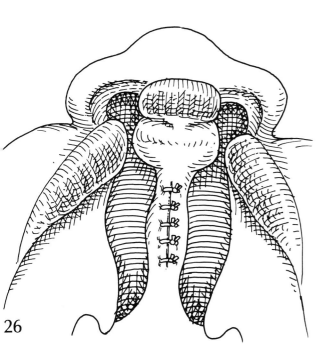

26

26

The incision is closed and the cleft lip repaired as previously described.

Postoperative care

As for bilateral cleft lip repair.

CORRECTION OF ASSOCIATED NASAL DEFORMITY IN UNILATERAL CLEFT LIP

Introduction

The features of unilateral cleft lip nasal deformity are: (1) deviation of the free inferior border of the nasal septum to the non-cleft side so that it presents in the nostril on the non-cleft side; (2) the dome (inter-crural angle) of the alar cartilage is at a lower level on the cleft side than on the normal side; (3) the nostril border on the cleft side is usually lower than on the normal side; (4) there is an oblique band in the vestibule on the cleft side associated with distortion of the lateral crus of the alar cartilage and an external groove over the nostril; (5) the alar base is frequently depressed on the cleft side and the nostril threshold is wider.

Many surgical approaches, testifying to the difficulty of the problem, have been described for correction of unilateral cleft lip nasal deformity. The method which has met with most consistent success in the author's hands, that of Tajima and Maruyama[1], will be described here.

Preoperative

Indication

Unilateral cleft lip nasal deformity is present.

Preoperative considerations

The patient must be free from nasal infection and fit for surgery.

Age

The operation is usually performed either at the age of 5 or 6 years to minimize deformity as a child enters the school years, or in adolescence as part of the correction of deviation of the whole nasal skeleton by rhinoplasty.

Anaesthesia

Oral endotracheal general anaesthesia with mid-line placement of the tube over the lower lip.

Local infiltration of the operative area with 0.5 per cent lidocaine with 1:200 000 adrenaline (epinephrine) for haemostasis.

Position of patient

Supine with the head on 'doughnut' and the neck extended with rolled towels under the shoulders.

The operation

27

The alar base on the affected side is pushed medially and upwards. An incision is marked to mimic the curve of the normal nostril from the lateral oblique nostril fold, upwards and externally over the nostril rim, and back into the vestibule to end halfway down the membranous septum.

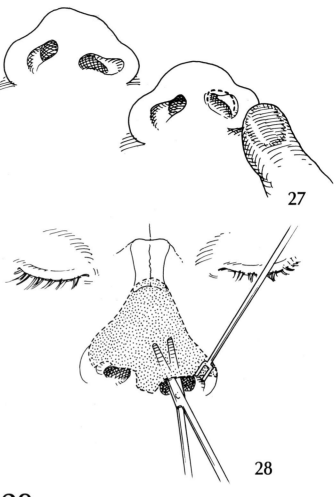

27

28

The skin of the nose is undermined widely in a plane superficial to the cartilaginous and bony skeleton of the nose. The undermining extends over the upper portion of the columella.

28

29

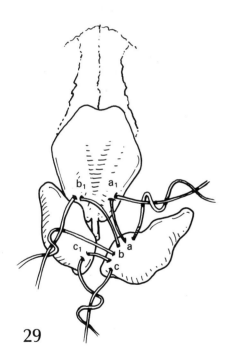

29

Three 5–0 clear nylon sutures are then placed: (a,a_1) from the upper border of the lateral crus of the alar cartilage to the lower border of the lateral cartilage on the cleft side; (b,b_1) from the intercrural angle (dome) of the alar cartilage on the cleft side to the lower border of the lateral cartilage on the normal side; (c,c_1) from the dome of the alar cartilage on the cleft side to the dome of the alar cartilage on the normal side. All three are placed before they are tied. When tied they draw the nasal tip on the cleft side forwards and upwards.

30

The skin flap is draped over the rim of the nostril and minor trimming of the free lower border of the lateral crus carried out if necessary. The skin is suitably trimmed and sutured and the nostril packed with gauze bolsters to obliterate the dead space and support the repair.

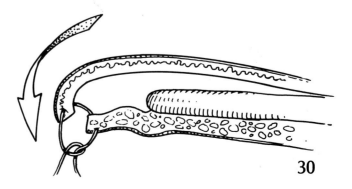

30

MINOR CORRECTIONS OF REPAIRED UNILATERAL CLEFT LIP

CORRECTION OF MISMATCHED CUPID'S BOW LINE

31

Primary repair of the lip has resulted in a step deformity along the while roll at the top of the Cupid's bow line. An incision is planned on either side of the lower portion of the skin scar line, extending around the mucosal repair line. On the high side of the skin repair this line is bowed; on the low side it is straight. On the mucosa the reverse is true. The white line is tattooed with a straight Keith needle dipped in methylene blue on either side of the incision to guide the subsequent placement of sutures.

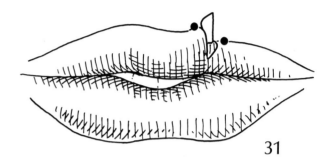

31

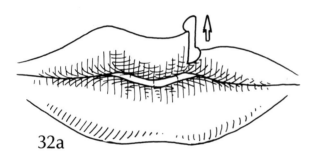

32a

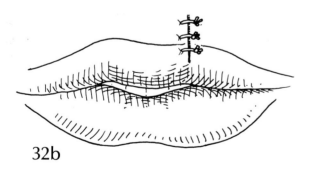

32b

32a & b

The delineated skin and mucosa are excised, the wound margins undermined to facilitate vertical movement of one side of the incision relative to the other and the wound closed with the two sides in correct alignment.

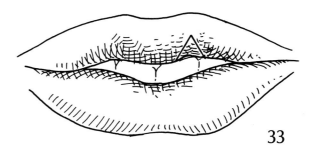

CORRECTION OF NOTCHING OF LIP BORDER

33

The notch is excised.

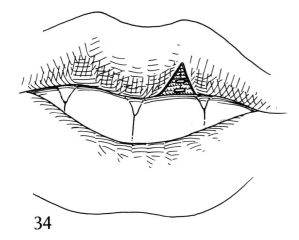

34

If the notch is deep, the muscle at the lip border is approximated with buried sutures.

35

Z-plasty flaps are marked, raised and transported.

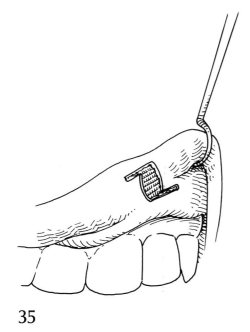

36

The incision is closed by suturing the flaps in place.

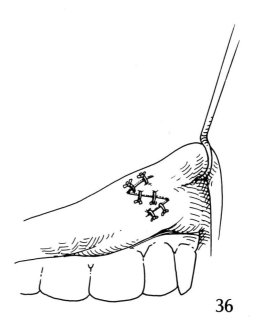

CORRECTION OF FULLNESS OF LIP MUCOSA ON REPAIRED SIDE OF CLEFT

37

A line is drawn on the lip mucosa to match the level of the lip border on the normal side and 1 or 2 mm below this an elliptical incision is planned. The size of the ellipse should be sufficient to allow the lip border to be rolled around to the correct level when the incision is closed.

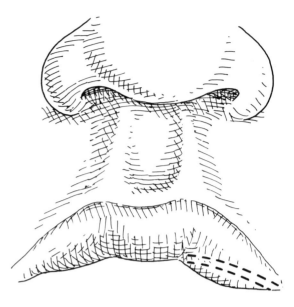

37

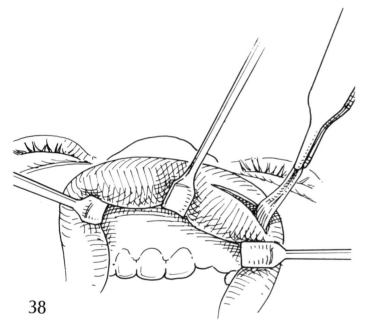

38

38

A horizontal wedge of tissue is removed.

39

The incision is closed, rolling the lip border inward to bring it to the correct level.

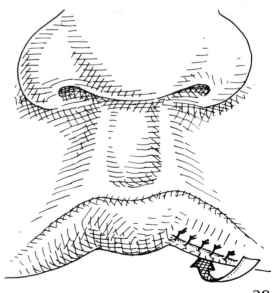

39

ELONGATION OF SKIN REPAIR LINE IN FORESHORTENED LIP

40

Minor degrees of foreshortening may be corrected by an elliptical scar excision, undermining of the skin margins and closure. Larger discrepancies in length are corrected by scar excision and wound closure incorporating a Z-plasty.

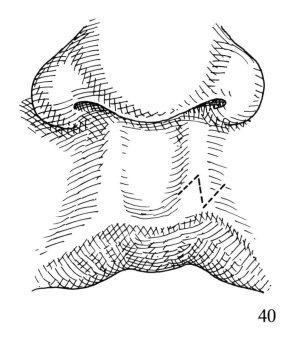

40

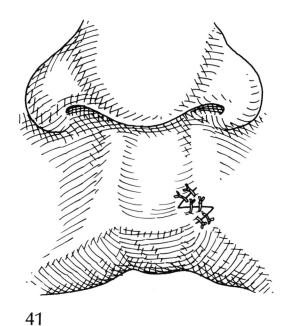

41

41

The Z-plasty flaps are transposed and sutured as shown.

SECONDARY PROCEDURES IN BILATERAL CLEFT LIP

ABBÉ (LIP-SWITCH) FLAP FOR AUGMENTATION OF UPPER LIP

Indications

A tight recessed upper lip following primary repair of cleft lip. The deformity occurs when too much tissue has been discarded at primary repair, when the premaxilla has been removed or when the prolabium has been used to form the columella rather than the centre of the lip. The use of the Abbé flap is most commonly confined to cases of bilateral cleft lip with or without cleft palate.

Anaesthesia

Nasal endotracheal anaesthesia which allows access to both the upper and lower lips without the anaesthetic tubing intruding in the field of operation. Distortion of the upper lip and nostrils should be avoided by careful placement and fixation of the tube.

Position of patient

Supine with the head on a 'doughnut' and rolled towels under the shoulders.

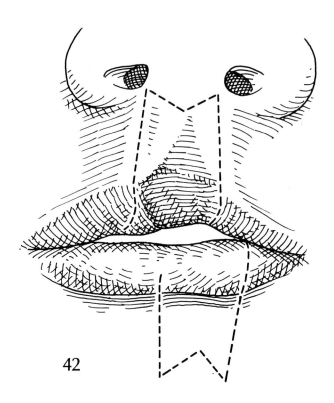

42

42

The flap consists of a full-thickness wedge of lower lip incorporating skin, muscle, mucosa and vermilion border. The flap is based on the inferior labial artery. For best results the flap should be set symmetrically into the centre of the upper lip and have sufficient vertical length to reach the base of the columella. To obtain adequate eversion of the repaired upper lip and an adequate buccal sulcus most cases require that more mucosa than skin is incorporated in the flap.

43

The flap is raised, the upper lip tissue is excised and the flap rotated into position. A thin pedicle incorporating the inferior labial artery on one side is the point of rotation.

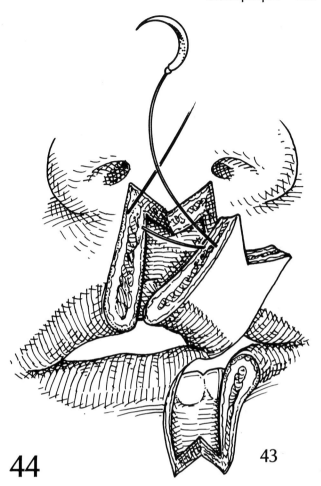

43

44

The flap is sutured in place in layers and the donor defect in the lower lip closed in the same fashion. Intermaxillary fixation is unnecessary. Postoperatively, the airway is maintained with a nasopharyngeal tube.

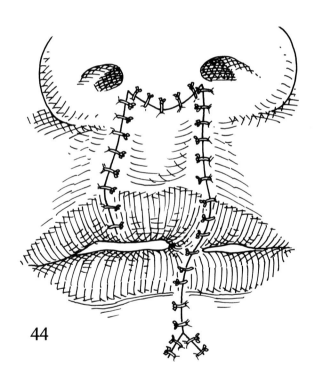

44

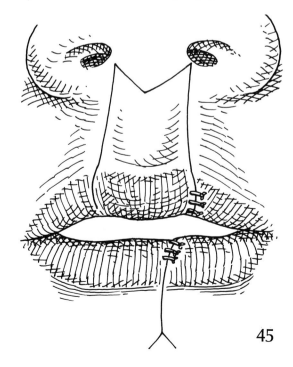

45

45

Seven to ten days later the pedicle of the flap is divided and its inset into the upper lip is completed. The donor defect on the lower lip is suitably trimmed and closed.

ADVANCEMENT OF NASAL TIP IN REPAIRED BILATERAL CLEFT LIP

Following repair of a bilateral cleft of the lip the columella is almost invariably short and the nasal tip is drawn backwards and lacks protrusion. A really satisfactory method of correcting this deformity has yet to be devised. The two most commonly accepted methods will be described. As regards the degree of forward projection obtained, the methods produce comparable results.

The operation is generally carried out around the age of 5 years and often revised in adolescence in combination with a rhinoplasty.

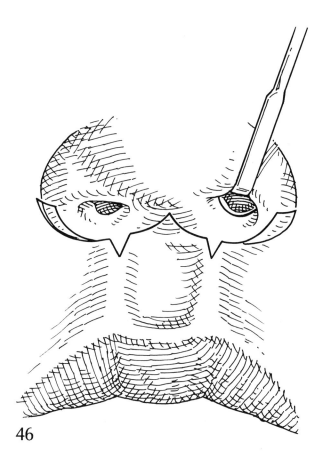

46

Columella advancement (Cronin method)[2]

46

The procedure consists essentially of creating bilateral bipedicle flaps in the columella, the floor of the nose and the alar, combined with a wedge excision of the alar bases and narrowing of the nostril floor by V-shaped excisions. The illustration shows the pre-operative markings.

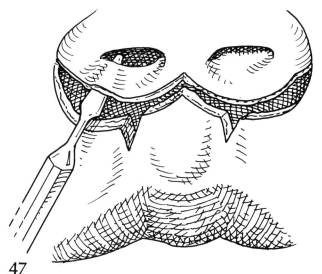

47

47

The flaps are incised and undermined widely as far medially as the nasal spine. The lateral wedge excisions extend through half the thickness of the alar base. Wide undermining of the flaps is necessary to achieve maximum advancement. V-shaped wedges are excised at the nasal floors.

48

Skin hooks in the nostril margin rotate the flaps medially and forward. Deep sutures are used to approximate the bipedicle flaps and the skin incisions are sutured.

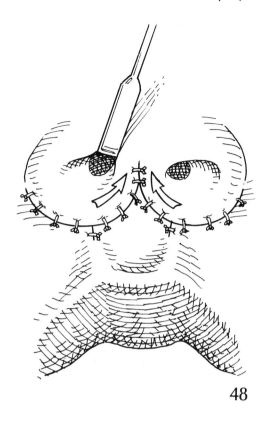

48

Columella advancement (forked flap (Millard) technique)[3]

49

Forked flap incisions incorporating the scars of the previous repair are marked out on the upper lip. From the lateral margin of the base of each flap the incisions extend laterally across the nasal threshold and around the alar bases.

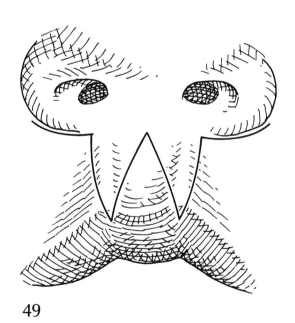

49

50

The flaps are raised and the dissection extended upwards in the membranous septum, mobilizing the flaps still further and finally leaving their bases on the nasal tip.

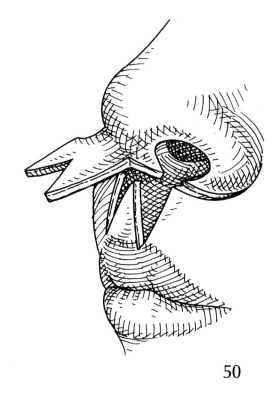

50

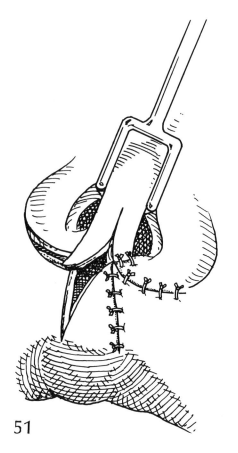

51

51

Traction is applied to advance the columella. The flaps are sutured to each other. The lip incisions are approximated and the alar bases drawn inwards.

CORRECTION OF CENTRAL NOTCH ('WHISTLE DEFORMITY') IN REPAIRED BILATERAL CLEFT LIP

The prolabium in the bilateral cleft lip is devoid of muscle and lacks bulk as compared with the lateral elements. As a result, the repaired lip, instead of showing a central tubercle, shows a central notch or 'whistle deformity'. Correction should aim at building up the central deficiency at the lip border and uniting the muscle from the lateral elements behind the prolabial skin to complete the continuity of the orbicularis oris muscle.

This can be accomplished by a V-Y advancement of the mucosa from the back of the lip, mobilization and joining of the lateral muscle and downward rotation of muscle flaps to form a central tubercle to the lip.

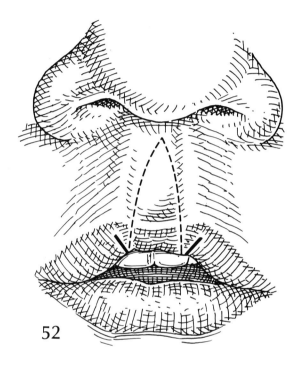

52

A V-shaped flap is marked out on the lip mucosa with its base anteriorly across the prolabium. The flap passes around the lip border and has its tip at the top of the buccal sulcus.

52

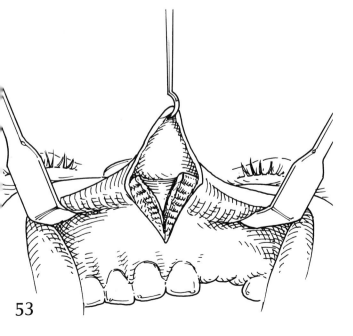

53

The flap is raised submucosally to expose the lateral muscle from its posterior aspect.

53

54

The muscle is undermined and freed from skin and mucosal insertions. A flap of muscle based below is dissected from the muscle bundle on each side.

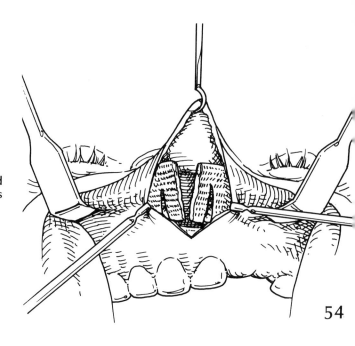

54

55

Muscle flaps are rotated downwards and medially, and sutured to each other to form the central tubercle of the lip. The superior muscle bundles are approximated in the midline.

55

56

The upper portion of the buccal sulcus is closed by approximation of the mucosa of the lateral lip elements (stem of the Y). The V-shaped flap is advanced around the lip over the tubercle created from the muscle flaps and sutured in place.

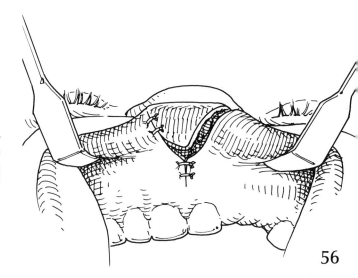

56

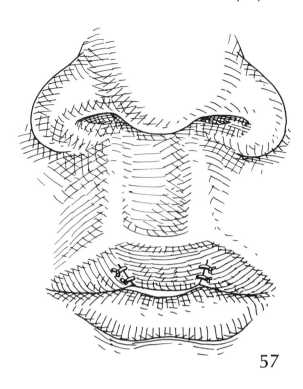

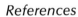

57

The closure is completed.

57

References

1. Tajima, S., Maruyama, M. Reverse-U incision for secondary repair of cleft lip nose. Plastic and Reconstructive Surgery 1977; 60: 256–261

2. Millard, D. R. Columella lengthening by a forked flap. Plastic and Reconstructive Surgery 1958; 22: 454–457

3. Cronin, T. D., Upton, J. Lengthening of the short columella associated with bilateral cleft lip. Annals of Plastic Surgery 1978; 1: 75–79

Illustrations by Kevin Marks

Repair of cleft palate

I. W. Broomhead   MA, MChir, FRCS
Consultant Plastic Surgeon, The Hospital for Sick Children and Guy's Hospital, London, UK

Introduction

The treatment of cleft palate malformations must be accepted as a multidisciplinary one, involving many specialities: plastic surgery, maxillofacial surgery and orthodontics, otorhinolaryngology, speech therapy and, in some cases, psychiatry. This is because disturbance of natural growth factors follows all types of cleft, being more severe in those which involve the whole of the primary and secondary palate.

Repair of secondary cleft palate has two objectives. The first is to suture the midline cleft, but the second and more important one is to obtain a push-back or retroposition of the soft palate in order to produce a competent nasopharyngeal sphincter. In other words, the soft palate must adequately reach the posterior pharyngeal wall on phonation. The operation is, therefore, described as a V to Y retroposition of the palate. The repair should be carried out before the child starts to speak, the ideal time being between 12 and 18 months of age.

Preoperative

The haemoglobin is checked preoperatively and routine antibiotics (penicillin) are given.

Anaesthetic

A general anaesthetic is required with endotracheal intubation, using an armoured tube or curved metal connection to prevent deformity of the tube with restriction of the airway from compression by the mouth gag, usually a Dotts gag.

Position of patient

The surgeon sits at the head of the table. The child's neck is extended by means of a small sandbag under the shoulders and by the headpiece of the operating table being lowered one notch. Once the gag is inserted and opened, the anaesthetist checks the airway. A small pack is then placed in the back of the pharynx and the airway rechecked.

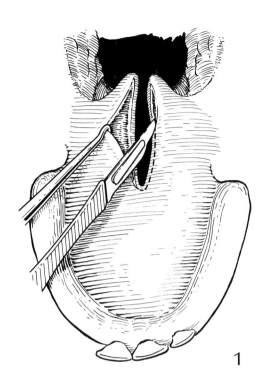

The operation

1

The edges of the cleft are incised using a No. 15 blade on a long handle. Incision of the edge rather than paring away tissue preserves tissue for the closure.

1

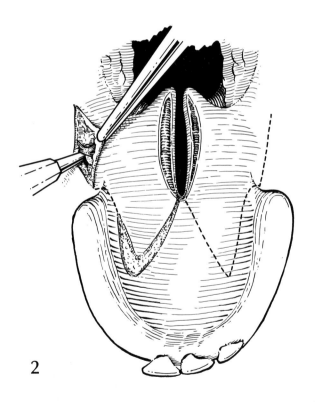

2

2

Dissection of the lateral palatal spaces and fracture of the hamular process

An incision just through the mucosa is made from the anterior pillar of the fauces to the centre of the posterior end of the alveolus. By blunt dissection the hamular process is identified, and a straight palate dissector is pushed vertically downwards just lateral to the process. The palate dissector is pushed medially to fracture the hamulus and is then swept towards the anterior pillar of the fauces, opening up the lateral palatal space between the medial pterygoid muscle laterally and the tensor palati muscle medially. A short piece of 2.5 cm ribbon gauze is inserted temporarily while a similar dissection is performed on the opposite side.

3

Raising of palatal mucoperiosteal flaps

The length of the posterior flaps will depend upon whether a two-flap or a four-flap repair is necessary. Bleeding is controlled by forceps pressure over the region of the greater palatine foramen. With a No. 15 scalpel blade firm incisions are made on to the bone of the hard palate. It is then possible to strip the posterior flap subperiosteally with a Mitchell's trimmer to the posterior edge of the hard palate and identify the posterior (greater) palatine artery. Small mosquito artery forceps are placed on the cut end of this vessel.

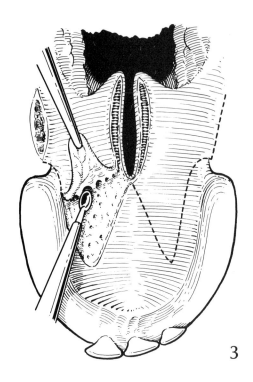

3

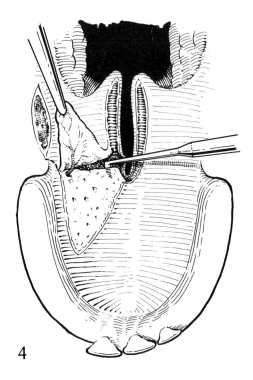

4

4

Mobilization of nasal mucosa

The attachment of the musculus uvulae is divided with fine iris scissors. Stripping free of the nasal mucosa is best commenced with the pointed end of the Mitchell's trimmer. This is followed by the sharp palatal hook from the posterior palatal spine, dissecting anteriorly keeping the instrument pulled upwards against the bone. The dissection is completed with the blunt palatal hook.

5

Mobilization of lateral pharyngeal wall

The remaining palatal mucosa between the two lateral incisions is incised. The soft tissues behind the greater palatine artery are freed with the sharp point of the Mitchell's trimmer. With the appropriate curved palate dissector, keeping this instrument dissecting on to the medial border of the medial pterygoid plate, that is on to bone, the lateral pharyngeal wall is freed from the bone. This area of dissection is joined to the freed nasal mucosa to allow full medial movement of the tissues.

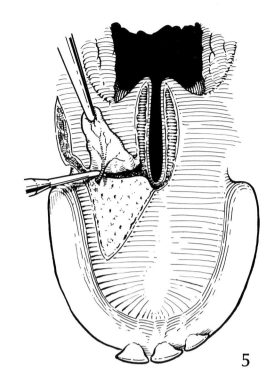

5

6

Release of greater palatine artery

This manoeuvre, described by Conway[1], allows posterior movement of the artery in the lengthening of the soft palate. A small wedge of bone is removed from the posterior part of the greater palatine foramen by making two cuts with a 5 mm nasal osteotome, the medial cut being made first. The artery can then be eased posteriorly with the Mitchell's trimmer.

6

Raising of anterior flaps

7

In the two-flap repair, the central part of the anterior palatal mucosa is stripped off the bone for a few millimetres, to ensure complete separation from the nasal layer.

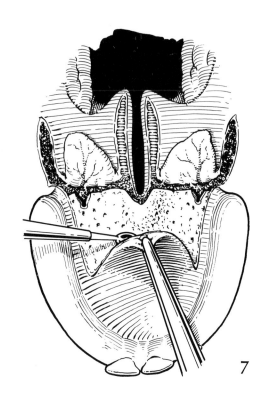

7

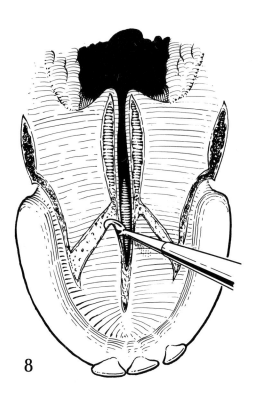

8

8

In the four-flap repair, two anterior mucoperiosteal flaps are stripped off the hard palate to the back edge of the alveolus. A right-angled knife is the ideal instrument for this dissection. In some cases, to allow adequate medial transposition of these flaps, a small back-cut is necessary into the lateral part of the base of the flap, but care must be taken not to destroy adequate blood supply to the flaps.

9

Completion of dissection

At this stage it will be found that the separation of the oral and nasal layers is inadequate at the junction of the hard and soft palate. Sharp dissection with a No. 15 scalpel easily opens up the tissues into the soft palate to separate these layers.

Similar dissection of opposite side

In midline palatal clefts a similar dissection is carried out in raising posterior and anterior flaps and freeing the lateral wall on the opposite side.

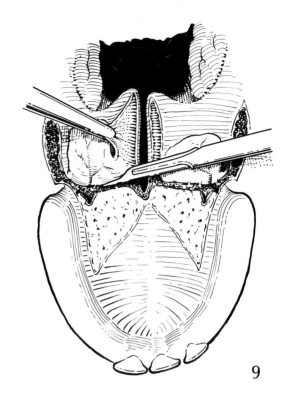

9

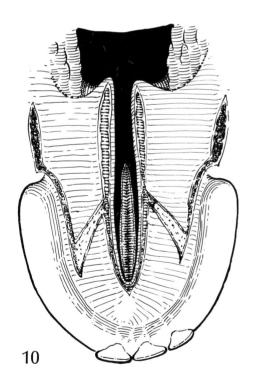

10

10

Septal flaps

If the cleft extends well anteriorly, closure of the nasal mucosa in the anterior part can only be achieved by freeing septal (vomerine) flaps. An incision is made down the midline of the free edge of the septum and the mucoperichondrial flap on each side is stripped off the vomerine bone and septal cartilage, first with a Mitchell's trimmer followed by more wide freeing with palatal raspatories.

In unilateral clefts of the palate, the anterior nasal flaps extend from the lateral palate on the side of the cleft and from the septum on the medial side. Prior to closure the cut end of the greater palatine artery is ligated with 3/0 catgut.

Closure of palate – nasal layer

11

Complete closure must be obtained on both the nasal and oral sides of the cleft. Closure of the nasal layer is first commenced anteriorly with either 2/0 plain or 3/0 chromic catgut. These sutures are placed so that, when tied, the knot is on the nasal side. Sutures are most easily inserted with a Reverdin needle.

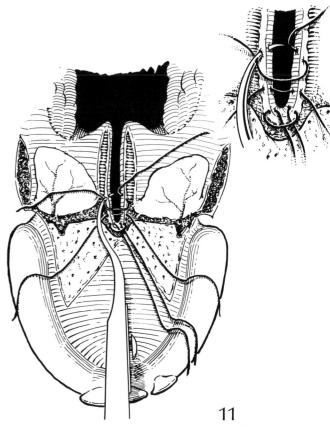

11

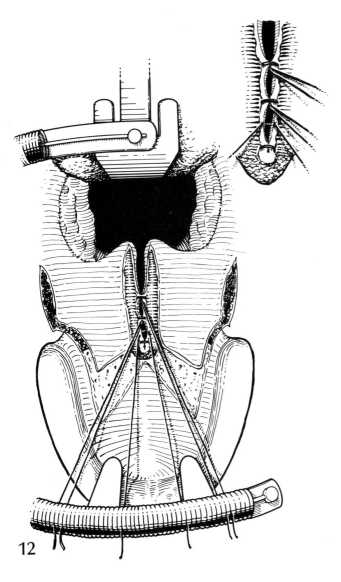

12

12

At the junction of the hard and soft palates an 0 plain or 2/0 chromic catgut stitch is used and inserted so that later it can be brought through the posterior oral flaps and tied on the oral side. This is an extremely important stitch as it approximates the nasal and oral layers – it is known as the 'A' stitch and is tied as a figure-of-eight. Some surgeons use a similar figure-of-eight stitch to approximate the nasal mucosa and the anterior flaps in a four-flap repair – 'B' stitch. Posterior to the 'A' stitch, suturing of the nasal layer continues with fine catgut (2/0 plain, 3/0 chromic) to the uvula. Technically it is easier to insert all the sutures posterior to the 'A' stitch before tying them, the loose ends of the stitches being conveniently held in the Kilner suture-carrier which is fixed to the mouth gag.

Closure of oral layer

13 & 14

This commences at the uvula. Atraumatic 6/0 nylon is perhaps a more reliable suture than catgut to use in the soft palate. These sutures do not have to be removed as they extrude spontaneously. More anteriorly, interrupted 3/0 plain atraumatic catgut stitches are used until closure to the 'A' stitch is reached. The end of this suture is crossed over (figure-of-eight) and passed through the posterior oral flaps with the Reverdin needle. It is wise to insert this stitch on the oral side as a vertical mattress suture to prevent inversion of the wound edges.

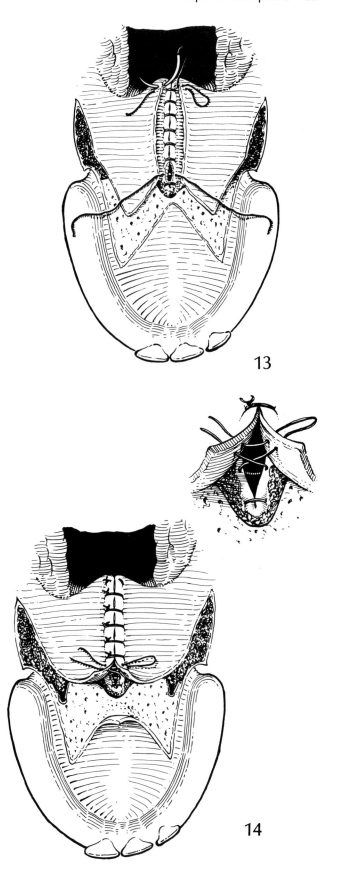

13

14

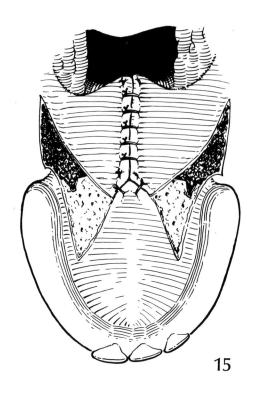

15

15

Anterior to the 'A' stitch, interrupted 3/0 catgut sutures are again used to approximate the posterior flaps. In a two-flap closure this is completed by diverging this closure on either side of the single anterior triangle or oral mucosa.

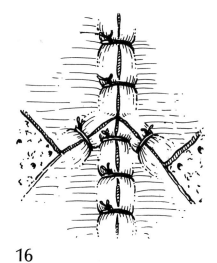

16

16

If a four-flap repair is necessary, the anterior flaps are approximated with 3/0 catgut sutures from before backwards with completion of the closure by interdigitating these flaps with the posterior ones, in whichever way they fit most comfortably. If a 'B' stitch has been inserted, this is now tied.

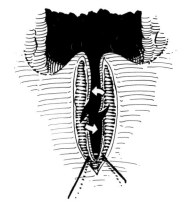

17

Minor modifications

Nasal layer

17 & 18

In some clefts, where the width of the cleft is not excessive, further lengthening of the nasal layer to obtain a greater push-back can be achieved by performing a Z-plasty in the nasal layer closure.

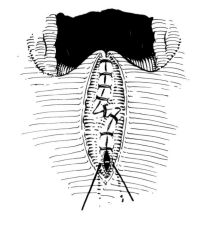

18

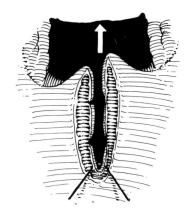

19

19 & 20

Alternatively, small lateral cuts, sutured longitudinally, may be equally successful.

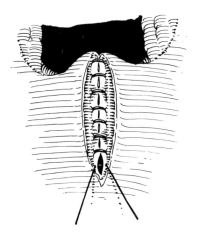

20

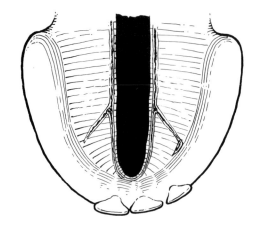

21

21, 22 & 23

Oral layer

Oral closure of the anterior palate can sometimes be achieved more soundly by crossing over the anterior flaps.

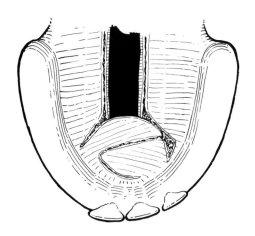

22

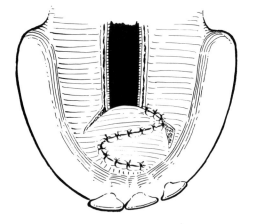

23

Lateral packs

24

Following the medial and posterior movement of the oral tissues, to obtain midline closure and an adequate push-back, a raw area is left laterally over the hard palate extending backwards into the lateral palatal space. Some surgeons leave this exposed.

An alternative is to pack the space lightly with 2.5 cm ribbon gauze soaked in either Compound Tincture of Benzoin or Whitehead's Varnish. One end is inserted deep into the lateral palatal space which is carefully packed except for the area over the hard palate; the second end is inserted into this space and then packing is completed. This prevents a free end of the ribbon gauze from becoming loose. The pack is removed on the seventh postoperative day, with forceps, without anaesthesia, using a posteriorly directed movement.

The advantages of using lateral palatal packs are:

1. haemostasis;
2. splinting of the palate and reduction of lateral tension on the suture line;
3. prevention of food entering the lateral space.

The only disadvantage is the possibility of slight infection, as a little fever may develop on the fifth or sixth postoperative day. This subsides the moment the packs are removed.

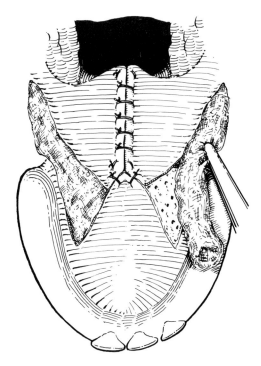

24

Final procedures

The small pack at the back of the throat is removed after ensuring that no bleeding is occurring. If there is some oozing of blood, the gag should be released slightly and digital pressure placed over the posterior flaps for a minute or so. The gag is removed and a suture of 2/0 silk. inserted into the posterior half of the tongue. Traction on this allows maintenance of an adequate airway and negates the use of an airway which could damage the suture line. The tongue stitch is removed after 24 hours.

The child is turned on to one side, the endotracheal tube removed, and any postoperative suction needed is carried out with great gentleness. The child should never leave the theatre or recovery area until the anaesthetist is satisfied with the airway.

Postoperative management

Postoperative sedation

These children do not suffer any severe postoperative pain. Restlessness is invariably due to failure to maintain an adequate airway. A full dose of any analgesic which depresses the respiratory centre is, therefore, dangerous. Only half doses of sedative may be given.

Postoperative care

Spoon-feeding can be started on return to full consciousness, first with sterile water or dextrose saline and rapidly returning to normal feeding. Water or dextrose saline is given after each feed and a soft diet maintained for 1 month after the operation.

Complications

Respiratory inadequacy

In the early postoperative period temporary tracheostomy may be wise in severe cases of micrognathia, or essential if endotracheal intubation is impossible. Emergency tracheostomy is rarely indicated.

Infection

This is very rare if routine antibiotics are used. The antibiotic used must be changed if the throat-swab culture reveals non-sensitive organisms.

Haemorrhage

Primary or reactionary haemorrhage is very rare and usually ceases with sedation and transfusion. Secondary haemorrhage is also rare, but if it occurs is usually from the anterior cut end of the greater palatine artery. Diathermy coagulation under general anaesthesia may be necessary if routine supportive therapy fails.

Breakdown or failure of healing

If perfect healing is not achieved, a further attempt at repair should be delayed for one year after the operation. The delay allows the tissues to improve and scar tissue to soften, making the subsequent operation more likely to succeed. To attempt surgery earlier is unrewarding.

Reference

1. Conway, H. Combined use of push-back end pharyngeal flap procedures in management of complicated cases of cleft palate. Plastic and Reconstructive Surgery 1951; 7: 214–224

Further reading

Kilner, T. P. Cleft lip and palate repair technique. St Thomas Hospital Reports 1937; 2: 127–140

Le Mesurier, A. B. Method of cutting and suturing lip in treatment of complete unilateral clefts. Plastic and Reconstructive Surgery 1949; 4: 1–12

Matthews, D. N. Premaxilla in bilateral clefts of lip and palate. British Journal of Plastic Surgery 1952; 5: 77–86

Millard, D. R. Complete unilateral cleft of the lip. Plastic and Reconstructive Surgery 1960; 25: 595–605

Tennison, C. W. Repair of unilateral cleft lip by stencil method. Plastic and Reconstructive Surgery 1952; 9: 115–120

Veau, V. Division palatine. Paris: Masson et Cie, 1931

Wardhill, W. E. M. Technique of operation for cleft palate. British Journal of Surgery 1937; 25: 117–130

Cleft palate – pharyngoplasty

James Calnan   FRCP, FRCS
Professor of Plastic and Reconstructive Surgery, Royal Postgraduate Medical School,
Hammersmith Hospital, London, UK

Preoperative

The term pharyngoplasty means 'plastic or reparative surgery of the pharynx', derived from the Greek words 'plassein' (to mould) and 'pharynx' (the throat). It therefore means little, but in patients with cleft palate the term pharyngoplasty has one object in view: to eradicate nasal escape of air during speech.

In English, only the sounds M, N and NG allow nasal escape during their pronunciation. All other vowels and consonants demand that the soft palate elevate to occlude the nasopharynx from the stream of air emitted through the larynx. If the soft palate is unable to do its job, then certain primary and secondary faults occur in speech. The primary faults, those dependent essentially on an incomplete nasopharyngeal mechanism, are the following:

1. Weak volume for all vowels and consonants.
2. Lack of clarity of articulation – a lack of crispness in speech.
3. Lack of adequate voice projection.
4. Nasal escape of air and frequently a clearly audible nasal breath sound or whistle, especially when the nasal septum is deflected.
5. Excessive nasal resonance, with a muffling effect on speech.

The secondary faults (as a result of certain adjustments to the disability) are the following:

1. Glottal stop sounds are substituted for P, T, K, B, D and G, because the necessary air pressure for the production of these plosive sounds cannot be built up or maintained in the mouth. The sound is therefore made further back, in the larynx.
2. Pharyngeal fricative sounds replace the consonants S, Z, SH, ZH and sometimes CH and J, for similar reasons.
3. Articulatory insufficiency occurs, that is, defective articulation due to insufficient use of the tongue, lips and jaws.
4. Unintelligible vocalization is produced, such as a snort, instead of a voice sound.
5. Harshness of voice attempts to overcome the effects of excessive nasal resonance.
6. Nasal grimace may be evident.
7. Breathlessness during conversation.

All these defects should be obvious to the alert clinician during consultation. Even so (and particularly if the examining surgeon was responsible for the original repair of the cleft palate) an independent assessment should clarify the defects in speech so that the surgeon is fully aware of them and knows that the success or failure of his operation can be so accounted.

1

All this assumes agreement that in the normal person the soft palate elevates easily to meet, and so occlude, the nasopharynx during speech; if it does not then either the soft palate should be lengthened or the depth of the pharynx narrowed. The accompanying illustration shows occlusion of the nasopharynx by a normal soft palate.

The first choice has been dealt with in the chapter on 'cleft lip and palate' (see pp. 000–000) and here we are only concerned with an operation to decrease the size of the pharynx. Again, there is a choice but each one depends on an accurate assessment of the function of the soft palate. Of necessity, the decision to carry out a pharyngoplasty will depend on the quality of speech of the patient. Because speech is an acquired characteristic, it is wise to defer a decision until the age of 5 years or later. However, it should be recognized that at about 12 years the learning of new speech sounds slows down considerably and hence the interval of about 8 years becomes important for the future prospects of the patient.

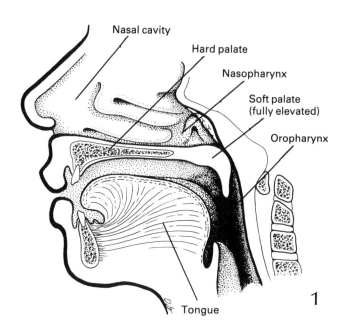

1

Timing and indications for pharyngoplasty

1. Speech is developing well, but nasal escape of air is a prominent feature.
2. An independent assessment indicates that nasal escape is preventing the development of normal speech sounds.
3. The palatal cleft has been adequately repaired, say 6–12 months before the speech assessment.
4. Intelligence and development of speech are not unduly retarded.
5. The patient is old enough to make speech assessment accurate.
6. Radiological evidence shows that the soft palate elevates normally (to above the level of the hard palate) yet there is an appreciable gap between it and the posterior pharyngeal wall during speech sounds. Alternatively, the soft palate may show poor elevation and the decision then is whether the soft palate or pharynx is primarily at fault.
7. The soft palate is of normal length for age. There are no published 'norms' for soft palate length and so experience must be the arbiter.

Contraindications for pharyngoplasty

These follow quite naturally from the above. (1) Doubt about the development of speech, either because this is slow or because the patient's mentality is retarded; any doubts about the diagnosis of cleft palate as the sole reason for poor speech should also be included. (2) General unfitness for an operation.

Preoperative investigations

Apart from the usual physical examination for fitness before any surgical operation, six specific investigations are advisable because the information is of importance for success.

Haemoglobin level It is unusual to find the haemoglobin below about 10 g/100 ml (Normal = 12.0–17.0 g/100 ml), but if it is then blood transfusion should be considered before or at the time of operation because occasionally there may be a marked blood loss during and after pharyngoplasty. Although late loss of blood is rare, when it does occur (as with tonsillectomy), urgent replacement is demanded.

In those patients from the Mediterranean area a blood film to detect the presence of sickle cells should also be carried out. A sickle-cell crisis after a non-urgent operation is an unnecessary complication and may be fatal.

Throat and nose smears To exclude the presence of B haemolytic streptococci (particularly Lancefield's group A), the only organism guaranteed to prejudice the outcome.

Speech assessment An accurate, detailed and written assessment of speech, preferably carried out by a speech therapist. Although the surgeon can do this himself such an assessment is likely to be biased. It is worth knowing the degree of nasal escape (the reason for pharyngoplasty) and the extent of defects in articulation so that the need for speech therapy after operation can be anticipated and planned for.

Assessment of expectations Some knowledge of the patient's job, expectations, education and level of intelligence is a useful guide as to the motivation to achieve normal speech and the likely prognosis. Few patients really understand that their speech is abnormal simply because we regard what we hear of our own voice as normal.

Hearing assessment An investigation of hearing is important because the cause of any hearing loss needs to be known. Indeed, treatment for this, such as the insertion of grommets or the removal of tonsils and adenoids, should precede the pharyngoplasty. A loss of 30 decibels in both ears may well account for the poor development of articulation, apart from the nasal escape.

X-rays Most important of all, in the author's view, are good X-rays to show the degree of elevation of the soft palate during a speech sound (the author prefers 'EE . . .' as it is easier to produce and can be held for long enough to allow the radiographer to take a picture). On the whole, most vowels and some consonants will suffice. Because the mouth is wide open when saying 'Ah . . .', the soft palate does not need to elevate fully to prevent nasal escape and so this particular vowel is unsuitable; the disproportion in size between the wide open mouth and the nasopharyngeal isthmus when saying 'Ah . . .' does not require the soft palate to elevate even in many normal people. On the other hand, most consonants are of such short duration that the radiographic film can easily miss the important moment.

Therefore two films – one taken at rest and another when saying 'EE . . .' – preferably with the head fixed in a cephalostat, provide important information and allow certain measurements to be made; most of the measurements are of interest only to those doing research, but they should answer two questions: Is the palate too short and does it elevate normally? Is the pharynx too deep? The decision for pharyngoplasty depends largely on the answers to these questions.

If the clinical observation that the soft palate is mobile (by inspection when the patient says 'Ah . . .', the only speech sound which allows direct observation from the mouth) conflicts with the radiological evidence of, say, an immobile palate, the clinical observation should be preferred and further radiological studies made. It may well be that poor communication or lack of coordination was at fault. In such patients cineradiography is a valuable aid. Movements during repeated sounds, preferably simple vowels or consonants contained in a short sentence but with words which require full elevation of the soft palate, can be photographed and studied at leisure.

The choice of the type of pharyngoplasty depends largely on the answers to two questions: What is the size of the gap between the elevated soft palate and the posterior pharyngeal wall? Does the soft palate elevate naturally and easily?

Measurement of the length of the soft palate (at rest and on elevation) and the depth of the pharynx depends entirely on the accuracy of the lateral radiographs. It is better to overestimate the gap between the soft palate and posterior pharyngeal wall than to be too precise; underestimation carries the risk of total failure (a 1 mm gap is hardly less disastrous than a 10 mm gap) while overestimation of the defect is of little consequence.

The choice of pharyngoplasty

There are, in general, three types of pharyngoplasty as follows:

1. A single flap from the posterior pharyngeal wall, united to the posterior edge of the soft palate. This decreases the area of the nasopharyngeal isthmus.
2. Bilateral mucomuscular flaps transposed from the lateral pharyngeal walls to a horizontal position on the posterior pharyngeal wall. These narrow the width and the depth of the pharynx.
3. An implant behind the mucosa of the posterior pharyngeal wall to narrow its depth.

The options are to some extent mutually exclusive and depend on the following factors:

1. The preference of the surgeon and his experience.
2. Whether the soft palate is immobile (an indication for single flap pharyngoplasty) or fully mobile (transposed flaps or implant).
3. The original cause of nasal escape. If poor speech followed adenoidectomy, it is reasonable to argue that an implant (to replace the bulk of the adenoids) would be the method of choice.
4. The size of the gap between the elevated soft palate and the posterior pharyngeal wall. In the author's experience a gap of more than 2.5 cm is unlikely to be overcome by an implant or transposed mucomuscular flaps. One then has either to decide on a single operation using a posterior pharyngeal wall flap or proceed in two stages: mucomuscular transposed flaps at the first stage and some months later an implant, when the size of the residual gap can be measured.

The operations

Anaesthesia

A general anaesthetic is preferred, but a skilled anaesthetist is more important than the type of anaesthesia, because the following features are very desirable.

An armoured oral endotracheal tube should be placed exactly in the mid-line of the mouth. Armoured because the cleft palate gag, which is used to provide adequate exposure and to keep the tongue out of the way, should not compress the endotracheal tube and reduce the airway; in the midline of the mouth so that the endotracheal tube will fit neatly under the slot in the tongue spatula with an equal amount of the tongue on each side so that the clasps of the gag fit correctly over the teeth when the gag is opened fully. Because a pharyngeal gauze pack will get in the way of the operation, the endotracheal tube should have a protective inflatable cuff. In addition, the neck of the patient will be extended and the operation table tilted head-down so that any blood will collect in the nasopharynx (and this can be easily removed) and not encroach on the trachea.

The level of anaesthesia should be such that the operation can be conducted comfortably. Occasional 'gagging' does not matter much, but consistently light anaesthesia will be annoying to the surgeon.

The patient should wake up within a few minutes of the end of the operation, so that he can protect his own airway. The operative site and the postnasal space will be sucked clear of blood clot and secretion before extubation, but because the wound may ooze later it is vitally important that the cough reflex and the swallowing reflex be fully competent. Pharyngoplasty should carry no mortality.

Instruments

The usual set of instruments may suffice but the following points are useful to remember:

1. Forceps, scissors and the needle-holder should be 18 cm (7 inches) long because of the distance at which the surgeon has to work. Waugh's forceps (toothed and non-toothed), Metzenbaum scissors and a Denis Browne needle-holder all make for a quicker, more satisfying and more efficient procedure.
2. The Kilner modification of the Dott gag (a modification of the Boyle-Davis gag) allows good exposure of the operative site, while the coiled spring around the periphery of the gag is convenient for holding sutures until they are tied.
3. Two soft rubber catheters (size 3 or 4) should be threaded down each nostril into the pharynx and sutured through the 'eye' of the catheter to the posterior edge of the soft palate on each side of the uvula. When the catheters are retracted and clipped to the head drapes, the soft palate will be retracted into the nasopharynx, allowing a good view of the operative site.
4. Good illumination is important. Some surgeons use a head-lamp, others a spot-light. Both carry the disadvantage that the field of vision may be good for the surgeon but poor for the assistant. If the patient has been positioned correctly the normal operating theatre light (of the shadowless type) suffices.
5. Efficient suction with a choice of sucker ends should be used.

2

Position of patient

The patient lies supine, with a sandbag under the shoulders so that the neck is fully extended and the head lies comfortably in a head-ring. The open mouth of the patient should now face vertically upwards.

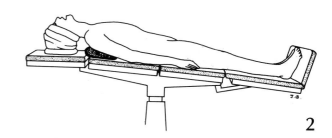

2

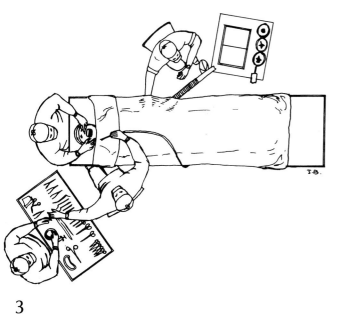

3

3

The surgeon stands at the head of the operating table so that he sees the patient upside-down. The assistant stands on his right, always with the sucker in one hand, and the scrub nurse stands behind the instrument trolley which is wedged between surgeon and assistant.

Preventive haemostasis

To reduce the amount of oozing it is advisable to infiltrate the tissues of the posterior pharyngeal wall (and the soft palate when necessary) with 1:200 000 adrenaline (epinephrine) solution – readily available with 0.5 per cent lignocaine (lidocaine). Only 1–2 ml are required, but the surgeon should identify the anterior tubercle of the arch of the atlas (an essential reference point) before injecting any solution. If the anaesthetist objects to the use of adrenaline (because he is using halothane) normal saline can be substituted.

IMPLANTATION PHARYNGOPLASTY

4

The surgeon identifies the upper edge of the anterior tubercle of the arch of the atlas (the most prominent point on the posterior pharyngeal wall) by inspection and palpation and makes a transverse incision of about 3 cm through the mucosa down to the anterior common ligament at this site. The anterior common ligament is recognized immediately as a pale structure and any oblique fibres of the palatopharyngeus muscle should be divided.

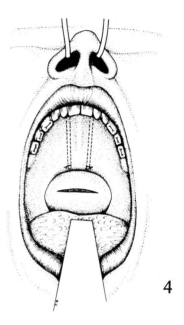

4

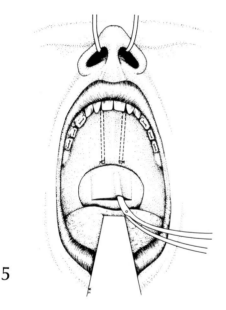

5

5

With curved scissors a pocket is made on this plane by blunt dissection up towards the nasopharynx so that the implant will lie over the basisphenoid. The pocket is expanded laterally until the resistance of the Eustachian cushions is felt.

The width of the submucosal pocket is now estimated (it is usually about 3 cm in the adult) and a small gauze pack is inserted into the wound to stop minor oozing. The author prefers to use autogenous costal cartilage with its perichondrium as a free graft, which is removed from the right sixth or seventh rib while the pharyngeal dissection is proceeding. If a single rib cartilage is of insufficient thickness, a second graft is removed through the same oblique chest incision (which is then closed in layers, with a corrugated drain left in for 24 hours, thus reducing the risk of a haematoma). If the pleura is punctured no attempt should be made to suture it, but the anaesthetist should inflate the lung before the final intercostal muscle suture is tied. A plain chest X-ray film should always be taken the following day to exclude the possibility of pneumothorax,

The importance of preserving the perichondrium on the cartilage cannot be stressed too much; without this covering, invasion of blood vessels occurs and the cartilage quickly disappears, whereas with its perichondrium cartilage will survive as a free graft. In one patient 17 years later there was spotty calcification on the X-ray, which is what normally happens to costal cartilage with age.

6

The cartilage graft is measured, trimmed to the correct length and inserted into the pocket made behind the posterior pharyngeal wall, to lie horizontally and snugly on the anterior common ligament and above the level of the atlas. A finger is used to push the graft finally into place, so that it is no longer in view. When a second graft is required to produce the necessary bulk, that too is laid horizontally over the first. There is no need to suture the cartilage graft to the anterior common ligament because, not having undermined the lower edge of the mucosal incision, wound closure will hold it in the correct position.

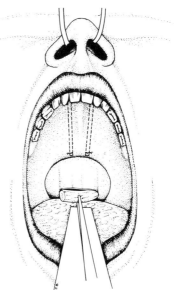

6

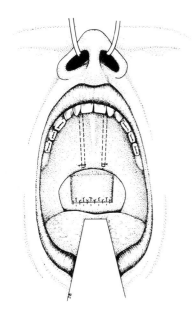

7

7

The mucosal wound is now closed by 3/0 chromic catgut mattress sutures. This is the first time during the operation that this delicate tissue has been handled by forceps; the upper wound edge contains no muscle and is commonly friable, although the lower edge may be thicker due to a few fibres of the superior constrictor muscle. Good deep bites are recommended but no suture is tied at this stage, the ends being left long enough to tie with ease when all have been inserted. Usually 3–4 sutures are required initially, the most lateral ones being tied first to reduce tension on the central sutures. If mucosal edges are over-everted some simple interrupted sutures can be placed between the mattress sutures. The tissues, however, are often very friable and excessive suturing may lead to unexpected tears.

The wound is now dabbed dry, a little tincture of benzoin applied, the nasopharynx sucked clean and the retraction catheters released and removed. The soft palate will most probably lie over the suture line and obscure it, especially if the uvula has become oedematous and swollen. A little sterile grease should be applied to both nostrils and to the corners of the mouth to alleviate the subsequent soreness (due mainly to drying during the operation).

The other material sometimes used for implantation is soft silicone rubber, because hard materials, whether bone or plastic, tend to be extruded within a few months.

PHARYNGOPLASTY BY MUCOMUSCULAR TRANSPOSITION

8

The operative technique is similar to that described above. Based on the Eustachian cushion, a vertical flap of as great a length as possible (usually 3–4 cm) is made on each lateral wall of the pharynx. It is usually easier to make the anterior incision first (just behind the posterior pillar of the fauces) and then to undermine, by blunt dissection using curved scissors, towards the midline of the posterior pharyngeal wall. The plane of dissection should be deep to the salpingopharyngeus muscle (which runs mainly vertically), but a branch of the ascending pharyngeal artery may be divided and cause temporary and marked bleeding: pressure from a swab will usually control this. Using scissors, the posterior vertical incision is now made of the same length and at the junction of the lateral and posterior pharyngeal walls – not an accurately identifiable anatomical site but rather an estimate so that the flap will be about 1.5 cm wide. The horizontal incision to release the flap is now made by joining the two vertical incisions as low down as is visible. The flap will immediately retract into the nasopharynx.

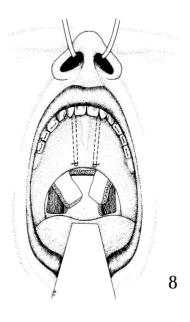

8

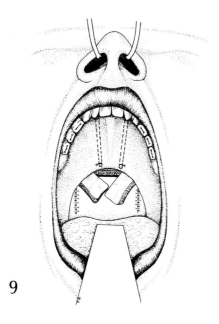

9

9

The defect in the lateral pharyngeal wall is sutured with 3/0 chromic catgut, again using mattress-type sutures. The same procedure is then carried out on the other side.

The nasopharyngeal isthmus is now markedly narrowed. A horizontal incision made high on the posterior pharyngeal wall, joining up the two lateral wounds, will gape to create a space into which the two vertical flaps can be sutured transversely.

10

It is advisable to suture the upper edge of one flap to the upper edge of the posterior pharyngeal wall incision before suturing the other flap to the lower edge of the same incision. Finally the two flaps are united with interrupted sutures which pick up mucosa and muscle at the same time. Because the flaps have retracted it is important to sew them together at their correct tension to produce a well-defined mucomuscular ridge across the whole width of the posterior pharyngeal wall.

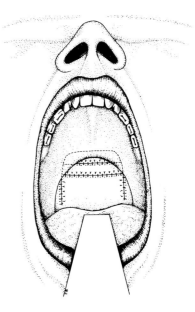

10

FLAP PHARYNGOPLASTY

11

The intention is to suture the posterior edge of the soft palate to the posterior pharyngeal wall for the maximum width possible, leaving only lateral openings of about 0.5 cm diameter to allow comfortable nasal breathing at rest.

The pharyngeal flap is raised by making a vertical incision on one side, at the junction of the lateral and posterior walls of the pharynx and starting from near the Eustachian cushion. Through this incision the whole of the posterior wall of the pharynx is undermined by curved scissors across to the opposite side, where a similar vertical incision is then made. The horizontal incision, joining the two verticals, is made as high as possible and the flap thus raised. Pressure is usually sufficient to stop bleeding from the defect on the posterior pharyngeal wall which is not sutured but left as a raw area to heal by secondary intention.

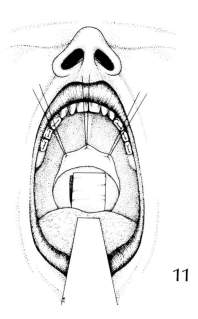

11

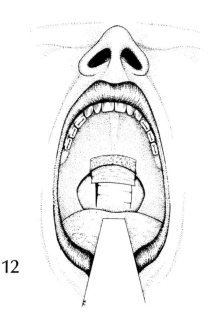

12

12

An incision is now made across the buccal surface of the soft palate, about 0.5 cm from its posterior margin, for its full width (that is from the anterior pillar of the fauces on each side). The posterior edge of the palate incision is undermined by sharp dissection so that it will turn back and up into the nasopharynx and thus create a raw area large enough to receive the pharyngeal flap and of at least 1 cm in depth to ensure primary union.

13

The pharyngeal flap is now sutured to the anterior edge of the raw area on the soft palate either by chromic catgut or 4/0 silk. Silk becomes shaken from the suture line some weeks later, so it does not have to be removed, and it also seems to provide cleaner healing in the adults. Again, sutures should be of the mattress type. Unless the soft palate is exceptionally long it is usually impossible to suture the posterior edge of the soft palate wound to the lower wound edge of the posterior pharyngeal wall – and so provide a two-layer flap closure which is less likely to contract in width later.

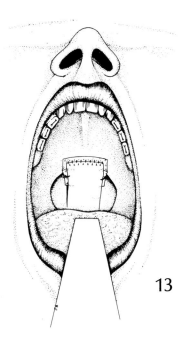

13

Postoperative care

Little in the way of special treatment is required. The diet should be soft and appetizing, with plenty of fluids for the first few days because swallowing will be painful. A drink of water after each meal is sufficient to keep the wound area clean.

Analgesics are required for 48 hours but morphia which depresses the cough reflex is best avoided. Antibiotics on the whole have no place unless clearly indicated and should not be used routinely to hide poor technique.

Explanation of what has been done is important, particularly because patients who have had an implant pharyngoplasty may suffer neck stiffness (on one or both sides, presumably from serous permeation from the operative site into the splenius and scalene muscles). This clears in 7–10 days, but the temporary 'wry-neck' is a little disconcerting for the patient and the relatives.

Some improvement in speech can be expected within a few days but the full effect of the operation should not be assessed for at least three months.

Further reading

Calnan, J. S. Surgery for speech. In: Calnan, J. (ed) Recent Advances in Plastic Surgery. London: Churchill-Livingstone, 1976; 39–57

Hynes, W. Results of pharyngoplasty by muscle transplantation in 'failed cleft palate' cases, with special reference to influence of pharynx on voice production. Annals of the Royal College of Surgeons 1953; 13: 17–35

Pigott, R. W., Makepeace, A. P. The technique of recording nasal pharyngoscopy. British Journal of Plastic Surgery 1975; 28: 26–33

Rosenthal, W. Zur Frage der Gaumenplastik. Zentralblatt für Chirurgie 1924; 51: 1621–1627

Accessory auricles and preauricular sinuses

Bard Cosman MD
Formerly Professor of Clinical Surgery, Columbia University College of Physicians and Surgeons, New York, USA

Introduction

The external ear arises from tissue derived from the first and second branchial arches. Errors in their development are the origin of accessory auricles and preauricular sinuses.

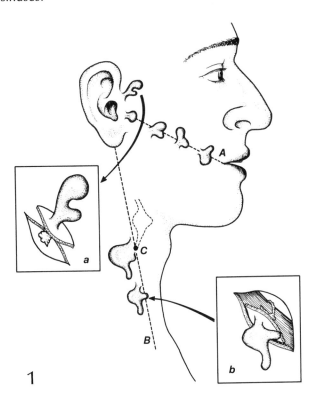

The operations

ACCESSORY AURICLES

1

These structures are soft tissue masses frequently containing cartilage of auricular type. They occur along two main axes: (a) on a line from the tragus to the lateral lip commissure, and (b) from the lobule to the clavicle along the anterior border of the sternomastoid muscle.

The immediate pretragal area is the most frequent location. Removal is for cosmetic reasons and is best carried out in the neonatal period by simple elliptical excision along the skin lines. Tying off the base without excision may leave the cartilage component behind and so lead to later growth and apparent 'recurrence' (Inset a).

Cheek accessory auricles, found in first and second branchial arch syndrome (hemifacial microsomia), are often larger and more complex than those in the pretragal area but their treatment is the same.

Neck lesions are termed 'cervical auriculars' and often have a fibrous band which extends over the medial aspect of the sternocleidomastoid muscle and is attached to the deep fascia (Inset b). Rarely they may be associated with the external opening of a second branchial arch sinus (C), in which case removal must be a part of total excision of the sinus and cyst; otherwise simple elliptical excision along the skin lines suffices.

1

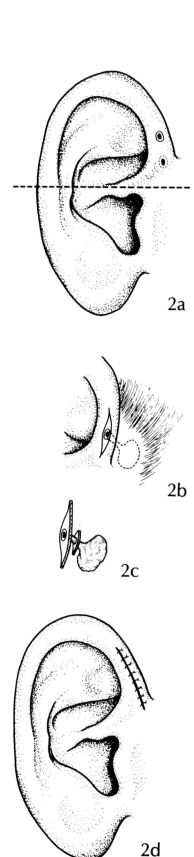

2a

PREAURICULAR SINUSES

2a–d

These lesions are epidermoid inclusions arising during the embryonic coalescence of the tissue forming the external ear. Often asymptomatic, their operative removal is indicated only when they become the site of recurrent infections. Characteristically, the sinus openings are on the ascending crus of the helix or just inferior and anterior to it (a). Openings located inferior to the dotted line are more likely to be the external openings of first branchial cleft sinuses.

Elliptical excision of the sinus opening and dissection of the tract usually leads to a small cyst lying on the temporalis fascia. The tract lies in apposition to the helical cartilage and a portion thereof should be taken with the specimen to avoid transecting the tract (b and c). Dissection is facilitated by preoperative injection of methylene blue into the sinus and/or by placing a probe in the tract. Simple wound closure in line with the helix is accomplished (d). Operation should be carried out in infection-free intervals if possible.

2b

2c

2d

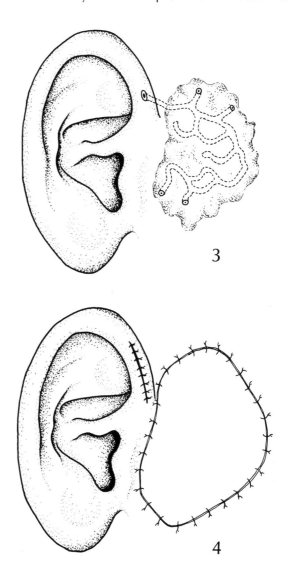

3

4

3 & 4

Multiple episodes of acute infection, spontaneous drainage, and surgical incision and drainage lead to the development of an area of ramifying epithelial lined tracts in the preauricular region.

Wide excision of involved skin and subcutaneous tissue, preserving the facial nerve and resurfacing with a skin graft, may be necessary. A small area may be covered by a retro-auricular full thickness graft for good colour match but large areas require other donor sites. Graft take is improved by the use of a tie-over dressing (bolus dressing).

Complications

Failure to remove associated cartilage may lead to apparent recurrence of accessory auricles. Residual epidermal elements will lead to preauricular sinus recurrence. Re-excision is the treatment for both complications.

Further reading

Brownstein, M. H., Wagner, N., Helweg, E. B. Accessory tragi. Archives of Dermatology 1971; 104: 625

Fabian, D., Lewin, M. L., Karlan, M. S. Cervical auriculars: congenital chondro-cutaneous appendages of the neck. Plastic and Reconstructive Surgery 1970; 45: 360

Sykes, P. J. Preauricular sinus: clinical features and the problems of recurrence. British Journal of Plastic Surgery 1972; 25: 175

Illustrations by Patrick McDonnell from originals by the author

Congenital deformities of the ear

Bruce S. Bauer MD, FACS, FAAP
Attending Plastic Surgeon, Division of Plastic Surgery, The Children's Memorial Hospital, Chicago;
Assistant Professor, Department of Surgery, Northwestern University Medical School, Chicago, Illinois, USA

Introduction

Congenital auricular deformities range from the most minor distortions of the helical rim and small auricular tags to the most severe malformations of skin and cartilage, as seen in microtia. Total absence of the external ear is extremely rare. These anomalies occur either in formation or during fusion of the auricular hillocks along the margin of the first branchial cleft during the 4th–12th week after conception. While it is beyond the scope of this text to describe the treatment of the whole spectrum of auricular deformities, a clear understanding of the more common deformities and their characteristic cartilaginous abnormalities will provide a foundation from which to develop a logical approach to ear reconstruction in all those cases which do not conform to a particular pattern. This chapter therefore concentrates on correction of the congenitally prominent ear, constricted ear and cryptotia, and on reconstruction of the microtic ear.

CONGENITAL PROMINENT EARS

Indication

The main indication for correction of this deformity is to remove the cause of the ridicule to which the affected child is subjected, particularly in early school years. The deformity is most prominent at this time because the ears approach adult size early in the growing face. However, this early attainment of near-adult size (by the age of 5–6 years) allows correction at any time from this age onward without harmful effects on ear development[1].

1 & 2

Anatomy

In the majority of cases the prominent ear lacks definition of the antihelical fold so that there is no definite angle between the concha and the scapha and the ear stands straight out from the side of the head. However, this is not invariably the case. Sometimes the antihelix is well defined and the prominence is due to an abnormally deep concha and a crus. Occasionally lack of antihelical definition and conchal overdevelopment exist together[2].

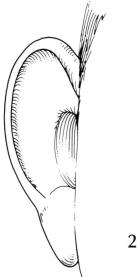

1

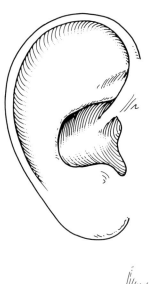

2

Goals of otoplasty

The goals of otoplasty as listed by McDowell[3] are correction of the protrusion, particularly of the upper pole; visibility of the helix and antihelix; a smooth helical line; maintenance of an undistorted postauricular sulcus; symmetry; and avoidance of a plastered-down look. In addition, there is increasing emphasis on avoiding the sharp antihelical fold commonly associated with techniques in which the cartilage is incised along the new antihelix (as in the Luckett procedure and its modifications).

Preoperative

Anaesthesia

General anaesthesia with endotracheal intubation is necessary in most children. Local anaesthesia is satisfactory for adults.

Preoperative preparation

While many surgeons have special preferences for draping the head and excluding the hair from the operative field, the major emphasis should be on preventing tension, which could distort the ears, and on both ears in clear view to ensure postoperative symmetry.

The operation

Regardless of the technique chosen it is imperative to tailor the procedure to the specific deformity present and not to rely on a single technique for treating all prominent ears. In the classic deformity where prominence is due to lack of development of the antihelical fold alone, I prefer the technique described by Stark and Saunders[4], as this seems to give the most consistent and pleasing results. This technique consists of folding and then retroposing the ear with mattress sutures between the scapha and the fascia over the mastoid.

3

The ear is first folded back to simulate the proposed new antihelical fold, and the superior and inferior crura of the antihelix and their junction are tattooed using a Keith needle and methylene blue. The tail of the helix is similarly marked.

4

The incision

After infiltrating the skin with 0.5% lignocaine (lidocaine) and 1:200 000 adrenaline (epinephrine) for haemostasis, a dumb-bell shaped ellipse of skin is excised. The medial side of the ellipse lies in the postauricular groove and the lateral edge just medial to the proposed new line of the antihelix.

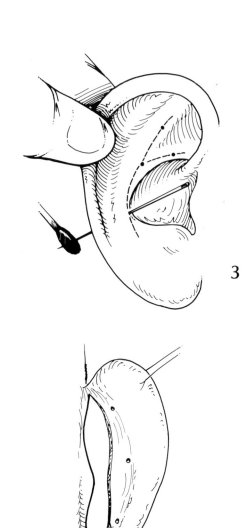

3

4

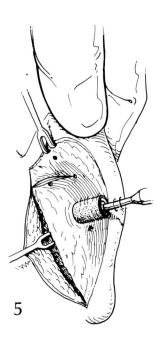

5

5

The soft tissue is elevated from the cartilage, revealing the tattoo marks. A small dermabrader head is used to create a wide groove along the line of the antihelix and its superior crus; this groove should weaken the cartilage enough to allow easy folding but not enough to give a sharp ridge when the ear is folded back. The line of the inferior crus can then be incised back to its junction with the superior crus, depending on the degree of development of this key landmark in the specific case. Attention may also need to be directed to the helical tail and antitragus. These may require trimming or reduction if the lobule is excessively prominent.

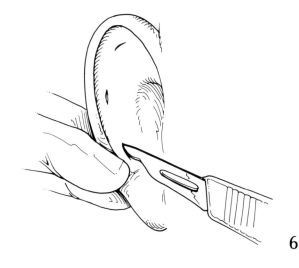

6

6, 7 & 8

Three 2–3 cm incisions are made in the scaphal skin and helical sulcus down to but not through the cartilage. Clear nylon sutures threaded on 1½-inch (approximately 4 cm) Keith needles are passed from these anterior incisions through the cartilage and out to the postauricular wound. A small curved needle is then threaded on each in turn and passed through the fascia over the mastoid. This technique allows firm suture fixation in cartilage and perichondrium without fixation to the overlying skin. Suturing of these anterior incisions is not required. Additional sutures can be placed if needed to ensure a smooth antihelical fold.

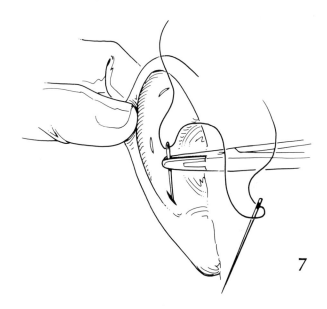

7

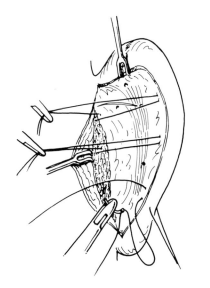

8

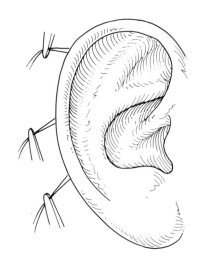

9

9 & 10

The three or more nylon sutures are tied, but only tight enough to pull the ear back into a natural position, the correct distance from the side of the head. The initial placement of a surgeon's knot allows setting of each suture at proper tension before final tying in the chosen position.

The skin is closed with a running subcuticular 4/0 pull-out nylon suture.

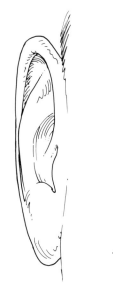

10

Postoperative care

Following wound closure the ear is splinted by careful packing with absorbent cotton soaked in mineral oil. A fluffed gauze and Kling bandage (Johnson and Johnson) is applied and the dressing left in place for 10 days. The dressings and sutures are then removed and no further dressing is required during the day. An elastic cloth headband is used at night for a further two weeks to prevent accidental forward traction on the ear.

THE CONSTRICTED EAR

The term constricted ear was suggested by Tanzer[5] to describe the full range of ear deformities previously classified as cup ear and lop ear. Cosman[6,7] mentioned four characteristic features of the deformity that vary with its severity. These are: (1) lidding, (2) protrusion, (3) decreased ear size, and (4) low ear position.

Anatomy

The four basic features of the deformity are caused by the following anatomical abnormalities. *Lidding* is due to helical overhang, arch shortening and flattening. *Protrusion* is secondary to shortening of the helical arch, vertical compression of the scapha and flattening of the antihelical crura. *Decreased ear size* results from the above changes as well as from a decreased skin envelope, conchal widening and angulation, and actual decreased auricular cartilage size. The *low ear position* is not unlike that seen in other severe auricular malformations and is of similar aetiology.

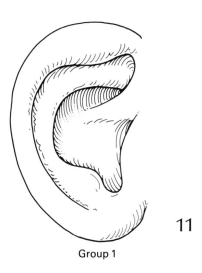

11

Group 1

Treatment

11, 12 & 13

Tanzer[5] subdivided these deformities in a manner that is particularly relevant to the choice of surgical repair. Group 1 have a minor deformity of the helix alone, giving a lidded appearance to the ear. Group 2 have a moderate to severe deformity involving the helix and scapha, and are further divided according to the need for supplemental skin at the margin of the auricle. Group 3 have extreme cupping, with the constriction almost producing a tubular form. These cases are often associated with deformities of the external auditory meatus and middle ear.

Group 1 constriction is treated by either readjusting the helix to gain greater height or reducing the lid by a full thickness excision. Group 2 constriction requires a combination of a V–Y advancement, a 'banner flap' or other method for helical lengthening, and cartilage scoring, dermabrasion or conchal mastoid sutures to correct the protrusion. In the more severe cases of group 2, the constricted segment can be split to produce a wedge-shaped defect which can be filled with a contra-lateral conchal graft. In these more severe cases, as well as in group 3 deformities, the anatomy is often best appreciated by degloving the ear to allow a direct view of the cartilage. After correction of the cartilage defect, any skin deficiency can be covered with local skin flaps.

Group 3 constricted ears are tubular in shape and often closely approach a microtic deformity. A conchal cartilage graft alone may be insufficient for auricular excision, and the ear can then be reconstructed using the techniques described for microtia reconstruction (see pp. 264–272). The tubular auricular vestige can be unfurled and spliced into the costal cartilage framework after this is placed.

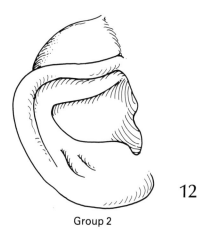

12

Group 2

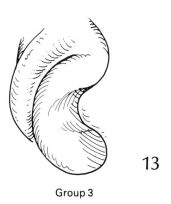

13

Group 3

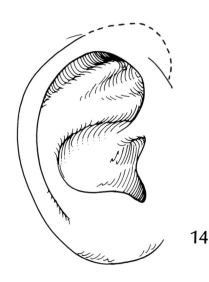

14

CRYPTOTIA

14, 15 & 16

While cryptotia is a rare anomaly in Whites, it is one of the more common congenital anomalies in Orientals (occurring in 1 in 500 Japanese). The deformity is bilateral in 40–50 per cent of all cases and the right side is affected more commonly in unilateral cases. The superior one-fourth to one-third of the auricle is buried under the temporal skin and the retroauricular sulcus is absent. There are varying degrees of scaphal underdevelopment and sharpening of the antihelical crura (particularly the superior crus) and there are often fibrous adhesions in the groove behind the superior crus. The degree of involvement varies considerably from case to case and may vary from side to side in bilateral cases[8–10].

In treating this type of ear deformity the emphasis, as in the treatment of the constricted ear, is on correction of the skin deficit and expansion or reshaping of the cartilage as indicated.

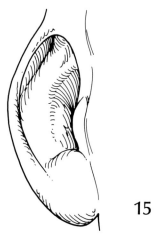

15

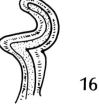

16

The operation

17

The superior pole of the ear is pulled forward with traction to allow placement of the incision superior and posterior to the helical rim, thereby ensuring an intact rim of skin over the superior pole of the ear. The incision illustrated lends itself well to coverage of the superoposterior cutaneous defect with an inferiorly based postauricular skin flap.

18

The dissection is carried down directly to the underlying cartilage and the adhesions in the groove behind the antihelical superior crus are lysed. Because of the inherent cartilaginous spring this alone may not be sufficient to allow the superior pole to come forward. Therefore an incision is made through and directly along the superior crus, and several mattress sutures are placed in the cartilage along this line to reverse the sharp angulation.

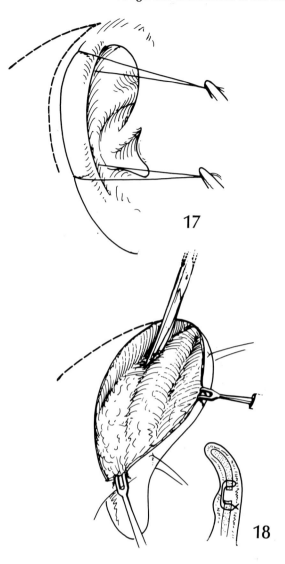

17

18

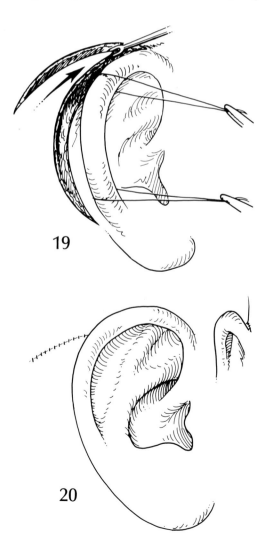

19

20

19

With the adhesions lysed and the superior crus reshaped, the superior pole of the ear will assume its normal position in relation to the side of the head, although this creates a postauricular skin defect requiring flap closure. This is most readily covered by elevating and advancing an inferiorly based postauricular flap in a V–Y fashion.

20

Following flap advancement and wound closure, the superior pole of the ear should remain in a normal relationship to the scalp, with a well-developed superoposterior auricular sulcus.

MICROTIA

Although microtia occurs in only 1:7000 to 1:8000 births, this major congenital ear deformity can result in significant psychological trauma to the affected child. It is no longer acceptable to offer these children the alternative of glue-on plastic prostheses or silastic implants that will be subject to later trauma, infection and loss, because consistently good results can be obtained with autogenous cartilage grafts[11, 12].

The staged reconstruction, which can begin at 5 years of age, involves (1) placement of an autogenous costal cartilage framework; (2) rotation of the lobule, formation of a conchal depression and tragal reconstruction; (3) limited elevation of the helical rim; and (4) minor final adjustments.

21

Anatomy

In classic microtia the sausage-shaped vestige is made up of a rudimentary lobule and various additional remnants. The external ear is usually absent. The deformity is usually unilateral, with the right side more commonly affected than the left. Microtia may present as only one manifestation of hemifacial microsomia, and a continuum exists from microforms of underlying bone and soft tissue deformity to hypoplasia involving all structures derived from the first and second branchial arches.

While the external and middle ear are deformed to varying degrees, the inner ear is essentially intact. If hearing is normal in the opposite ear it is not necessary to reconstruct the middle ear or external canal on the affected side since these procedures may compromise the result of the external ear reconstruction. However, future middle ear surgery, if deemed advisable, is not obstructed or complicated by the microtia reconstruction.

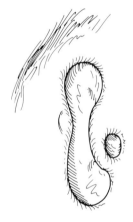

21

The operation

First stage

The cartilage framework is placed during the first stage to make maximal use of the non-scarred elastic skin in the area of the skin pocket. This also allows more accurate splicing of the lobule in the second stage.

The cartilage is dissected extraperichondrially and an attempt is made to preserve as much perichondrium as possible during the framework carving. This appears to play a significant role in maintaining long-term cartilage integrity by enhancing its vascularization.

22

X-ray film templates are used to mark the correct position and size for the reconstructed ear. By transposing the normal ear outline over the microtic vestige and cutting out the pattern of the vestige, an X-ray film template is obtained which can be correctly positioned over the microtic ear at the time of operation without further reference to the normal side.

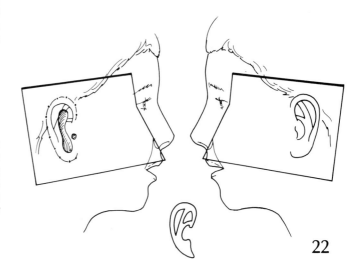

22

23

23

The cartilage graft, which is carved to exaggerate the helical and conchal rims, inferior crus and posterior conchal wall, is shaped from the costal cartilage of the contralateral 6th–8th ribs because the contralateral cartilage has a natural curve which is more conducive to obtaining maximal framework projection.

In most cases the antihelical–crural complex is carved from the 6th costal cartilage and the helix from the entire 7th costal cartilage. Using the full width of the 7th cartilage for the height of the helical rim gives greater projection than the layering techniques of framework building and also simplifies the framework carving. A small segment of the free end of the floating 8th costal cartilage may be used for the helical crus or to add depth to the posterior conchal wall, but this is not always required. By maintaining the major portion of the 8th costal cartilage the postoperative deformity along the costal margin is minimized.

24

Using the previously fashioned template for the cartilage framework, the cartilage for the antihelix and its crura is cut from the 6th costal cartilage. Again, it should be emphasized that perichondrium is preserved wherever possible.

The helical rim is shaped by carving a trough with a metal gouge from what was previously the visceral or inner surface of the 7th costal cartilage. This hollowing not only mimics the helical lip and scapha but also helps to break the spring in the cartilage so that it can take the curve of the full helical rim.

The projection of cartilage at the site of the synchondrosis between the 6th and 7th costal cartilage always falls at a point along the posterior (or under) surface of the midhelical rim, thus allowing adjustment of the finished framework to gain symmetry with the opposite ear, however great the projection required from the mastoid and scalp.

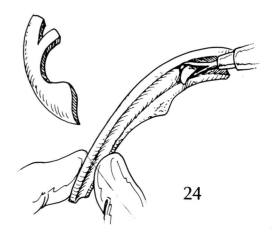

24

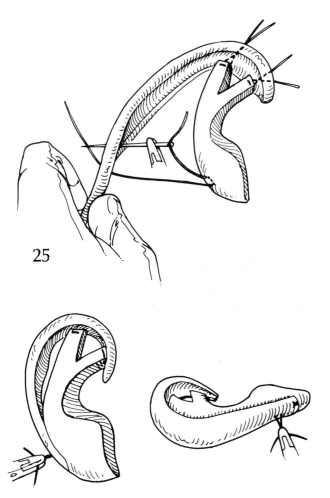

25

25 & 26

Again using the template, the segments of the cartilage are spliced together with 5/0 stainless steel wire passed through the cartilage with fine straight Keith needles. Once the splicing is completed, adjustments can be made by further carving of the inferior crus and posterior conchal wall and by trimming of the undersurface of the helical rim until the final height of the framework is established.

26

27

After completion of the framework, attention is turned to creation of the pocket for cartilage placement. The position of the reconstructed ear is tattooed with methylene blue, using the pre-made template. Through a small preauricular incision (which can be planned to lie just behind rather than across the lateral reconstructed tragus) a pocket is created for the graft. All cartilage remnants are excised from the auricular vestige. However, in patients lucky enough to have a microtic deformity in which a portion of the cartilage of the concha, antitragus or other key landmark is normally shaped, this can be preserved and spliced into the costal cartilage framework.

The dissection of a very thin skin flap enhances definition of the underlying cartilage detail, allows better skin–cartilage coaptation and appears to play a significant part in preventing late deformation of the reconstructed ear.

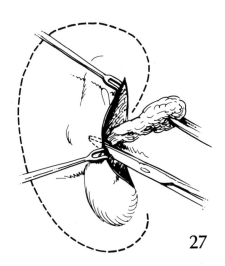

27

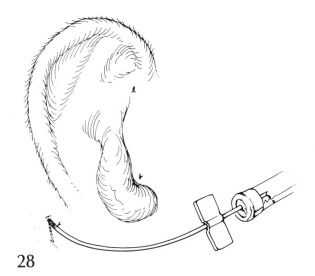

28

28

With the very thin skin flap and excision of cartilage remnants there is ample skin to both cover the cartilage framework and drape it down into all the folds of the cartilage. This is aided by the use of continuous suction drainage after skin closure. The skin is closed in layers and suction is applied using a 19-gauge butterfly needle reversed so that the needle end is stuck into a vacuum blood drawing tube or connected to another source of continuous suction. Additional holes are cut in the drain end. Nursing staff must be instructed to monitor the suction closely in order to ensure that it is continuous for 3–5 days postoperatively. By this time there should be good adhesion between the cartilage and overlying skin. The use of suction drainage eliminates the need for any bolster sutures between skin and cartilage and also eliminates the need for any elaborate dressings postoperatively other than a soft bulky dressing of fluffed gauze and Kling bandage. The patient is given prophylactic broad spectrum antibiotics intraoperatively and this is continued for 4–6 days postoperatively and during the two subsequent stages of reconstruction.

Second stage

The second stage of reconstruction is carried out 2–3 months after the first. During this stage the lobule is rotated and spliced into position with the helical rim, the tragus reconstructed and the concha deepened if required.

Lobular transposition

29

After careful planning to ensure that the lobule is transposed sufficiently inferiorly to produce an ear of equal length to the normal ear, the vertically oriented lobular remnant is dissected downward and transposed to its horizontal position and spliced into line with the helical rim cartilage. While it is often necessary to free the lobule extensively and carry it on a thin inferior skin pedicle, its blood supply can be safeguarded by leaving a fairly thick layer of subdermal fat.

The technique of lobular transposition depends on the size and position of the lobular remnant. In the majority of cases the skin from most of the posterior surface of the lobule is left as a flap based along the conchal rim and used to line the concha as the lobule is dissected downward from its vertical position. The site along the helical rim on to which the lobule will be spliced is marked and de-epithelialized, and the lobule is then transposed and sutured in that position. At this point the exposed concha can be further excavated by removing any remaining subcutaneous fat or pieces of cartilage to provide maximal depth.

In some cases the lobular remnant may be too small to allow sufficient skin to be transposed with the lobule and to line the conchal depression. In these cases the lobule is transposed and spliced in a Z-plasty fashion, and additional skin for lining the concha is obtained as a full thickness graft from the postauricular surface of the contralateral ear. The choice of procedure for lobular transposition should be based on whichever offers the best prospect of restoring maximal fullness and roundness to the lobule while maintaining symmetry with the normal ear.

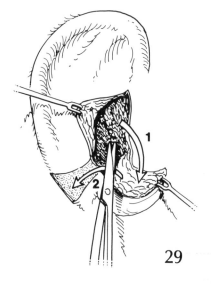

29

30 & 31

Tragal reconstruction

The tragus is reconstructed with a chondrocutaneous graft taken from the concha of the contralateral ear. The graft is excised as an ellipse from the anterior surface of the concha, including anterior skin and the underlying cartilage. The donor area is closed with interrupted and running 6/0 nylon sutures.

A small anteriorly based skin flap is then elevated at a previously marked position for the tragus. This flap is backed with the composite graft, giving a thin delicate reconstructed tragus. The graft is sutured in place with nylon along its outer margin and chromic catgut along its deeper conchal edge. Bolster sutures are placed to ensure close coaptation of graft and the tragal skin flap.

The harvesting of the composite graft from the contralateral concha and closure of the donor site will bring about some decrease in the projection of the normal ear. A contralateral otoplasty may be completed at this time to ensure symmetry between the reconstructed and normal ear or it can be delayed until the third stage of reconstruction. If it is planned to use a full thickness postauricular graft during the elevation of the helical rim of the reconstructed ear, the otoplasty should definitely be delayed until the graft is taken.

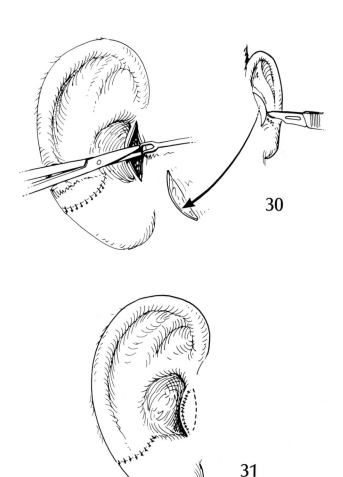

30

31

Third stage

Using the above techniques, the height of the helical rim and symmetry between the two ears may be excellent on completion of the second stage and the third stage may be delayed indefinitely. However, a limited elevation of the helical rim is necessary to highlight the shadow behind the rim of the helix and thus give it a more natural appearance. This stage may be carried out as early as three months after the second stage. The elevation is more limited than in techniques previously described in order to preserve as much as possible of the well-vascularized tissue surrounding the cartilage graft and some sensory innervation to the skin overlying the reconstructed ear.

32

The elevation begins with a W-plasty like incision from the point where the lobule is already free from the mastoid to a point along the superoanterior helix that will allow formation of a superior auricular sulcus. The extent of this elevation is dictated by the degree of sulcus formation accomplished in the previous stages. The incision is placed far enough from the helical rim to allow a collar of skin to be folded just around and over (posterior to) the auricular rim.

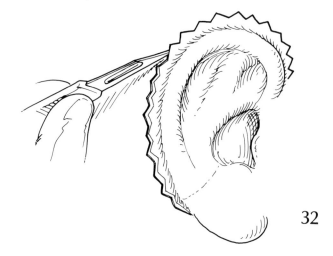

32

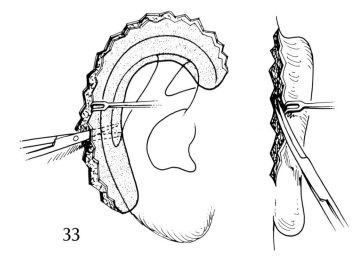

33

33

Limited undermining is carried out posterior to the cartilage framework, keeping the skin flap thin along the ear margin. Care is taken to preserve some vascular tissue over the cartilage graft.

34

The anterior skin flap is advanced around the helical rim by first placing a running suture through the points of each of the triangular flaps and then pulling this suture tight. This effectively decreases the radius of the curve as the points come together and the skin is drawn posterior to the rim. Several interrupted clear nylon sutures placed into the posterior surface of the cartilage framework will further secure the flap around the ear margin.

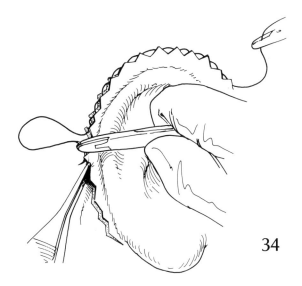

34

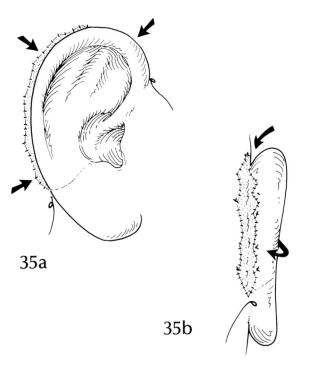

35a

35b

35a & b

The third stage is completed with grafting of the postauricular defect. When little elevation is required this may be accomplished with a full thickness postauricular graft from the contralateral ear. More often, however, a larger graft is required and a split thickness graft is harvested either from the inner surface of the upper arm or from the buttocks.

Great care must be taken to place several sutures deep into the sulcus to avoid tenting of the graft and a less than satisfactory sulcus formation. The graft is best secured with a bolus tie-over dressing packed well into the sulcus.

36

Further stages of reconstruction generally involve only minor touch-ups to improve conchal definition, deepen selective areas of the postauricular sulcus or touch up scars at the junction of the helical rim and lobule. Efforts should be made to get as perfect a symmetry as possible between the two ears and further limited otoplasty may be required on the contralateral ear.

In general, the major reconstruction is completed well within a year of its beginning. However, the need for final touch-ups is probably best judged after a full year of scar maturation.

Patients are reviewed once a year to assess the long-term results of reconstruction. Efforts should continue, as in all other major reconstructive procedures, to modify and refine the existing techniques as long as it seems possible to improve helical definition and appearance.

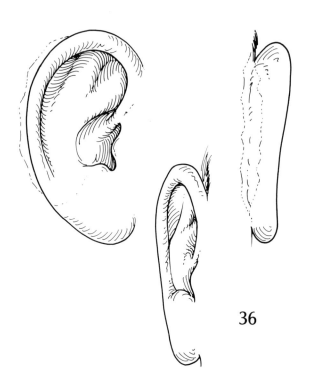

36

References

1. Adamson, J. E., Horton, C. E., Crawford, H. H. The growth pattern of the external ear. Plastic and Reconstructive Surgery 1965; 36: 466–470

2. Kernahan, D. A., Bauer, B. S. Congenital ear deformities other than microtia. In: Kernahan, D. A., Thomson, H. G., eds. Symposium on pediatric plastic surgery, pp. 203–214. St. Louis: C. V. Mosby Co, 1982

3. McDowell, A. J. Goals in otoplasty for protruding ears. Plastic and Reconstructive Surgery 1968; 41: 17–27

4. Stark, R. B., Saunders, D. E. Natural appearance restored to unduly prominent ears. British Journal of Plastic Surgery 1962; 15: 385–397

5. Tanzer, R. C. The constricted (cup and lop) ear. Plastic and Reconstructive Surgery 1975; 55: 406–415

6. Cosman, B. Repair of moderate cup ear deformities. In: Tanzer, R. C., Edgerton, M. T., eds. Symposium on reconstruction of the auricle, pp. 118–133. St. Louis: C. V. Mosby Co, 1974

7. Cosman, B. The constricted ear. Clinics in Plastic Surgery 1978; 5: 389–400

8. Fukuda, O. Cryptotia (Discussion of Simons, J. N.). In: Tanzer, R. C., Edgerton, M. T., eds. Symposium on reconstruction of the auricle, pp. 145–149. St. Louis: C. V. Mosby Co, 1974

9. Washio, H. Cryptotia: pathology and repair. Plastic and Reconstructive Surgery 1973; 52: 648–651

10. Ohmori, S., Takada, H. Cryptotia. Aesthetic Plastic Surgery 1979; 3: 15–28

11. Brent, B. The correction of microtia with autogenous cartilage grafts. II. Atypical and complex deformities. Plastic and Reconstructive Surgery 1980; 66: 13–21

12. Bauer, B. S. Reconstruction of the microtic ear. Journal of Pediatric Surgery 1984; 19: 440–445

Illustrations by Patrick McDonnell from originals by the author

Reconstruction of major acquired auricular defects

Bruce S. Bauer MD, FACS, FAAP
Attending Plastic Surgeon, Division of Plastic Surgery, The Children's Memorial Hospital, Chicago;
Assistant Professor, Department of Surgery, Northwestern University Medical School, Chicago, Illinois, USA

Introduction

While there is a considerable amount of literature devoted to reconstruction and correction of congenital deformities of the ear, there is far less on repair of acquired auricular defects. Brent[1] has described the treatment of acquired auricular deformity using a variety of techniques depending on the level (upper, middle or lower) of the defect and the need for supplemental skin and/or cartilage. In his summary he stated that 'case individualization is necessary, and a systematic assessment of the residual tissue is a requisite when planning an appropriate reconstruction'. However, the surgeon is often faced with large defects due to trauma or tumour resection that cannot readily be reconstructed with composite grafts, conchal cartilage grafts or local skin flaps. This chapter concentrates on reconstruction of major auricular defects with the temporoparietal fascia flap, describing in detail the use of this versatile and extremely reliable technique.

Indications

Major auricular defects can result from traumatic avulsion of the ear, resection of large tumours, direct thermal injury or the consequence of post-burn chondritis, and from repeated unsuccessful attempts at reconstruction of acquired or congenital ear deformities. In each of these cases the surgeon is faced with a cartilage defect which is too large to be reconstructed with the remaining auricular cartilage (contralateral or contralateral plus ipsilateral) as well as a deficiency of local hairless skin. Even if local skin is available, it may lack sufficient pliability because of excessive local scarring. Reconstruction under these circumstances requires replacement of skeletal support, pliable vascularized tissue coverage and non-hairbearing skin coverage. These requirements are all fulfilled by the temporoparietal fascia flap[2–6].

1

Anatomy

The anatomy of this subcutaneous axial fascial flap has been clearly described by Byrd[1,2]. The temporoparietal fascia arises from the fascia of the temporalis muscle beneath the zygoma and becomes contiguous with the galea aponeurotica at the crest of the temporal fossa in the region of the temporoparietal suture. From its point of origin the temporoparietal fascia becomes distinct from the superficial to the fascia of the temporalis muscle. Superiorly, it is superficial to the pericranial tissues. Throughout its course it remains deep to the subdermal fat.

In general, the flap is raised with its blood supply based on the superficial temporal vessels although it can also include or be based on the postauricular vessels alone. If absolutely necessary it can be used as a random pattern flap.

The superficial temporal vessels course anterior to the helical crus at the root of the ear and at this level lie deep to the subdermal fat and on the surface of the subcutaneous fascia. There are numerous perforating vessels to the overlying subdermal plexus. The superficial temporal vessels maintain their relationship to the temporoparietal fascia and subdermal fat until approximately 10 cm above the helical crus. Here the vessels take a more superfical course and emerge into the subdermal fat. Examining the flap from its deep surface, the vessels can be seen easily until they make the transition to this more superficial plane. The vascular territory of the fascia ends approximately 12 cm above the helical crus, where the vessels become contiguous with the subdermal plexus.

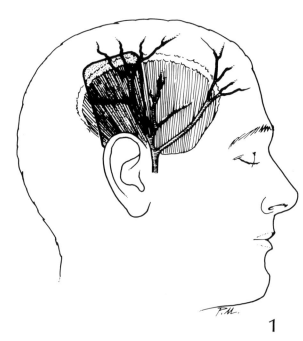

1

The operation

2

The incision most commonly used is an inverted H, with the vertical limb placed over the midportion of the required flap and the horizontal limbs placed along the root of the ear inferiorly and just beyond the superior extent of the flap dissection. This incision allows the dissection to be begun and the correct plane to be entered without the risk of inadvertent injury to the vessels that could occur if the incision were placed directly over the vessel. The hair need only by shaved in a thin strip directly over the incision – if one prefers to shave the hair at all.

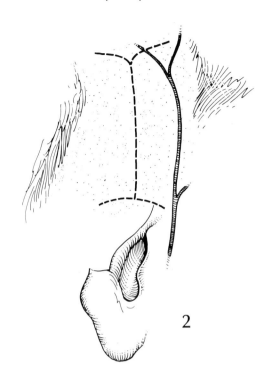

2

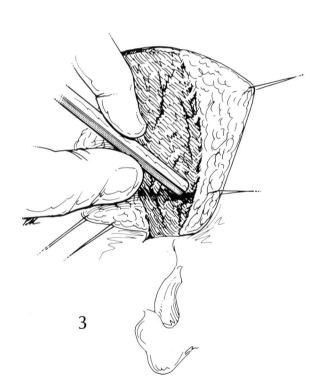

3

3

A Doppler probe is used to trace the course of the superficial temporal artery and postauricular artery and these are marked. The incision, begun distally, is made through the dermis to a level just beneath the hair follicles and then, as the flaps are raised, the plane of dissection can be deepened through the subdermal fat until it immediately overlies the temporoparietal fascia and axial vessels. The dissection can be resumed in the plane just deep to the hair follicles when the area directly over the superficial temporal artery is reached, in order to minimize the risk of injury to the pedicle. However, with increasing experience this change in the plane of dissection is not necessary. Elevation of the scalp flap continues on either side of the incision until the necessary width and length of temporoparietal fascia is exposed. The Doppler probe can be used intermittently throughout the dissection to ensure correct design of the flap and assess the extent of flap dissection about the axial vessels.

4

Flap elevation

The galea is divided distally and this division is carried down on either side of the flap through the temporo-parietal fascia to the level of the ear. The postauricular skin flap can also be dissected at this time to expose the fascia along the whole superoposterior root of the ear remnant together with the remains of the auricular cartilage.

The extent and location of the defect to be reconstructed determine whether the flap will have a broad pedicle, including both superficial temporal and post-auricular vessels, or a narrow pedicle with the superficial temporal vessels alone. If the flap is to be carried on a single vessel care should be taken in narrowing the pedicle, leaving it about 2 cm wide and hugging the cartilaginous margin of the ear as a back-cut is made along the inferior border of the flap.

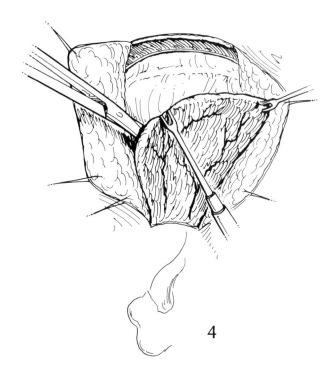

4

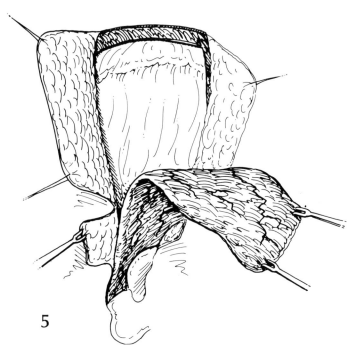

5

5

The flap is now elevated with the plane of dissection deep to the galea and superficial to the pericranial tissues and the anterior fascia of the temporalis muscle. This dissection is in an avascular loose areolar plane and the vessels within the flap substance are readily identified.

6

Placement of cartilage graft

Once the flap has been elevated and a competent vascular supply confirmed, the costal cartilage is harvested from the contralateral chest and the framework constructed as described in the chapter on 'Congenital deformities of the ear', pp. 256–272. The framework is modified in order to splice it into place with any useful remaining auricular cartilage.

At this time several interrupted nylon sutures can be placed to begin the scalp closure behind the temporoparietal fascia flap. The graft is then spliced into place and its position confirmed by using a previously drawn template. The cartilage is sutured to the exposed fascial bed and remaining cartilage with interrupted 4/0 clear nylon sutures.

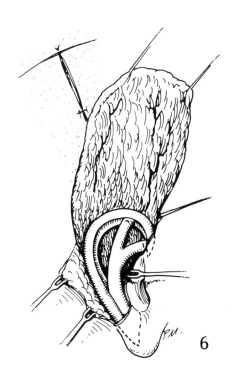

6

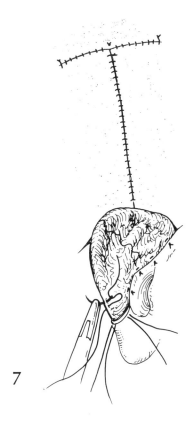

7

7

Coverage of cartilage graft

The thin pliable fascia flap is draped over the cartilage graft and trimmed lightly, making sure to leave adequate tissue to fold down into the interstices of the cartilage graft. Anteriorly the available skin is sutured to the flap in a vest-over-pants fashion, using 5/0 chromic catgut sutures. Posteriorly great care is taken to establish a postauricular sulcus as the flap is sutured to the margin of the postauricular skin in a similar fashion to that used anteriorly.

8

The exposed fascia is then covered with a skin graft, using either split thickness skin alone or a full thickness postauricular graft on the anterior surface of the ear and a split skin graft in the sulcus. If the patient is agreeable, the scalp offers an ideal donor site for the split thickness skin graft. The graft is held in place with a running 5/0 chromic suture. No sutures are placed from the graft directly into the fascia flap in order to avoid any vascular compromise.

Before completing the wound closure of the scalp and ear, a fine suction drain (or drains) is placed, again keeping in mind the importance of establishing a strong vacuum beneath the flap to ensure close coaptation of flap and cartilage (*see* chapter on 'Congenital deformities of the ear', pp. 256–272).

The graft is dressed with a layer of non-adhesive greasy gauze covered with moulded sheets of cotton soaked in water and mineral oil. Fluffy gauze and a Kling bandage (Johnson and Johnson) are then applied over the head and the drain(s) connected to continuous suction.

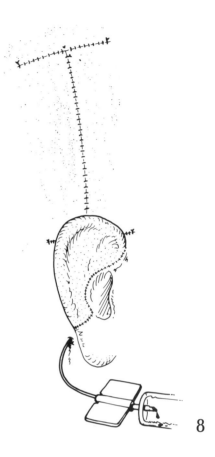

8

Postoperative care

The dressing is first changed about 5 days postoperatively to check graft take and uncomplicated healing. The drains are left in place for 4–5 days unless significant drainage is still present, in which case they are left longer.

In all cases there is significant swelling of the flap overlying the cartilage and in the early postoperative period it is often difficult to distinguish the underlying cartilage detail. The major swelling gradually resolves over the first 4–6 weeks after reconstruction, but improvement in contour and detail of the ear continues for as much as one year after surgery. For this reason, further touch-ups on the ear are best delayed for at least 6–9 months.

Summary

The temporoparietal fascia flap is an extremely reliable, as well as versatile, flap which affords ample thin pliable cartilage coverage where surrounding skin is either absent or excessively scarred. In addition it can be used as a microvascular free flap from the contralateral side when auricular and surrounding tissue losses are so great as to obviate the use of ipsilateral tissue.

References

1. Brent, B. The acquired auricular deformity: a systemic approach to its analysis and reconstruction. Plastic and Reconstructive Surgery 1977; 59: 475–485

2. Brent, B., Byrd, H. S. Secondary ear reconstruction with cartilage grafts covered by axial, random and free flaps of temporoparietal fascia. Plastic and Reconstructive Surgery 1983; 72: 141–152

3. Byrd, H. S. The use of subcutaneous axial fascial flaps in reconstruction of the head. Annals of Plastic Surgery 1980; 4: 191–198

4. Fox, J. W., Edgerton, M. D. The fan flap: an adjunct to ear reconstruction. Plastic and Reconstructive Surgery 1976; 58: 663–667

5. Ohmori, S. Reconstruction of microtia using the Silastic frame. Clinics in Plastic Surgery 1978; 5: 379–387

6. Tegtmeier, R. E., Gooding, R. A. The use of a fascial flap in ear reconstruction. Plastic and Reconstructive Surgery 1977; 60: 406–411

Illustrations by Michael Carroll

Restorative surgery of the nose

Gary C. Burget MD, FACS
Plastic Surgeon, Chicago, Illinois, USA

Introduction

An open wound of the nose is most easily closed by excising exposed bone and cartilage, and lining the defect with a skin graft. However, certain fastidious patients wish not only to have the defect closed but also want to 'look normal'. This chapter outlines an approach that aims to restore the nose to a normal appearance. The depth and location of the defect determine which materials and techniques are used.

Defects that involve only skin and superficial fat may be repaired with a full-thickness skin graft. Where bare bone or cartilage is exposed a flap is required. If a defect extends through cartilage or bone to mucosa, then a cartilage graft must be used also to achieve normal contour and prevent contracture. Full-thickness defects of the nostril margin demand a thin composite flap of skin and cartilage identical to the normal nasal lining and another flap for cover. Bilateral subtotal or total losses of the nose are infrequent deformities. Millard has described the use of the seagull flap for these large defects[1-4].

Certain principles are unique to aesthetic reconstruction of the face, that is, reconstruction where the aim is to recreate the missing part in its original shape, colour, texture and movement.

1. Raw materials for the reconstruction should exactly match missing materials.
2. Missing tissue should be restored in three dimensions using appropriate materials for each layer.
3. An exact pattern of the missing part should be employed using the contralateral normal as a template when it is available.
4. Donor scars should be placed in normal contour or wrinkle lines where they will not be seen.
5. Scars at flap margins should be placed so that they mimic the shadowed valleys or lighted ridges of the normal nasal surface.
6. Topographic subunits of the nasal surface (i.e. tip, dorsum and alar lobule) should be replaced *in toto* so that as a centripetal, or 'trapdoor', contraction occurs the bulge of the flap will resemble the normal convexity of the tip, bridge or alar lobule.

The operations

REPAIR OF SHALLOW NASAL DEFECTS

When a defect of the nose extends only through the skin and superficial subcutaneous tissue, only skin need be replaced to achieve a normal contour. Postauricular skin grafts are too red for the nose. Supraclavicular grafts become shiny and wrinkled. The forehead skin is a good match for the nose, but makes a risky graft. Preauricular skin is a good first choice for it is reliable as a free graft, matches the nose well and can cover a defect as large as 2.5 × 4 cm.

When a defect covers a large area, such as half of the nasal tip, bridge or ala, it is often wise to excise the remaining skin of such a topographic subunit and replace it with a single piece of skin. In this way, border scars do not cross smooth surfaces such as the tip, dorsum or alar lobule but lie in the normal shadowed valleys of the nasal surface where they are not easily seen.

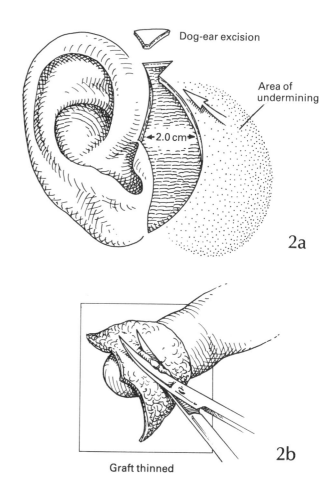

1

1

Excising entire skin of nasal tip

The remaining skin of the nasal tip is excised following the borders of the lateral crura of the alar cartilages. The perichondrium is carefully preserved. The line of excision is kept slightly above the nostril margin in the soft triangle, to prevent postoperative upward contracture of the nostril margin.

2a & b

Obtaining skin graft

A full-thickness piece of skin measuring 2.0 × 5.0 cm is excised as a vertical pointed ellipse in the hairless region just in front of the ear. The graft is obtained from the right side so that telephone use will not be compromised. The excised skin is thinned with high-quality Joseph scissors down to the dermis. The donor site is undermined anteriorly for 2.5 cm and advanced toward the ear. Small holes are cut in a No. 19 butterfly (scalp vein) infusion catheter and this, attached to a vacuum tube (Vacutainer) acts as a drain. The donor wound is closed with 5/0 white or clear inverted subcuticular sutures and 6/0 skin sutures. The final scar should lie just in the preauricular skin crease.

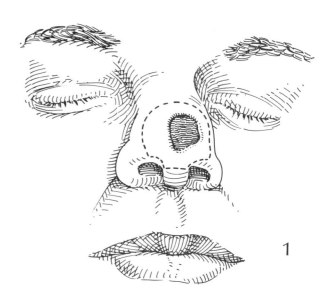

Dog-ear excision

Area of undermining

←2.0 cm→

2a

Graft thinned

2b

3

The preauricular skin graft is sutured onto the nasal defect with four key 5/0 sutures. Using a fine scissors the graft is trimmed to fit the defect and sutured in place with interrupted 6/0 sutures under slight tension. A bolus dressing of sterile foam rubber is placed over a piece of petrolatum gauze and held in place with peripheral 5/0 sutures. This dressing is removed in three days and all sutures are removed.

In patients with sebaceous hypertrophy or mild rhinophyma, the smooth preauricular skin graft may contrast with the pitted skin of the nose. A dermabrasion of the nasal skin at three months will improve the match of skin textures.

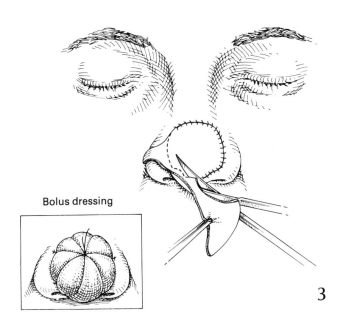

Bolus dressing

3

REPAIR OF DEEP DEFECTS OF NASAL TIP AND BRIDGE

A free skin graft cannot be used to resurface areas of bare bone or cartilage larger than a few milimetres. For such deep defects of the nasal tip or dorsum, a midline forehead flap provides a good match of skin colour, surface texture and pliability.

In the patient illustrated here, a deep defect extends through the perichondrium of the alar cartilages. The dome of the left alar cartilage is missing.

4

Excising remaining skin of tip and dorsum

In this case a large part of the nasal tip and dorsum are missing. The remaining normal skin of these two topographic subunits is excised so that they may be replaced with a single flap. The excision crosses the soft triangle, skirts the nostril margin and follows the slight depression that surrounds the two domes of the nasal tip and the ridges which mark the edges of the nasal dorsum. This places the final scars in shadowed depressions rather than on smooth lighted surfaces of the nose. Furthermore, since the entire nasal tip and dorsum are replaced as a single flap, postoperative contraction in the flap will cause it to bulge slightly, resembling the normal convex surfaces of the nasal tip and dorsum.

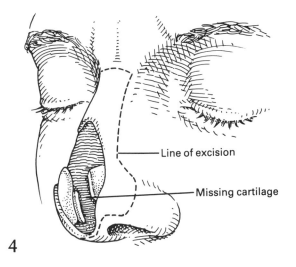

Line of excision

Missing cartilage

4

5

Replacement of missing alar cartilage

The lining skin of the vestibule is dissected from the upper half of inner surface of the right alar cartilage. Great care is required to prevent perforation of this thin lining. The upper half of this normal contralateral cartilage is excised paralleling the nostril margin. It is sutured into the defect in the dome of the left alar cartilage as a graft with 6/0 mattress sutures and will give a normal bulge and light reflection to the left side of the nasal tip. An exact three-dimensional pattern of the nasal dorsum and tip subunits is made from heavy aluminium foil.

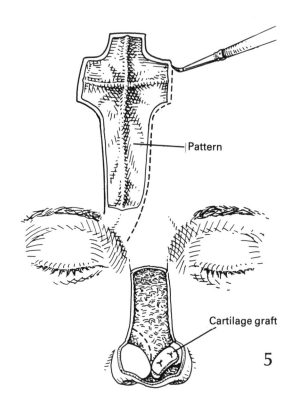

Pattern

Cartilage graft

5

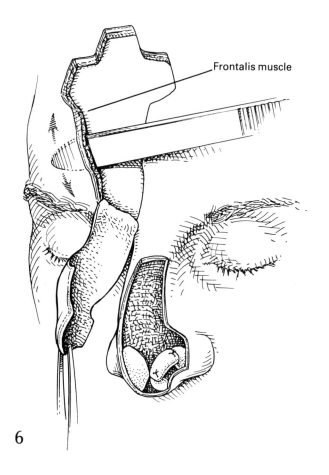

Frontalis muscle

6

6

Design of median forehead flap

The pattern is flattened, turned upside down, and exactly traced at the hairline above the vertical frown crease medial to the eyebrow. No extra margin of skin is included in the flap. The base of the flap is only 1.2–1.5 cm wide to prevent strangulation. The flap is incised, elevated off the frontalis muscle and thinned nearly to dermis around its distal margins with a high-quality Joseph scissors. Frontalis muscle is included with the base of the flap. Care is taken not to injure the supratrochlear vessels lying just superficial to this muscle. If the forehead is vertically short (less than 6 cm) the pedicle can be lengthened by extending it across the eyebrow and supraorbital rim. In this way nearly all midline forehead flaps can be made to cover the upper half of the columella.

Closing the forehead donor site

7

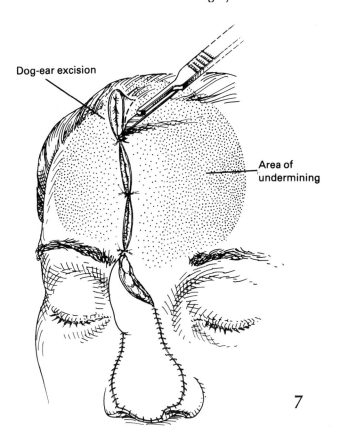

Dog-ear excision

Area of undermining

7

Twisted 180° and transposed 180°, this thin flap is set with 6/0 sutures into the defect for which it was exactly designed. The frontalis-galea layer of the forehead and scalp is lifted off the periosteum for about 7 cm laterally and superiorly using blunt dissection with a scapel handle or the index finger. The frontalis-galea layer should not be scored as this will result in arterial bleeding. A dog-ear excision superiorly extends the wound into the hair-bearing scalp. The forehead defect is then closed with two key 3/0 sutures, 4/0 clear or white subcuticular sutures and 5/0 skin sutures.

A transverse wrinkle line of one side can be matched with the other. If a gap remains in the donor wound it should not be closed under tension or with a skin graft but packed with gauze and allowed to heal by wound contraction as this gives a superior result.

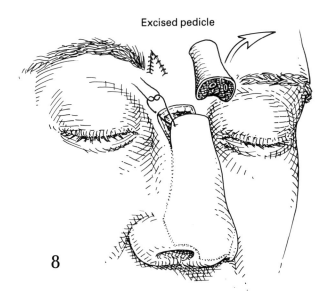

Excised pedicle

8

8

Excision of the pedicle

After 21 days the pedicle is excised, using local anaesthesia. Frontalis muscle and scar tissue are removed from the proximal stump and it is inset just medial to the eyebrow as an inverted 'V', 8–10 mm high. The distal pedicle is inset along a transverse wrinkle line at the level of the canthi. Four months must pass before the skin of the flap assumes its normal colour and softness.

REPAIR OF ALAR DEFECTS

The term 'ala' will refer here to the fleshy part of the lateral wing of the nose below and lateral to the alar groove, the alar lobule. The soft fat of a nasolabial flap contracts into a ball postoperatively, limiting its usefulness in repair of the nasal dorsum and tip. But a superiorly-based nasolabial flap is ideal for replacement of the fleshy ala: postoperatively it contracts into a fleshy blob that looks like a normal alar lobule. For large and deep defects of the fleshy ala, a cartilage graft is required to prevent notching of the nostril margin.

9

Excision of remaining alar skin

In the patient illustrated here, a wound through the ala had been closed three weeks earlier by suturing the covering skin to the lining skin of the vestibule. The remaining surface of the fleshy ala is excised following the alar groove and skirting the nostril margin. Small skin flaps based on the edge of the defect are preserved and turned inward and sutured together to supply the lining of the defect. A three-dimensional pattern of stiff aluminum foil is constructed, using the contralateral normal ala as a template.

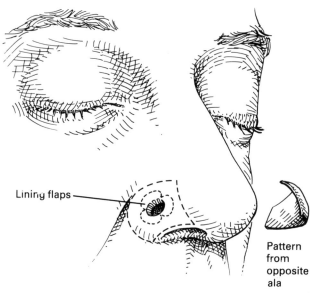

Lining flaps

Pattern from opposite ala

9

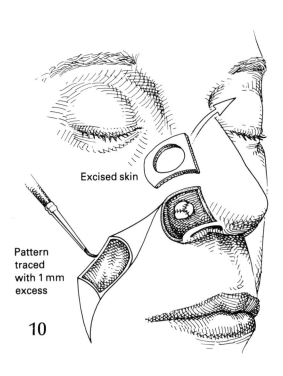

Excised skin

Pattern traced with 1 mm excess

10

10

Design of a nasolabial flap

The pattern is flattened, reversed, inverted and traced with a 1 mm additional margin of skin just above the nasolabial crease. A nasolabial flap based on perforating vessels from the facial artery[5] is outlined around this larger-than-normal design of the ala. A dog-ear excision is added distally, and the skin component of the flap is narrowed proximally so that the final donor scar will lie exactly in the nasolabial crease.

11

Mobilization and placement of a nasolabial flap

The flap is elevated and thinned to between 8 and 10 mm in thickness. The base of the flap is thicker. Great care is used in dissecting the base of the flap so as not to injure the fine vessels perforating the *levator labii alaeque nasi muscle.* Using magnifying loupes, fibrous attachments at the base of the pedicle are severed to allow easy transposition of the flap into the alar defect, but all blood vessels are preserved. A thin cartilage graft measuring 0.5 × 1.0 cm obtained from the nasal septum or from the concha of the ear is fixed in place with 6/0 mattress sutures. This graft will prevent alar margin notching. The nasolabial flap is then sutured into place under no tension with interrupted 6/0 sutures.

Closure of nasolabial donor site

The skin of the cheek is undermined for 3 cm supero-laterally. A suction drain (*see Illustration 2*) is placed in the donor wound and the wound is closed with 5/0 white or clear inverted subcuticular sutures and 6/0 skin sutures. The drain is removed in 36 hours. All sutures are removed by the fourth postoperative day.

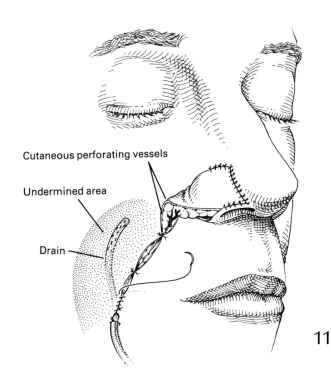

Cutaneous perforating vessels

Undermined area

Drain

11

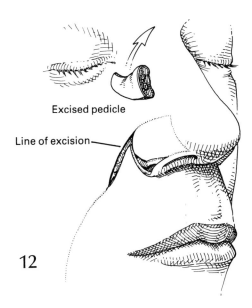

Excised pedicle

Line of excision

12

12

Division of pedicle and repair of alar base

Three weeks following the initial surgery the nasolabial pedicle is divided close to the cheek. The donor site is closed so that the scar lies exactly in the alar groove and nasolabial crease. The distal skin of the flap attached to the ala is thinned, trimmed and inset with fine interrupted sutures along the alar groove and nostril margin. Over the following months the flap contracts to form a bulge that resembles a normal nasal ala.

REPAIR OF A SMALL NOTCH OF NOSTRIL MARGIN

13

This small full-thickness defect of the alar margin calls for new lining and cover only. The scarred tissue which surrounds a healed defect of the nostril margin may be elevated as three small 'turnover' flaps based on the edge of the defect. These are sutured together with the skin side inside for nostril lining. These flaps are composed of scar tissue and their length is limited to 5 mm by the avascularity of the tissue. (When normal skin surrounds a defect these flaps can be made much larger.) These tiny flaps of scar tissue make a stiff, delicate nostril margin.

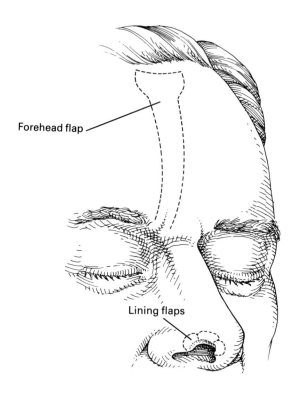

Forehead flap

Lining flaps

13

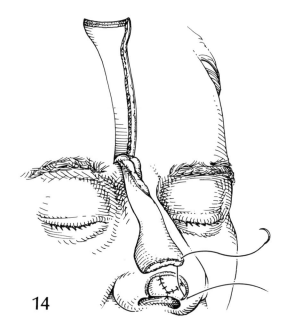

14

14

The external skin cover is provided by a midline forehead flap (see *Illustration 6*). A nasolabial flap is less satisfactory than a forehead flap for covering the nasal tip or dorsum because of its propensity to contract into a blob.

REPAIR OF A LARGE FULL-THICKNESS DEFECT OF NOSTRIL MARGIN

Aesthetic repair of a full-thickness defect of the nostril margin aims for the ideal: a delicate, yet rigid, nostril margin which will not contract upward during healing nor collapse inward on inspiration. Chondrocutaneous grafts from the ear, placed under a forehead flap weeks before it is transposed, make a satisfactory nostril margin, but require an additional stage of surgery and frequently fail to survive. The operation described here is a highly reliable technique for reconstructing a nostril that approaches the normal ideal.

15

The alar cartilage occupies the tip of the nose. The thin lining skin of the nasal vestibule is closely adherent to its inner surface. A sizeable remnant of the alar cartilage and its lining skin usually remains just superior to defects of the lower third of the nose. These are ideal materials for repair of the nostril margin, for they are thin, yet rigid, and are, indeed, the very tissues which line a normal alar margin.

16a, b & c

To bring the new nostril lining down to its proper position, a bipedicled flap 7–10 mm wide and 3 cm long is designed horizontally just superior to the defect. The flap is based medially on the dorsum of the septum and laterally on the nostril floor.

This flap with its backing of alar cartilage is incised, freed from the overlying nasal skin and allowed to move inferiorly to the level of the nostril margin. Often the lateral crus of the alar cartilage is divided, preserving the mucosa of the flap. As it swings down, a dog-ear forms at each base.

A 5/0 stitch in each dogear holds the bipedicled flap in its proper position. The fragment of alar cartilage on the flap may be sutured to the normal contralateral alar cartilage to hold it in proper position. Though this flap is long and thin it is highly vascular, and its survival can be relied upon.

A secondary lining defect remains above the bipedicled nostril margin flap. This defect can be repaired with a superiorly based nasolabial flap (see *Illustration 10*), but this may cause sun-damaged facial skin to be placed inside the nose as lining where, at a later time, a carcinoma may develop undetected. For patients with such sun-damaged facial skin, a composite flap of contralateral septal mucosa and cartilage is used to line this secondary defect.

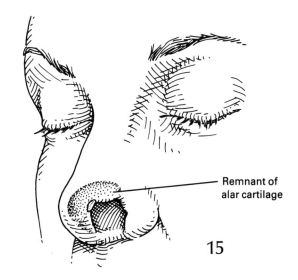

Remnant of alar cartilage

15

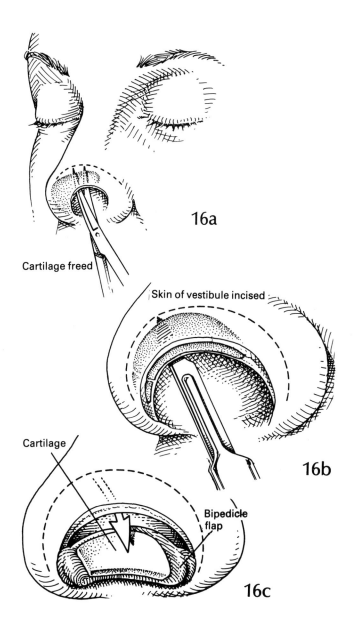

16a

Cartilage freed

Skin of vestibule incised

16b

Cartilage

Bipedicle flap

16c

17a & b

Access to the septal flap is achieved by incising and reflecting the ipsilateral septal mucosa. The flap of septal cartilage and contralateral septal mucosa based anteriorly is incised and swung laterally like the page of a book, hinged on the dorsum of the septum (a). A 1 mm strip of cartilage is removed at the base of the flap to allow easier hinge action. This flap is sutured to the lining sidewall of the nose laterally and the delicate nostril margin flap inferiorly with 4/0 gut sutures. The cartilage of the flap is scored vertically so that it may be bent in the shape of a vault (b). These two lining flaps of vestibular skin and septal mucosa, backed by cartilage, form a rigid, yet delicate, nostril lining which resists postoperative scar contraction and will not collapse on inspiration.

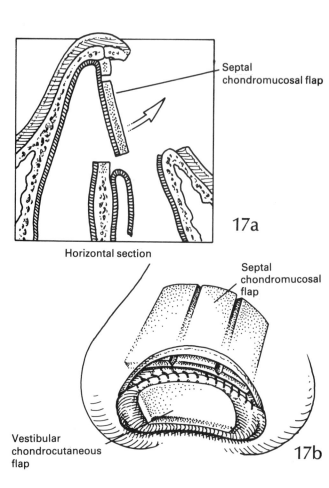

Septal chondromucosal flap

17a

Horizontal section

Septal chondromucosal flap

Vestibular chondrocutaneous flap

17b

Adding auricular cartilage graft to nostril margin flap

If the remnant of alar cartilage attached to the bipedicled nostril margin flap is too small to support the nostril rim, an auricular cartilage graft from the wall of the concha is used to lend support. A strip of cartilage 4 mm wide and 3.0–3.5 cm long can be removed from the concha. This strip of cartilage is inserted into a pocket in the nasal tip and another in the nostril floor, and is sutured to the nostril margin flap with 6/0 mattress sutures. The bipedicled nostril margin flap is vascular enough to support this free cartilage graft.

18

The completed nasal lining is covered with a thin midline forehead flap based on the supratrochlear vessels (see *Illustration 6*) and designed from an exact pattern of the nasal defect. The forehead donor defect is closed by advancement (see *Illustration 7*). When a large forehead flap has been used, the upper one third of the donor defect may be difficult to close. This should be packed with petrolatum gauze and allowed to heal by wound contraction since the result will be superior to a skin graft. Three weeks later the forehead pedicle is excised (see *Illustration 8*).

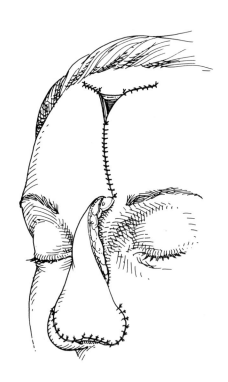

18

RECONSTRUCTION OF LARGE BILATERAL DEFECTS

When both sides of the nose are missing and only a part of the nasal bones remain, Millard[1-4] has used a septal strut as a central support, adjacent skin as lining for the vestibules, a seagull shaped midline forehead flap to cover the dorsum, tip and alae and a strut of rib cartilage to raise the tip and define the dorsum. This requires three surgical stages plus several additional operations to shape the alae and sidewalls and thin the nostril margins.

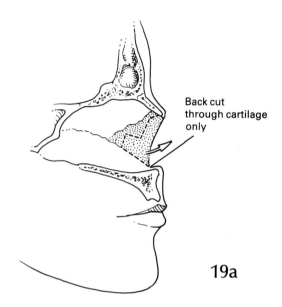

Back cut
through cartilage
only

19a

19a & b

Stage I: Advancement of an L-shaped septal strut and delay of lining and cover flaps

If the nasal septum has been amputated flush with the maxilla, it can be advanced to serve as a central support for the nose. The septum is freed from the septovomerine groove using a scalpel for the mucosa and an osteotome for the cartilage. The L-shaped flap of mucosa and cartilage is incised, rounding the inner angle of the L to preserve blood supply. A back-cut in the cartilage only may be necessary to allow this L-shaped chondromucosal strut to swing forward and rest on the nasal spine. The flap is incised in such a way that a cuff of mucosa can be closed over the exposed cartilage along its posterior edge (a). A split-thickness skin graft is applied along the inferior edge of the L-shaped flap with interrupted 6/0 sutures since an insufficient mucosal cuff is present along this edge (b). The edge of the septal donor site within the nose is closed by removing exposed cartilage and suturing both sides of the septal mucosa over it.

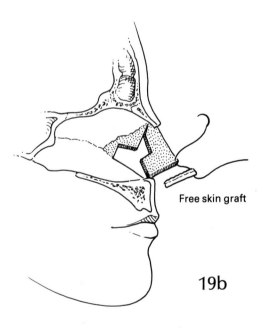

Free skin graft

19b

20

At the same stage that the septal strut is advanced, lining flaps are delayed by incision and slight undermining. The remaining skin of the nasal dorsum is delayed as a lining flap based on the superior edge of the defect by incising the margins, undermining partially and suturing the flap back in place. Bilateral nasolabial flaps designed as wide as local skin laxity will allow are delayed in the same fashion.

The forehead flap is traced from a three-dimensional pattern cut from heavy aluminium foil in the shape of the nasal surface which is to be replaced. It resembles a soaring gull with wings to resurface the alae, a head to cover the upper third of the columella and a narrow body for nasal dorsum and tip. The wings and head of this seagull flap are incised and sutured, but not undermined, as this will cause stiffness in the flap.

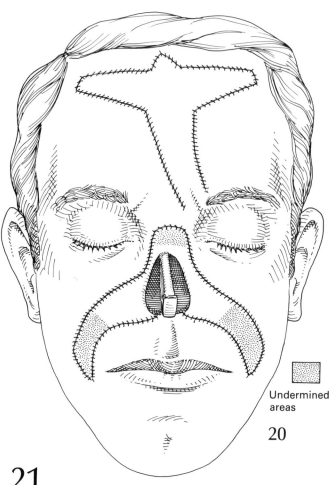

Undermined areas

20

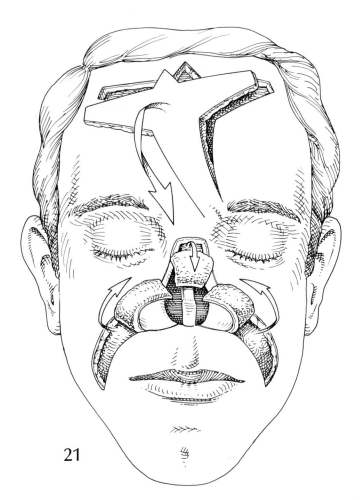

21

21

Stage II: Bringing together lining and cover flaps

Six weeks later the superior lining flap is elevated with the periosteum of the nasal bones and turned inferiorly, hinging on the edge of the defect. A central strip is denuded so that this flap can be attached to the pared edge of the septal strut. Bilateral nasolabial flaps are elevated. Dissection with loupes is employed at the base of each flap so that the small perforating vessels from the levator labii muscles are not injured. The nasolabial flaps are sutured to the columella, to the superior lining flap and to the septal strut to create overly large nasal vestibules.

The edges of the seagull flap are elevated off the frontalis muscle. Frontalis muscle is left attached to the central axes of the body, head and wings. The base of this flap is kept narrow (1.5–2.0 cm) and is centred on the vertical frown crease which overlies the corrugator muscle. Dissection with loupes is employed at the base of the pedicle so that corrugator muscle fibres can be selectively divided, preserving branches of the supratrochlear vessels and nerves. The edges of the seagull's wings and body are thinned nearly to the dermis, but the entire thickness of the frontalis muscle is left in its central axes. The flap is twisted 180°, transposed 180° and sutured into place under no tension. Special attention should be given to the points of the wings or alae. If they cannot be sutured without tension they should be left hanging and sutured at a later time.

Closure of forehead defect

22

The edges of the donor defect are elevated bluntly with a scapel handle or finger for 7 cm laterally and superiorly between the frontalis-galea level and the periosteum (*see Illustration 7*). It is inadvisable to score the galea as arterial bleeding may result. The defect is brought together with key 3/0 sutures. Dog-ear excisions may be necessary at the ends of the wings and head. The horizontal and vertical defects are then closed with 4/0 white or clear subcuticular sutures and 6/0 skin sutures.

On most occasions a central defect will resist closure. This should not be dragged together under great tension nor should a skin graft be applied. If the residual defect is packed with gauze it will contract during the next several weeks and the result will be superior. A fine suction drain (*see Illustration 2*) is placed beneath the seagull flap and attached to a vacuum tube to pull lining and cover flaps together.

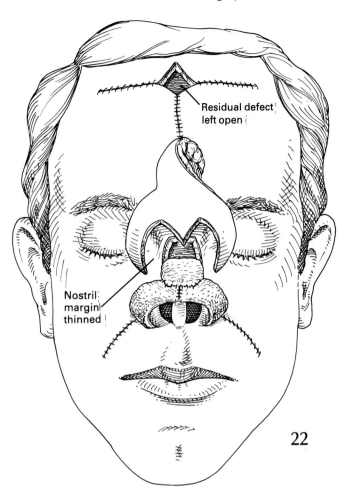

Residual defect left open

Nostril margin thinned

22

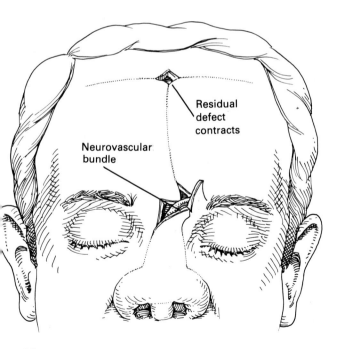

Residual defect contracts

Neurovascular bundle

23

23

Stage III: Excision of pedicle

Three weeks after the skin flaps are brought together the pedicle is excised. Since the base of the forehead pedicle was designed narrow, there is no need to replace it on the forehead at the time of division in order to keep the eyebrows separated. The bundle of subcutaneous tissue and frontalis muscle containing the supratrochlear vessels and nerves is preserved. The proximal stump of skin is elevated off the bundle for 1 cm, thinned, trimmed to the shape of an inverted 'V' between 8 and 10 mm high and inset at the medial end of the eyebrow. The distal pedicle is elevated off the frontalis muscle and trimmed to a rectangular shape. It is inset into the superior end of the nasal bridge along a transverse wrinkle line. The neurovascular bundle, which may cause a bulge under these flaps, is preserved in this way and ensures a good vascular supply to the flap tissue. It also preserves sensation in the reconstructed nose.

TWO OPERATIONS TO REFINE A RECONSTRUCTED NOSE

After 4 months have passed it will often be seen that three features of the reconstructed nose are not up to the normal standard. First, the nasal sidewall does not flow into the cheek as a continuous concave slope; second, the alar groove is not present separating the nasal sidewall from the ala; third, the nostril margin is not thin and sharp, but is thick and blunt and obstructs the nostril airway.

Contouring nasal sidewall and alar groove

After nasal lining and cover flaps have been brought together, at least 4 months should elapse to allow the reconstructed tissue to become soft and pliable.

24a & b

The forehead tissue that has been used to reconstruct the nasal dorsum and sidewall will usually bulge and be separated from the cheek (which is deficient in subcutaneous tissue) by an indented vertical scar (a). To correct this, the scar is excised and the skin of the nasal sidewall and cheek are elevated off the underlying subcutaneous tissue for 1.5 cm. If the cheek is deficient of tissue, Millard's flip-fat-flap is used to turn a layer of fat 0.5 cm thick from the region of excess on the nose to the deficient region on the maxilla. This flap is secured with half-buried 6/0 mattress sutures tied on the surface of the cheek skin. This will create a smooth continuous slope of nasal sidewall and cheek.

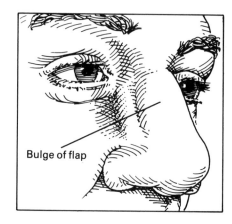

Bulge of flap

24a

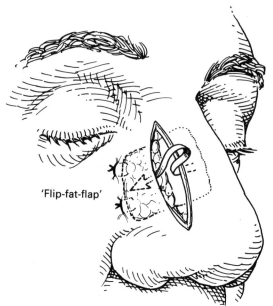

'Flip-fat-flap'

24b

25

The flap skin is also elevated off the nose inferiorly in the region of the ala. The concave slope of the nasal sidewall and the gentle curved valley of the alar groove are then carved in the subcutaneous tissue and scar of the nose. This sculpturing is best done by making a series of parallel cuts 1 mm apart in the tissue under the flap. Each strip of subcutaneous tissue may then be picked up with a fine forceps and excised with a very fine curved scissors until the normal contour of sidewall and alar groove is achieved. The skin of the nasal flap is then anchored into the alar groove with four sutures of 6/0 white or clear material. A fine suction drain (see *illustration 2*) is introduced and the skin incision is closed with 6/0 sutures.

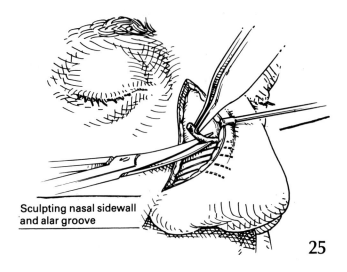

Sculpting nasal sidewall and alar groove

25

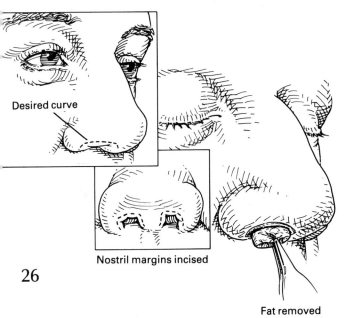

Desired curve

Nostril margins incised

26

Fat removed

26

Thinning nostril margin

When a nasolabial flap is used to restore the lining of the nasal vestibule, the result is always a thick, blunt alar margin. Four months or more after the initial operation a thinning procedure is carried out through the marginal scar. The normal level of the nostril is marked on the reconstructed nostril margin. The marginal scars are excised. (Only when the nostril margin is to be lifted is a wider strip of tissue excised.) The cover skin is elevated as a thin flap off the underlying subcutaneous tissue for 1 cm superiorly. The lining tissue is elevated in the same way and the intervening wedge of subcutaneous tissue is excised. The marginal excision is closed with 6/0 sutures. The lining flap is held in place with a bolus of foam rubber placed inside the nostril.

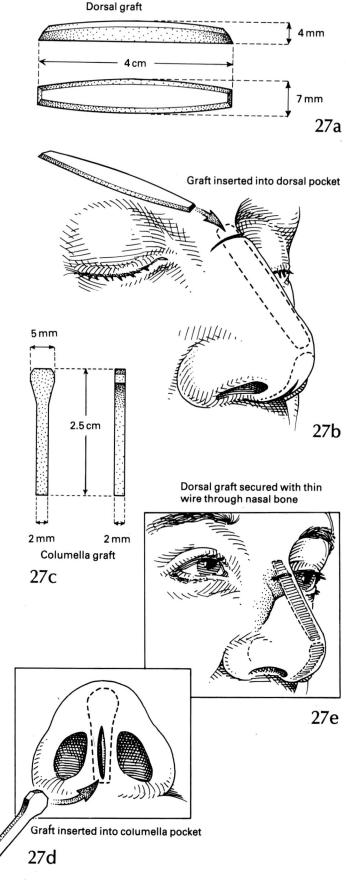

Dorsal graft

4 mm

4 cm

7 mm

27a

Graft inserted into dorsal pocket

27b

5 mm

2.5 cm

2 mm   2 mm

Columella graft

27c

Dorsal graft secured with thin wire through nasal bone

27e

Graft inserted into columella pocket

27d

Costal cartilage grafts to dorsum and columella

As a final step in nasal reconstruction, cartilage grafts may be added to lift and narrow the dorsum and give more point to the nasal tip. These grafts are obtained from the seventh or eighth costal cartilage. These grafts do not support the nose, but rather add a sculptured volume which changes the surface contour.

27a–e

A 1.5 cm transverse incision is made at the level of the medial canthi. A pocket, 1.2 cm wide, is dissected with a No. 67 knife blade or curved Joseph scissors down to the supratip region. A dorsal rib cartilage graft approximately 4 × 7 ×40 mm is carved for this pocket, shaving from all sides symmetrically to prevent warping (a and b). A second incision 1.2 cm long is made vertically in the midline of the columella and a pocket is dissected from the columellar base to the nasal tip. A tip graft patterned after Sheen[6], 2.5 cm long with a head 5 mm wide and a columellar stem 2 mm wide, is carved for this columellar pocket (b and c). Each graft is grasped along its entire length with a long narrow smooth forceps to aid in sliding it into the pocket (b and d). Occasionally a 5/0 wire suture is required to fix the dorsal graft to the nasal bones (e). Care must be taken that the loop of this fixation suture is submucosal and does not pass through the nasal cavity. Usually neither graft requires fixation for they are held snugly in the pockets created for them. The wounds are closed with 6/0 sutures.

References

1. Millard, D. R. Reconstructive rhinoplasty for the lower half of a nose. Plastic and Reconstructive Surgery 1974; 53: 133–139

2. Millard, D. R. Reconstructive rhinoplasty for the lower two-thirds of the nose. Plastic and Reconstructive Surgery 1976; 57: 722–278

3. Millard, D. R. Aesthetic aspects of reconstructive surgery. Annals of Plastic Surgery 1978; 1: 533–541

4. Millard, D. R. Aesthetic reconstructive rhinoplasty. Clinical Plastic Surgery 1981; 8: 169–175

5. Herbert, D. C. A subcutaneous pedicled cheek flap for reconstruction of alar defects. British Journal of Plastic Surgery 1978; 31: 79–92

6. Sheen, J. H. Aesthetic Rhino-plasty. St Louis, Mosby, 1978

llustrations by Helen McIlhenny

Repair of nose with distant flaps

Norman C. Hughes OBE, FRCS, FRCSI
Consultant Plastic Surgeon, Royal Victoria Hospital, Belfast, Royal Belfast Hospital for Sick Children
and The Ulster Hospital, Dundonald, Belfast, Northern Ireland

Introduction

When a nasal defect is too large to repair with free composite grafts or local flaps, a forehead flap generally gives the most satisfactory result. However, when the skin of the forehead has been destroyed or when a secondary defect in that area is unacceptable, tissue for the reconstruction has to be obtained from further afield.

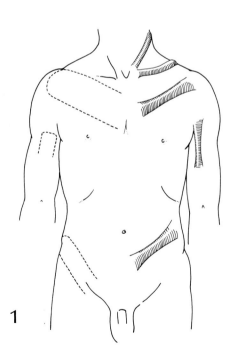

1

1

Alternative sources

1. Neck tubed pedicle flaps raised along the line of the sternomastoid muscle or transversely in the supraclavicular region are suitable for small defects. They provide skin of a texture and colour similar to that of the face and, owing to the excellent blood supply, a length to breadth ratio of 4:1 is acceptable. Secondary scarring is a disadvantage, particularly with the sternomastoid flap.
2. The deltopectoral axial flow flap has the advantage that it can be transferred directly to the nose without the necessity for any preliminary delay procedure.
3. The acromiothoracic tubed pedicle flap has somewhat similar alignment to the deltopectoral flap but is swung on its outer attachment 3–6 weeks after it has been raised and tubed.
4. The classical Italian flap from the upper arm is rarely used. As it is distally based a preliminary delay is essential, and when the flap is attached to the nose the position is difficult to maintain and uncomfortable for the patient.
5. Extensive scarring resulting from burns may necessitate the transfer of flaps from the abdomen or elsewhere, making use of the wrist or forearm as an intermediate carrier.

The acromiothoracic tubed pedicle nasal reconstruction illustrates the principles involved in any tubed flap procedure.

295

Acromiothoracic tubed pedicle flap

FIRST STAGE

2

Planning

Two oblique parallel lines outlining the flap are marked on the anterior surface of the thorax. Staggering of these lines assists both closure and the later upward swing of the tubed pedicle to the nose. The incision markings should extend to the anterior border of the deltoid muscle, as the mobility of the point of the shoulder facilitates attachment of the flap to the nose. A length to breadth ratio of 3:1 is permissible, and in planning an extra 5 mm width should be allowed for loss which will occur when the scar is excised on opening up the tube. The amount of skin required to reconstruct the lower part of the nose must not be underestimated. The distance from one alar base to the other measured around the tip is from 7 to 8.5 cm, which is greatly in excess of the length of the nose.

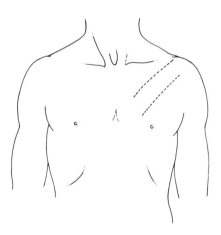

2

3

Raising and thinning of flap

The parallel incisions are carried through skin and full thickness of subcutaneous fat to the fascia overlying the muscles, and the bipedicle flap is raised by sharp dissection. Excess fat is then carefully removed, leaving the flap a uniform thickness. In an obese patient fat removal must continue until the flap tubes readily without showing any sign of tension. In a lean individual marginal trimming of fat to facilitate suturing may be all that is required. Complete haemostasis must then be achieved.

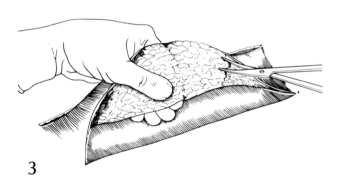

3

4

Tubing of flap

An interrupted suture is inserted close to each end of the flap at a point where it still tubes without tension. The ends of these sutures are clamped and act as stay sutures, while the intervening part is tubed using either continuous suture or fine interrupted stitches.

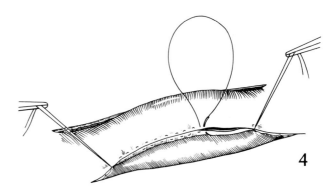

4

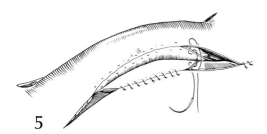

5

5

Closure of the donor site

After undermining the skin edges between fat and fascia the donor site is closed by interrupted sutures. The triangular defects at each end are approximated to corresponding defects on the undersurface of the tube, a special suture being used to achieve accurate approximation at the apex of each triangle.

For a very wide defect the application of a split-skin graft is preferable to direct closure.

6

Application of dressings

Non-adherent dressings are applied to the suture lines, and gauze rolls or pieces of thick plastic sponge are strapped in position on each side of the tube. These protect the tube from pressure, while leaving it exposed so that its circulation can be observed.

In cases where the donor site has been grafted, great care must be taken to ensure that the graft dressing in no way obstructs the circulation through the tubed pedicle.

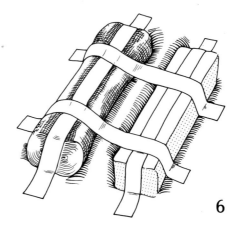

6

SECOND STAGE

Detachment of pedicle and preparation of recipient site

Provided healing has progressed satisfactorily the medial end of the pedicle may be detached after 3 weeks and the chest defect closed by direct suture.

7a & b

For the larger nasal defects it is generally advisable to resurface the entire nose. Local flaps are turned downwards or inwards to provide the essential lining for the reconstructed nose. As these lining flaps are based on scar tissue and are being swung through up to 180°, they must be elevated with care and fully mobilized from the underlying nasal bones or nasal septum. They are maintained in the correct position with interrupted sutures of fine absorbable material.

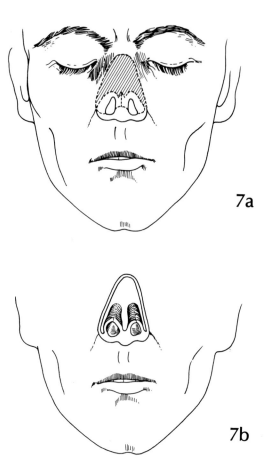

7a

7b

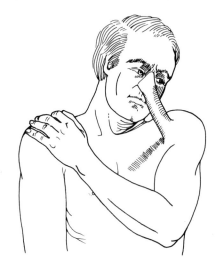

8

8

Implantation of end of tubed pedicle

The central scar is excised so that an adequate amount of the tube is opened up. Carefully executed, this procedure does not in any way jeopardize the circulation in the flap. The flap is then sutured into the nasal defect, generally in an up and down position, although in some cases a transverse attachment may be more suitable.

Care must be taken to avoid tension on the tube, close observation being necessary particularly in the immediate postoperative period while the patient is recovering from the anaesthetic.

THIRD STAGE

9

Separation of pedicle

Aftrer 3 weeks the pedicle is divided and the flap is inset on the nose. Thinning of the flap must not be overdone at this stage. If the inset is complicated it is advisable, when dividing the pedicle, to leave a generous amount of flap and to defer the final detailed adjustment to a later date. The unused portion of the tube is generally opened up and returned to its original site.

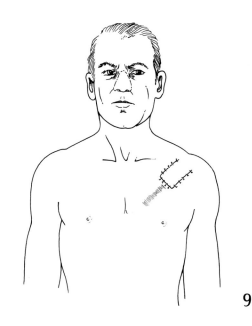

9

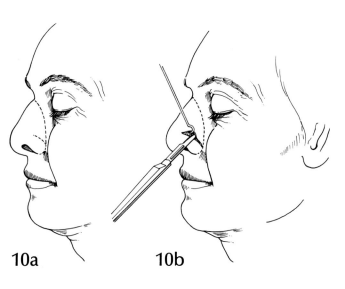

10a   10b

10a & b

Later adjustments

Small curved incisions are made on each side of the reconstructed nose, at a level corresponding to the upper border of the alar cartilage, and the subcutaneous fat is removed. The incisions are closed with interrupted sutures, one or two of which pick up the deeper tissues. This results in a great improvement in the conformation of the reconstructed nose. Any other minor adjustments are carried out at the same time.

Editor's note

A common error in the planning of an acromiothoracic pedicle for repair of the nose is to base the tube on the acromiothoracic arterial axis. Unless the tube is based on the point of the shoulder, its mobility will be restricted and the tube too short for a position of reasonable comfort to be maintained. Some form of restraint, e.g. extension strapping from head to deltoid region and outer arm, is perhaps advisable if only as a reminder to the patient to avoid putting tension on the tube.

Illustrations by Robert N. Lane

Structural support in forehead flap rhinoplasty

John Watson FRCS, FRCS(Ed)
**Formerly Consultant Plastic Surgeon to The London Hospital;
The Queen Victoria Hospital, East Grinstead, Sussex, UK**

The problem of the provision of adequate support for a forehead rhinoplasty where there is total or subtotal destruction of the nose is formidable and remains to some extent unsolved. When the defect is mainly a skin loss, with perhaps part of the cartilaginous nasal tip missing, simple application of a forehead flap (see chapter on 'Restorative surgery of the nose', p. 279–294) gives a very acceptable result, the turning-in of local lining flaps from the margins of the defect, together with the terminal infolding of the forehead skin, giving sufficient lining and rigidity to create the contours of the tip, nostrils and columella.

In more extensive defects, however, serious difficulties arise from lack of available skin for adequate lining and loss of bony and cartilaginous supporting structures. The method to be described provides skin lining for the nasal tip and alar vestibules. Fortunately, there is usually sufficient skin available to provide lining for the upper part of the nasal cavity, if necessary using inturned nasolabial flaps. On rare occasions, in cases of complete nasal loss, it is possible to use a lined (infolded) tube pedicle from elsewhere to provide lining skin and crude preliminary closure of the defect, subsequently sacrificing the outer layer which is replaced with the forehead rhinoplasty. Certainly, the provision of adequate lining is essential in reconstruction if the new nose is not to become shrivelled and retracted.

Failure to provide structural support in these extensive nasal losses tends to lead to progressive loss of the shape of the new nasal tip, which tends to sink downwards towards the upper lip, and to flattened collapse of the whole nose. The incorporation of autogenous cartilage to form the alar domes as an integral part of the forehead rhinoplasty is a great help in overcoming these difficulties.

The operation

Stage I

1

The lining and support for the new nostrils is secured by the removal of composite chondrocutaneous grafts from the anterior surface of the conchal hollows of each pinna. The shape of the hollows is almost correct for the purpose and the rolled external border of the hollow is taken, as this will form the new nostril rim. Grafts measuring approximately 20 mm × 10 mm can normally be obtained. The defects are repaired with small split skin grafts after trimming back any marginal exposed cartilage. An overtied wool bolus is applied to maintain pressure between the graft and the preserved postauricular layers, and the ultimate defect is minimal.

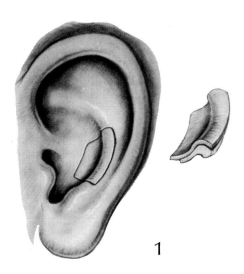

1

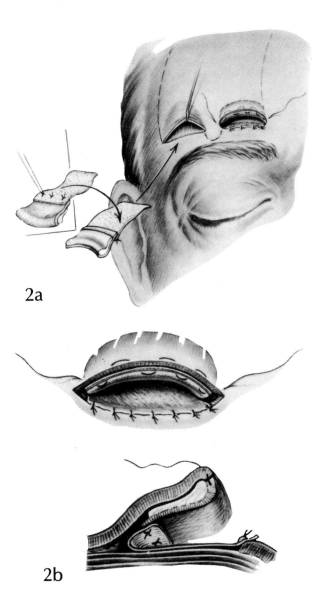

2a

2b

2a & b

The exact position and size of the proposed flap is then delineated on the forehead. This will normally be not less than 7.5 cm wide. Two incisions are made at the site of the new nostril margins and, by undermining the skin subdermally and superficial to the frontalis muscle, two tunnels are created. After suturing two small split skin grafts to the distal borders of the chondrocutaneous grafts, these are thrust into the tunnels with the cartilage lying beneath the forehead skin, the attached skin graft forming a skin lining for the apex of each tunnel and the exposed frontalis muscle. The junction of forehead skin and chondrocutaneous rim is closed with a fine nylon intradermal suture and the cavity carefully packed with wool. The wool is retained in the tunnel with adhesive strapping, but pressure should not be applied over the outer surface of the chondrocutaneous grafts. In this way the two nostrils are performed on the forehead. Full vascularization of the grafts takes some time, and it is important not to shift the complex downwards for 6 weeks, as premature performance of the second stage may lead to necrosis of the grafts beneath an intact skin cover.

Stage II

3 & 4

Marginal lining flaps are elevated and inverted across the nasal defect. The whole forehead complex is then elevated and the chondrocutaneous nasal tip brought down. Good vascularization of the apex of the flaps is essential and for this reason mobilization of the whole forehead on both temporal and supraorbital arteries is preferred. Anaesthesia with induced hypotension is a great boon in avoiding blood loss. The apex of the flap tends to form itself naturally into the contours of a nasal tip and is sutured into position within and without. The forehead defect is grafted with split skin.

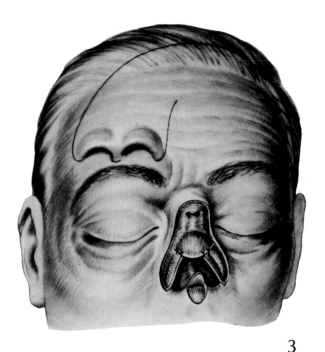

3

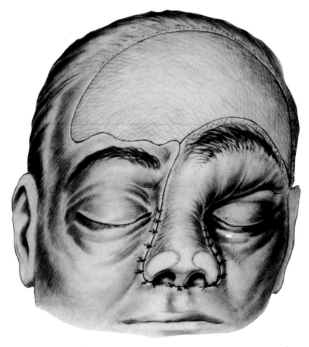

4

Stage III

After 3 weeks the flap is divided at subglabellar level and the margin inset. The residual forehead and scalp skin is returned after excision of redundant free graft. The potential unsightliness of the grafted forehead is to some extent mitigated by the fact that the frontalis muscle has been preserved and, at a later date, appearance can be improved by the substitution of a full thickness skin graft.

5

It is possible to carry out a similar repair for half the nose by using a lateral (Gordon-New) sickle scalp flap so that only the temporal forehead is marked, but in this case the flap *must* be delayed. Distances are deceptive when using this flap and special care is necessary in planning to ensure that it will reach its destination without tension.

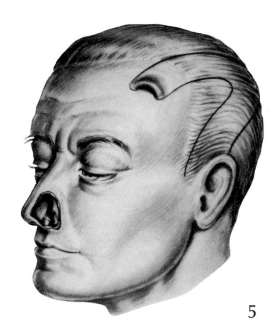

5

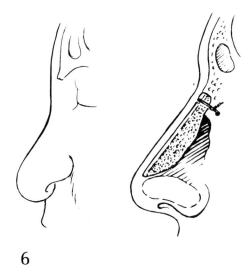

6

6

With the distal end of the rhinoplasty supported in this way, no additional measures may be necessary if some distal septal bony support remains. When, however, this is lacking, with development of a saddle deformity, a dorsal bone graft taken from the inner table of the ilium can be inserted via the subglabellar scar. Its upper end is fixed by wiring, the external loop of which should be submucosal and not penetrate the nasal cavity. Attempts to insert an L-shaped graft with columellar strut tend to be ineffective and greatly broaden the columella and nasal tip.

Illustrations by Kevin Marks

Cosmetic rhinoplasty

R. L. G. Dawson FRCS
Formerly Consultant Plastic Surgeon, Mount Vernon Hospital, Northwood,
and Royal Free Hospital, London, UK

Introduction

Very careful selection of patients for cosmetic rhinoplasty is essential, but discussion of this large subject is outside the scope of this book. Once the need for hump reduction and narrowing, with shortening, and reduction of the bulbous tip has been established, the patient is prepared for operation as follows.

Preoperative

Premedication is given. General anaesthesia is preferred, with an endotracheal tube through the mouth. The anaesthetist packs off the pharynx firmly. A solution of 10 per cent cocaine and 1:1000 adrenaline is applied to the nasal mucosa of each nostril, using three cottonwool swabs on orange sticks. These are left in place for 10 minutes. Some surgeons use hypotension and then there is no need for adrenaline and cocaine.

The operation

The patient is placed on the operating table with the head elevated to 30°. The head is draped with two head towels. An injection of 1.25 per cent lignocaine (Xylocaine) with 1:100 000 adrenaline is used: 2 ml are injected into the columella and nasal bridge, and 2 ml subcutaneously on each side of the nose. A further 10 minutes should elapse to allow the injections to take effect.

The future nasal shape is outlined in Bonney's blue on the skin of the nose, and excess intranasal hairs are removed.

1

The nostril is lifted up with a rake retractor, and a Joseph's double-edged knife, curved on the flat, is inserted at the fold between alar and lateral nasal cartilages. The knife is passed up on each side superficial to the lateral cartilage and nasal bones, as high as the frontal bones.

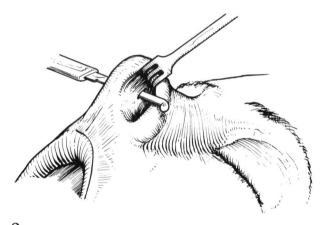

1

2

A blunt-ended Bistoury knife is inserted over the bridge-line to free the skin and is brought downwards over the septum, separating the columella from the lower end of the septum.

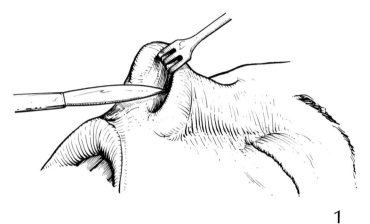

2

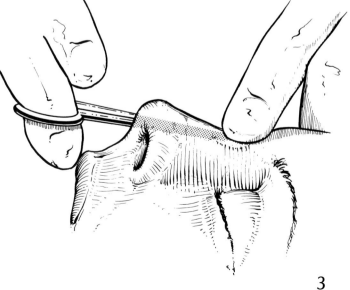

2

3

Small scissors are used to separate the procerus and corrugator muscles from the skin, and these muscles are scraped off the nasal bones with a Howarth elevator. In this way the full hump deformity becomes apparent.

3

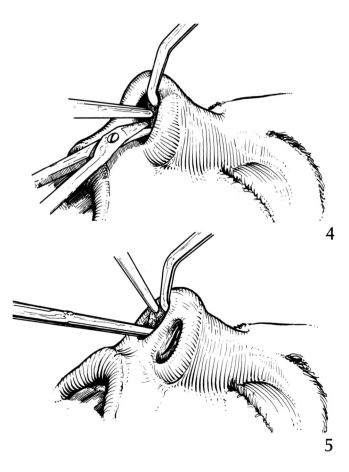

4

5

4 & 5

The amount of lateral cartilage to be excised is estimated and appropriate incisions made through the lateral cartilage along the septum. Th excess septum along the bridge is also excised.

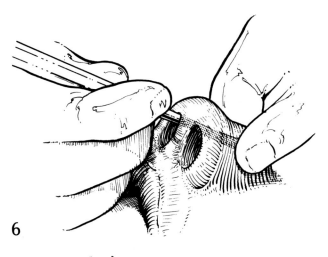

6

6

A McIndoe nasal chisel is inserted beneath the three pieces of cartilage so incised to remove the bony hump in continuity, upwards. The freed bony hump is then removed together with the three prongs of cartilage.

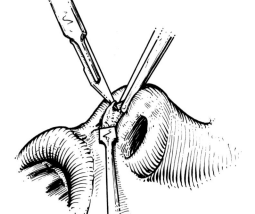

7

7

The lower end of the septum is removed to shorten the nose and tilt the tip up a little. Care must be taken not to remove too much. If the anterior nasal spine is very prominent, with the upper lip drawn upwards towards the nasal tip, this spine must be removed by chisel at the same time.

8

The lateral infracture and narrowing must now be performed through a separate small incision on both sides, the periosteum being separated with a Joseph's elevator, anterior to the canthal ligament. Either a Joseph's saw or a 5 mm osteotome is used to cut the bones coronally as far as the frontal bone. Subsequent out-fracture with a small chisel across the frontonasal process separates the nasal bones and frontonasal process from the rest of the skeleton, so that they can be brought together to narrow the bridge-line.

The columella is now reattached to the lower end of the septum, and any excess lateral cartilage, prolapsing into the shortened nose, is trimmed off. Three through-and-through catgut sutures suffice to reattach the columella

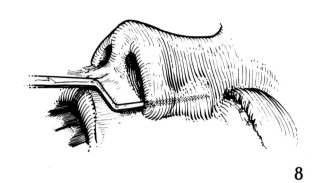

8

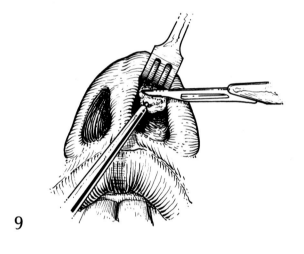

9

9 & 10

The bulbous nasal tip must now be thinned. This is done by everting the nasal rim on both sides, making an incision in line with the new septal height, through the dome cartilage and its lining skin, but stopping short of the rim of the cartilage. The cartilage and its lining skin are pulled out with a hook and the covering skin is separated from them by blunt scissor dissection. The lining skin is then dissected off the everted cartilage, and the appropriate amount of cartilage is removed on either side to obtain a narrower, symmetrical tip.

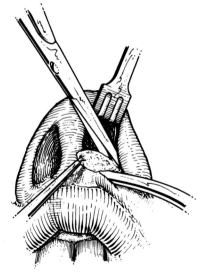

10

11a & b

If the tip still stands up too much, because of the strength of the medial crura, a portion, appropriate to the amount of correction needed, can be removed from the base of the columella. The resulting scar abutting on the upper lip is practically invisible after about 2 months.

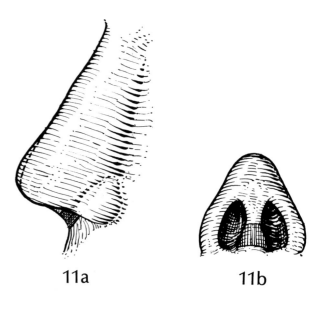

11a   11b

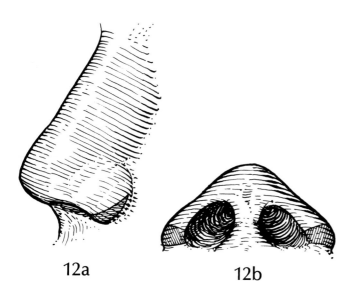

12a   12b

12a & b

When the resulting set back of the nose results in flared nostrils, a wedge must be removed from the alar bases on both sides. The back incision must be made about 1 mm in front of the alar crease, otherwise a small, ugly, depressed scar will result.

The bifid nasal tip can be corrected in two ways. If the deformity is small, then the soft tissue can be removed between the two medial crura and the crura sutured together with fine catgut. If the deformity is large, then it is best to remove an ellipse of skin between the two medial crura as well. The resulting small vertical columella scar becomes virtually invisible in the course of time.

The 'hanging tip', where too much columella and lower septum is seen from the lateral view, needs additional removal of the lower end of the septum, and the columella sutured back to a higher level. If the lower edges of the medial crura are still too prominent, these can be removed directly through a small incision over them. The resulting sutured scar is only temporary.

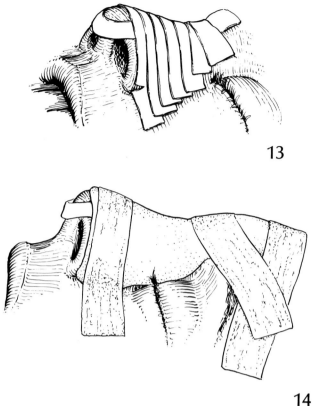

13

14

13 & 14

When the operation has been completed, the nose is draped with strips of 13 mm (½ inch) zinc oxide strapping, one strip being split to surround the actual nasal tip. A closely moulded plaster of Paris, eight sheets thick, is applied after petroleum jelly has been put on the eyes and eyebrows. This is fixed to the forehead and face with 2.5 cm (1 inch) Elastoplast. A small tulle-gras pack is inserted into each nostril, into the actual vestibule of the nasal tip to pack the lining skin against the nose tip skin.

Postoperative care

The patient is nursed sitting up as much as possible, with ice-packs on the eyes for the next 24 hours. The nostril packs are removed in 48 hours and the patient is sent home. Alar base and columella sutures are removed in 7 days and the plaster fixation in 2 weeks. Some swelling of the nasion, and a numbness of the nasal tip may persist for a few weeks, but sensation always returns. Residual swelling may take 6 months finally to disappear.

Illustrations by T. Tarrant

Injuries of the eyelids

John C. Mustardé   FRCS(Eng.), FRCS(Glas.)
Consulting Plastic Surgeon, West of Scotland Regional Plastic Surgery Centre, Canniesburn Hospital, Glasgow, and Royal
Hospital for Sick Children, Glasgow, UK

Introduction

Injuries of the eyelids are particularly important because
of the ever-present risk to the underlying eye, either at the
time of the injury or at a later date when, due to scar
contraction, the cornea may be exposed and damaged.

Because the eyelids have a 'skeletal' structure – the
tarsal plate – which imparts their normal curved shape,
injuries of the lids may be considered as either *partial-
thickness*, i.e. involving skin and orbicularis oculi only, or
full-thickness, i.e. involving skin, orbicularis, tarsal plate
and the closely subjacent conjunctiva.

As with all surface tissues, there are three categories of
injury.

1. *Wounds without loss of tissue.*
2. *Wounds with loss of tissue.*
   Either of these wounds may affect either only part or
   the whole of the thickness of the eyelid.
3. *Scars.*

Partial-thickness injuries

Wounds

1a & b

Injuries caused by glass or cutting instruments may run in any direction. If the wound lies in the line of the fibres of the underlying orbicularis muscle a continuous 6/0 intradermal suture may be used, fixing both ends to the skin with squares of adhesive. Such sutures are pulled out in 5 days.

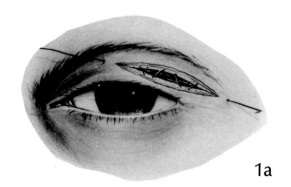

1a

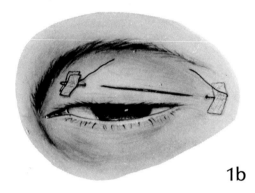

1b

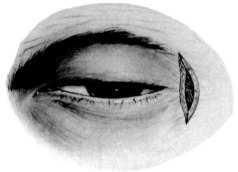

2a

2a & b

If, however, the wound lies *across* the line of the orbicularis fibres there will be retraction of the wound edges and interrupted 5/0 Prolene or silk sutures should be used to close the skin wound.

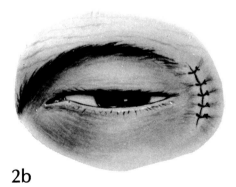

2b

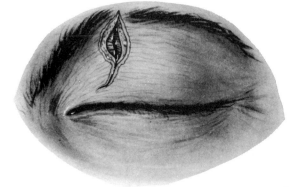

3a

3a, b & c

If the orbicularis has also been divided across its fibres it must be united with interrupted sutures of 6/0 chromic catgut. The skin sutures are removed in 5 days.

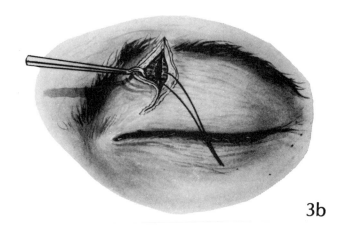

3b

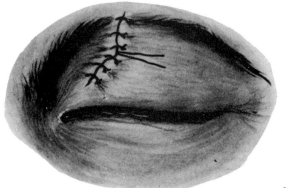

3c

Loss of tissue

Central

4a, b & c

Partial-thickness loss of tissue of the lids may result from injury by cutting instruments, by animal or human bites, by resection of tumours or by burns. Such loss of tissue on or close to the eyelids should be dealt with by application of a skin graft. When the defect is on or close to the lower lid, in the medial canthal or the lateral canthal regions, or in the pretarsal area of the upper lid (the region immediately superficial to the tarsal plate), a full-thickness skin graft should be inserted. The most suitable skin to use, from the point of view of colour, texture and thickness is postauricular. Upper eyelid skin is too thin to produce a satisfactory result, except in the upper lid, and, even if it is available, it is not the best material to use.

Full-thickness skin grafts should be cut to fit the defect so that edge-to-edge apposition is obtained, and there should be no overlapping of graft edges with subsequent necrosis and production of a thicker scar. In the absence of deep scarring such grafts will contract very little, but an additional amount (about 15 per cent) should be inserted to counteract the slight contraction which will take place. The whole graft is put on the stretch by leaving the sutures long and 'overtying' them under slight tension across a pad of cotton wool. The overtied sutures are removed in 1 week, and the graft may be lightly smeared with petroleum jelly or any oily preparation for about a week.

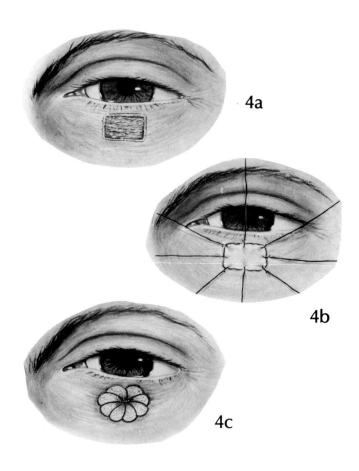

4a

4b

4c

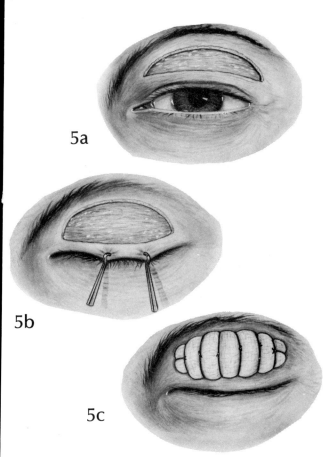

5a

5b

5c

5a, b & c

In the upper lid above the pretarsal zone, loss of tissue should be made good by using a split-skin and not a full-thickness graft. This is because split skin is more supple and will produce the normal eyelid folds more readily than the full thickness of the skin. However, as a skin graft contracts in direct proportion to its thickness the thinner split-skin graft will contract by about a third of its area and additional skin must be inserted, being kept on a slight stretch during healing by tying the sutures joining the graft and the wound edges over a suitably large cottonwool pad.

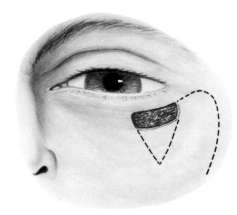

6a

Peripheral

6a–d

If the loss of tissue involves the peripheral parts of the orbit, e.g. the malar prominence, where the skin is thicker and there is a layer of subcutaneous fat, insertion of even a full-thickness skin graft into the defect will result in a sunken appearance of the graft. In resurfacing peripheral areas of the orbit, flaps of skin and subcutaneous tissue should be brought into the site and skin of a similar texture, colour and thickness should be used. Therefore local flaps, such as rotation flaps, should be used wherever possible.

Such flaps are usually obtainable in regions below, lateral to and above the orbit, but if local rotation flaps are not for some reason available a flap may have to be transferred from another area.

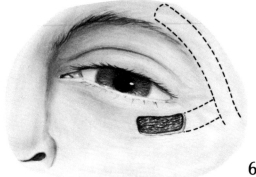

6b

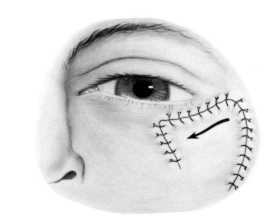

6c

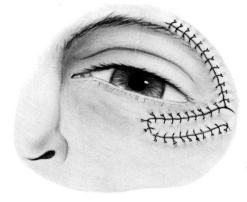

6d

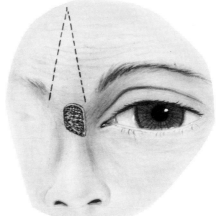

7a

7 & 8

For defects in the peripheral part of the medial canthal region it is best to bring down some skin and sub-cutaneous tissue from the centre of the forehead, either by using the V–Y procedure or by turning down a long flap on a pedicle, the latter being divided after a 2-week interval.

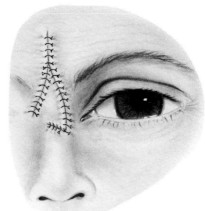

7b

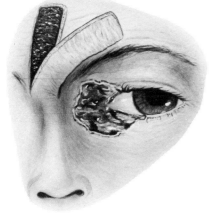

8a

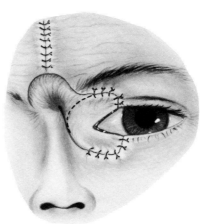

8b

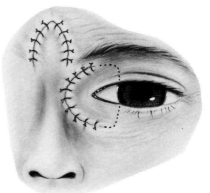

8c

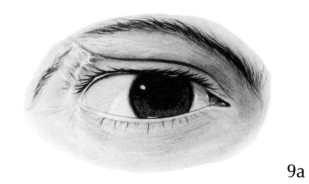

9a

9a, b & c

Scars

Contraction of partial-thickness scars running between the lid margin and the periphery of the orbit may cause the margin to turn out, producing ectropion. Scars of the eyelid skin are seldom thick enough to require excision, and any tight line or scar causing such an ectropion should, after scar contraction has ceased some 6–9 months after injury, be broken up by the use of a Z-plasty confined to the skin. There is seldom troublesome scarring in the orbicularis layer so that it is usually unnecessary to include it in the Z.

Gross superficial scarring of a lid may need to be resected *en bloc*, producing a loss of tissue – which may have been the original clinical condition. The defect is then treated as described above.

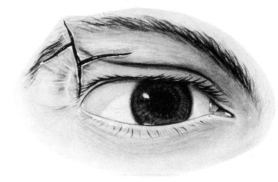

9b

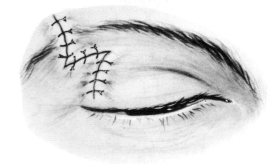

9c

Full-thickness injuries

Wounds

10

Full-thickness injuries of the eyelids caused by cutting instruments may run in any direction but generally speaking they are oblique because the lids are protected from vertical slashes by the more prominent eyebrows and cheeks. With such injuries there is always a possibility that the underlying cornea has been damaged so it must be examined carefully, after inserting a drop of 1 per cent fluorescein.

The essential requirement in closing a full-thickness wound of the eyelid is to re-align the divided tarsal plate. If this alignment is carried out accurately there will be no deformity of the lid margin, but if it is incorrectly carried out a deformity will result no matter what normally unnecessary adjuncts, such as intermarginal sutures, are used.

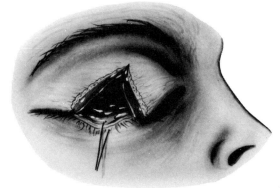

10

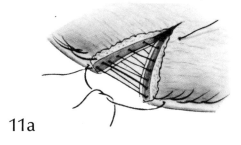

11a

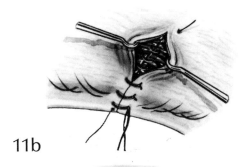

11b

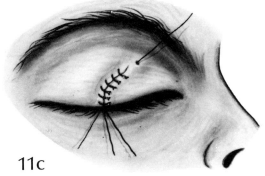

11c

11a, b & c

The two edges of the tarsal plate (and its closely applied layer of conjunctiva) are carefully approximated using a 6/0 running suture of monofilament material such as Prolene, commencing by passing the suture through the skin peripheral to the wound and bringing it out at the top of the conjunctival wound. The suturing is carried over-and-over until the margin is reached. A separate 5/0 silk suture is inserted exactly in the grey line on each side to give accurate approximation of the margin and if need be a similar suture is inserted at the lash line. These sutures are left about 2.5 cm (1 inch) long so that they can be held down onto the lid skin by a square of adhesive and so kept away from the cornea. The skin and orbicularis oculi of the rest of the wound are closed in two layers. Except for the marginal ones, the skin sutures are removed in 5 days. The marginal suture or sutures, as well as the pull-out sutures are removed after a week.

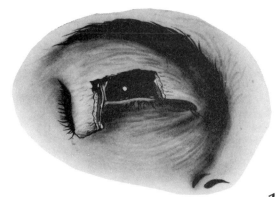

12a

Lacerated wounds

12a, b & c

There is a type of laceration of the eyelids which is caused by a blow on the lid directed away from the nose. If the force is strong enough the lid tears through at its weakest point. In the upper lid this is at first vertically through the large tarsal glands which run up in the tarsal plate. If the force continues, the tear then runs horizontally across the top of the tarsal plate through Müller's muscle and the levator aponeurosis, producing an L-shaped wound. These wounds are closed in layers as already described, but separate continuous, pull-out sutures should be used for the horizontal and the vertical components of the tear.

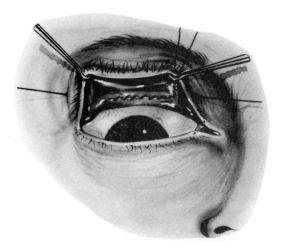

12b

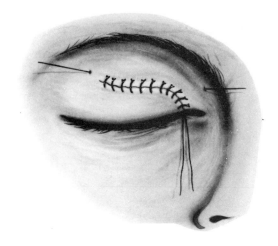

12c

13

In the lower lid the weakest point is where the various heads of the orbicularis oculi are becoming small tendons but have not yet united to form the strong medial canthal tendon. This is 1 or 2 mm medial to the punctum with the result that the lacrimal canaliculus is torn across.

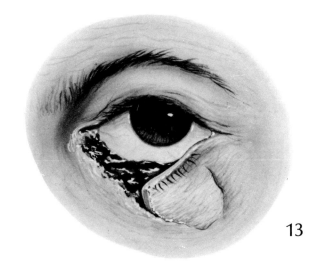

13

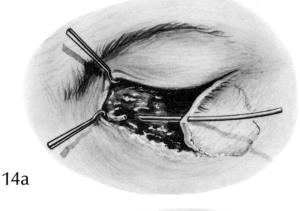

14a

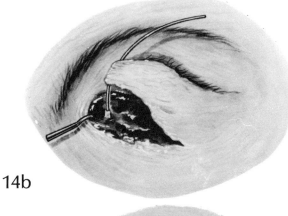

14b

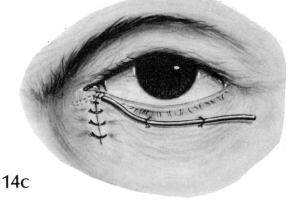

14c

14a, b & c

An attempt must be made at the time of injury to locate the medial divided end of the canaliculus, which usually shows up as a paler structure if normal saline is used to cleanse the wound. A 1 mm silicone tube is passed via the punctum and the peripheral part of the canaliculus into the medial opening and thence into the lacrimal sac. The tube is lashed along the lid margin by sutures, and the conjunctiva is closed with 6/0 chromic catgut. A permanent suture of 5/0 Prolene or nylon is used to approximate the medial end of the tarsal plate to the medial canthal tendon. If this is not done, the powerful action of the orbicularis oculi will drag the lid laterally and the scar will stretch considerably. Finally, the orbicularis muscle is closed with 6/0 chromic catgut and the skin with 5/0 silk or Prolene. The tube is left in place for 2 weeks, and thereafter gentle probing weekly should help to ensure that at least about 60 per cent of these repaired canaliculi will remain patent. Even if the canaliculus does not remain patent, only a small proportion of patients will complain of troublesome epiphora, such as might call for more drastic surgery to produce a channel between the conjunctiva and the lacrimal sac.

Loss of tissue

Full-thickness loss of tissue involving an eyelid may on rare occasions result from an injury such as a bite but is most often due to resection of an eyelid affected by cancer. A through-and-through defect is left which will require full-thickness reconstruction of the eyelid, a subject which is dealt with in the Chapter on 'Reconstruction of eyelid defects', pp. 321–331.

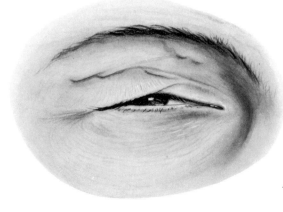

15a

15a–d

Scars

Full-thickness scars of the lids produce centrifugal contraction in all layers of the lid, which becomes notched and is not everted as with partial-thickness scars. It is unusual for the scars themselves to have to to be excised, and once an interval of 6–9 months has elapsed to allow all contraction of the scar to cease, a Z-plasty is carried out through *all* thicknesses of the lid. The various flaps are transposed and sutured in layers, using 6/0 pull-out Prolene to approximate as one layer the conjunctival and tarsal edges; these pull-out sutures are held under light tension by squares of adhesive tape. The orbicularis muscle and the skin are closed in layers as described previously. The skin sutures are removed on the fifth day and the pull-out sutures on the seventh.

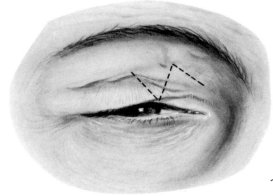

15b

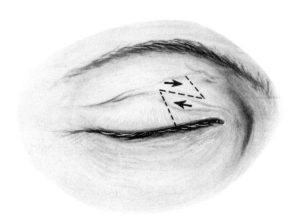

15c

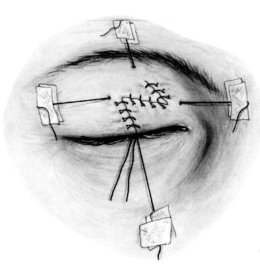

15d

Reconstruction of eyelid defects

John C. Mustardé FRCS, FRCS(Glas.)
Consulting Plastic Surgeon, West of Scotland Regional Plastic Surgery Centre, Canniesburn Hospital, Glasgow, and Royal Hospital for Sick Children, Glasgow, UK

Preoperative

Indications

Reconstruction of full-thickness defects of the eyelids may be required in patients with congenital colobomas or in whom there is a loss of a part, or all, of an eyelid as a result of trauma or following resection for extirpation of a neoplasm. To reconstruct an eyelid it is necessary to provide a mucus-secreting lining and a skin covering layer. Of equal importance is the construction of a stable margin, with mucosa along the border, to avoid any possibility of rubbing on the cornea by the skin layer. Small, wedge-shaped defects of up to a *quarter* of the lid length can be closed directly, perhaps after division of the appropriate crus of the lateral canthal ligament, but in more extensive lid losses a new sector of eyelid tissue must be provided. In the *lower* lid this is done by rotating the lateral part of the eyelid, and the skin overlying the zygomatic region, towards the nose to close the gap. In defects up to a third of the original lid length, lining for the new sector may occasionally be obtained from the conjunctiva of the lateral part of the fornices, but in larger defects lining and tarsus (the latter to prevent sagging) are provided by the use of a free composite graft of mucosa and cartilage taken from the nasal septum. A fringe of mucosa can be turned back over the top edge of the cartilage so as to produce a stable margin.

Defects affecting only the *margin* of the lid may be reconstructed, as far as the skin is concerned, by means of a bipedicle flap of skin from the upper lid.

In the *upper* lid the missing sector of the lid tissue is replaced by turning up a full-thickness wedge of the corresponding lower lid. Repairing the resulting lower lid defect by a cheek rotation is described above. This, of course, provides the all-important stable margin.

Special contraindications

Congenital coloboma should not be corrected until the child is at least 1 year old, as the lid remnants may be very tiny in these patients, but careful watch must be kept to ensure that the cornea is not becoming endangered by drying out. Extensive neoplasms of eyelids, where the pathological process is found to be involving the orbit, must be treated by radical ablation of the orbital contents – and this should include the whole of both eyelids. No reconstruction should be carried out, and a prosthesis should be worn.

Preoperative preparation

An antibiotic cream should be used for a few days to clear up an infected ulcerating lesion where the conjunctiva has become involved. In cases in which it is expected that nasal mucosa and cartilage will be required, the mucosa of the anterior nares should be shrunk and rendered ischaemic by the application of equal parts 10 per cent cocaine and 1:800 000 adrenaline applied either on ribbon gauze or on cottonwool-charged orange sticks for 5 minutes.

Anaesthesia

Local infiltration anaesthesia may be used in closing minor defects where nasal septal cartilage and mucosa will not be used; otherwise general inhalation anaesthesia, using an oral endotracheal tube, is preferable.

Position of patient

The patient should be supine, with a 20° tilt to the table, and the neck itself should be extended. The surgeon stands at the head of the table, or to one or other side of the head. Towelling should be draped to leave the whole of the affected side of the face, including the nose and the cheek (and the ear in extensive cases), exposed. The skin and nostrils are cleansed with 1 per cent aqueous solution of Hibitane.

The operation

THE LOWER LID

1

The incision

The affected sector of the lid is excised in all thicknesses, along with an additional triangle below: at least 5 mm clearance must be given all round the tumour. The line marking the cheek flap is drawn; it should curve upwards above the canthus and then down in front of the ear.

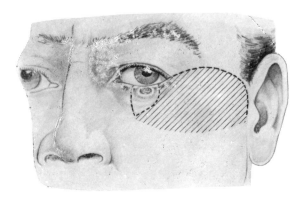

1

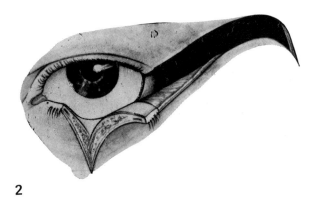

2

2

Splitting of lateral canthal ligament

This is done horizontally, the lower crus being divided from the orbital margin, and any remaining lid margin lateral to the defect is mobilized by dividing the conjunctiva in the lower fornix. A start is made to outline the cheek flap, undermining it thoroughly in the layer of fat beneath the skin as shown in the shaded area in *Illustration 1*. By trial and error it will be found how far the cheek flap must be rotated to allow the lid defect to close.

3

Closure of defect

The defect in the lower lid is closed vertically in three layers, and if there is insufficient conjunctiva in the lower fornix to line the new sector of the lid a free composite graft of mucosa and cartilage from one side of the nasal septum is inserted to provide lining and tarsal plate. The cartilage of the septal graft should be trimmed to about 1.5 mm thickness and should leave a fringe of mucosa exposed around its periphery; the graft is sutured using a pull-out monofilament suture.

The subcutaneous tissue of the cheek flap (point XI) is hitched to the periosteum of the orbital margin above the lateral canthal ligament (point X) with a non-absorbable buried stuture to take the main weight of the cheek flap.

3

4

Closure of cheek wound

The upper edges of the septal graft and the cheek flap are sutured to form the margin of the new lid sector, and the wound in the cheek is closed in two layers, inserting a drain if there has been extensive undermining.

An antibiotic cream is introduced into the lower fornix and a light dressing should be applied for 48 hours over any undermined cheek flap. Where a free septal graft of either mucosa or mucosa and cartilage has been used the whole orbital area should be kept covered by a light pressure dressing for 72 hours.

In total reconstruction of the lower lid the technique is essentially the same, with the exception that no remnants of lid margin will exist to be sutured together and conjunctiva should not be mobilized in the lower fornix.

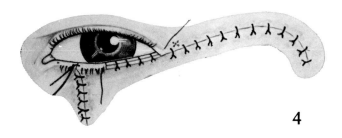

4

Marginal defect of lower lid

Where a defect of the lower lid is confined, or will be confined, to the margin but is extensive in width – for example, following trauma or over-treatment by radiotherapy to marginal lesions – the following procedure may be adopted.

5

Outline of flap

A double-pedicle flap (skin-orbicularis) is outlined in the loose skin in the orbital part of the upper lid.

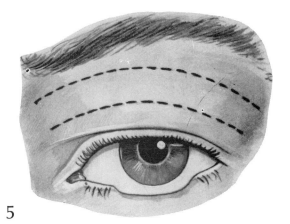

5

6

Undermining of flap

The flap is undermined and, if necessary, the edges of the defect are excised. When the defect is very shallow and adequate conjunctiva can be obtained from the lower fornix, a flap is dissected up to the new lid margin. If the conjunctiva is at all deficient, a free composite graft of nasal septal mucosa and cartilage should be used for lining.

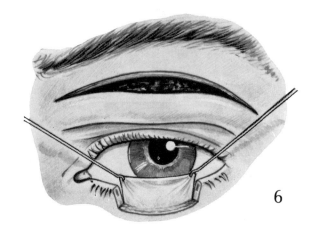

6

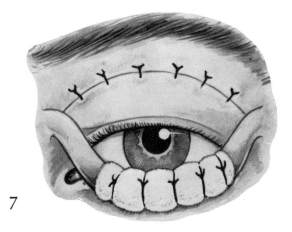

7

7 & 8

Closure of wound

The wound in the upper lid is closed and the flap brought down to be sutured over the lining layer of the new lower lid margin. The sutures may be tied over a roll of cotton wool to prevent the skin flap from curling inwards. Two weeks later the unused pedicles of the flap are returned to the upper lid.

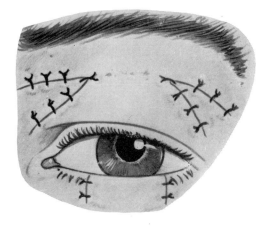

8

THE UPPER LID

Defects of less than half the lid length

9

Excision of tissue

A margin of 5 mm of unaffected tissue is excised with all tumours. A flap of all thicknesses of the lower lid will be rotated up into the defect, and the pedicle of the flap should be sited beneath the midpoint of the defect. The flap should lie on the *lateral* side of the pedicle if possible, to avoid disturbing the drainage apparatus of the lower lid, and its length should be between a half of the defect and a quarter of the normal lid length.

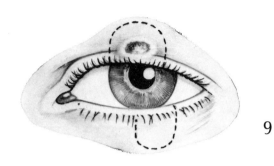

9

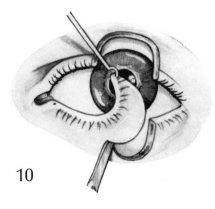

10

10

Dissection of flap

The lower lid flap should be dissected in all its thicknesses, using scalpel and scissors, taking care not to approach closer to the margin in the area of the hinge than 5 mm in order to preserve the comparatively large arcade of marginal vessels running 3 mm from the margin.

11 & 12

Closure of defect

The defect in the lower lid is closed in three layers, thus drawing the base of the lid flap into a position that will allow the flap to lie in the upper lid defect without tension on the hinge. The flap is sutured into the upper lid in three layers – conjunctiva, orbicularis muscle and skin – being careful to avoid damage to the marginal vessel by sutures. No dressing need be applied.

Two weeks later the vascular hinge is divided and the lid margins are revised.

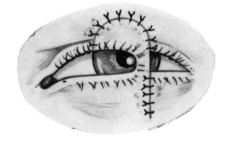

11

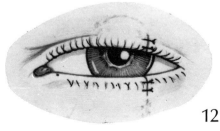

12

Defects of more than half the lid length

13 & 14

Outline of flap

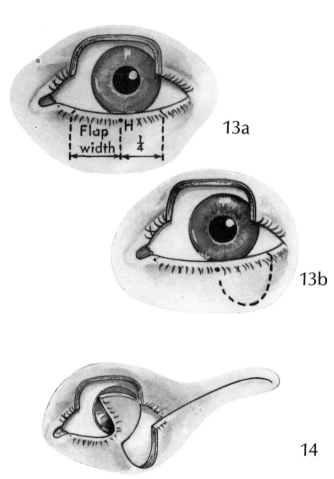

13a

13b

14

Where a defect exists which is greater than a half, the siting of the pedicle and the size of the lower lid flap to be used must be determined in a more accurate manner. The limits of the defects are marked on the lower lid and the equivalent of a quarter of the full lid length is marked off from the *lateral* side. This point indicates the site of the pedicle hinge and the remainder of the marked margin represents the width of the flap to be used to rotate into the defect (the reduction in size of the flap to be used to fill the defect is compensated for by the stretching of the lid tissues).

As in the case of smaller defects, the flap should be outlined on the *lateral* side of the hinge.

The secondary defect which will be created in the lower lid cannot be closed directly as it is over a quarter of the normal lid length and the remaining lid tissues will not stretch to this extent. A cheek flap of suitable size is outline and undermined, as described in lower lid reconstruction.

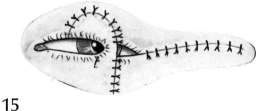

15

15

Closure of defect

The lower lid defect is first closed, lining the small lateral sector of lid constructed from the cheek flap with existing conjunctiva – or nasal septal mucosa where necessary. The lower lid flap is sutured in place, but care must be taken to search for and attach the remnants of the levator muscle to the connective tissue of the lid flap close to the tarsal plate. A light dressing may be applied to the cheek flap for 48 hours to prevent haematoma.

After 2 weeks the vascular hinge is divided and the lid margins reconstructed, as with smaller defects.

TOTAL OR SUBTOTAL DEFECTS

16 & 17

Outline of flap

In very large upper lid reconstructions it will be impossible to locate the lower lid flap on the *lateral* side of the pedicle because it would encroach on the cheek. In such cases it should be retained on the *medial* side of the pedicle hinge.

The lid flap must be carried across on this pedicle towards the nose when the cheek flap is rotated medially to reconstruct the lower lid. The cheek flap should be adequate and should be extensively undermined (as indicated in reconstruction of the lower lid).

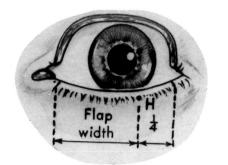

16

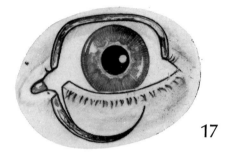

17

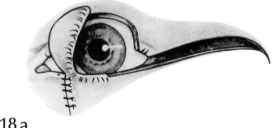

18 a

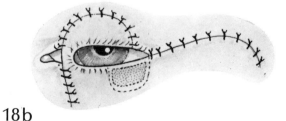

18 b

18a & b

Closure of defect

Lining and tarsus for the new lateral sector of the lower lid should be provided by a free graft of nasal septal cartilage and mucosa, as previously described. The conjunctiva of the upper lid remnant is sutured to the lower lid flap, and the stump of the levator muscle (identified at the time the defect is created) is sutured to the connective tissues of the lid flap to provide elevation. A light pressure dressing is applied for 72 hours over the lower lid and cheek flap, care being taken to avoid pressure on the vascular pedicle of the lid flap.

Two and a half weeks later the pedicle is divided and the lid margins revised.

Note The punctum and canaliculus of the lower lid should always be spared, and the outline of the lower lid flap should be moved a few millimetres laterally to avoid them when necessary.

SIMPLIFIED UPPER LID RECONSTRUCTION (MODIFIED SWITCH FLAP)

Outline of flap

19

If any upper lid remnant is present, the base of the flap should lie on the same side. (Where the upper lid is totally absent, or the defect is central, the base should be on the lateral side.)

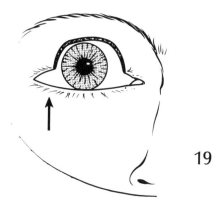

19

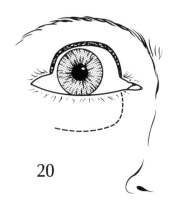

20

20

Avoiding the punctum, a flap long enough to fill the defect is designed on the lower lid. The pedicle is 7–8 mm in width.

21

Inset of flap

The free end of the flap is rotated up and inset into the defect, only as far as this can be done without tension. The levator muscle should also be sutured to the flap as far as possible. All remaining raw edges should be closed temporarily – skin to conjunctiva – to minimize infection and scarring.

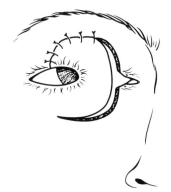

21

22

Completion of upper lid reconstruction

After 2 weeks the pedicle is divided and the rest of the flap is inserted in the upper lid. The remainder of the levator attachment is carried out.

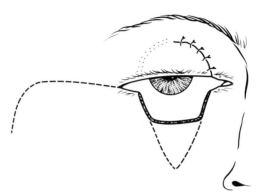

22

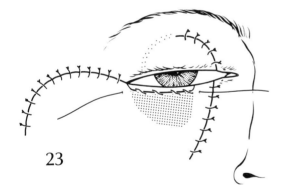

23

23

Reconstruction of lower lid defect

A cheek flap is rotated to close the lower lid defect and the lateral part of the lower lid is reconstructed using a composite graft of nasal septal mucosa and cartilage to provide lining, support and a stable margin.

TOTAL RECONSTRUCTION OF UPPER LID
(MODIFIED SWITCH FLAP)

24

The base of the lower lid flap lies on the lateral side.

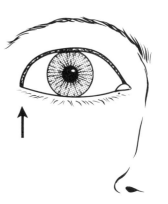

24

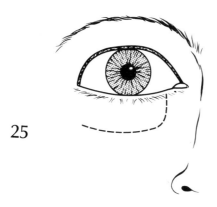

25

25

Three-quarters of the lower lid is raised as a full-thickness flap.

26

The medial end of the flap is inset.

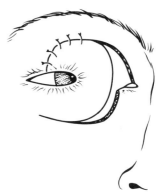

26

27

After 2 weeks the remainder of the lower lid is freed and inset.

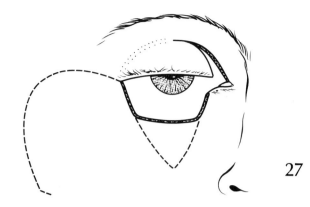

27

28

The full-cheek rotation flap is lined with a chondromucosal graft.

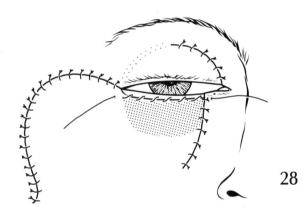

28

Special postoperative care and complications

Lower lid

The dressings, where present, are removed at the times recommended. The lids are cleansed with Hibitane 1 per cent aqueous solution daily and an antibiotic cream applied.

Haematoma beneath the cheek flap must be watched for and dealt with.

All skin sutures are removed at the fifth or sixth day and the monofilament pullout sutures used in closing conjunctival wounds on the sixth day.

The nasal cavity is packed with tulle gras at the time of operation, and this may be removed in 7 days. The septum will shortly heal spontaneously.

Upper lid

Careful planning of the flap of lower lid tissue and exact positioning of the site of the vascular pedicle should eliminate tension on the marginal vessels; but in the event of damage to these a white avascular flap may be produced. Or it may be that, because of undue kinking,

the flap becomes intensely congested; should the colour of the flap not improve in 5 to 6 hours, the whole flap should be released from the upper lid defect and allowed to lie free, in an unrotated position, for several days until a good colour has returned to it. The flap can then be re-inserted into the upper lid defect, and any exposure and drying out of the cornea which might be present during the intervening period can be avoided by covering both lids with a watchglass, which is sealed to the tissues with adhesive tape.

Further reading

Hueston, J. T. Abbe flap techniques in upper eyelid repair. British Journal of Plastic Surgery 1961; 13: 347

Hughes, W. L. Reconstructive Surgery of the Eyelids, London: Kimpton, 1943

Manchester, W. M. Simple method for repair of full thickness defects of lower lid with special reference to treatment of neoplasms. British Journal of Plastic Surgery 1951; 3: 252–263

Mustardé, J. C. Repair and Reconstruction in the Orbital Region, Edinburgh: Livingstone, 1966

Smith, B. Eyelid surgery. Surgical Clinics of North America 1959; 39: 367–378

Illustrations by T. Tarrant from originals by R. Callender

Contraction of the eye socket

John C. Mustardé FRCS, FRCS(Glas.)
Consulting Plastic Surgeon, West of Scotland Regional Plastic Surgery Centre, Canniesburn Hospital, and Royal Hospital for Sick Children, Glasgow, UK

Preoperative

Indications

Contraction of the eye socket is generally a chronic process and in most instances affects the lower fornix first of all. It may continue as a submucosal fibrous tissue reaction until both fornices are affected, and in severe degrees of contraction, the cavity of the socket may be almost obliterated. Treatment involves the enlargement of the affected contracted fornices by insertion of a graft of mucosa or skin.

Preoperative preparation

The socket should be as free from infected discharge as possible and a regimen of instillation of antibiotic eyedrops, such as 10 per cent sulphacetamide sodium (Albucid), thrice daily for a week before operation should be instituted if there is any discharge from the socket.

Anaesthesia

Local infiltration anaesthesia can be used if skin is to be used as a graft material, but if oral mucosa is being used and also in severe degrees of contraction, general inhalation anaesthesia is preferable.

Position of patient

As for reconstruction of eyelids (see p. 321).

The operations

CONTRACTION OF LOWER FORNIX

1

The incision

An incision is made across the whole width of the back of the socket, *not* in the depths of the fornix, so that a flap of conjunctiva may be draped down behind the lid in order to minimize turning in of the lid margin at a later date due to contraction of the inserted graft.

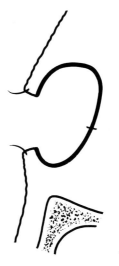

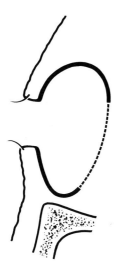

2

Dissection of fornix

Using curved, blunt-pointed scissors, a dissection is made close to the orbital septum of the lower lid and in a direction downwards towards the orbital margin. The free edge of the conjunctiva is draped down behind the lower lid and may be tacked down to the back of the lid in the depths of the dissection.

3

Insertion of graft

If the contraction is moderate, a graft of mucous membrane taken from inside the lower lip may be draped over the lower half of an extra-large prosthesis, and by this means it will be retained in the lower fornix where it will create a deep pocket. The prosthesis should remain in position for a minimum of 6 weeks, but the socket can be irrigated daily around the prosthesis after 1 week in order to keep the socket clean.

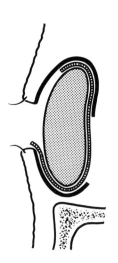

3

Insertion of normal prosthesis

The grafted fornix will be excessively large to begin with after the over-large prosthesis is removed but will contract down fairly rapidly. A blank prosthetic eye of normal size should be used until contraction is complete as there may be some change in the position of the pupil during this process.

4

Retention of prosthesis in severe contraction

If the contraction of the lower fornix is severe a larger graft will be required. In such cases thin split skin from the inner aspect of the arm should be used. It will be necessary to hold the over-large prosthesis or mould to prevent its extrusion as the graft contracts. This is done by incorporating a stainless steel pin in the mould and attaching this by universal joints and bars to an upper oral cap splint, to a pin screwed into the frontal bone at the eyebrow or to a plaster of Paris headcap. Management is otherwise as already described above.

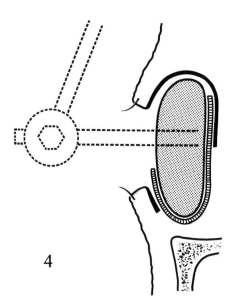

4

CONTRACTION OF UPPER AND LOWER FORNICES

5

The incision

When the contraction involves both upper and lower fornices the incision should be made across the centre of the posterior surface of the socket. It should stretch from canthus to canthus.

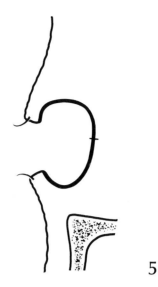

5

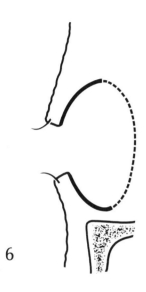

6

6

Dissection of fornices

The lower reflection of conjunctiva and formation of a fornix is carried out as in *Illustration 2*. The upper conjunctival flap is reflected in a similar manner, but care must be taken to avoid damaging the levator muscle.

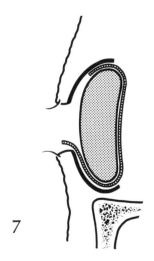

7

7

Insertion of graft

A skin graft is wrapped round a large mould which has a pin incorporated and the mould and graft are inserted into the socket. It may be advantageous to make a lateral incision for 1 cm to split open the lateral canthus in order to facilitate the insertion. This wound is sutured. The pin is attached to a skeletal fixed point as shown in *Illustration 4*.

Removal of large prosthesis

A minimum of 8 weeks should elapse before any attempt is made to remove the large prosthesis (or mould) and fit a normal-sized blank prosthesis. A lateral canthotomy may again be required.

SEVERE TOTAL SOCKET CONTRACTION

8 & 9

Resection of scarred conjunctiva

When contraction of the socket is severe and involves both fornices, for instance following failed socket surgery, the whole of the scarred conjunctiva should be excised to within 2–3 mm of the lid margin.

Dissection of fornices

The fornices are now created as in *Illustration 2* (lower) and *Illustration 6* (upper).

10

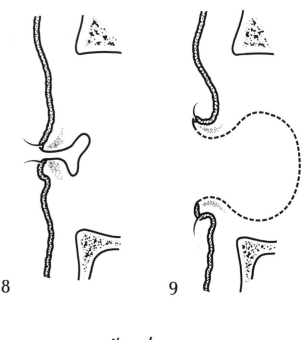

8   9

Insertion of graft

The extra-large prosthesis should be totally covered by skin graft and the free edge of the graft should be gathered together by a 4/0 chromic catgut suture. This will allow the lid margins to be sutured together with a pull-out suture thus burying the graft. A lateral canthotomy will be required. The steel pin which is incorporated (and is fixed to a skeletal point as in *Illustration 4*) should be hollow to permit irrigation through connecting holes in the mould and should be placed at the medial edge so that it will not obstruct formation of a subtotal tarsorrhaphy.

Removal of large prosthesis

This is carried out after 3 months by incising along the line of the tarsorrhaphy and by opening up the canthus as described in *Illustration 7*. If there are more than 2–3 mm of raw surface left on the lids along the margin, a small skin graft should be applied.

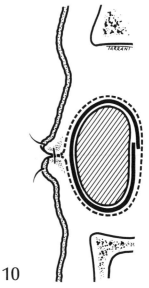

10

Special postoperative care and complications

The socket should be irrigated twice daily, commencing one week after surgery, with a solution containing some mild detergent agent.

In all socket-grafting procedures haemostasis must be complete, otherwise haematoma formation may lead to loss of graft and further contraction. In total reconstruction for severe contraction, irrigation can be carried out by means of the hollow fixation pin. For other cases, a length of fine tubing fixed to a syringe nozzle can be inserted around the prosthesis and irrigation carried out through this.

Continuous redness and inflammation of the lids will indicate the probability that there has been slough of part of the graft due to haematoma. The inflammation should be carefully watched and if becoming obviously worse, the lids must be opened and the granulating area scraped and grafted. The large prosthesis is again inserted but the lids are not sutured.

When the large primary mould which holds the skin graft extended in the socket is removed the initial blank prosthesis should be slightly larger than normal – about midway between the primary mould and the final prosthesis.

The mixture of skin and conjunctiva should not lead to undue socket discharge unless a thick split skin graft has been used, and toilet two or three times a day should keep the socket clean.

Illustrations by Robert N. Lane and T. Tarrant

Ptosis of the upper lid

John C. Mustardé FRCS(Eng.), FRCS(Glas.)
Consulting Plastic Surgeon, West of Scotland Regional Plastic Surgery Centre, Canniesburn Hospital, and Royal Hospital for Sick Children, Glasgow, UK

Preoperative

Indications

In congenital ptosis, levator muscle function may vary from good to clinically undetectable. Except in the latter case, conventional shortening of levator structures by an anterior or a posterior approach may improve the function of the muscle. The anterior approach is simpler, especially in severe cases, but leaves a visible scar: 4 mm of aponeurosis is resected for every 1 mm of ptosis. In paralytic ptosis the upper lid is hitched to the frontalis muscle by fascia lata or other substances.

The author's own more recently developed technique of ptosis surgery, involving preservation of the whole levator muscle complex and especially the sympathetically innervated Müller's muscle, is described after the conventional techniques.

Special contraindications

Where a squint is present, this should be dealt with before the ptosis to avoid diplopia. In third cranial nerve palsy the eye is turned downwards and outwards, and the cornea may remain exposed if the eyelid is raised before the position of the eye is corrected. Absence of Bell's phenomenon – by which the eye rolls upward during sleep – is a contraindication to operation in paralytic ptosis.

Preoperative preparation

Some surgeons cut the lashes short, but this is quite unnecessary; the eyebrow should never be shaved.

Anaesthesia

Local infiltration anaesthesia, with instillation of 4 per cent cocaine into the conjunctival sac, may be used in adults (unless fascia lata must be obtained from the thigh), but in children general inhalation anaesthesia is essential, using an oral endotracheal tube.

Position of patient

The patient should be supine with the neck extended. The surgeon stands directly above the head of the patient and towels are draped to leave the forehead, eyes and nose exposed. The skin is cleansed with 1 per cent aqueous solution of Hibitane.

337

The operation

POSTERIOR APPROACH

1 & 2

Insertion of sutures

A silk traction suture (omitted in subsequent illustrations for clarity) is inserted into the proposed highest point of the upper lid margin and, by traction on this, the lid is everted over a suitable instrument such as Desmarre's (or the author's own) retractor. The conjunctiva is ballooned off from the underlying superior tarsal muscle by injection of 1:80 000 adrenaline in saline or 1 per cent local anaesthetic.

The conjunctiva is incised in a curving line immediately proximal to the superior edge of the tarsal plate and is carefully dissected away from the superior tarsal muscle. Three double-armed 4/0 white silk sutures are inserted in mattress fashion from the raw surface.

Once the conjunctiva has been completely dissected free from the superior tarsal (Müller's) muscle and the underlying levator aponeurosis, these latter are picked up at two sites (X – X) 3–4 mm from the superior edge of the tarsus and about 7 mm on each side of the line of the traction suture. The tissues so grasped are held by 4/0 silk sutures (black to distinguish them) which are knotted (*inset*).

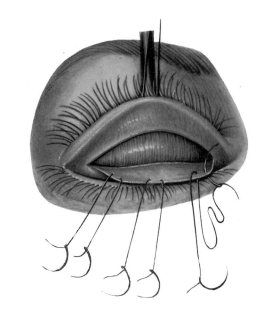

1

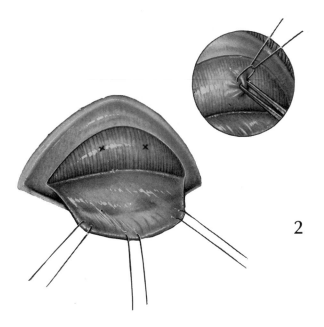

2

3

Separation of layers

Using these black sutures for traction, the superior tarsal muscle and levator aponeurosis are separated from the tarsal plate with a scalpel (some surgeons prefer to hold the muscle in a clamp which is passed beneath it before sectioning).

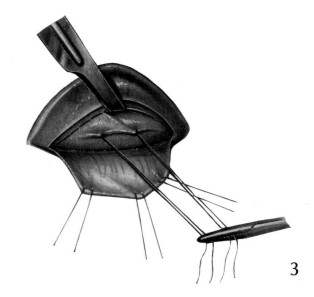

3

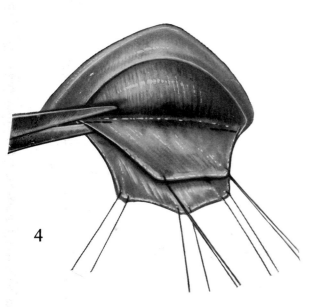

4

Division of aponeurosis

4

Blunt dissection with scissors, in the layer between the levator structures and the orbital septum, will allow the former to be drawn down as a separate sheet, but the fibrous lateral and medial horns of the aponeurosis must be divided to permit full and free extension.

When this has been done the elastic recoil of the levator muscle can usually be demonstrated.

5

Resection of aponeurosis and muscle

The amount of aponeurosis and muscle to be resected having been calculated (4 mm must be deducted from the total to account for the tissue lying between the black silk traction sutures and the final line of section of the tarsal plate), an indicating mark is made on the muscle in line with the margin stuture, and the central double-armed white suture is brought up through the levator muscle at this spot, embracing 3–4 mm of muscle. The other two white sutures are passed through the levator, but should be 2–3 mm closer to the peripheral cut edge to provide a curve to the lid. The excess muscle and aponeurosis are excised as shown by the dotted line.

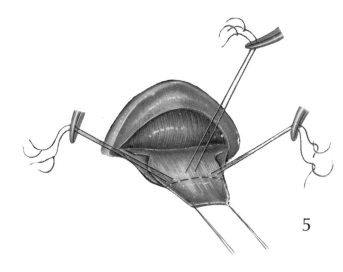

5

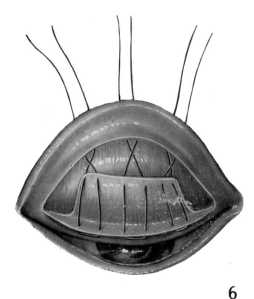

6

6

Excision of superior tarsal border

A narrow strip of the superior tarsal border, 1.5 mm in width, is excised (not shown in illustration) to provide firm attachment for the levator muscle. Each double-armed suture is crossed over to grasp the muscle more tightly, and the points of the needles, having been inserted through, or close to, the cut edge of the tarsal plate, are brought out through the skin of the lid.

7

Closure

The double-armed sutures are brought on to the surface of the skin so that one end is about 6 mm and the other, vertically above it, about 8 mm from the lid margin. The ends are tied firmly over a short length of rubber tubing or a catheter, 3 mm in diameter. The level of the lid should lie just above the centre of the pupil at the end of the operation. The lower lid is drawn up to protect the cornea by means of a suture inserted at the centre of the margin and which after antibiotic ointment is inserted, is fixed with adhesive to the forehead. The traction stitch in the upper lid margin is removed.

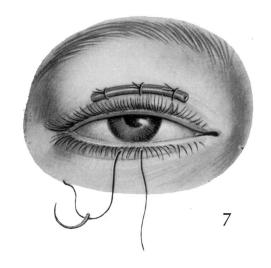

7

ANTERIOR APPROACH

8

The incision

The upper lid is grasped in suitable forceps or held by a traction suture. An incision is made through the skin along the line of the lid fold (as determined from the normal side) and the incision is deepened into the orbicularis muscle, by a spreading action, with scissors.

The muscle is gently dissected upwards and downwards from the orbital septum for a distance of several millimetres and is retracted. The exposed orbital septum is divided in the same line and is similarly retracted, revealing the levator aponeurosis.

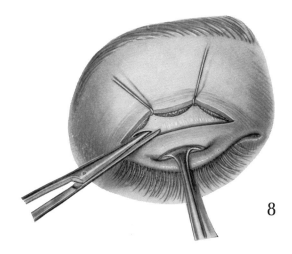

8

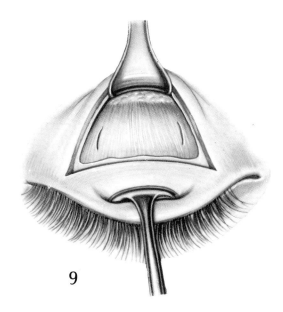

9

9

Separation of orbital septum

The orbital septum is separated upwards from the levator aponeurosis for 20–25 mm and two small vertical incisions are made through the levator, superior tarsal muscle and conjunctiva, into the upper fornix. These incisions should be at either extremity of the tarsal plate and immediately above it.

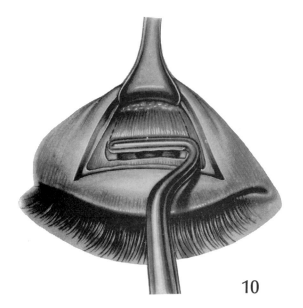

10

10 & 11

Introduction of muscle clamp

A ptosis muscle clamp is passed through these incisions to grasp the tissues, and all three structures are divided along the distal edge of the clamp immediately proximal to the tarsal plate and again vertically from either end of the clamp (as in the dotted lines) for some 15 mm. The composite flap is turned upwards and the conjunctiva is carefully stripped away from the superior tarsal muscle, leaving a small fringe within the grasp of the muscle clamp. The levator structures are dissected from the orbital septum on one surface and from conjunctiva on the other, and, when the lateral horns are severed at each side, they can be freely drawn down. Orbital fat may tend to herniate between the arcus marginalis of the septum and the levator, but it should not be excised unless it is troublesome, to avoid a hollow appearance of the lid postoperatively.

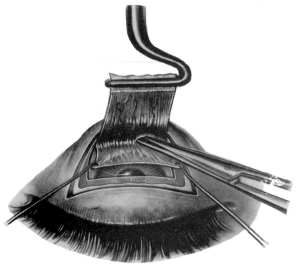

11

12

Suture of conjunctival flap

The conjunctival flap is sutured to the conjunctiva at the edge of the tarsal plate. The amount of levator to be resected is marked, and three 4/0 catgut sutures are used to anchor the levator at this level to the surface of the tarsal plate 4 mm below (distal to) the exposed upper edge. The excess levator tissue is excised.

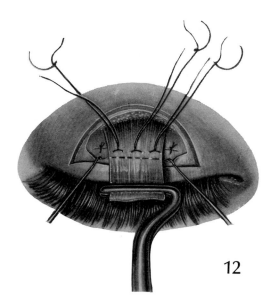

12

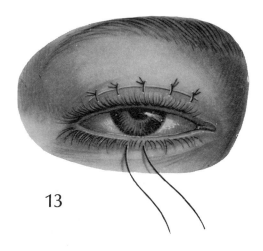

13

13

Closure

The skin and orbicularis muscle are closed by four or five 5/0 silk sutures which are passed right through all layers of the lid into the upper fornix in order to anchor the skin to the levator structures and so produce a lid fold. A suture in the lower lid margin permits the lower lid to be raised to protect the cornea.

FRONTALIS–TARSUS SLING

14

Incisions

Two small stab wounds are made within the eyebrow, 12 mm from a small central incision which is carried down close to the underlying periosteum. A curved central incision, 1.5 cm long, is made through skin and orbicularis muscle 8–10 mm above the lash line, depending on the age of the patient.

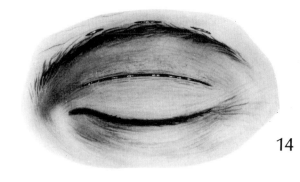

14

15

Fixation of fascia

The lower flap of skin and muscle is dissected away for 3–4 mm from the tarsal plate, and a strip of autogenous fascia lata, 3 mm wide and 15 mm long, is sutured to the anterior surface of the tarsus using 6/0 non-absorbable monofilament nylon or Prolene at two points, 8 mm apart and 5 mm above the lash line.

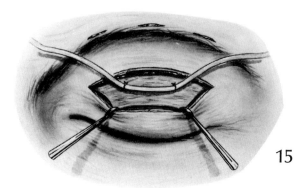

15

16

16

Connection to frontalis

The ends of the fascia are threaded on wide-eyed needles and passed up through the lid to emerge from the medial and lateral stab wounds. They are then passed back through the latter and emerge at the central wound where they are tied tightly enough to raise the lid margin to 1 mm above mid-pupil level. The knot is secured by a 6/0 nylon suture and buried deep in the wound. As the fascia is threaded vertically in the lid it should lie between the orbicularis muscle and the deeper orbital septum, except at the upper margin of the pretarsal lid wound where it should pick up a small portion of orbicularis muscle so as to anchor the wound edge to the tarsus and produce a supratarsal sulcus.

17

Closure

The skin wounds are closed with 6/0 catgut which need not be removed as it sloughs off in about 3 weeks. A traction (Frost) suture is inserted into the lower lid to lift it up for 24 hours.

17

SPLIT LEVEL LID RESECTION (MUSTARDÉ)
(For moderate ptosis with 7 mm or more levator action)

18

Superficial resection

An ellipse of skin and underlying orbicularis muscle is resected from the upper lid. It should be about 6–8 mm in width, depending on the age of the patient, and should extend along and above the line of the upper edge of the tarsal plate (i.e. 8–10 mm from the lash line at its centre), almost from canthus to canthus.

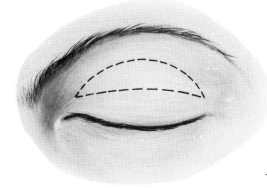

18

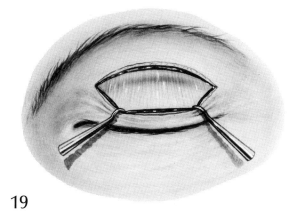

19

19

Exposure of tarsus

The skin and muscle is dissected free from the anterior surface of the tarsal plate almost to the lash line.

20

Conjunctival-tarsal resection

The lid is everted over a lid spatula and, apart from a strip 3 mm wide at the lid margin, the whole of the tarsal plate with overlying conjunctiva is resected.

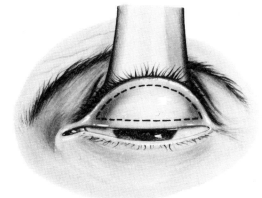

20

21

A full-thickness ellipse of the lid has now been resected, but at two levels in order to preserve the blood supply to the margin.

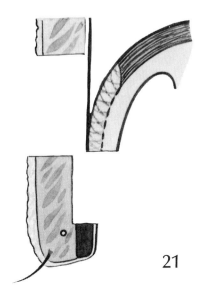

21

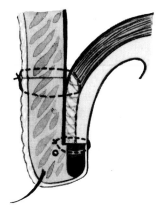

22

22

Closure

Finally, 6/0 catgut sutures are inserted through the free edge of the triple layer of levator aponeurosis, Müller's muscle and conjunctiva and then are carried back through the remainder of the conjunctival-tarsal plate at the margin. The skin sutures, also of 6/0 catgut, pick up the underlying levator aponeurosis so as to create a supratarsal fold. These sutures will gradually slough away and need not be removed.

SPLIT LEVEL RESECTION WITH LEVATOR HITCH (MUSTARDÉ)
(For severe ptosis with less than 7 mm levator action)

Initial steps

This operation is commenced exactly as for split-level lid resection described above but at the stage shown in *Illustration 19* the orbital septum is divided above its junction with the levator aponeurosis, so as to free the latter from it. When the lid is everted over the spatula, as in *Illustration 20*, the conjunctiva is incised immediately above the tarsal plate and separated from the underlying Müller's muscle for about 8–10 mm. This conjunctival flap is resected.

23

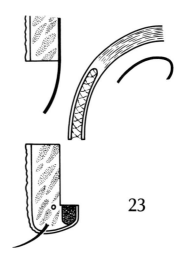

23

Isolation of levator complex

After resection of the tarsal plate the levator complex, comprising the levator aponeurosis with the closely applied Müller's muscle on its undersurface, now lies completely free inferiorly and can be drawn gently forward to expose the levator muscle.

24

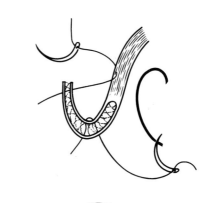

Formation of levator loop

Three small mattress sutures of 6/0 chromic catgut are passed through the levator complex from its undersurface so as to establish a hinge about which the lower end of the complex can be turned up and sutured on to itself. The mattress sutures are placed 5 mm from the free edge if there is 4–7 mm of levator action, but at 8–9 mm from the edge if there is less levator function than 4 mm. The free lower edge of the levator complex is sutured to levator muscle under slight tension.

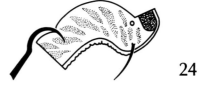

24

25

Closure

The three mattress sutures now pick up the cut edge of the conjunctiva above and the edge of the tarsal remnant below and are tied so that the knots will be buried in the tissues. The skin wound is closed with 6/0 chromic catgut sutures which pick up the underlying levator complex or its plication. As before, the sutures will not require removal.

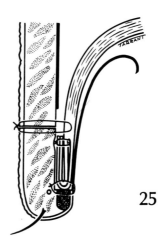

25

Special postoperative care

Unless there is much oedema present, or in the case of very young children, dressings and bandages are not required. The lower lid suture may be relaxed after 48 hours but, until it is seen that the cornea is being covered during sleep, the suture must be fixed again to the forehead each evening. Antibiotic cream is inserted between the lids twice daily.

In the posterior approach operation the mattress sutures over the tubing should not be removed before 12 days, but in the anterior approach technique and in the frontalis-sling operation, the sutures can be removed in 6 days.

Very rarely, it may be obvious shortly after operation that there has been an excessive degree of levator shortening, and in these cases firm traction on the upper lid, after injection of local anaesthetic into it, will allow the levator insertion to be torn away sufficiently to overcome the overcorrection. Treatment must be carried out early and with moderation.

In all cases of ptosis repair the final improved muscle function will not be fully obvious until 3–4 weeks after operation.

Further reading

Berke, R. N. Blepharoptosis. In: Hughes, W. L. ed. Ophthalmic plastic surgery. Rochester, Minnesota: American Academy of Ophthalmology, 1964

Iliff, C. E. Surgical management of ptosis. Somerville, N. J.: Ethicon, 1963

Jones, L. T. The anatomy of the upper eyelid and its relation to ptosis surgery. American Journal of Ophthalmology 1964; 57: 943–959

Mustardé, J. C. The treatment of ptosis and epicanthal folds. British Journal of Plastic Surgery 1959; 12: 252–258

Mustardé, J. C. Ptosis: epicanthus and telecanthus In: Mustardé, J. C. Repair and reconstruction in the orbital region. Edinburgh: Livingstone, 1966

Mustardé, J. C. Problems and possibilities in ptosis surgery. Plastic and Reconstructive Surgery 1975; 56: 381–388

Mustardé, J. C. The orbital region. In: Mustardé, J. C. ed. Plastic surgery in infancy and childhood, 2nd edn. Chapter X. Edinburgh: Churchill Livingstone, 1978: pp. 221–259

Rycroft, B. W. Blepharoptosis – congenital and traumatic – the transconjunctival and transcutaneous approach of levator resection in the treatment of ptosis. In: Troutman, R. C., Converse, J. M., Smith, B. eds. Plastic and reconstructive surgery of the eye and adnexa. Washington: Butterworths, 1962

Eyelid burns

A. J. Evans FRCS
Consultant Plastic Surgeon, Westminster Hospital, London,
Queen Mary's Hospital, Roehampton, and Croydon General Hospital, UK

Preoperative

Eyelid burns usually occur as part of a facial burn. Fortunately most thermal injuries in this area tend to be superficial or at worst deep dermal, whether due to scalding accidents in children or brief exposure to flash or flame in adults. The deepest burns are encountered in the unconscious patient, classically the epileptic or alcoholic, or when the victim is trapped in a burning building or vehicle.

Initial examination

The eyes should be inspected as soon as possible before swelling of the lids makes this difficult or impossible. Gross oedema of the lax tissues of the eyelids will be found in quite superficial burns, or even when the lids themselves are spared in a facial burn. In deep burns with coagulation in depth of the tissues little swelling can occur but the conjunctiva may be everted over the eyelid margins.

Early treatment

Burns of the face and eyelids are best treated by exposure and a dry coagulum develops quite rapidly. After oedema has subsided lid closure may become incomplete and the cornea should be protected by the frequent application of chloramphenicol ointment.

The coagulum of the superficial burn will start to separate at about 12–14 days postburn and in the deeper burn necrotic tissue should be excised at about the 14th day. The resulting raw areas will require a thin split-skin graft cover to secure healing but no attempt is made at this point to correct the developing ectropion. About 3 or 4 weeks later when stable healing has occurred, formal onlay grafting can be carried out on the upper eyelids. The lower lids can be left safely until later as they are not involved in the important task of covering the cornea. Upper and lower lids should never be repaired at the same time as this does not permit the necessary over-correction of the skin shortage.

Tarsorrhaphy is rarely necessary in the management of eyelid burns but may be indicated when part of the whole thickness of the upper eyelid has been destroyed.

Repair of upper eyelid

A thin split-skin graft is essential in this repair to permit elevation of the lid. Thin grafts shrink considerably and over-correction is therefore necessary to allow for this.

1

Two skin hooks, with points directed away from the cornea, exert downward traction on the eyelid margin. With a No.15 blade an incision is made 2mm from the eyelashes and carried medially for 1.5cm on to the side of the nose and laterally for about 2cm beyond the outer canthus.

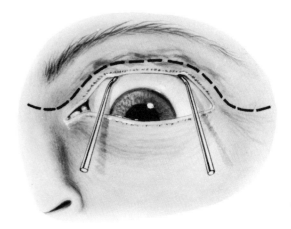

2

With the knife at an angle, undermining is carried out away from the lid margin to free the underlying tethered orbicularis muscle from the contracted scar tissue.

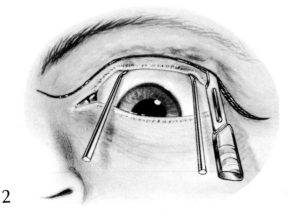

3

This process is continued, with scissor dissection of any deep scar bands, until gross over-correction is achieved with wide overlap of the upper lid over the lower. Silk sutures (4/0) are inserted along the margins of the defect and are left long.

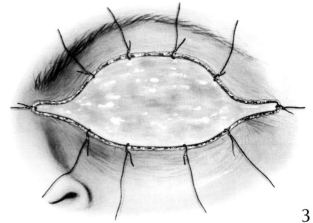

4

Dental stent is softened in hot water and a sausage-shaped portion is moulded into the defect, the long sutures bringing the margins up over the edge of the mould. After hardening in cold water the mould is conveniently spiked on a No.11 blade and a thin split-skin graft, preferably taken from the hairless inner aspect of the upper arm, is then draped, raw surface outwards, over the mould. Mastisol may be painted over the surface of the mould to help the graft adhere.

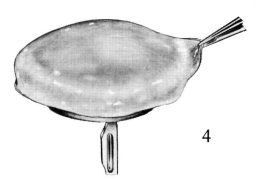

4

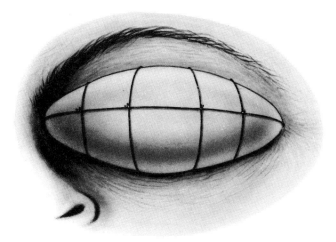

5

5

The long sutures are tied over the mould to hold the skin graft firmly against the raw surface of the eyelid. Small grooves are cut in the surface of the mould to prevent the sutures from slipping.

Chloramphenicol ointment is instilled into the eye and a pad and bandage are applied.

Postoperative care

The mould is kept in place for 7 days and then removed by cutting through the tie-over sutures. It is extremely rare for graft loss to occur.

Contraction of the grafted lid follows fairly quickly, and, although the early over-correction appears grotesque, the lid margin reaches its normal level in 2–3 weeks.

In deeper burns with some loss of orbicularis fibres contraction may continue, and the operation may have to be repeated after 3–4 months.

Repair of lower eyelid

The lower eyelid has a static role to play and is best repaired with a full-thickness Wolfe graft. The postauricular area provides the best colour and texture match.

6

Two skin hooks, with points directed away from the cornea, exert upward traction on the eyelid margin. With a No.15 blade an incision is made 2mm from the eyelashes and carried about 1cm beyond each canthus.

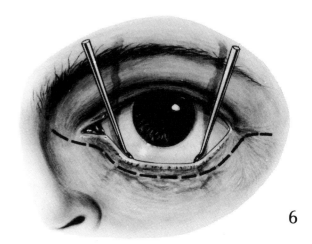

6

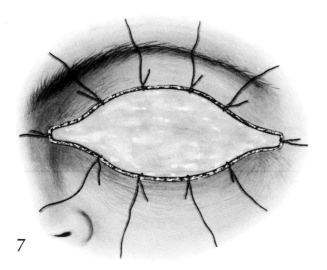

7

7

Undermining is carried out away from the lid margin until the eyelid is completely freed from scar tissue. Silk sutures (4/0) are inserted along the margins of the defect and are left long.

8

A pattern is made of the raw area in jaconet, transferred to the back of the ear and outlined in ink. The ear is held forward by a traction suture through the rim and the graft dissected free with a No.15 blade.

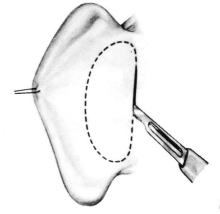

8

9

The postauricular defect is closed with a subcuticular nylon or catgut suture.

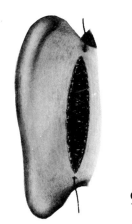

9

10

The graft is accurately sutured into the defect with 5/0 silk sutures and the long 4/0 sutures are then tied over paraffin-flavine pressure wool.

Chloramphenicol ointment is instilled into the eye and a pad and bandage are applied.

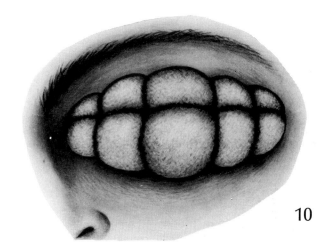

10

Postoperative care

After 7 days the tie-over sutures are cut through and the pressure-wool pack lifted off. Sutures around the periphery of the graft and the postauricular suture, if of nylon, are also removed.

Contraction of the graft is rare, but recurrence of ectropion may occur if there is much heavy scarring of the cheek below the graft. Further insertion of skin at eyelid margin level may then be needed, whether or not the cheek is to be repaired.

Editor's note

The vital importance of ensuring adequate corneal cover in facial burns cannot be over-emphasized. War experience has shown that sight is far more commonly endangered by corneal exposure from eyelid destruction than by burning of the globe itself. The grafting of eyelid burns, therefore, has first priority in the treatment of the facial burn, and, should corneal exposure occur early, it may be necessary to intervene before the coagulum spontaneously separates.

Illustrations by Kevin Marks

Blepharoplasty

Bernard L. Kaye MD, DMD
Clinical Professor of Surgery (Plastic), University of Florida College of Medicine, Jacksonville, Florida, USA

Preoperative

Indications

Aesthetic blepharoplasty is indicated for correction of one or more of the following eyelid deformities:

1. excess eyelid skin and muscle;
2. protrusions of fatty compartments against a weakened orbital septum ('bags'); and
3. hypertrophy of lower lid orbicularis muscle causing the appearance of transverse bulging near the ciliary margin at rest, or when the patient partially closes the eyes forcefully ('squinches' – Oxford English Dictionary).

Other special indications include the oriental eyelid and the exophthalmic eyelid, topics which are beyond the scope of this chapter but are well covered elsewhere[1,2].

Preoperative evaluation

Preoperative evaluation is not confined to the anatomical deformities, but also includes evaluation of visual acuity, visual fields, tear production, fundus examination and other examinations which may be done by the operating surgeon or by an ophthalmologist. General health as well as the patient's goals and attitudes must also be taken into consideration[3].

Choice of anaesthesia

Blepharoplasty may be performed under local or general anaesthesia. Although we do most of our blepharoplasties under local anaesthesia with sedation, we prefer general endotracheal anaesthesia supplemented with local anaesthetic containing adrenaline for patients who are very apprehensive, for severe cases of fatty protrusion and for prolonged procedures, when blepharoplasty is done with other facial operations. General anaesthesia provides advantages of complete patient comfort and improved blood oxygenation. The surgeon can work more rapidly and efficiently because the anaesthetist assumes responsibility for the overall care of the patient, allowing the surgeon to concentrate on the surgery[4].

The operation may be done as an outpatient or in-hospital procedure. All outpatients are required to remain under observation for at least 3 hours postoperatively.

Preparation

An intravenous infusion is started through a large vein (usually the anticubital vein) with a large-bore angiocatheter, for delivery of fluids and intravenous medications. Patients are monitored with a cardiac monitor and an automatic blood pressure monitor. We use benzalkonium chloride (Zephiran) and isopropyl alcohol as our skin cleansing agents, taking care to prevent these solutions from getting in the eyes. Surgical draping exposes the entire face.

Administration of local anaesthesia

If the operation is done under local anaesthesia we use mepivacaine (Carbocaine) 2 per cent with adrenaline 1:100 000 because of the rapid onset of anaesthesia. It is infiltrated with a 1 ml glass tuberculin syringe equipped with metal finger rings and a 30 gauge disposable needle for maximum delicacy of control and minimum patient discomfort. The addition of hyaluronidase (Wydase) 1 ml (150 turbidity-reducing units) per 5 ml of anaesthesia solution hastens the onset of anaesthesia and vasoconstriction, but it also shortens the duration of anaesthesia. Near the end of the operation we infiltrate with bupivacaine (Marcaine) 0.5 per cent with adrenaline. This infiltration is usually painless because anaesthesia is still present from the mepivacaine. Bupivacaine, because of the prolonged duration of anaesthesia, decreases or prevents postoperative pain for a long time. We do not use it initially, only because of prolonged onset of anaesthesia.

Preoperative medication

We have abandoned our previous practice of administering multiple preoperative medications intramuscularly or orally at some fixed time prior to the operation. Instead, all preoperative medication is given intravenously immediately before the procedure. If the operation is being done under local anaesthesia, we use diazepam (Valium) titrated in 0.5 ml (2.5 mg) increments until the patient is adequately sedated, supplementing the initial sedative dose with additional 0.5 ml increments of diazepam as needed during the procedure. If the operation is to be done under general anaesthesia, the anaesthetist gives the preoperative medication intravenously just before fully anaesthetizing the patient. We have found that gradual titration of premedication drugs by the intravenous route is safer and more reliable than giving a fixed intramuscular dose at a specific time preoperatively.

The operation

To minimize the duration of corneal exposure, our sequence of procedures is first to do all of the lower lid blepharoplasty except the skin-muscle trim, then do the entire upper lid blepharoplasty and, finally, return to the lower lid to trim the skin-muscle flap and close the lower lid.

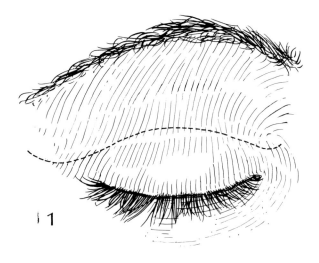

1

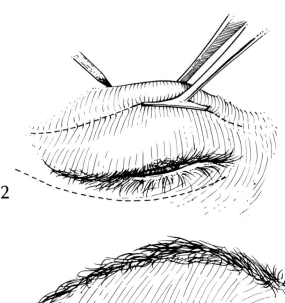

2

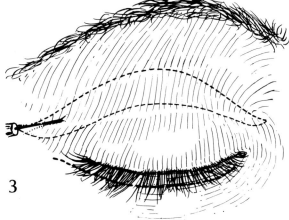

3

Infiltration of the lower lid includes the lateral canthal region, the inferior border of the lower lid, and the area just below the ciliary margin, where the incision will be made. The subciliary margin infiltration must be done very slowly to minimize patient discomfort.

1

In the upper lid the incision lines are marked prior to infiltration to avoid distortion. The inferior incision line is usually made in the natural tarsal fold if the crease is sufficiently cephalad to the ciliary margin. If the crease is low, we mark arbitrarily the inferior incision line approximately 10 mm cephalad to the ciliary margin. The level of the superior incision line depends on the amount of excess upper lid skin, and how much of the apparent skin ptosis is due to excess upper lid skin as opposed to ptosis of the forehead and eyebrows. If there is severe overhang of skin lateral to the external canthus, it is more likely to be due to brow ptosis rather than excess upper lid skin, and should be treated with a forehead lift[5]. Too frequently we have seen patients who were treated for this problem by upper lid blepharoplasty. A forehead lift with or without an upper lid blepharoplasty would have been a more appropriate operation.

2 & 3

The location of the superior upper lid incision is determined by gently pinching the excess skin horizontally with smooth Adson forceps or T-shaped Green forceps. The lid should close completely when the excess skin is pinched between the jaws of the forceps. We rarely make the superior skin incision line higher than half the distance between the inferior incision line and the lower margin of the eyebrows. If, after marking the planned upper lid skin excision to this level, there is still excess upper lid tissue, a forehead-brow lift should be considered. The superior and inferior upper lid incision lines are joined medially and laterally, outlining the area of upper lid skin to be excised, and the upper lid is then infiltrated with local anaesthetic solution.

The lower lid incision is marked, starting medially just below the lacrimal punctum, about 2 mm caudal to the ciliary margin, and continued laterally 2 mm below and parallel to the ciliary margin, until just below the lateral canthus. The marking line is then carried slightly superiorly and laterally into one of the natural crow's feet wrinkles, preferably one that extends in a horizontal direction, for 2–4 mm, depending on the amount of excess skin.

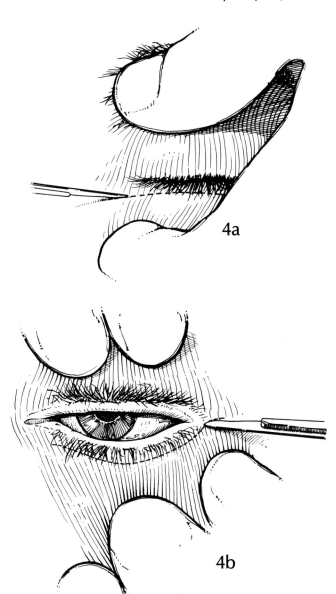

4a

4a & b

To cut this incision effectively, the lower lid skin must be stretched caudally by using the fingers of the non-dominant hand. For the right lower lid a right-handed surgeon can use his left hand crossed over his right, instrument-holding hand to stretch down the lower lid skin (a). For the left lower lid, the same surgeon can apply left-handed caudal traction without crossing over and covering his instrument-holding hand, making his incision in full view of the assistant (b).

4b

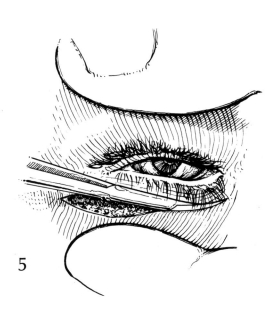

5

5

The skin incision is started lateral to the lateral canthus with a No. 15 blade. It is continued medially with curved blepharoplasty scissors (Storz N5066 or Stille 6202-10) below the ciliary margin to a point just caudal to the punctum. To avoid cutting the lower eyelashes the rounded points of blepharoplasty scissors are inclined slightly into the skin, pushing the cilia away from the skin with the outer edges of the blade.

6

The most important holding suture of the lower lid procedure is now inserted. This is a 6/0 Prolene suture inserted through the centre of the ciliary margin, not tied, and left long. The ends are clamped with a small needle-holder or haemostat and allowed to drape backwards and downwards over the forehead and scalp region. This weighted traction suture provides excellent cephalad counter-traction on the ciliary margin of the lower lid. It also protects the cornea by drawing the lower lid up over it.

After making the skin incision we do the rest of the dissection almost entirely with a battery-powered blue Concept cautery*[6]. This low-powered thermal cautery reduces bleeding significantly by giving off just enough heat to penetrate the orbicularis muscle and dissect the periorbital tissues without sparking or damaging adjacent structures, providing it is applied for very brief periods of time (less than one-second sweeps for dissection; less than 4 seconds for coagulation of stumps of fat compartments, as they are held in haemostats which act as heat sinks). The location of the actuating button, very near to the working tip of the instrument, allows the instrument to be held very close to its tip, with maximum precision of motion and minimum leverage, unlike the larger, more powerful and unwieldy electrosurgical instruments.

Once the skin has been incised an incision is made through the orbicularis muscle with the Concept cautery, parallel to the skin incision and 1–2 mm caudal to it, thereby creating a small step in the incision. Once the deep side of the orbicularis is reached, the skin-muscle flap can be elevated easily and quickly.

We use the skin-muscle flap technique exclusively for our lower lid blepharoplasties[7]. The results from this method are indistinguishable from those obtained by the more difficult skin-flap technique[8]. Moreover, the orbicularis muscle is intimately adherent to the overlying skin, and it is logical to treat both as a single layer.

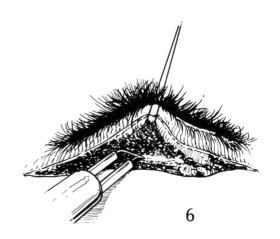

6

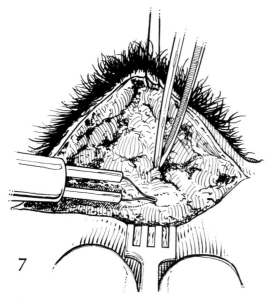

7

* The Concept ACCU-Temp Surgical Cautery, catalog No 4200, may be obtained from Concept Inc, 12707 US 19 South Clearwater, Florida 33516, USA

7

A practical aid to dissection at this point is to have the assistant provide traction on the superior edge of the skin-muscle flap in two directions simultaneously: anteriorly (ventrally) away from the globe, with a small rake retractor; and caudally by drawing the skin of the lower lid and cheek downward with the fingers. Meanwhile, the surgeon grasps the orbital septum with forceps and applies traction in a cephalad direction. These manoeuvres effectively open up the skin-muscle flap, revealing the areolar tissue deep to the orbicularis and superficial to the orbital septum. Although this plane is relatively avascular, we like to dissect it with the cautery, which immediately seals the few vessels that are encountered, preventing staining of the areolar tissue with extravasated blood and keeping the dissection clean and essentially blood free.

8

After the dissection has been carried down to the level of the orbital rim the fatty protrusions become immediately apparent, particularly in the central and medial compartments. The lateral compartment of the lower lid may not be as obvious, because it usually protrudes less, and, more importantly, it is located significantly cephalad to the level of the other two compartments. Gentle pressure against the globe will usually reveal the location of the lateral compartment. If the lateral compartment is small, either we do not treat it, or merely lightly cauterize its overlying orbital septum with the Concept cautery. We believe that this simple manoeuvre provides enough orbital tightening for minor protrusions through immediate shrinkage and subsequent scarring of the septal tissue.

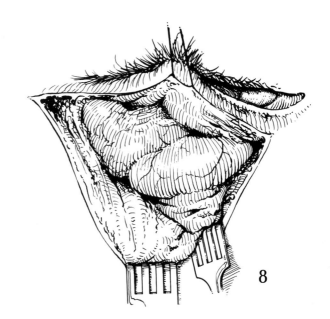

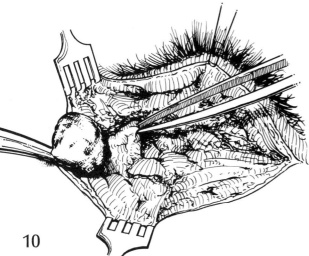

9

If there is significant protrusion of the lateral compartment the Concept cautery is used to cut into the apex of the protrusion.

10

The fat is allowed to extrude as far as it will without undue traction, and the surrounding tissues are gently wiped away from it with a small 'peanut' dissector.

11

The fatty protrusion is then infiltrated with a small quantity of local anaesthetic solution prior to cross clamping and amputation.

The fatty protrusions in all three lower lid compartments are quite sensitive and require infiltration with additional local anaesthetic solution prior to clamping and cutting, if the procedure is being done under local anaesthesia. The upper lid central compartment and the upper lateral compartment (if there is one) are relatively insensitive and usually do not have to be infiltrated. The upper medial compartment, however, requires supplementary infiltration of anaesthetic for clamping and cutting.

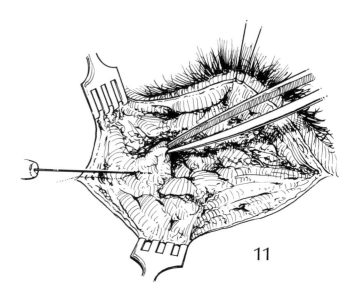

11

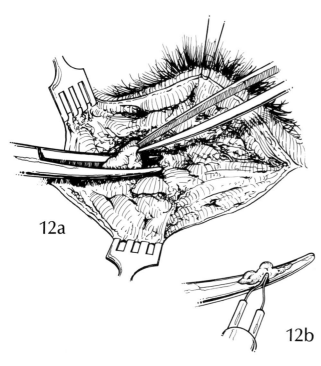

12a

12b

12a & b

The base of the protruding fat compartment is clamped with a lightweight mosquito haemostat at the level of the orbital septum (a) and the portion protruding superficial to the jaws is amputated with scissors or scalpel blade, leaving a generous cuff of tissue which is thoroughly cauterized to ensure adequate haemostasis (b).

13

During the clamping, amputating and cauterizing of the fatty compartment, it is preferable for the surgeon to hold the haemostat himself rather than risk excessive traction on it due to movement of the assistant's hand or the patient's head. By holding the mosquito haemostat between the ring and middle fingers, and resting the ulnar side of the little finger against the temple (when working on the right eyelid), or against the malar arch when working on the left eyelid, the left, haemostat-holding hand remains securely locked in the same relative position, even if the patient's head moves. The forceps which hold the fat for trimming are held between the thumb, index and long fingers of the left hand, leaving the right hand free to hold the scissors or scalpel blade[6].

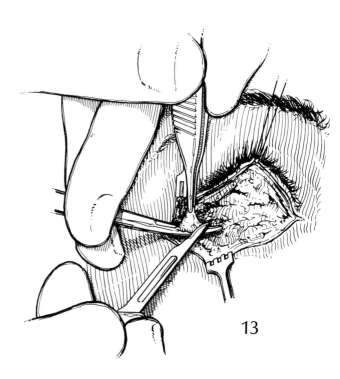

13

14

The central and medial lower lid compartments are dissected out and amputated in the same way as described for the lateral compartment. When dissecting between the central and medial compartments the pink belly of the inferior oblique muscle, which separates them, may be encountered. It should be protected from injury.

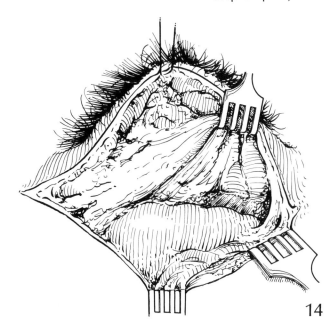

14

After the exesss fat has been excised from the lower lid compartments the entire operative field is inspected and any bleeding points are coagulated. The lower lid traction suture is then removed.

Trimming of the lower lid skin-muscle flap is postponed until the upper lid blepharoplasty has been completed and closed. This is because closure of the upper lid skin defect causes the lateral lower lid skin margin to be drawn cephalad, enlarging the apparent width of the lateral lower lid defect and therefore reducing and occasionally eliminating the amount of trimming required. Trimming of the lower lid flap before closing the upper lid defect could cause ectropion, or excessive pull on the lateral canthus, producing a 'cocker spaniel' look. Also, excised eyelid skin should not be discarded until after the entire operation has been completed, for obvious reasons. Some surgeons refrigerate the excised skin, saving it for a few days after the operation, in case some has to be restored. Conservative trimming of the lower lid should obviate the need for such frugality (see below).

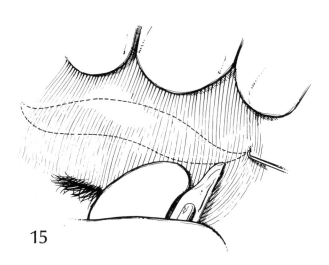

15

15

The upper lid skin is then excised within the previously marked out lines (which usually benefit from some reinforcement at this stage because of fading or 'bleeding' of the markings). It is difficult to make accurate incisions in the loose, mobile skin of the upper lid unless it is made taut by adequate traction in all directions. The assistant exerts medial traction on a single, fine skin hook placed at the medial end of the proposed excision. On the right side, the right-handed surgeon draws the brow superiorly with his left fingers. While holding the scalpel in the right hand between the thumb and first two fingers, the tip of the right ring finger, resting on the upper lid skin overlying the tarsal plate, can exert caudal traction as long as the eyelid skin and the surgeon's glove are dry. Alternatively, caudal traction may be exerted with the assistant's fingers.

When drum-like tautness has been achieved, the inferior and superior incisions can easily be made through the full thickness of the skin down to the orbicularis muscle.

16

After both the upper and lower skin incisions have been completed, the assistant withdraws the medial traction hook and applies traction hooks laterally to the superior and inferior cut edges of the skin. The surgeon grasps the lateral point of the incised segment of the skin with forceps or small haemostat for better grip and, by a combination of sharp dissection and gentle avulsion, separates it from the underlying orbicularis muscle. Multiple punctate bleeding vessels in the orbicularis can be controlled by cauterizing with the Concept cautery or by using adrenaline compresses.

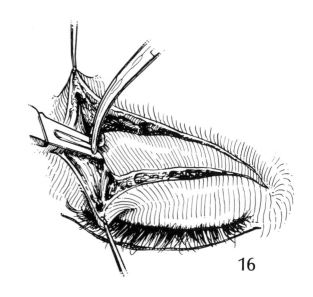

16

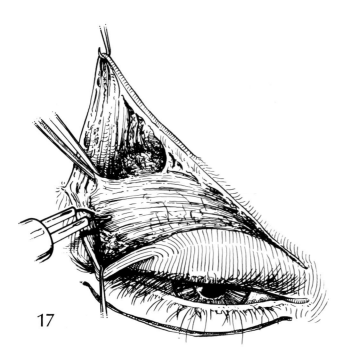

17

17

The upper fatty compartments can be excised by one of two methods. For optimum exposure the space deep to the orbicularis may be entered and the fatty compartments dissected out individually. To prevent injury to the underlying levator muscle and tendon when entering the suborbicularis space, the assistant inserts fine skin hooks into the superior and inferior cut edges of the skin at the lateral end of the dissection and exerts traction anteriorly, away from the globe, thereby lifting the orbicularis away from the levator. The orbicularis is penetrated laterally, but not too far, to prevent injury to motor nerves in this area[9].

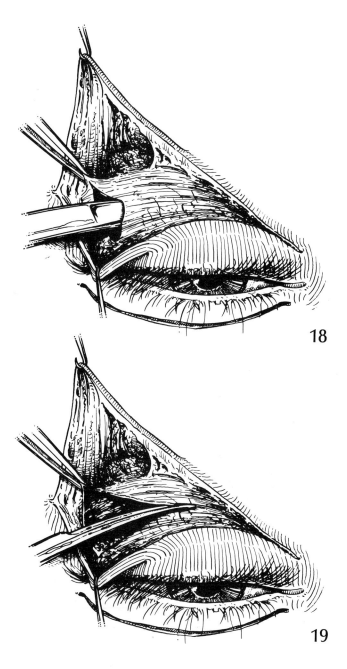

18 & 19

The orbicularis is undermined medially with blepharo-plasty scissors at a level 2 mm cephalad to the inferior skin incision margin and split horizontally at the same level from the lateral to the medial end of the eyelid.

18

19

20

20

After elevating and freeing up the superior flap of orbicularis slightly, a 2–3 mm strip of muscle is excised from its inferior edge. This helps to emphasize the superior tarsal fold postoperatively by encouraging adhesion of the lower, cut end of the orbicularis to the underlying levator tendon[10]. Anchoring procedures to suture the cut edge(s) of the orbicularis to the underlying levator aponeurosis are indicated only occasionally, such as where there is a true, total absence of the tarsal fold, as in the oriental eyelid (see below).

21a, b & c

After the suborbicularis compartment is entered and the muscle strip excised, additional blunt or cautery dissection will reveal the fatty compartment lying on the levator (a). Occasionally, what appears to be a lateral fatty compartment may be encountered (b). The lateral compartment and the central compartment often comprise a single sheet of fat, extending out from the depths of the supraorbital sulcus (c).

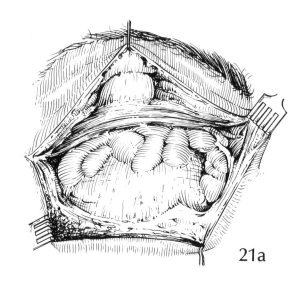

21a

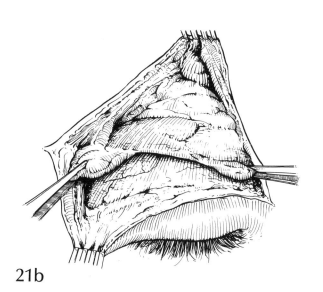

21b

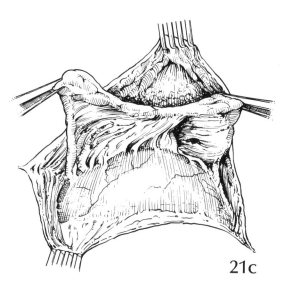

21c

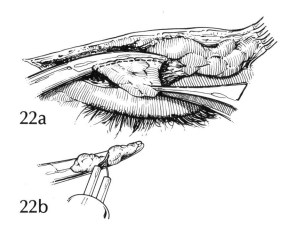

22a

22b

22a & b

This sheet of fat is clamped near its base, amputated, and the residual cuff coagulated, as described for the lower lid fatty protrusions. The upper lid fat should not be excised over-zealously, especially in the male, for fear of creating an empty, hollow-eyed look.

23

The central upper lid fatty compartment is found easily, but sometimes the upper medial compartment may be difficult to identify. To reveal it, the assistant applies single-hook traction superiorly and inferiorly at the medial end of the dissection, while the surgeon presses gently on the globe, causing the medial compartment to protrude.

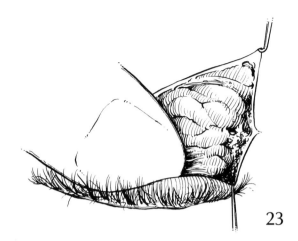

23

24

If it is of any significant size, it is incised and the excess fat allowed to extrude. The fat is injected with local anaesthetic, clamped, amputated, and the residual cuff electrocoagulated. We prefer electrocautery for this step, rather than the smaller Concept cautery, because of the large vessels characteristically found in the medial compartment. This is true for the lower lid as well.

If there is total absence of a supratarsal fold, as in the oriental eyelid, we perform a supratarsal fixation procedure[11], attaching the inferior cut edge of the orbicularis to the underlying levator aponeurosis with interrupted 6/0 plain catgut sutures.

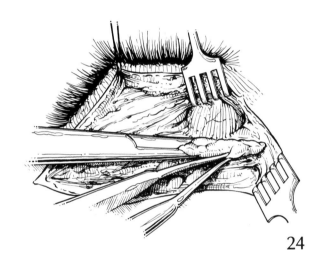

24

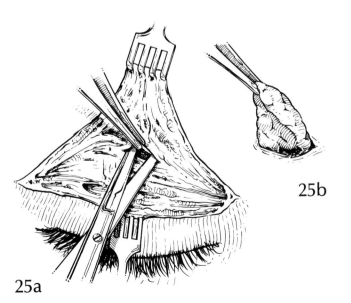

25b

25a

25a & b

If there is relatively little excess upper lid skin and muscle, with a good tarsal fold, an alternative method of treating the upper lid fat compartments without dissecting the suborbicularis space is simply to apply pressure on the globe to see the protrusions of the fatty compartments against the underside of the intact orbicularis. Small stab incisions made with scissors directly over these protrusions will allow the underlying fat compartments to protrude, after which they can be clamped and excised.

26

After careful inspection for haemostasis, the lateral third of the upper lid defect is closed. Closure of the medial two-thirds is deferred until after the lower lid flap is trimmed and sutured (to minimize the intraoperative duration of corneal exposure). As stated above, closure of the lateral part of the upper lid defect elevates the lateral portion of the inferior lid incision and should be done before the lower lid skin-muscle flap is trimmed, to prevent excess lower lid flap excision and resulting ectropion. If a strip of orbicularis has been removed to create a deeper tarsal fold, skin sutures should only engage the skin and not the orbicularis muscle, to allow the cut muscle edges to adhere to the underlying levator aponeurosis.

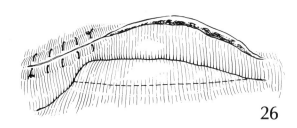

26

The skin-muscle flap is draped over the underlying tissue in a strictly cephalad direction, with no lateral vector. It should be compressed gently into place with forceps or a cotton applicator, ensuring that the flap does not bridge over any underlying hollows, but conforms closely to them. The flap is then marked for trimming, slightly cephalad to the cut edge of the ciliary margin, erring on the conservative side.

Although many surgeons close eyelid incisions with continuous intracuticular sutures, we prefer continuous vertical mattress sutures of 6/0 Prolene for upper lid closure. We find that this method of suturing provides secure, precise coaptation and insures against inversion of

wound edges. All sutures that penetrate eyelid skin must be removed early, usually 48 hours (but no more than 72 hours) postoperatively, to avoid cyst formation. After the upper lid incision is closed and the lower lid field reinspected for haemostasis, the lower lid skin-muscle flap can be trimmed.

Precautionary measures to prevent excess lower lid skin removal include opening the patient's mouth, and, if the patient is conscious, having him look upwards. Under general anaesthesia the patient's mouth is already open by virtue of the traction of the endotracheal tube. The assistant can provide additional caudal finger traction on the cheek.

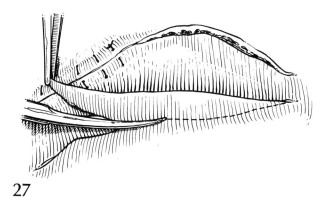

27

27

The portion of the flap which will fit between the medial and lateral canthi is trimmed from lateral to medial with blepharoplasty scissors, which have serrated edges and can cut minute slivers of tissue without slipping.

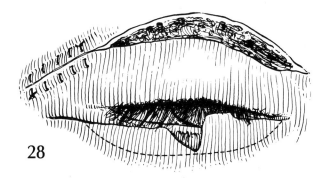

28

28

To ensure further against excess removal of skin, the excision is made on the cephalic side of the marked incision line. Alternatively, the flap may be split vertically down into its proper new level in one or two places; these pilot incisions can then be sutured, and the rest of the tissue trimmed at the same level.

29

To reduce transverse bulging of the orbicularis muscle (which may have been apparent preoperatively at rest or when the patient 'squinched'), an additional strip of orbicularis muscle (1–2 mm wide) is excised from the lower lid skin-muscle flap. This results in some brisk bleeding from four or five discreet vessels.

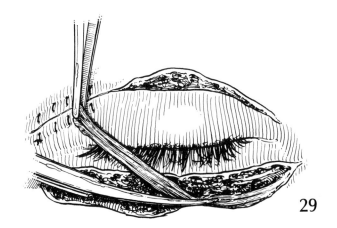

29

30

These are easily exposed by applying two fine hooks to the edge of the skin flap medially and laterally and turning down the flap. The bleeding vessels are sealed with the cautery.

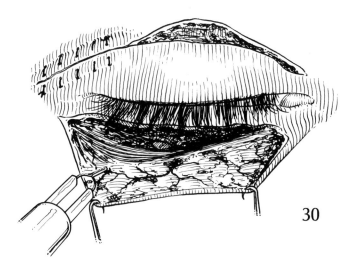

30

31

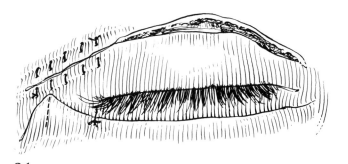

31

The flap is then returned to its place and sutured to the upper cut edge at the region of the lateral canthus with a single interrupted suture of 6/0 Prolene. Outside the lateral canthus there is usually a triangle of excess skin and muscle, pointing superiorly, which may be trimmed conservatively by gradually making a vertical, splitting incision in the flap, precisely to the level of the opposing skin edge.

32

The pilot incision is sutured to the opposing skin edge and the remaining excess tissue flaps can be trimmed with scissors or scalpel. One or two brisk bleeding vessels may be encountered in the cut edges and are readily controlled by cautery.

32

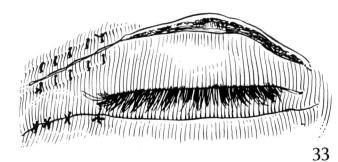

33

33 & 34

The lower lid is then sutured. We like to suture the lower lid securely, although some surgeons do not think this is necessary. At this point sensation may have started to return, particularly near the ciliary margin, and it is helpful to infiltrate additional bupivacaine solution along the ciliary margin.

The lateral-most portion of the incision, beyond the lateral canthus, is sutured with a few interrupted vertical mattress sutures of 6/0 Prolene. The rest of the lower lid, from the medial to lateral canthus, is closed with a continuous, very fine, over-and-over suture of 6/0 Prolene. The ends are not tied, but left long at each end of the wound. There is no need to knot the ends or even secure them with tape. They will stay where they are, and removal is easier if the ends are not secured.

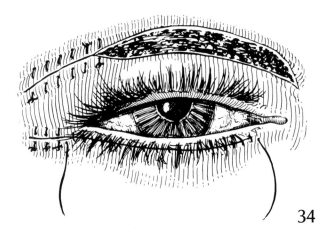

34

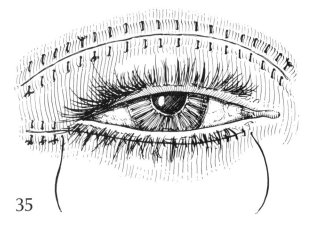

35

35

The remaining unsutured portion of the upper lid (medial two-thirds) is then closed with a continuous vertical mattress suture of 6/0 Prolene, as was the lateral third. At the end of the operation we instil protective ophthalmic ointment (Lacri-Lube S.O.P.) into the conjunctival fornix.

Postoperative care

We do not use dressings. Instead, chilled saline compresses are placed over the lids for comfort, control of oedema and absorption and dissolution of clots and crusts. Sutures are usually removed in 2 days, and after no more than 3 days, to avoid cyst formation. The lateral aspect of the lower lid incision is reinforced with sterile supporting tape (Steri-strips) for 3–4 more days.

Female patients are allowed to wear cosmetic make-up 4 days after the sutures are removed. Beginning 5 days postoperatively, patients are instructed in massage of the lower lids, moving (but not rubbing) the lower lids gently in a rotary upward and outward motion to milk out oedema and help prevent deep, underlying scar contracture.

Patients usually wear sunglasses during the initial healing period for comfort and camouflage. They are asked to remain very quiet for the first 2–3 days, to refrain from effort, to avoid bending their heads down, and to abstain from smoking, in order to avoid coughing and skin healing problems that smokers may be prone to. Normal, non-athletic activity is permitted, starting 5 days postoperatively, and strenuous activity may be resumed after 3 weeks.

References

1. Zubiri, J. S. Correction of the oriental eyelid. Clinics in Plastic Surgery 1981; 8: 725–737

2. Smith, B., Lisman, R. D. Cosmetic correction of eyelid deformities associated with exophthalmos. Clinics in Plastic Surgery 1981; 8: 777–792

3. Gradinger, G. P. Preoperative considerations in blepharoplasty. In: Kaye, B. L. and Gradinger, G. P., eds. Symposium on problems and complications in aesthetic surgery of the face. St. Louis: Mosby, 1984: 195–207

4. Kaye, B. L., Kruse, J. C. General anaesthesia for rhytidectomy: a review of 100 consecutive cases. Plastic and Reconstructive Surgery 1977; 60: 747–751

5. Kaye, B. L. The forehead lift: a useful adjunct to face lift and blepharoplasty. Plastic and Reconstructive Surgery 1977; 60: 161–171

6. Kaye, B. L. Two helpful technical aids in blepharoplasty. Plastic and Reconstructive Surgery 1983; 71: 714–715

7. Beare, R. Surgical treatment of senile changes in the eyelids: the McIndoe-Beare technique. In: Smith, B., Converse, J. M., eds. Proceedings of 2nd international symposium of plastic and reconstructive surgery of eye and adnexa. St. Louis: Mosby, 1967: 362–372

8. Spira, M. Lower blepharoplasty – a clinical study. Plastic and Reconstructive Surgery 1977; 59: 35–38

9. Zide, B. M. Anatomy of the eyelids. Clinics in Plastic Surgery 1981; 8: 623–634

10. Baker, T. J., Gordon, H. L., Mosienko, P. Upper lid blepharoplasty. Plastic and Reconstructive Surgery 1977; 60: 692–698

11. Sheen, J. H. A change in the technique of supratarsal fixation in upper blepharoplasty. Plastic and Reconstructive Surgery 1977; 59: 831–834

Illustrations by Ian Ramsden

The lips – repair of losses

Ian A. McGregor   ChM, FRCS
Director, Plastic and Oral Surgery Unit, Canniesburn Hospital, Glasgow, UK

Introduction

The difficulties of upper lip reconstruction are increased by the fact that, in addition to having symmetry derived from its Cupid's bow, the upper lip has symmetry in relation to the nose. Because of this it is only possible to close small defects without producing a cosmetic deformity sufficiently obvious to be unacceptable. The upper lip in the normal face also protrudes in front of the lower lip and any postexcisional tightness which reduces or eliminates this normal relationship is undesirable.

In contrast, the lower lip has no structure at its centre or shape to draw attention to asymmetry. It can also sustain a loss of one-third of its breadth before tightness or asymmetry begins to show.

Because of these facts the lower lip can be used as a source of tissue to reconstruct resections of the upper lip and a common practice is to transfer a full thickness wedge of the lower lip into the upper lip on a narrow pedicle containing the inferior labial vessels.

Anatomy

1

The bulk of the lip substance, upper and lower, is provided by the orbicularis oris muscle which acts as a sphincter. Although it normally works in concert with the dilator muscles which radiate from each angle it is its function as a sphincter which the surgeon works to restore in his reconstructive techniques. The lip muscle has the unusual and fortunate characteristic from the viewpoint of motor and sensory function that, when a wedge of its circumference is transferred from one lip to the other, losing its nerve supply in the process, it becomes reinnervated, with restoration of both its motor and sensory functions.

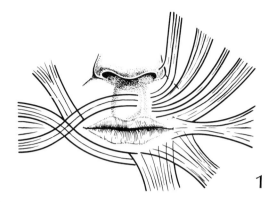

1

2

The vascular anatomy of the lips is also exploited for reconstruction purposes. In addition to a rich vasculature each lip generally has a constant artery which runs parallel to the margin. It arises on each side from the facial artery and meets its fellow in the midline. The labial arteries lie between the orbicularis muscle and the mucous membrane, approximately at the level of the junction between ordinary skin and the red margin. Their calibre and vascular efficiency allow large volumes of lip tissue to be transferred on a pedicle which contains little more than the vessels themselves.

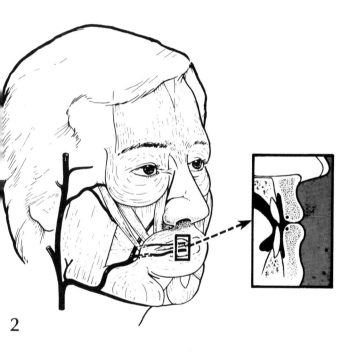

2

3a & b

Suturing techniques

The method used to approximate the limbs of a full thickness V-excision can be used in the closure of all full thickness incisions of the lips and is therefore applicable to many of the reconstructive procedures to be described.

When the closure is straightforward it can be made a two-layer one, treating the muscle and mucosa as a single layer. The precision of the manoeuvre can be increased if the skin is mobilized from the muscle for 2–3 mm back from the wound edge. This has the effect of formally defining the layers. A row of interrupted mucomuscular mattress sutures using chromic catgut is inserted to take the strain of the reconstruction, allowing the skin to be closed without tension or tendency to invert.

In some centres, the three layers, mucosa, muscle and skin, are individually closed. Such a closure is certainly preferable at certain sites in some reconstructions. It is not always obvious at first sight what the most advantageous position of the mucous membrane and, more importantly, the muscle layer is going to be. Independent suture of the mucosa, in addition to giving a more watertight closure, may give the surgeon a clearer idea of how best to close the muscle layer. This is particularly so when, despite the efforts of the surgeon, there is some tension present.

Two-layer closure can also be unwise when it seems possible that use of the necessarily larger mucomuscular suture may have the effect of strangulating blood vessels in a particularly sensitive site from a vascular point of view, for example close to one of the labial vessels.

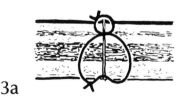

3a

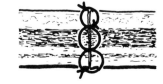

3b

The operations

The lower lip

VERMILIONECTOMY

In this, the so-called 'lip-shave', the red margin of the lower lip is excised with a small, variable amount of underlying muscle. The method is used in treating premalignancy and early malignancy of the red margin and the amount of underlying muscle excised depends on the estimated depth of invasion. If deep infiltration is present, the method is not suitable.

Resurfacing of the denuded red margin can be carried out by advancing the mucous membrane from the inner surface of the lip or using a tongue flap. Which method is appropriate depends on several factors. Mucosal advance-

ment tends to pull the lip margin backwards. If the lip has previously been well everted this is of no importance, but otherwise it produces an indrawn lip. If the lip shave has included much of the underlying muscle the convexity of the lip margin is lost and this is not restored by mucosal advancement. The tongue flap can be designed to include enough thickness of tissue to restore the roundness of the vermilion. Whichever method is used the excision of vermilion should be from angle to angle if the best cosmetic result is to be achieved.

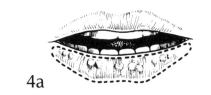

4a

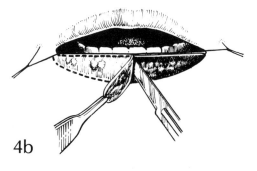

4b

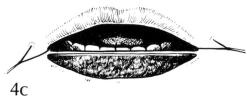

4c

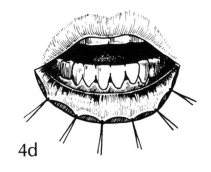

4d

4a–d

Mucosal advancement

As a rule in 'lip-shaves' that are suitable for this procedure the margin of the vermilionectomy anteriorly is the junction between red margin and skin proper; the margin posteriorly is the line of contact between upper and lower lip. Descriptions of how to advance mucosa vary in their recommendations concerning mucosal mobilization. The author has seen necrosis follow mobilization and advancement and has not found mobilization necessary. There seems to be enough mucosal mobility to allow advancement readily wihout formal mobilization. If mobilization is unavoidable it should be in the natural and relatively avascular plane between the submucosa and the muscle so that the minor salivary glands of the lip are mobilized with the mucosa. The sutures should be evenly spaced along the suture line so that tension is distributed properly.

Use of tongue flap

The site used on the tongue is the part closest to the lip. It is parallel to the line which demarcates the papillated dorsum from the smooth mucosa of the side and undersurface of the tongue. The precise site in relation to this line varies. The surgeon can use smooth mucosa or accept the rougher surface of the papillated tongue.

The method is used most often after 'lip shave' but it can also be used to provide a red margin after the completion of certain reconstructive techniques of the lips. These will be discussed later as appropriate.

5a–d

Use of dorsal mucosa (a)

The tongue is incised along the line which demarcates the two surfaces, dorsal and ventral, symmetrically on each side of the midline, for a length which corresponds to the length of the lip defect. The incision is deepened into the tongue muscle for approximately 1.5 cm in a direction that will give the flap substance and roundness to match the requirements of the reconstruction.

Use of ventral mucosa (b)

The tongue incision is made parallel to the rim and approximately 1.5 cm below it. A flap of mucosa and muscle based anteriorly is raised and rotated forward on its anterior hinge. The amount of muscle it contains is designed to match the loss of lip substance.

Suturing of the flap (c & d)

The tongue flap, dorsal or ventral, is sutured to the skin side of the lip defect. Accurate suturing, of a quality appropriate for skin closure, is not feasible owing to the absence of dermis in the tongue. The sutures tend to cut through the tongue muscle and a good 'bite' is desirable. It is wise to leave the sutures in position for a longer period than average. The resulting suture marks are of no consequence and indeed mimic effectively the vertical wrinkling usual at the vermilion border of many older patients.

Only the line between lip skin and the tongue mucosa should be sutured. The raw surface of the flap must abut directly on the raw margin of the lip and this will only happen if skin and flap mucosa alone are sutured.

Care of the flap

If the patient has teeth it is wise to fit a shield over the incisor teeth to ensure that the flap is not bitten through, particularly during recovery from the anaesthetic. A dental acrylic splint can be made to overlay the teeth and hold the mouth open. There is a surprising lack of discomfort from the attachment of tongue to lip.

Division of the flap

The flap can safely be divided in 2 weeks and inset into the lip. An absolute minimum of undermining to allow insetting is desirable or else necrosis of the flap rim may occur.

Behaviour of the flap

In its new dry environment the mucosa, papillated or smooth, tends to develop a scaly surface. This can be controlled by using an emollient cream. The tendency often diminishes with time.

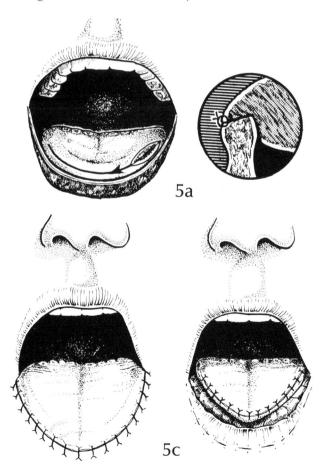

5a

5c

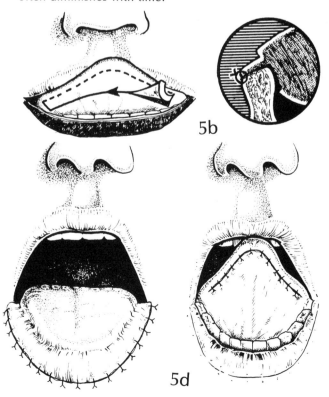

5b

5d

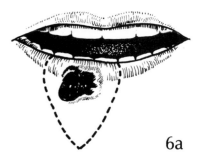

6a

V-EXCISION AND SUTURE

6a–d

This method is used for lesions whose excision does not remove more than one-third of the red margin of the lower lip. The defect is made in the form of a V-shaped wedge and is closed by approximating the two sides of the V. The method can be used at any site along the lip margin. In constructing the V it is clearly desirable to make the two limbs equal in length.

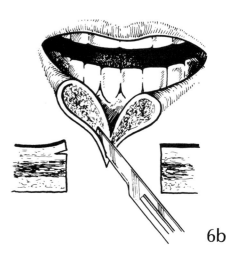

6b

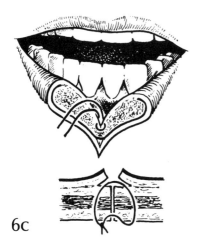

6c

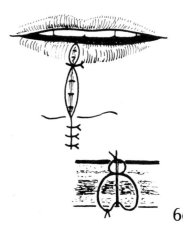

6d

7a–d

A small V is unlikely to reach the lower buccal sulcus and closure is easy. It can be more difficult when the V extends beyond the mucosa on to the chin. The difficulty arises in approximating the mucosa and muscle at the lower buccal sulcus. At this point the mucosa, as it reflects on to the alveolus, becomes more firmly anchored deeply and advancement becomes difficult. An incision along the buccal sulcus on both sides allows advancement and closure without tension.

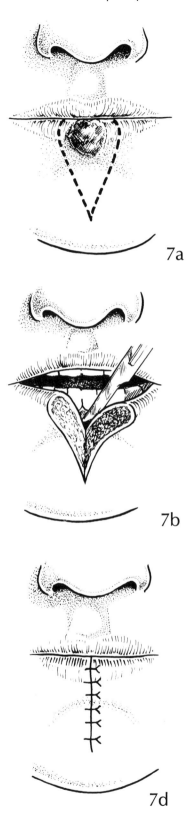

7a

7b

7d

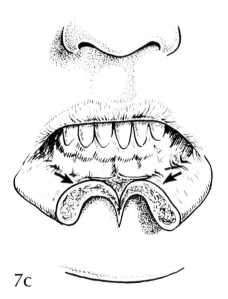

7c

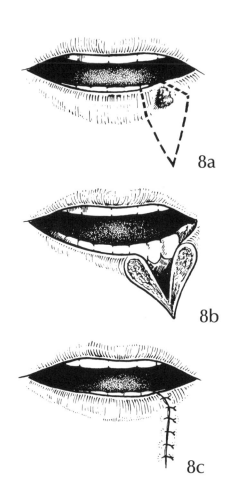

8a

8b

8c

8a, b & c

Near the angle of the mouth a minor problem can arise because the red margin, as it narrows to the angle, is likely to have grossly unequal widths on each side of the V to be sutured together. The two widths can be at least partially equalled by cutting the vermilion on the narrower side obliquely, thus lengthening it. The inequality of width can also be corrected by using a Z-plasty and this has the added use of eliminating any tendency to notching. It is necessary to make the point, however, that this device, while it is frequently desirable in non-malignant contexts, is positively contraindicated in malignancy since it will have the effect of spreading the line of potential recurrence.

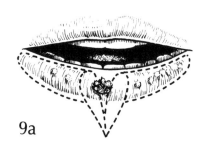

9a

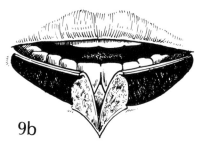

9b

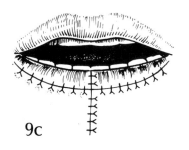

9c

9a, b & c

V-EXCISION AND VERMILIONECTOMY

This procedure is required when an invasive squamous carcinoma is associated with diffuse premalignant change in the remaining red margin. The red margin is excised as for a lip shave and this is combined with a V-excision. Closure of the V component is exactly as for the basic V-excision and suturing converts the defect into that of the simple lip shave. The defect of the red margin can then be managed, using mucosal advancement or tongue flap. The tongue flap gives a better cosmetic result. Extending from angle to angle, it bridges the suture line of the closed V and avoids the notch of lip margin which is almost inevitable if mucosal advancement is used.

10a–e

EXTENDED V-EXCISION AND BILATERAL ADVANCEMENT

This method can be used to reconstruct a defect which has the form of a broad V even if the defect extends from angle to angle. The tissue lateral to the angle on each side is advanced medially in order to close the two limbs of the V.

The apex of such a broad V has to be brought well down on to the chin if a 'dog-ear' is not to be produced when the V is closed.

To allow advancement of the tissues it is necessary to mobilize the soft tissues of the lip off the mandible and allow advancement without tension. Advancement must, of course, avoid damaging the mental nerve.

From each angle of the mouth an incision is made through the full thickness of the cheek, the line of incision curving slightly upwards and passing laterally as far as a little beyond the nasolabial fold.

With the tissue below the incisions on each side advanced medially, the two limbs of the V are sutured together and this reconstitutes the lower lip. The effect is to create a redundancy on each side of the upper lip. This shows as a 'dog-ear' approximately along the line of the nasolabial fold. The redundancy is of all the lip tissues - skin, muscle and mucosa, each corresponding to half of the original lower lip resection. The mucosal redundancy adjusts spontaneously but the skin and muscle redundancy is excised to leave a scar along the line of the nasolabial fold. It is not always necessary to excise muscle – skin excision alone may be adequate.

A new vermilion may be provided by advancing mucosa or by incorporating a tongue flap. Mucosal advancement tends to produce a lip that lacks a full vermilion. A central notch is also common. A tongue flap gives a more adequate red margin and avoids a notch.

This method of reconstruction works best when the patient has a thin face and there is marked nasolabial redundancy of tissue. Even so, it tends to produce a tight lower lip associated with an apparent fullness of the upper lip. This tightness, coupled with the inevitable scar running laterally from the angle, can also make insertion of dentures difficult.

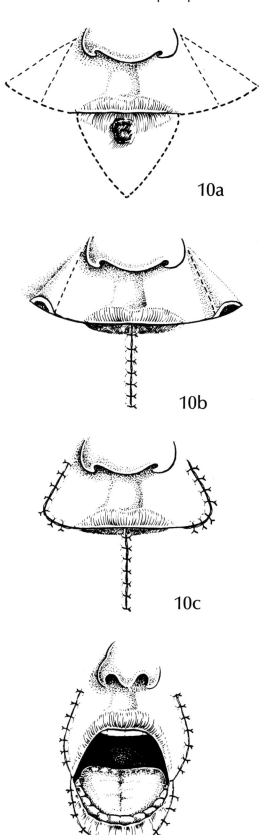

10a

10b

10c

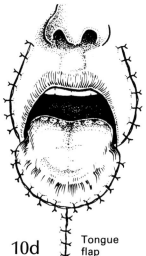

10d   Tongue flap

10e   Mucosal advancement

THE FAN FLAP

11a, b & c

For a defect of up to one-half of the lower lip that can be converted into the shape of a rectangle a full thickness flap can be fashioned in the shape of a fan on the cheek lateral to the defect. This flap, mobilized, is 'rolled' round to fill the defect of the lip.

In its 'classic' form a full-thickness incision is made extending in the arc of a circle around the angle of the mouth on to the upper lip at a distance from the vermilion equal to the depth of the defect of the lip. At about the level of the nasolabial fold a back-cut is brought almost to the red margin. This leaves the flap pedicled on the labial vessels and capable of being mobilized and advanced to meet the opposite side of the lip defect, to which it is sutured. Suture in this way restores the oral sphincter and the flap is sutured along its margin in layers. Initially, of course, the two sides of the defect along the margin of the 'fan' are of different lengths. The inequality is made good by suturing under different tensions on the two sides, by closure of the back-cut and sometimes by incorporating a Z-plasty at a suitable point in its circumference.

The effect is to roll round the angle of the mouth and reduce its total width. Because of this the method is not recommended for defects of more than two-thirds of the lip; it works best when the defect is towards the lip centre and a cuff of vermilion is available on both sides to suture together.

The fan flap constructed in this way can cope only with a defect limited in size and site. The inevitable denervation of the flap is regarded by some as a disadvantage. Two modified versions of the method are available, each of which eliminates one of the disadvantages and adds to the versatility of the principle.

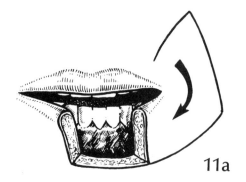

11a

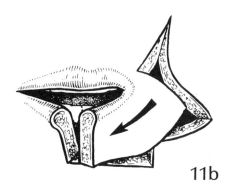

11b

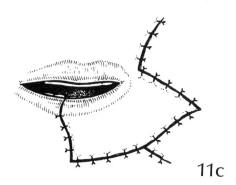

11c

12a & b

THE NEUROVASCULAR FAN FLAP

In this modification an attempt is made to preserve the nerves and arteries of the orbicularis muscle in the flap. This reduces the amount of advancement possible and the limit on advancement is added to by the absence of a back-cut at the base of the flap. To compensate, two flaps are routinely designed, one on each side, and both are advanced to meet centrally.

As in the standard fan flap, skin incisions from each side of the defect parallel to the lip margin are carried round each angle into the upper lip as far as the level of the alar base. These are deepened carefully, dividing the muscle, but at the same time taking every care to preserve any motor and sensory nerves met in the process as well as blood vessels. The mucosa is left intact except where it has to be defined for suturing towards the margin of each flap.

The effect is to redistribute the muscle and vermilion and to provide a complete sphincter, without at the same time losing significant motor or sensory function. Like the standard fan flap the method reduces the circumference of the mouth and this in turn limits the amount of lip which can be removed to two-thirds. The retention of sensory and motor function does make it a better method than the standard fan flap, though neither method can readily be combined with a lip shave and this limits their use to the patient without significant dysplasia of the vermilion adjoining the main lesion.

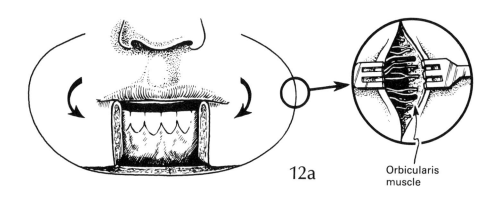

12a

Orbicularis
muscle

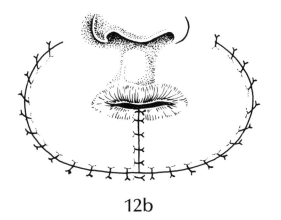

12b

THE MODIFIED FAN FLAP

When the resection extends to the angle of the mouth and involves half of the lip an alternative modification of the classic fan flap design is possible.

13a–e

The defect is almost square and for repair a flap similar in essence to that used in the classic fan flap is outlined on the cheek immediately lateral to the lip defect. The difference in technique rests in the fact that the flap instead of being rolled medially to fill the defect rotates around the angle of the mouth. The effect is to leave the angle at approximately the same site as preoperatively and the width of the mouth consequently remains unchanged. The flap rotated into position has no red margin as such on its free border and the vermilion can be reconstituted as in the 'lip shave' by advancing the mucosa. In many instances the red margin adjoining the actual excision merits removal as a lip shave and when this has been done the entire lip margin – stripped segment and reconstructed segment – can be covered effectively with a tongue flap.

The method shares the denervation disadvantages of the standard fan flap, but the lack of nerve supply is not a significant disability when only half the lip has been excised. Possibly its main advantage is that the flap rotates round the angle, which remains in its original position, compared with the standard fan flap.

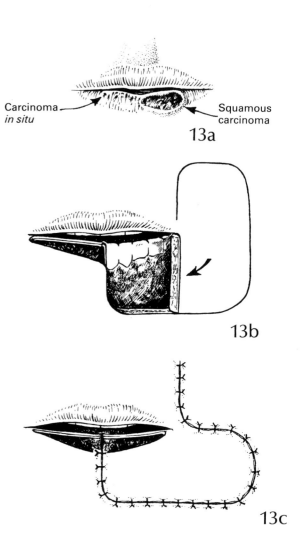

Carcinoma *in situ*

Squamous carcinoma

13a

13b

13c

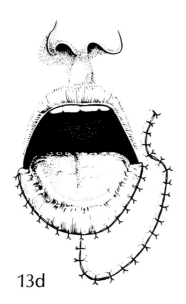

13d

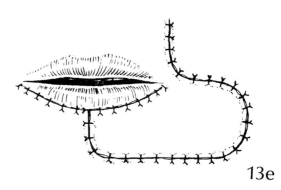

13e

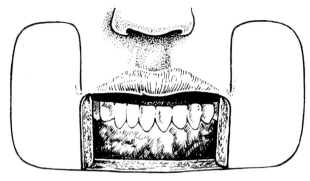

14a–d

The method can be applied equally well to the totally excised lower lip. The defect can be regarded as having two parts, each half of the lip, with each being reparable by a fan flap. In other words, the total reconstruction uses a double fan flap. The two flaps meet in the midline of the reconstructed lip and are there sutured together. All that has been said of the design of the single fan flap applies to the double. It has the same virtues and defects but does in addition have two minor defects of its own. First, the reconstituted red margin of advanced mucosa is a poor substitute for the normal vermilion; second, at the midline where four points meet in suture, two of skin and two of mucosa, minor breakdown is so common as to be virtually inevitable. In healing, a small notch remains to mark the spot. These deficiencies can be virtually eliminated by incorporating a tongue flap in the repair. Both motor and sensory re-innervation of the reconstructed lip take place with time.

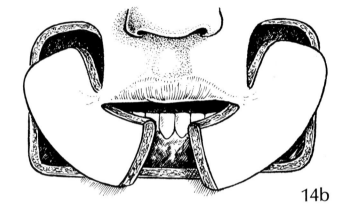

14a

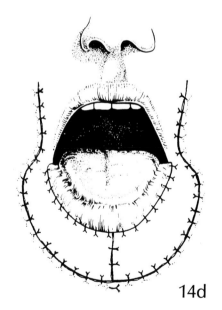

14b

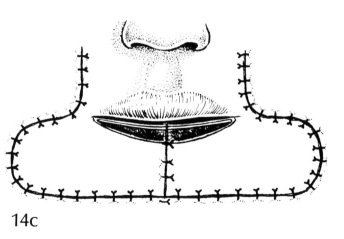

14c

14d

The upper lip

Excision of the upper lip for malignancy of its red margin is much less frequently required than that of the lower lip and as a result the methods of repair are less well standardized.

Partial-thickness defects

These can be managed either by using a *graft* or a *flap*, usually a local flap. The graft is usually a postauricular Wolfe graft. It is preferred because it matches the surrounding skin well in colour and texture though, of course, it does not grow hair, which can be a disadvantage in males. In addition it does not contract and thus the contour of the lip remains as originally designed at the time of grafting.

The local flap used is usually a transposed flap of nasolabial skin. The nasolabial line is usually capable of providing an adequate area of skin and the secondary defect can still be closed by direct suture. Most nasolabial flaps used for this purpose are superiorly based.

Full-thickness defects

The simplest procedure is the V-excision and repair, but it is less satisfactory than its lower lip counterpart. Compared with the lower lip, the upper lip is able to stand much less loss of tissue before tightness is clinically apparent and the normal overhang of upper on lower lip is lost. In addition the anchorage of the soft tissues around the nostrils to the underlying bony skeleton is so firm that no compensatory movement of the remaining lip is possible. Even a minor loss of tissue therefore quickly leads to a very obvious asymmetry of the two sides of the lip. Symmetry of the Cupid's bow is an obvious point of normality in any lip and this is very easily lost with even a minor excision in the region of the philtrum. The vertical length of the lip is a further feature which is readily altered by an excision and with its upper end fixed deeply at the alar base it is difficult to camouflage.

THE ABBE FLAP

15

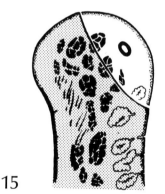

15

The point has already been made that one-third of the full thickness of the lower lip can be excised without increasing its tightness unduly and this makes the lower lip an available area for transfer of tissue to the upper lip. With its structure corresponding virtually absolutely to any defect of the upper lip it is ideal for the purpose. The large and highly effective artery near the lip margin means that such a flap can be raised with an extremely small pedicle and this makes it relatively easy to swing from one lip to the other without causing circulatory embarrassment to the flap despite its bulk relative to the pedicle.

The lack of significant anchorage of the lower lip over its width, angle to angle, means also that a wedge of lip required for a particular part of the upper lip can be taken with little or no regard to the demands of symmetry of the lower lip. The V of the lower lip excised for tumour can be removed from virtually any site and the same holds for the V used to provide tissue for the upper lip.

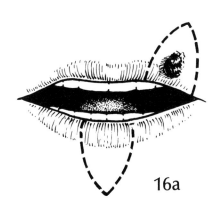

16a

16 & 17

Such a flap is therefore available to fill any defect of the upper lip up to one-third of its width. The procedure is commonly referred to as an Abbe flap. The basic shape of an Abbe flap is a V but this can be modified to fit an oddly shaped defect of the upper lip, provided the defect of the lower lip left by the transfer is either a V or a shape equally easy to close directly. The usual modification of shape is a W and it is required for fitting into the philtral area of the upper lip with its two nostril floors above. A W defect can either be closed as such or converted into a V by excising its central part, whichever will produce the better scar.

The flap, rotated through 180°, is sutured to the upper lip defect. The most important point of suturing is to make sure that in the vicinity of the pedicle the sutures are so placed as not to encroach on the vessels crossing it.

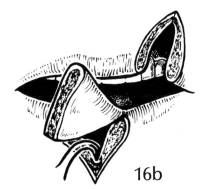

16b

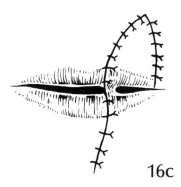

16c

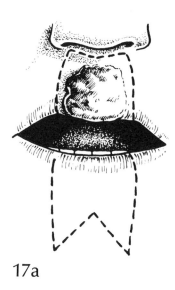

17a

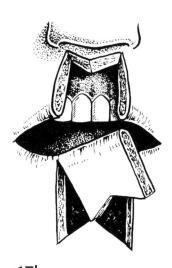

17b

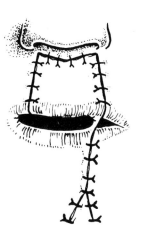

17c

18a & b

The labial vessels lie within the convexity of the vermilion between the muscle and mucosa. The lip is thus sectioned at its mucosal level to just below the line of the vermilion border; the skin is incised on the red margin for 0.5 cm. The muscle is divided almost completely but some is left intact to protect the vessels behind it. Constructing the pedicle in this way leaves it inside the red margin and mucosa and allows each skin-vermilion border to be matched at the time of the initial transfer. This makes subsequent division of the pedicle very straightforward.

When the flap is relatively short the lower lip defect can be closed directly but when the suture line extends on to the chin the incorporation of a Z-plasty with cross limb to correspond to the chin hollow gives a more pleasing result generally. A W can either be closed directly or converted into a V for closure.

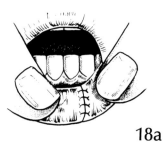

18a

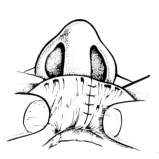

18b

ADVANCEMENT METHODS

19 & 20

Small upper lip defects can be dealt with by undermining and advancement (19a & b). When a defect of the upper lip too large to be filled with an Abbe flap is present it can be reduced in size by employing the rotation advancement principle, merely narrowing the upper part of the rectangle when this is central. This *crescentic peri-alar check excision advancement* can also be employed either bilaterally or unilaterally according to need and also uses the nasolabial area of availability but in a slightly different way. From the upper border of the rectangular excision an incision is made round the alar margin along the nasolabial groove (20a). Lateral to this a deep crescent of tissue is removed; the tissue lateral to the rectangle is mobilized, if necessary incising the upper buccal sulcus. Advancement of the lower cheek and upper lip medially simultaneously closes the peri-alar defect and reduces the rectangular defect. Advancement is most marked at the upper part of the rectangle and converts it into a shape more suitable to accept an Abbe flap.

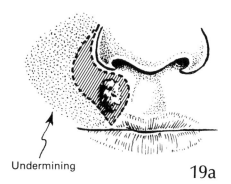

Undermining

19a

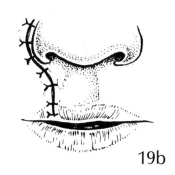

19b

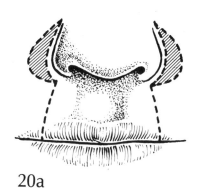

20a

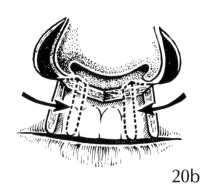

20b

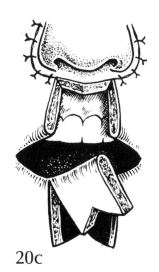

20c

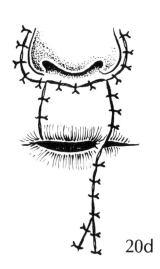

20d

The angle of the mouth

Most defects in the region of the angle are actually of one or other lip which, though they extend to the angle, do not actually involve the other lip.

Such a defect of the lower lip, if suitably square in shape, can, as already described, be reconstructed using a modified fan flap. The V-shaped defect can be managed either by using an *Abbe-Estlander* flap or an *Abbe* flap.

In the Abbe-Estlander flap a V-shaped flap similar in all respects to the Abbe flap is raised on the intact lip at its lateral extremity, with the lateral limb of the V meeting the red margin at the angle and the medial limb reaching to the margin of the vermilion. The flap is rotated 180° to fill the defect of the opposite lip and the pedicle becomes the new angle of the mouth. The defect left by the lip-switch is closed by direct suture.

The Abbe-Estlander flap, possibly because of the higher incidence of squamous carcinoma of the lower lip, tends mainly to be used for defects of the lower lip. Used in this way it very obviously narrows the mouth because the upper lip, which is the source of the flap, cannot provide much tissue without itself becoming narrow, possibly because in contrast to the lower lip the nose anchors it centrally. Loss of tissue to the other lip becomes very obvious as an asymmetry and certainly the asymmetry following transfer of an Abbe-Estlander flap tends to be apparent even to the casual observer.

A solution to this asymmetry is to open up the new angle to equate the two sides of the lip. This is seldom completely satisfactory. The new angle tends to gape and the red margin is unduly narrow. The minor deformity of narrowing is exchanged for that of the slightly gaping angle and despite the modifications of technique designed to prevent this it still tends to occur.

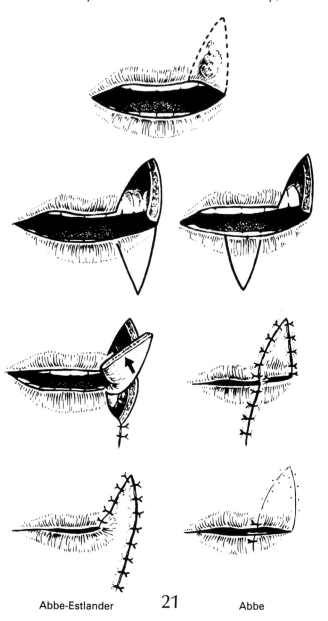

21

This problem of asymmetry is probably inescapable when the transfer is from upper to lower lip. The transfer from lower to upper is less prone to this and the Abbe-Estlander can be transferred in this direction with good result. A much better cosmetic result can however be achieved in such a situation by using a standard Abbe flap and rotating it in the opposite direction from the Abbe-Estlander. This, though it requires as a second stage the minor procedure of dividing the pedicle, leaves a more normal angle in the long run.

Abbe-Estlander   21   Abbe

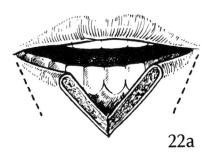

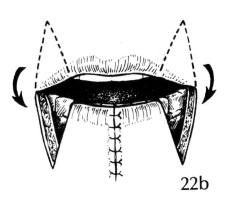

22a, b & c

A further application of the Abbe-Estlander principle has been to the central V defect of the lower lip. In this an incision made downwards from one angle through the full thickness of the lip, parallel and equal in length to the adjoining limb of the V, allows closure of the central V by moving across the rectangular flap so established and replacing it by a V defect of the angle. This defect can then be closed by the Abbe-Estlander flap. The method does not seem to offer any significant advantage over the others described and it suffers from the defects of Abbe-Estlander flaps in general.

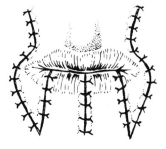

Illustrations by Pam McMaghie, Hooker Goodwin and William Schwarz

Surgical treatment of fractures of the upper and middle face

Richard Carlton Schultz MD
Clinical Professor of Surgery and Chief, Division of Plastic Surgery,
University of Illinois College of Medicine, Illinois, USA

Introduction

A high percentage of patients coming to the accident and emergency department with multiple injuries have sustained them in automobile accidents. Of these patients, approximately two-thirds will have significant facial trauma. Typically, there are injuries to the soft tissues and fractures of the facial bones.

The early management of facial injuries plays an important role in their final outcome, but the extent of the early treatment is dependent upon the nature of the associated injuries. Sometimes there are complications even after the most competent treatment and these may eventually require complex, multistaged reconstructive procedures.

Triage

In terms of timing, definitive treatment of most facial fractures ordinarily deserves low priority in the total care of the patient. With the exception of animal bites and accidental tattoo, treatment of soft tissue trauma can usually be safely delayed up to 24 h if the wound is given proper preparatory care. Most facial fractures are best treated several days after resorption of oedema. Whether the delay is mandatory or elective, neurological, abdominal, thoracic, orthopaedic and urological injuries should be evaluated first.

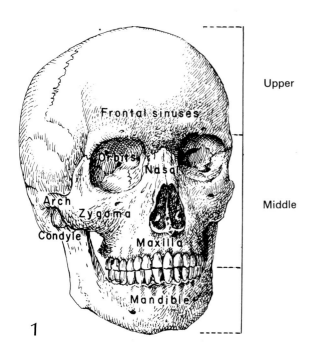

Upper

Middle

1

1

Classification of injuries

Although facial bones are some of the most complex bones in the body, injuries to them can be classified according to functional zones: upper face, middle face and lower face (mandible).

Diagnosis and treatment can be outlined according to these classifications. The diagnosis of bony injuries must sometimes result from clinical evaluation alone, as the initial X-ray examination may not always demonstrate facial fractures. Poor dental occlusion may be the first clue of mandibular or maxillary fracture. Diplopia may be the only positive finding of a fractured orbital floor.

2a–f

Careful observation can disclose depressed frontal sinuses, a deviated nasal complex, a depressed zygoma, enophthalmos, an asymmetrical mandible or a malaligned dental arch. Systematic bimanual palpation will help to avoid missing less obvious fractures. Palpation of the bony parts can usually elicit tenderness and sometimes motion and crepitus at the fracture sites. Palpation of the supraorbital ridge (2a) and infraorbital ridge and zygoma (2b) may reveal irregularities. The malar eminences should be examined for a discrepancy in height (2c) and palpation of the zygomatic arch may reveal a depression (2d). The dental occlusion should be examined for gross irregularities (2e) and after stabilizing the head the maxilla should be checked for motion (2f).

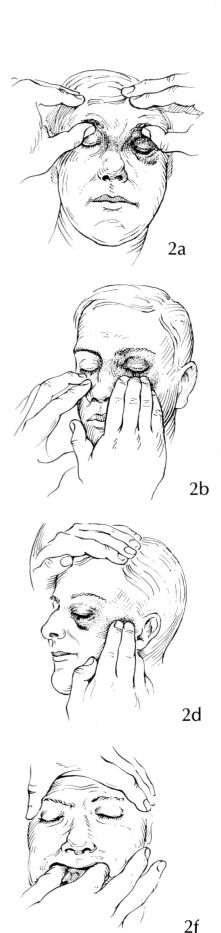

2a

2b

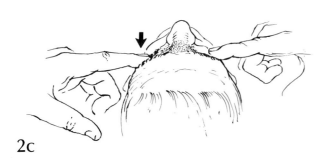

2c

2d

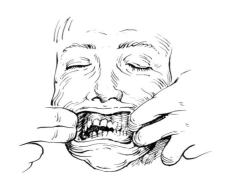

2e

2f

The operations

FRACTURES OF THE UPPER FACE

Fractures of the frontal area usually involve the thinner bones of the frontal sinuses or the supraorbital ridges. Because of the close proximity to the brain, injuries in this area are more likely to be accompanied by greater morbidity and to be more life-threatening than any other facial fractures. Positive physical findings usually appear in the ocular region because of extravasation of blood into the orbital area. Periorbital ecchymosis is observed in nearly all cases. Nasal fractures and overlying lacerations of the forehead are often found in association with fractures of the upper face. Treatment of these fractures involves reduction of the bony fragments by either the direct or indirect approach and interosseous fixation when required for stabilization.

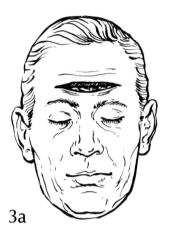

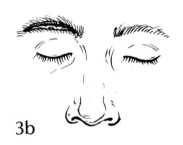

3a

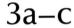

3a–c

Elective incisions for exposure of glabellar and supraorbital fractures are shown. A bitemporal (coronal) forehead flap can also be used.

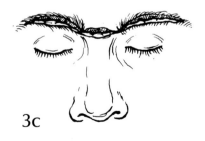

3b

3c

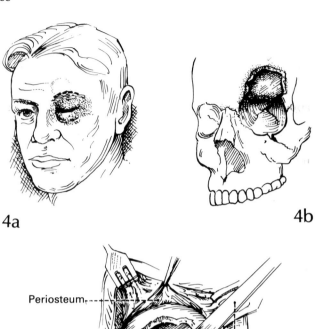

4a–c

Depressed supraorbital fractures are approached through a brow incision (4a). The fracture fragment is depressed into the orbit (4b) and is elevated gently by a wedging manoeuvre with a flat osteotome to avoid over-reduction and tearing of the orbital roof lining (4c).

4a

4b

4c

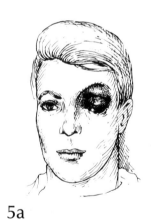

5a

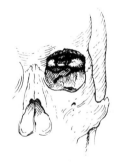

5a & b

The physical findings of comminuted supraorbital fractures include a flattened brow with displaced orbital contents due to the depressed fragment from the roof of the orbit, anaesthesia of the forehead and periorbital ecchymosis (5a). Postero–anterior X-ray may confirm the diagnosis (5b); however, tomograms or CT scan will give more detailed information on the extent of displacement of the fracture(s).

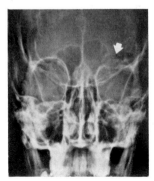

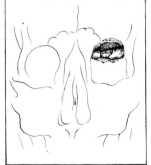

5b

6a–c

Fractures in the supraorbital, ethmoid, upper nasal and frontal sinus areas are best exposed through a bicoronal incision and turning down the forehead ('open sky approach'). This allows detailed examination and reassembling of the comminuted fragments in accurate anatomical alignment. A comminuted supraorbital fracture can be reduced with a tracheal hook. When bony fragments are unstable, they must be wired directly to adjacent solid bone. Periosteum must be incised and elevated to expose the fracture in a manner that will preserve maximum adherence to comminuted fragments and provide additional support for these fragments when repaired (6a). The fragment is reduced by placing an upward–forward thrust on the tracheal hook and fixation is achieved with interosseous wire (6b). The supraorbital ridge is thus restored and the periosteum repaired (6c).

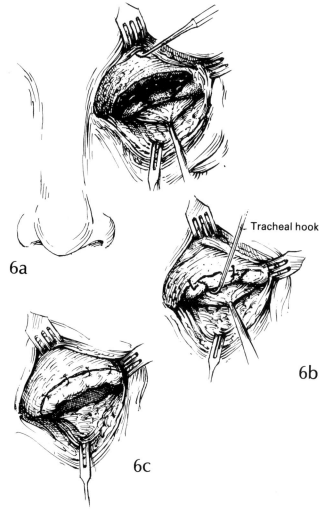

6a

Tracheal hook

6b

6c

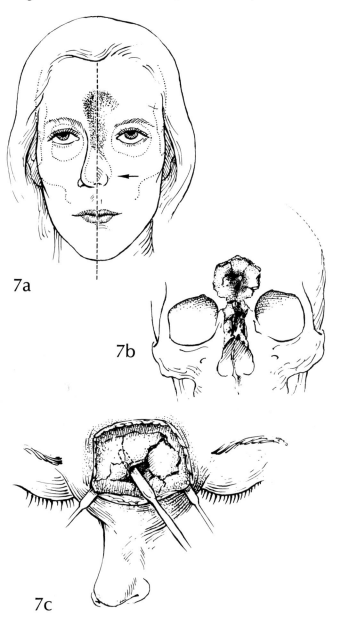

7a

7b

7c

7a–c

A depressed fracture of the frontal sinus is associated with a depressed and asymmetrical deformity of the forehead and nose (7a) due to the comminution (7b). To elevate the fracture, a central fragment is removed. Maximum periosteal contact with the fracture fragments should be preserved. Depressed bone fragments must then be elevated delicately, also preserving any attachments between the fragments. Often a large, depressed central fragment can be removed to provide access to the sinus so that the other depressed fragments can be elevated together. The central fragment is then simply replaced if there is reasonable stability. When more rigid support is necessary, it is fixed into position with fine (28 gauge) stainless steel wire threaded through small holes, carefully drilled into the central fragment and adjacent stable fragments. Even with complex injuries, there is seldom an indication to discard the large, contour-forming bone fragments. Cerebrospinal rhinorrhoea, when present, will sometimes stop spontaneously when posterior wall fractures are reduced. Even though reduction is not perfect anatomically, if a sufficient amount of glabellar prominence is reconstructed, the replaced thick forehead flap and the effects of subsequent healing will usually restore features to their normal appearance (7c).

8a–c

An indirect approach can be used to elevate depressed glabellar fractures. An incision is made superior to or within the medial aspect of the eyebrow and, by careful dissection, the roof of the medial orbit is exposed. Located in this area are three branches of the sensory frontal nerve: the supraorbital, the frontal proper and the supratrochlear. Care must be taken to preserve these nerves, as they provide sensation to the forehead and scalp, to the frontal sinus and the skin and conjunctiva of the upper eyelid. Next an incision is made in the periosteum of the supraorbital roof and the periosteum is reflected from the medial orbital area of the frontal bone (8a). With a power drill, directed medially and superiorly, a hole approximately 1 cm in diameter is made through this small area into the frontal sinus (8b). A small angled raspatory or Joseph periosteal elevator is then introduced into the frontal sinus. With care taken to keep the mucous membrane lining and periosteal covering intact, the depressed fragment of the anterior wall of the frontal sinus can be elevated and reduced, with the opposite hand on the forehead for counter pressure and control. The periosteum covering the orbital roof is then replaced, sutured when possible and the incision closed in layers (8c).

Packing or draining of the frontal sinuses has not been found necessary in any of these techniques. Excision of the lining membranes is necessary only when marked tearing and displacement of the mucous membranes occurs. Cysts of the lining membrane (mucopyocele) have been reported. However, with the preservation and gentle handling of the mucous membrane, such cysts should occur rarely if the ostia draining the frontal sinuses into the nose remains functional.

Appropriate debridement of avascular or pulped sinus mucosa, accurate replacement of soft tissue and systemic antibiotic therapy should accompany the bony reduction. Some surgeons advocate removal of the comminuted bone fragments and extirpation of the sinuses, but this bone loss results in gross deformity. These deformities require extensive secondary reconstructive procedures to correct, whereas primary bony reconstruction, as outlined, gives excellent functional and aesthetic results without complications.

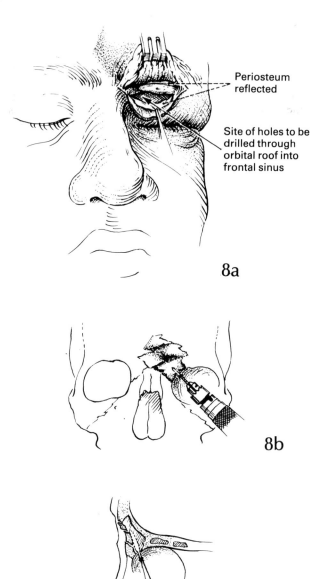

Periosteum reflected

Site of holes to be drilled through orbital roof into frontal sinus

8a

8b

8c

FRACTURES OF THE MIDDLE ZONE OF THE FACE

Fractures in this region of the face often result from injury to unrestrained passengers within an automobile. They range from the nasal fracture, which is the simplest, to the maxillary fracture, which is the most complex of all facial fractures. Because of the prominence of the nasal complex and the thickness of the bone supporting it, nasal fractures are the most common of all facial fractures. Other fractures frequently seen in the middle third of the face involve the maxilla, the zygoma, the zygomatic arch and the bones making up the orbit.

Nasal fractures

Clinical findings are the most reliable means of making the diagnosis of a nasal fracture. The radiological appearance may be normal even when the nose shows gross traumatic deformity. A history of a nosebleed following injury, deviation of the nasal pyramid and crepitus on palpation are the most important clinical findings.

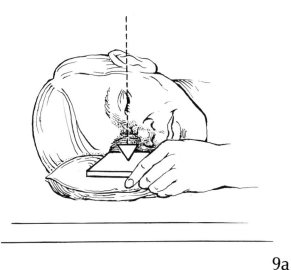

9a

9a & b

Lateral and occlusal X-ray projections of the nasal bones may document these fractures precisely, but often they will not do so even when repeated attempts are made. The history of a previous fracture or nasal deviation is important, since a healed displaced nasal fracture often cannot be reduced by the usual closed reduction techniques.

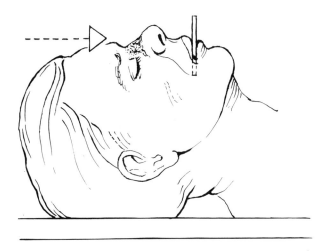

9b

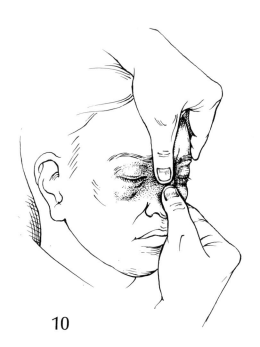

10

10

Laterally angulated fractures of the nasal pyramid, when seen before the onset of oedema, can sometimes be reduced by digital pressure with or without the aid of local anaesthesia. If the entire pyramid is laterally displaced and the patient is seen shortly after injury, a quick push of the pyramid towards the midline with both thumbs will sometimes achieve anatomical reduction with only momentary discomfort to the patient. In such instances, external splinting is usually unnecessary; if reduction is complete, the repositioned nasal fragments should be stable unless forcibly displaced. Otherwise, closed reduction should be delayed 5–7 days to allow for resolution of the swelling. Reduction can be delayed up to 2–3 weeks if necessary. The need for reduction can best be determined after the oedema has resorbed. Undisplaced nasal fractures require no reduction.

11a–f

Anaesthesia of the nose is accomplished by insertion of intranasal packs soaked in a 5 per cent cocaine solution accompanied by an external block using 1 per cent lidocaine with epinephrine. Excess cocaine solution is pressed out of the cotton rolls (11a) and the rolls are inserted into the nares (11b). The external block is achieved by injecting from above (11c), blocking the infraorbital nerves (11d), injecting below (11e) and submucosally (11f).

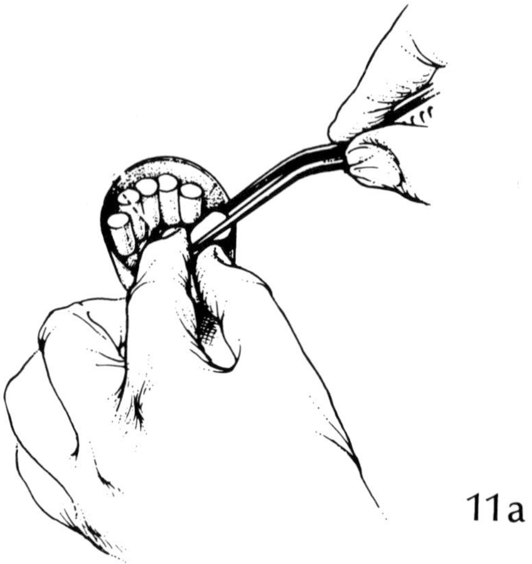

11a

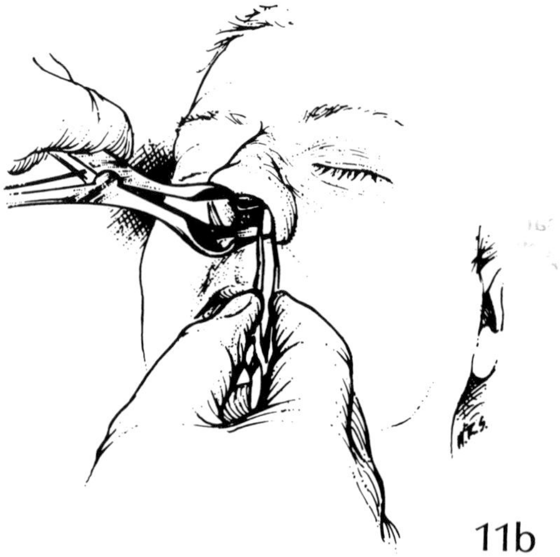

11b

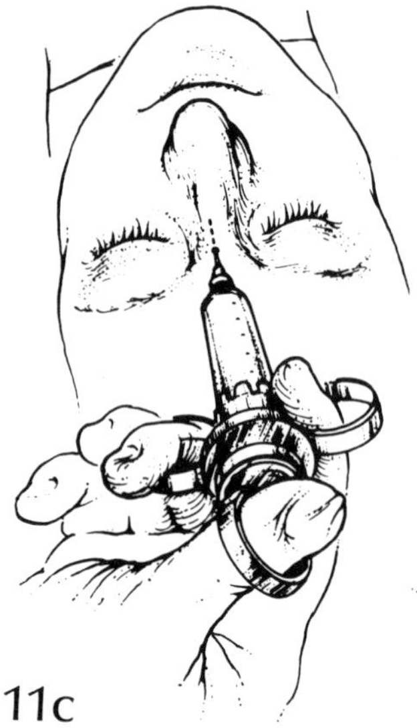

11c

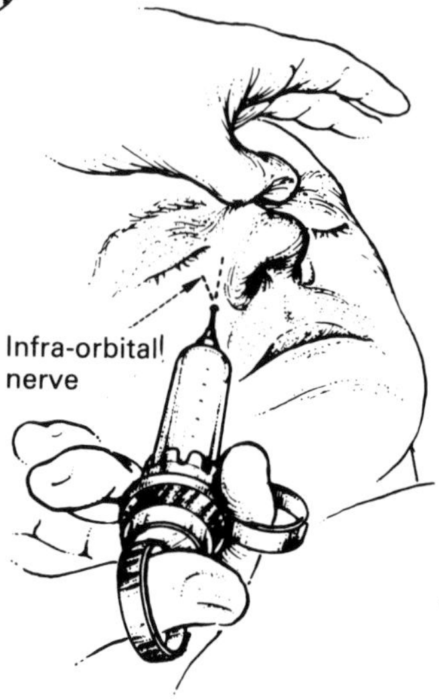

Infra-orbital
nerve

11d

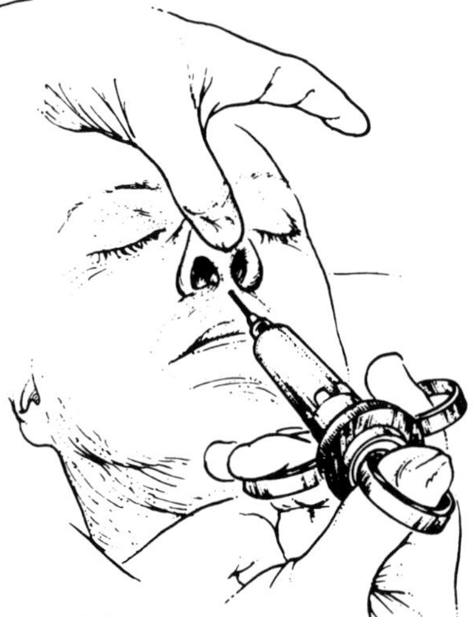

11e

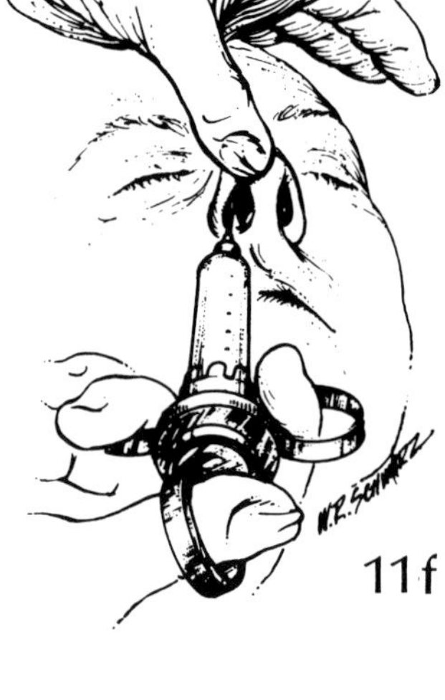

11f

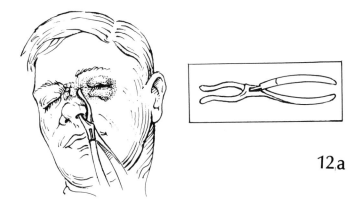

12a

12a–c

After the nose has been anaesthetized, disimpaction and reduction can be accomplished utilizing Walsham forceps for the nasal pyramid (12a), Asch forceps to replace the nasal septum in the midline (12b) and Salinger reduction instrument to further shape and contour the nasal pyramid and tip (12c).

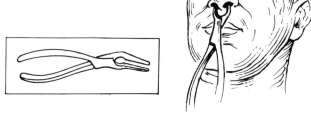

12b

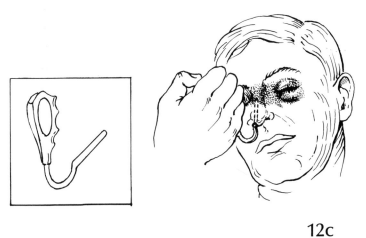

12c

13a–e

Following reduction of the fracture the fragments are
immobilized by the application of a plaster of Paris splint.
The splint is first grossly cut (13a), further trimmed to the
nasal contour while wet (13b), further moulded to the
nose before the plaster sets (13c) and held in place using
micropore tape, contoured to the cheek (13d). The dry,
rigid but contoured splint is easily removed at 1 week
(13e).

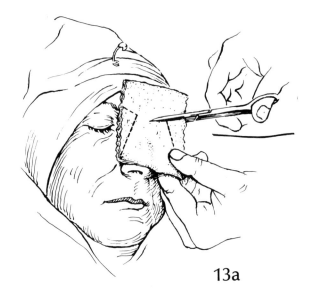

13a

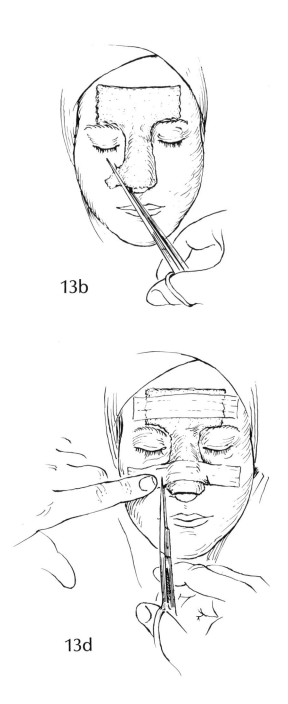

13b

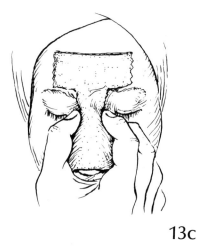

13c

13d

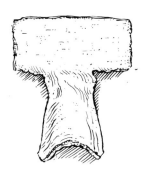

13e

14a–f

Although a severely displaced nasal fracture may be reducible by closed techniques for several months, a minimally displaced fracture will often become fixed by fibrous union within 3–4 weeks. Efforts to correct the deformity after such healing often require open reduction and osteotomies. An intracartilaginous incision is made (14a) and the membranous septum is separated from the columella (14b). With further dissection, the anterior dome is exposed (14c). The membranous lining is reflected from the septal angle (14d), the periosteum is elevated with a Joseph elevator (14e) the cartilagenous dorsum can then be lowered with sturdy Ragnell scissors (14f).

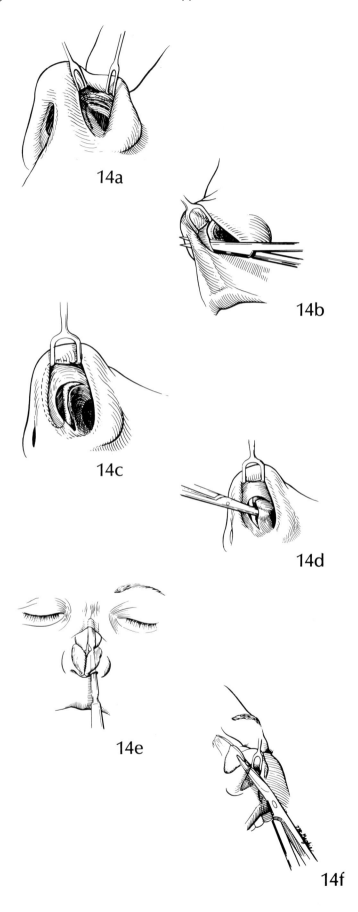

15a–d

Lowering of the bony dorsum is accomplished with a double-guarded osteotome (15a). Shortening of the caudal septum is done, as needed, with scissors (15b) and further contouring of the bony dorsum is achieved with a sharp rasp (15c). The nasal bridge can be narrowed with resection of small triangles of bone (15d).

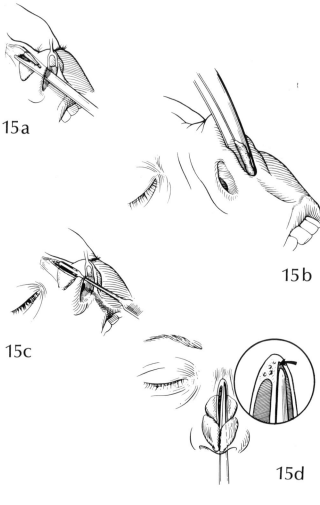

15a

15b

15c

15d

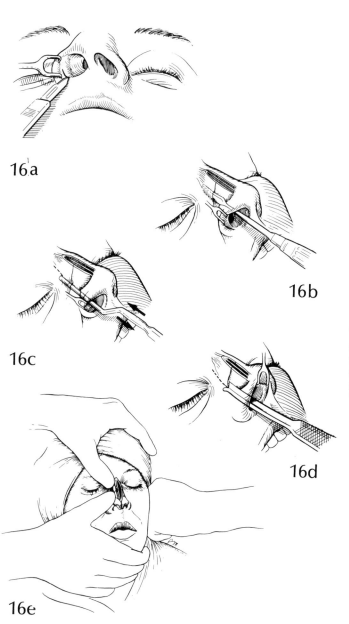

16a

16b

16c

16d

16e

16a–e

Through lateral piriform incisions (16a) the periosteum is elevated from the lateral aspects of the nasal bones and frontal processes of the maxillae (16b). The lateral osteotomies are begun with a rhinoplasty saw (16c) and completed with a guarded Silver's cartilage chisel (16d). The bones are repositioned with digital pressure (16e).

17a–d

When severely comminuted displaced nasal fractures heal, significant bone loss may occur from absorption. In such cases, reconstruction of the nasal profile is often best accomplished by bone grafting the dorsal ridge with a shaped graft taken from the iliac crest. A nasal plaster splint is similarly applied following these two reconstructive procedures, just as after closed reduction of an acute nasal fracture (*see Illustrations 13a–e*).

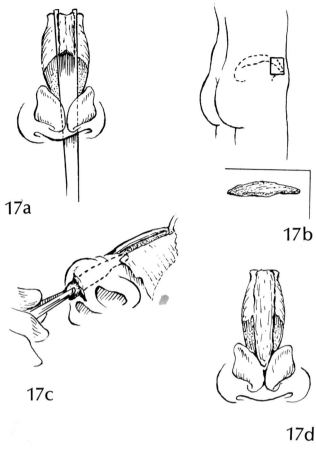

17a

17b

17c

17d

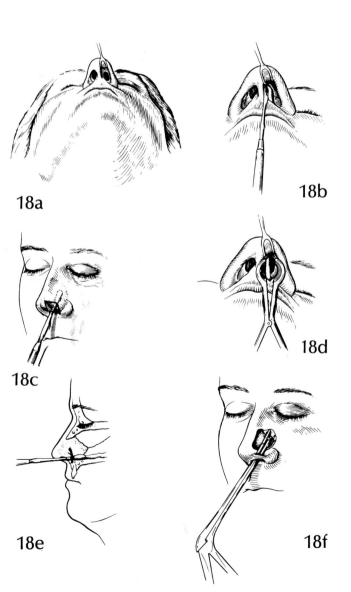

18a

18b

18c

18d

18e

18f

18a–f

When nasal airway obstruction occurs following septal trauma and cartilage deviation, this should be corrected by submucosal septal resection. An inverted J incision is made through the septal mucosa (18a), the mucosa elevated (18b) and a submucosal dissection performed (18c). The mucosa is retracted bilaterally with a nasal speculum (18d) and the base of the septal cartilage and boney spur prised free with a Freer elevator (18e). The portion of bony septum causing the obstruction is then resected with a rongeur (18f).

Maxillary fractures

The mechanism of injury in maxillary fractures is usually direct impact to the mid-face. Fractures of the maxilla may go unrecognized in the cursory physical examination and in routine skull X-rays. They are best diagnosed clinically by the manual demonstration of motion in the maxilla (*see* *Illustration 2f*).

19a–e

Maxillary fractures occur with great variety, even in the same maxilla when one side is compared to the other They can be best understood by considering them as originally described by LeFort: I, transverse; II, pyramidal; III, craniofacial disjunction.

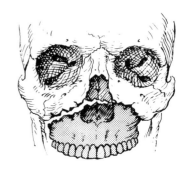

19a

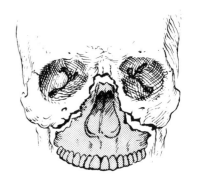

19b

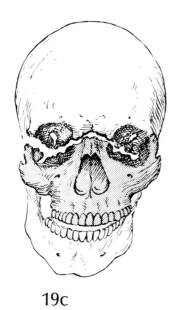

19c

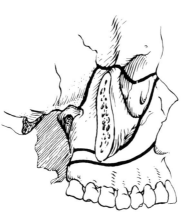

19d

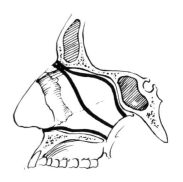

19e

Transverse maxillary fractures (LeFort I)

The fracture is often associated with a blow to the upper lip. The detached portion is often a single segment made up of the alveolar process, the palate and the pterygoid process. Inspection of the dental arches usually demonstrates an open bite with superior displacement of the maxillary incisors. With this fracture, motion of the entire upper dental arch and palate may be detected by grasping the upper teeth (see *Illustration 2f*). An isolated alveolar ridge fracture may also permit motion of the upper dental arch.

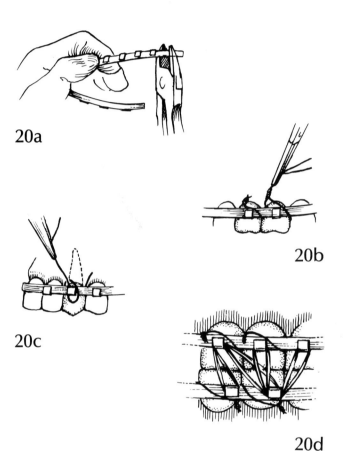

20a

20b

20c

20d

20a–d

Treatment of a transverse maxillary fracture consists of reduction and immobilization. This is a accomplished best by intermaxillary fixation with prefabricated metal arch bars which are first cut and shaped to fit the dental arch (20a) and then ligated with fine wire to the upper and lower dental arches (20b). Care should be taken to loop the wire around the arch bar to prevent loosening of the canine tooth (single root) (20c). Intermaxillary fixation is then achieved with dental elastics or wire ligatures (20d). In some cases, interosseous wire fixation at the fracture site, combined with intermaxillary fixation, may be required for stabilization.

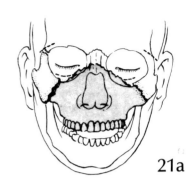

21a

21a–c

Pyramidal fracture (LeFort II)

An impact higher on the mid-face may result in a fracture that passes from the alveolus posteriorly along the nasal process of the maxillary bone, across the root of the nose and posteriorly through the lacrimal bones, the floor of the orbit and the pterygoid process. The isolated maxillary fragment is pyramid-shaped. Unless the blow has impacted the maxilla posteriorly or superiorly, motion can be detected at the medial portion of the orbital floors by grasping the upper teeth and rocking them back and forth. This fracture is quite unstable and tends to displace posteriorly. Incisions for exposure are made in the supraorbital (brow) and infraorbital regions (21a). Suspension wires are then passed behind the zygoma with a trochar (21b) and reduction and immobilization accomplished with wire suspension from the frontal bone or intact zygoma and intermaxillary fixation. Direct wiring at the infraorbital rim may add to the stability of the repair. Comminution is sometimes found at these points, however, and makes interosseous wiring difficult (21c).

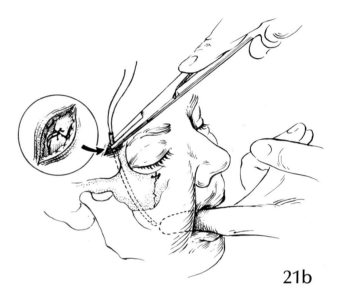

21b

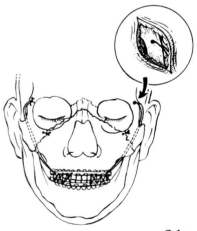

21c

Craniofacial disjunction (LeFort III)

Powerful forces delivered to the maxilla may completely separate the facial bone structures from the base of the skull. The only remaining attachment of the face to the skull is soft tissue. This injury is more severe than the pyramidal fractures because the fractures extend transversely across the nasal bridge, both posterior orbital walls, the lateral orbital rims and the zygomatic arch, separating the face from the cranium. Patients with this facial fracture often have an associated intracranial injury.

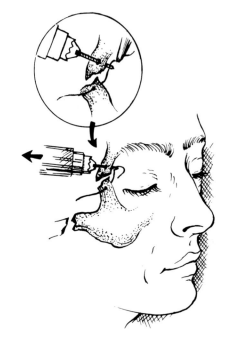

22a

22a & b

Treatment consists of reduction and immobilization of the fracture, using techniques similar to those used in LeFort II fractures (see *Illustrations 21a–c*) with the addition of interosseous wiring at the zygomatic frontal suture to provide greater immobilization. Two techniques of retrieving the wire outward through drilled holes involve fixing the wire threaded through the hole in the drill bit (22a) or using a smaller wire loop to retrieve the fixation wire (22b). Cerebrospinal fluid rhinorrhoea is not a contraindication to operative reduction of this fracture. In some instances, this reduction will stop the rhinorrhoea. The deformity that results from inadequate treatment of a severe maxillary fracture is a flattened, elongated or depressed mid-face.

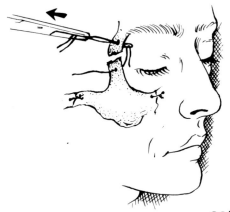

22b

23

Because of severe associated injuries, significant delay in the definitive treatment of maxillary fractures may be necessary. When this delay exceeds 3 weeks, there is often sufficient fibrous union to prevent mobilization of the maxillary fragments. When this occurs, either surgical refracture or application of external disimpacting forces becomes necessary. The latter can often be accomplished with a 3–5 lb (1.5–2.3 kg) weight applied to an arch bar, using pulleys on a Balkan frame, during the 24 h preceding surgery.

Numerous special appliances and instruments have been developed for the treatment of maxillary fractures and special metal and plaster headcaps devised for external support. Despite mechanical refinements, these skull-supported traction devices (Visor-Halo and Diadem) fall

short of their intended function. They are difficult to apply, uncomfortable for the patient to wear and require constant adjustment. They usually do not remain in place for the length of time required to accomplish their purpose. The preferable method of treatment of most maxillary fractures is open reduction and internal wire fixation, along with the use of intraoral acrylic splints and dental cap splints. Late treatment of healed displaced LeFort II and III fractures, as described by Tessier, consists of monoblock repositioning of the displaced bony mass and filling the resulting bone defects with bone grafts.

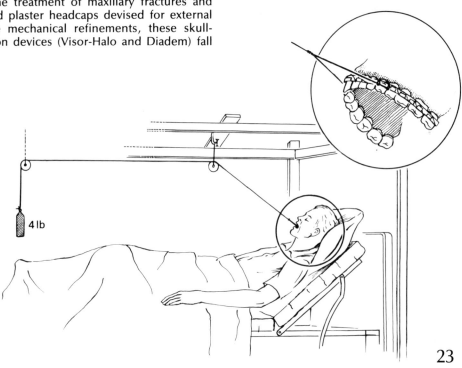

4 lb

23

Zygomatic fractures

24a & b

The zygoma has two components: the malar eminence and the zygomatic arch. Fractures may occur at either segment, separately or in both, but an isolated arch fracture is uncommon. The most common fracture of the zygoma involves depression of the malar eminence. This type of fracture consists of three parts – hence, the terms 'tripod fracture' and 'trimalar fracture'. The fracture sites are usually found at the zygomaticotemporal and zygomaticofrontal suture lines and the infraorbital foramen (24a). The fractured zygoma may undergo varying degrees of rotation and depression, depending upon the mechanism of injury and displacement of the lateral palpebral ligament may be seen.

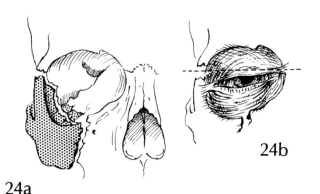

24b

24a

25a–f

Treatment usually requires open reduction and internal interosseous fixation at two of the three fracture sites. A steplike incision in the lower eyelid is made (25a) and the periosteum along the inferior orbital rim and orbital floor is raised (25b). The zygoma is elevated by passing a sturdy curved instrument (such as curved Mayo scissors or Dingman elevator) behind the zygoma through a lateral rim incision and placing an upward-forward force on the zygoma to disimpact it and position it anatomically (25c). The reduction is ascertained by observing the inferior orbital rim fracture line and the zygomaticofrontal suture line. Direct observation of the inferior orbital rim and orbital floor is made and after drill holes are made, the fractures are wired appropriately (25e). When comminution or depression of the orbital floor is present, a thin (0.02–0.04 inch) sheet of alloplastic material, dimethylpolycyloxaine (Silastic), shaped to fit over the orbital floor, or a thin piece of autogenous bone, can be placed beneath the periosteum (25e,f). The implants are usually well tolerated and provide support for the orbital contents. This procedure prevents subsequent 'entrapment' of the inferior extraocular muscles into the fracture site. Failure to effect an anatomically stable reduction often results in a flattened and depressed malar eminence after the swelling has resorbed.

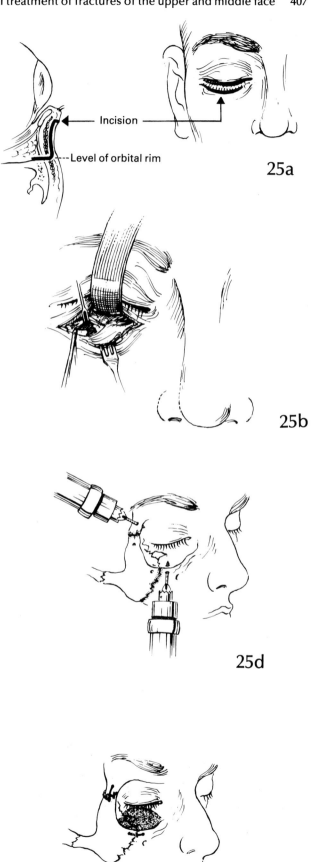

Incision

Level of orbital rim

25a

25b

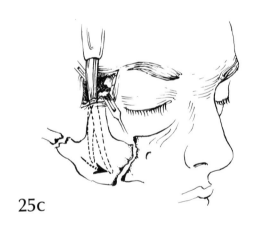

25c

25d

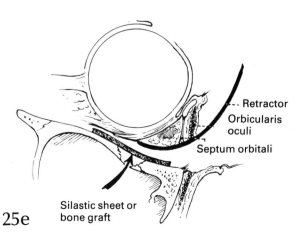

Retractor

Orbicularis oculi

Septum orbitali

Silastic sheet or bone graft

25e

25f

26a–d

Some authors have advocated semiclosed reduction through a Caldwell-Luc incision into the maxillary sinus. The reduction is performed through the sinus through an anterior antrostomy site (26a). The sinus is then packed with Iodoform gauze to maintain reduction. As the pack is inserted, the surgeon palpates the inferior orbital rim with his free hand and, thus, controls the fracture fragments and prevents overcorrection in the reduction or angulation of the zygoma (26b–d). This technique is somewhat hazardous; blindness has been reported secondary to compression and thrombosis of the ophthalmic vessel or from injury to the optic nerve by bony fragments at the time of manipulation. If packing of the maxillary sinus is necessary to maintain reduction, it should be done with the orbital floor under direct vision.

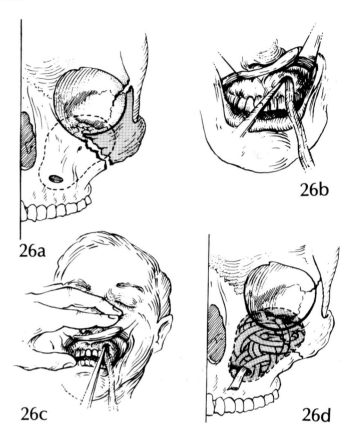

26a

26b

26c

26d

27a–c

Zygomatic arch

The zygomatic arch is fractured by a direct force. Considerable force is required to depress this arch, which must be fractured centrally and at both ends for depression to occur. Swelling over the zygomatic arch is seen initially, but depression or flatness characteristically follows resorption of the oedema and haematoma. Unilateral orbital ecchymoses are common, and tenderness, with occasional crepitation, can be elicited by palpation. Interference with mandibular excursion from impingement of the depressed fragments on the mandibular condyle or coronoid process occurs infrequently, but it is most important to ascertain. Zygomatic arch fractures can often be visualized on X-ray in the Waters projection, but special tangential (submental/vertical) views are best.

To reduce zygomatic arch fractures, the arch is restored by a force opposite in direction to the fracturing force. This is most simply accomplished by a semi-open method known as the Gillies technique. An incision is made in a vertical direction through the scalp and temporalis fascia, avoiding injury of the superficial temporal vessels (27b). The Kilner elevator can then be passed through this incision, deep to the zygomatic arch following the course of the temporalis muscle. With a lifting force, the bone fragments are reduced, restoring the arch. A snapping sensation is often felt by the surgeon as the arch is restored (27c). The architectural nature of arch construction obviates the need for support from below or internal fixation. The small opening in the temporalis fascia need not be sutured, but the scalp incision is closed with a single layer of silk sutures. Pressure dressings are contraindicated.

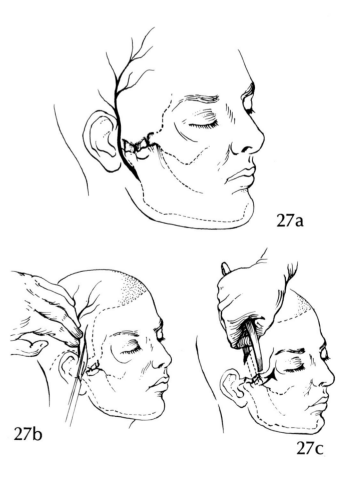

27a

27b

27c

Orbital floor fractures

28a & b

The forces of blunt trauma to the globe can be transmitted in various directions to cause 'blow-out' fractures to the orbital floor. The air-filled maxillary sinus below the orbital floor offers no support and comminuted fracture segments, periorbital fat and portions of the inferior rectus and inferior oblique muscles can be depressed into the maxillary antrum. Orbital floor fractures are most commonly seen in association with fractures of the zygoma. Isolated 'blow-out' fractures of the orbital floor resulting from the mechanism described above are rare.

Initially, there are orbital ecchymoses involving the lids, conjunctiva and sclera. Sometimes there is depression of the pupil on the involved side, although in other cases there is elevation due to compensating haematoma and oedema within the orbit. Enophthalmos following orbital fracture can result from enlargement of the orbital cavity, restriction of the eye from entrapment of the inferior rectus and inferior oblique muscles and loss of intraorbital fat by herniation and fat necrosis.

Such fractures are difficult to demonstrate by X-ray. A suggestive X-ray finding in a routine Waters projection is antral clouding due to haemorrhage.

These fractures are reduced as soon as the periorbital swelling subsides, since comminuted fracture fragments are more easily reduced before fibrous union takes place. An incision is made just inferior to the palpebral margin of the lower eyelid as described in the open reduction method for zygoma fractures (*see Illustration 25a*).

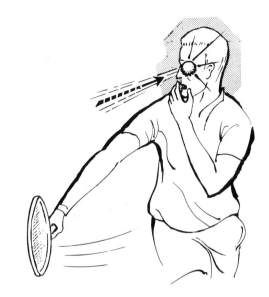

28a

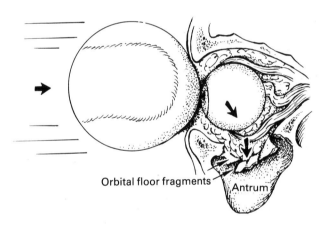

Orbital floor fragments   Antrum

28b

29a & b

To avoid infraorbital fat, the dissection is carried subcutaneously to the level of the inferior orbital rim, then deep into the rim periosteum through the orbicularis muscle. The periosteum of the orbital floor is then incised at the rim and carefully elevated with a delicate, angled raspatory. All comminuted bone fragments of the orbital floor are preserved and herniated orbital fat and entrapped muscles returned into the orbit. A shaped piece of Silastic of appropriate thickness, or thin piece of autogenous bone, is inserted subperiosteally for support. Occasionally, when marked depression has taken place or when late healing has occurred with absorption of comminuted fragments, the floor can be built up with layered, contoured Silastic implants or bone grafts. The periosteum is then allowed to fall back into its normal position, and the periosteal incision is closed at the orbital rim with catgut sutures when possible. The skin incision is then closed and the eye is dressed using antibiotic ophthalmic ointment in the conjunctiva.

There is a growing tendency among some ophthalmologists to treat many 'blow-out' fractures conservatively; however, the risks involved in exploration of the orbital floor are minimal compared to the hazards of failing to reduce significantly depressed fractures, particularly when associated with herniation of intraorbital contents into the maxillary antrum. Unfortunately, direct observation is still the only certain means of determining the extent of orbital floor injury.

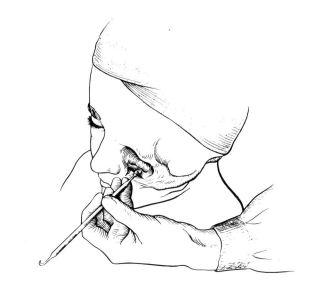

29a

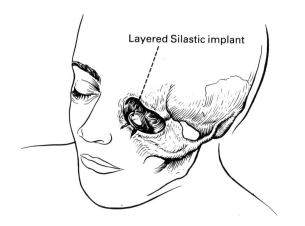

Layered Silastic implant

29b

Illustrations by K. Joy Graham

Fractures of the mandible

Michael Awty MRCS, LRCP, FDSRCS(Eng)
Consultant Oral and Maxillofacial Surgeon, Queen Victoria Hospital, East Grinstead, Sussex, UK

While the principles of the reduction and fixation of mandibular fractures are essentially the same as those of the treatment of any other fractured bone, certain features are peculiar to the mandible.

1. The presence of teeth allows very accurate reduction – by placing the mandibular teeth in occlusion with those of the maxilla. At the same time, this accurate reduction is essential for proper mastication and to ensure that there is no uneven stress which would impair healing. Good alignment is also necessary for the edentulous jaw, to enable dentures to be constructed.
2. The tooth-bearing portion of the mandible is covered only by mucoperiosteum, and a fracture in this region is frequently compound into the mouth and therefore prone to infection.
3. Lost teeth and pieces of denture must be accounted for, as they may be inhaled. A chest X-ray should be taken if there is any doubt. Dentures, however broken, should be kept, as they may be useful as splints or in the making of splints.
4. Fixation must be sufficiently strong to counter the muscle pull on the fragments which will occur in speech and swallowing; the method chosen will depend on the site of fracture, the number and state of teeth present and the age and general health of the patient.

Preoperative

Investigations

The history will suggest the fracture site and the position of possible secondary fractures; for example, a blow to the left of the mid-line of the mandible may fracture the underlying canine region and also the opposite angle of the jaw or the opposite condyle.

The most important investigation is the clinical examination, and palpation is necessary both extra- and intra-orally. Note should be taken of: (1) difficulty in jaw movement; (2) anaesthesia or paraesthesia of the lower lip, indicating a fracture involving the inferior dental canal; (3) tenderness over the fracture site, which may be swollen; (4) condylar movements; (5) ecchymoses in the floor of the mouth or buccal sulcus; (6) step deformity in the dental occlusion.

Displacement may occur in the direction of the blow, but also in the direction of muscle pull; for example, the anterior segment is pulled downwards by the depressor muscles with bilateral body fractures, particularly in the elderly.

Pressure on the point of the chin and compression across the angles of the jaw will reveal complete mandibular fractures, and frequently crack fractures, by producing pain at the site of the fracture.

Bilateral fracture in the anterior part of the mandible may leave the symphysis unstable; this makes the anterior segment likely to be drawn backwards by the action of the tongue and floor-of-mouth muscles, which can lead to inability to control saliva and may even produce obstruction of the airway. For this reason, the patient should always be nursed in the cardiac position, that is semi-upright or lying on his side – *never lying on the back.*

Radiography

Posteroanterior jaw and right and left lateral oblique visualizations of the mandible are the minimum, giving views at right angles to one another, and more specialized views may be necessary for fractures in the anterior part of the mouth and to establish whether or which teeth are involved in the fracture. The pan-oral film on its own, while a useful screen, is not adequate for diagnosis, as overlapping fractures sometimes do not register and it only shows malalignment in one plane.

Methods of fixation

Eyelet wiring

1

This method is the simplest and one of the best, provided that there are enough occluding teeth in both jaws for accurate reduction and immobilization. It may also be used when the fracture is in the ramus or the condylar neck, when stabilization is all that is necessary.

The eyelets are made of soft stainless steel wire, 0.35 mm in diameter, prestretched 10 per cent of its length. The eyelet can be formed by making a loop around the shaft of a dental burr, leaving the two ends about 10 cm long for ease of handling.

Eyelets are arranged in pairs, one in the upper and one in the lower jaw, roughly opposite one another, and with the chosen teeth coming into stable occlusion. The two ends are passed between two teeth so that the eyelet is on the buccal side, and they are then passed one around each tooth. For good retention the wire is kept low down on the gum, below the greatest diameter of the tooth crown, and the posterior wire is brought towards the front of the mouth and through the eyelet, to be twisted up on its fellow on the anterior buccal surface of the tooth nearer the midline. All twists should be clockwise and laid towards the midline, thus allowing any later adjustments to be made from the front. Tie wires, of thinner gauge than the eyelet wires, join the upper and lower eyelets, forming the intermaxillary fixation (IMF). The tie wires are thinner so that if an emergency arises (such as obstruction) the tie wires can be cut by a nurse with scissors.

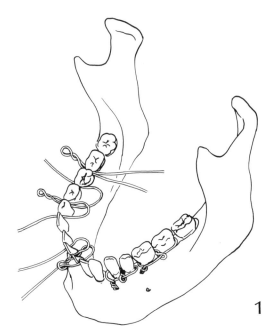

1

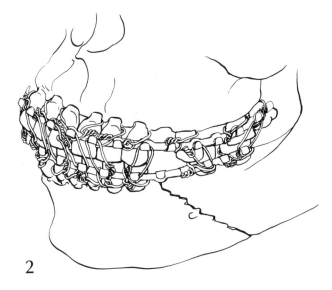

2

Arch bars

2

These provide an equally readily available method of fixation and have the advantage that they can be used when fewer teeth are present and when gaps between teeth need to be bridged. The bars are wired to the teeth and then tie wires are used for IMF.

Round-section arch bars are the most versatile because they allow the dental arch to be followed accurately; but when vertical displacement is troublesome, flat-section strip bars (as in the illustration) are useful.

Silver cap splints

3

When particularly strong fixation – as, for instance, part of fixation for a middle third injury – is necessary, cap splints are indicated. Splints allow more rigid fixation and can be easily incorporated in extra-oral support for more extensive facial injuries. The splints are prepared from impressions taken of the patient's teeth and need an experienced maxillofacial technician for their production. One splint is made for the maxilla and a separate splint for each segment of the fractured mandible. IMF of soft stainless steel wire is applied, using cleats. The separate portions of the lower jaw may then be joined by a bar, which is made from an impression taken after fracture reduction, and then screwed to locking plates previously soldered to the splint.

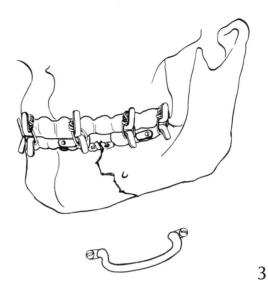

3

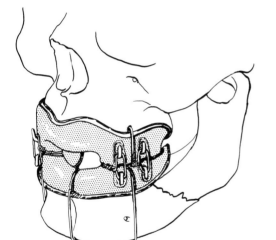

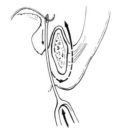

4

Gunning splints

4

These splints are used when one or both jaws are edentulous. In principle they are dentures, with flat blocks instead of teeth, and it is very useful to keep a patient's denture, as this may be able to be modified and used as the splint, or it may provide some of the necessary preliminary technical measurements, so saving clinical time. The fit surfaces of the splints are lined with black gutta percha to prevent pressure ulceration. The upper splint, which does not have a complete palate, is fixed to the maxilla by peralveolar wires passed through the bone in the premolar region. The lower splint is held in place by two circumferential wires around the body of the mandible. To pass the wire, a Kelsey Fry awl is pushed up through the skin below the body of the mandible, into the lingual sulcus, close to the bone. The stainless steel wire is then threaded through the eyelet of the awl and drawn down, around the lower border, keeping close to the bone, and then into the mouth again (in the buccal sulcus). Cleats, provided on the buccal aspect of the blocks, enable tie wires to be applied for immobilization in the usual way.

METHODS OF INTERNAL FIXATION

Direct bone wiring or interosseous wiring is used where fracture sites are unstable because of angulation or muscle pull. Internal wiring may also be used if, for reasons of poor general health (for example chronic respiratory infection), IMF is inadvisable.

Upper border wiring

5

This method is used to maintain reduction of unstable fractures – commonly at the mandibular angle and sometimes at the symphysis – and is used in conjunction with immobilization of the jaw by one of the methods already described. A wire is fixed across the fracture by an intra-oral approach. An alveolar flap giving adequate access is raised and holes are drilled with a dental round burr (size 6) in a right-angled handpiece. The holes should be at least 0.5 cm from the fracture ends. Where a tooth is to be removed from the fracture line (for example a wisdom tooth in a fractured angle), the holes may only need to be drilled into the socket, as the outer plate is thick, compact bone which gives adequate strength. This avoids raising the mucoperiosteum on the lingual aspect, which, of course, itself provides valuable splinting. However, in the symphysis the holes must go right through the bone. The wire should not be finally tightened until the teeth are in occlusion, and the twist is then cut short and turned in to the anterior burr hole.

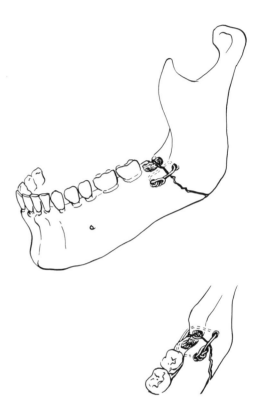

5

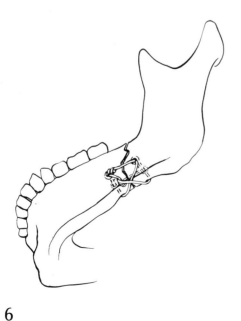

6

6

Lower border wiring

This method is used when reduction of the fracture is difficult to maintain and for unilateral fractures if for other reasons it is undesirable to wire the jaws of the patient together postoperatively. The fracture is exposed by a short submandibular incision and the wire is fixed across the fracture site at the lower border of the mandible. Two separate wires are commonly used: first a butt wire for initial stability and then a 'figure-of-eight' wire to give greatly enhanced stability. The first wire is passed through the anterior hole and back through the posterior hole, and then, with the fracture reduced and the teeth in occlusion, the two ends are twisted firmly together. The twist is not turned down, as the second wire is then passed through the anterior hole from the lateral aspect, brought round beneath the fracture and passed from the lateral aspect again through the posterior hole. The two free ends are then twisted together beneath the jaw, forming a figure-of-eight over the fracture site. Each twist can then be turned down.

7

Plating

This method is used when it is important to avoid intermaxillary fixation for medical or economic reasons.

It has several disadvantages: it leaves an external scar; the plate may have to be removed if there is subsequent infection or ulceration into the mouth; it can only be used when the fracture is in such a position as to allow the plate to lie flat against either the lateral side or the lower border of the mandible.

The fracture is exposed through a submandibular incision and reduced, while marks are made corresponding to the screw holes of the plate. The holes are then drilled through the compact bone, two on each side of the fracture. Care should be taken to avoid the neurovascular bundle; screws and plates should be of the same material.

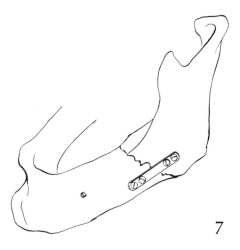

7

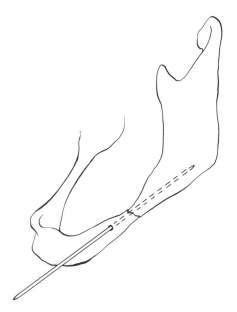

8

8

Bilateral fractures in the thin mandible

Control of reduced bilateral fractures in the elderly and infirm is often difficult, and Gunning splints are frequently inadequate. Yet it is just this type of patient in whom wiring is often inadvisable for general medical reasons (for example chronic respiratory infection). Internal fixation is sometimes indicated to facilitate apposition of the small fracture surfaces and to overcome the pull of the mandibular depressor muscles. It is vitally important not to raise the periosteum in this type of fracture because the main blood supply to the bone is by this route and not by the neurovascular canal.

A Steinmann pin is introduced into the mandibular canal in the region of the mental foramen and passed backwards, with the fracture segments held in correct alignment. The pin may either be cut off flush with the bone and the skin closed, so leaving the pin there permanently, or it may be left protruding through the skin incision for subsequent removal. In this case the pin end should be protected (by a small cork for example), and the pin-skin junction sealed with a wick of narrow ribbon gauze impregnated with Whitehead's varnish and tied around the pin to prevent local infection. Ideally both fractures should be pinned, but one side will counter the muscle pull and the other side can then be wired or plated *supra*periosteally.

9

Bone pins

These are used to control unstable fractures in which simple methods of internal fixation involving the introduction of a foreign body are inappropriate, for example when there is infection at the fracture site or poor bone apposition. Pins are also used to maintain fragments in correct position at the time of bone grafting. Toller's maxillofacial screw-pins with self-tapping thread, 7 cm × 3.2 mm in diameter and made of titanium, are very suitable (Down Bros., England).

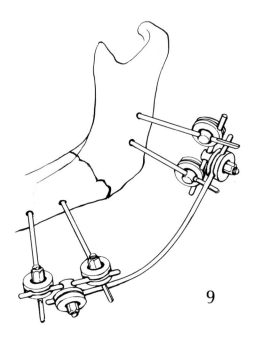

9

Postoperative care

Antibiotic cover is desirable for the incision to consolidate rapidly, especially in cases where internal fixation has been used. If general anaesthesia has been used, particular care must be taken to guard the airway during the recovery period. Wire-cutters should be kept near the patient and staff instructed as to which wires to cut to release the intermaxillary fixation. Feeding, which will be fluid or semisolid, should be high in protein and nutrients, and given in small quantities at frequent intervals. Oral hygiene should be carried out after each feed.

Immobilization time for uncomplicated mandibular fractures is 3 weeks in fit young adults, a little less in children, and more in older patients and those with multiple injuries or debilitating illness. In nearly all cases a period of intermaxillary fixation, resting the part, reduces the incidence of postoperative complications.

An upper border wire very occasionally ulcerates through the oral mucosa some time after treatment, and must then be removed, but this is usually a simple matter, using local analgesia.

EPITHELIAL INLAY

This is used to help restore the external contour of the face.

It is contraindicated when there is inadequate soft tissue cover over supporting bone.

10 & 11

A suitably sized pocket is created by a supraperiosteal dissection over the underlying bone. This pocket, when large enough to take the 'plumping' prosthesis, is lined with a thin free skin graft taken from the hairless area of the inner upper arm. The skin is held in position by draping it raw surface outwards on a temporary black gutta percha bung fixed to a previously constructed tray attached to cap splints. After 10 days the bung is removed briefly for cleaning, and 4 weeks later an acrylic bung is made to provide the desired amount of contour. Once the pocket is stable the silver splints are removed and the bung is maintained in position by a dental appliance. Cleaning the pocket initially must be swift, as skin contraction takes place rapidly. The services of a skilled maxillofacial technician are necessary.

Postnatal inlays are introduced in a similar fashion. Bungs may be in sections to aid retention or facilitate withdrawal for cleaning.

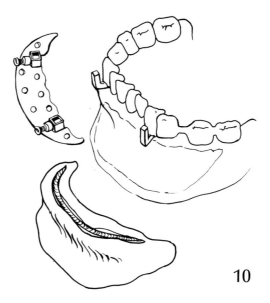

10

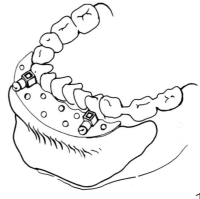

11

Illustrations by K. Joy Graham

Facial palsy – its management with static support and muscle transfer

Nicholas M. Breach FRCS, FDS, RCS
Consultant Surgeon, Head and Neck, The Royal Marsden Hospital, London, UK

Introduction

Paralysis of the muscles of facial expression, due to damage to the VIIth cranial nerve results in exposure of the cornea, epiphora, oral incontinence and facial asymmetry. Each of these symptoms is of major importance.

Surgical techniques are aimed at reanimation, but where this is not possible static support is offered, either to achieve resting symmetry or for protection as in the case of corneal exposure. It has been said that it is never possible to restore natural spontaneous expression and that when reanimation does occur following surgery the patient must learn to imitate emotional expression.

Eyelid closure

The levator muscles of the upper eyelid are not paralysed in facial palsy, so that when techniques which close the eyelids are used the normal levator mechanism generally enables the patient to open them.

GOLD WEIGHTS

Preoperatively a wax mould of the correct size and weight to produce eyelid closure is made. This specific mould can then be cast in fine gold, which is an inert material in the tissues.

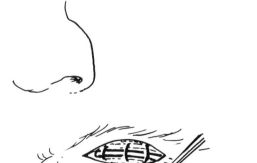

1

1

A transverse incision is made in the lateral upper eyelid skin. A pocket is developed superficial to the tarsal plate, but deep to the remnant of the orbicularis oculi. The gold weight is inserted into the pocket–as close to the eyelid margin as possible at the midpoint of the lid.

Lid magnets are sometimes used in a manner similar to that described for the insertion of gold weights, the opposing magnet being inserted into the lower lid. The disadvantage of this technique is that the metal is relatively non-inert and consequently likely to ulcerate the overlying skin.

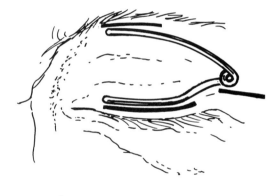

MOREL-FATIO SPRING

This light spring of stainless steel wire is implanted into the upper eyelid to produce closure.

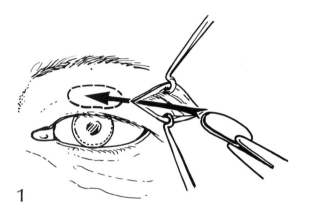

2

2 & 3

A lateral upper eyelid incision enables a pocket to be made in the eyelid margin, superficial to the tarsal plate, and inferior to the supraorbital rim. The spring is inserted and its limbs sutured to the tarsal plate at the eyelid margin and to the periosteum of the supraorbital rim.

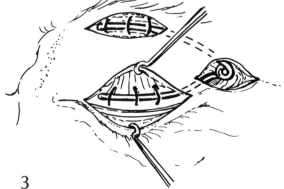

3

TEMPORALIS TRANSFER

The transfer of slips of the temporalis produce eyelid closure when the teeth are clenched.

4

The temporalis fascia is exposed through an extended preauricular incision. Transverse medial and lateral canthal incisions allow access to develop pretarsal pockets at both eyelid margins.

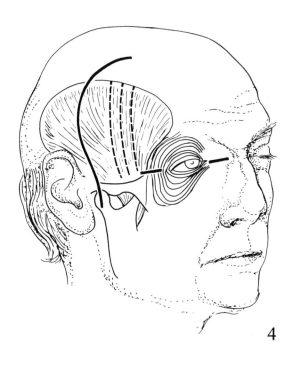

4

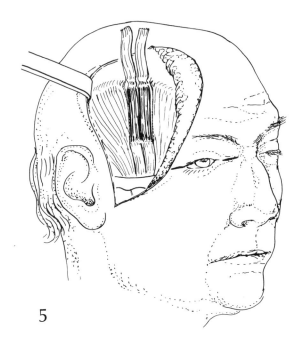

5

5

Two musculofascial slips are raised based on their origin from the temporal line. The slips must be teased apart, taking care not to divide the nerves supplying the muscle fibres.

6

The posterior musculofascial slip is introduced into the tunnel developed in the upper eyelid and the anterior slip into the lower lid. The distal parts of the tendon are crossed at the inner canthus and sutured to the canthal ligament using a non-absorbable suture. A similar suture is placed at the lateral canthus.

If regular training is undertaken, satisfactory eyelid closure can be readily achieved by clenching the teeth; with practice it will become a reflex habit.

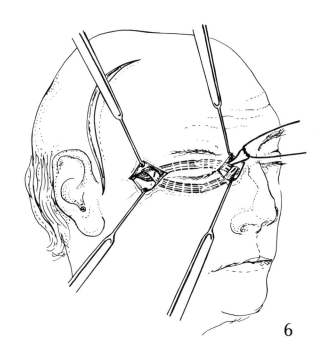

6

'THREE-SNIP' OPERATION

Provided that the lower eyelid is correctly positioned against the globe and that there is no damage to the canaliculi or the lacrimal drainage system, epiphora is rarely a problem. When through loss of eyelid tone, i.e. in facial palsy, the lower eyelid is displaced from its normal position tearing can become a serious problem. Improvement in the symptoms of epiphora can be achieved with the use of the 'Three-snip' technique. This technique opens the canaliculus by eliminating the punctum.

7a & b

The punctum and canaliculus of the lower eyelid are dilated with a 'Nettleship' dilator. One blade of a pair of fine iris scissors is placed in the vertical component of the canaliculus, the opposing blade is placed on the overlying conjunctiva and a cut is made.

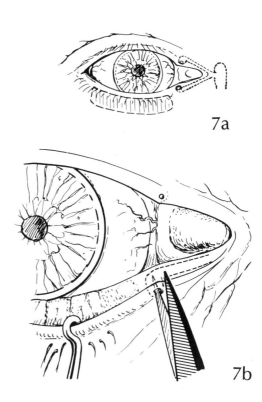

7a

7b

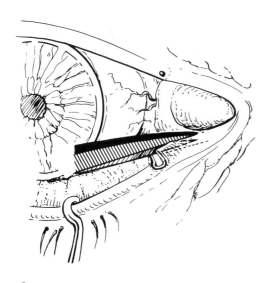

8

8

The second snip is made by placing one blade of the scissors in the horizontal component of the canaliculus and the opposing blade on the free eyelid margin. The cut is made to split the free margin of the eyelid.

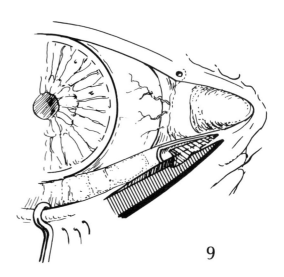

9

9 & 10

The third snip joins the two extremes of the former cuts; in this way a triangle of tissue which includes the conjunctiva is removed, leaving a canalicular trough into which tears drain. The inner canthal region is kept well lubricated during the first few days of healing; epithelialization of the raw surface rapidly occurs.

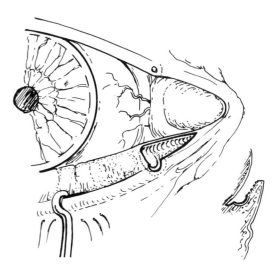

10

Operations on the angle of the mouth

11 & 12

EXCISION OF NASOLABIAL SKIN

Excision of an ellipse of nasolabial skin reduces the apparent skin excess and elevates the droop of the angle of the mouth.

When the edges of the surgical wound are approximated to close the defect the medial margin is advanced in an upward and medial direction, thereby raising the angle of the mouth.

A similar and more profound result can be achieved with a face-lift approach from a preauricular incision. The facial and cervical skin is undermined to the nasolabial crease. The skin is lifted upwards and backwards and the skin excess is trimmed.

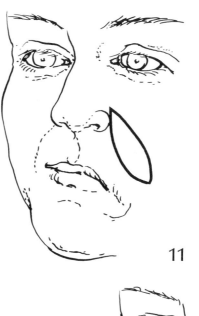

11

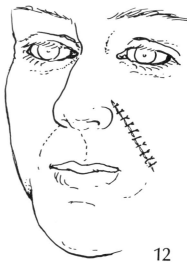

12

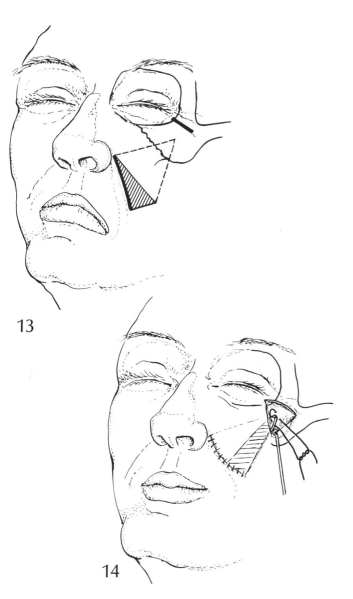

13

14

NASOLABIAL DERMOFAT SLING

13 & 14

Rather than discard nasolabial skin, a triangular area (shown as the shaded triangle in *Illustration 13*) is de-epithelialized and divided from the surrounding skin except for along its lower border. A pocket is created deep to the subcutaneous fat towards the malar prominence. The apex of the dermofat flap is then rotated into the pocket and sutured with a non-absorbable stitch to the malar periosteum using the incision shown. The residual nasolabial wound is then closed primarily.

Although the early results of this adjustment are satisfactory there is some relapse as gravity takes its toll.

STATIC SUPPORT FOR THE ANGLE OF THE MOUTH

Two strips of fascia lata measuring 18 cm ×1 cm are required. These may be obtained by a lateral thigh incision, in which case the defect can be closed to prevent muscle herniation. However, strips are most easily obtained with a fascial stripper – handling of the strips must be kept to a minimum as infection readily occurs.

15

Three incisions are made to give the access necessary to develop tunnels in the upper and lower lips from the angle of the mouth.

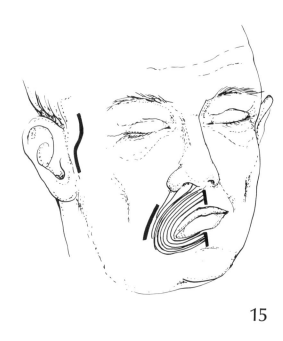

15

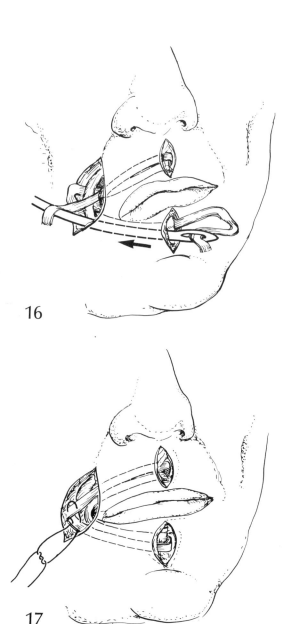

16

17

16 & 17

The fascia is inserted in a figure-of-eight manner. This is best done with a fascia needle (Blair-Reverdin). Once the two loops have been inserted the ends are crossed and sutured with a non-absorbable stitch. The tension should be adequate but not excessive as bunching of the lips will make it difficult to open the mouth.

18 & 19

The most efficient support for the angle of the mouth is made by placing the second fascial loop around the zygomatic arch. Once again this is best accomplished with a fascia needle. A preauricular incision is used to gain access to the zygomatic arch; alternatively the loop may be stitched to the temporalis fascia. The needle is passed through the temporalis fascia deep to the zygomatic arch and tunnelled deep to the masseter muscle towards the incision at the angle of the mouth, passing deep to the two bands of the loop previously inserted. A non-absorbable stitch is used to suture the two ends of the fascia. The loop must be placed under tension, thereby over-correcting the position of the angle of the mouth.

Wound drainage should not be required, but a pressure dressing and a course of antibiotics will reduce postoperative complications. When there is gross skin excess this sling procedure can be accompanied by either a unilateral face lift or an elliptical excision of nasolabial skin.

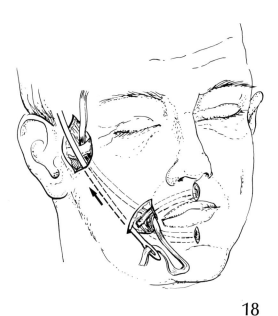

18

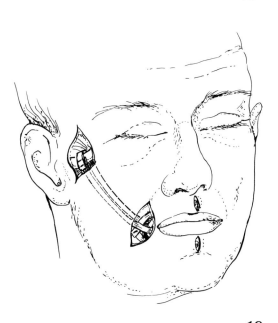

19

MUSCLE TRANSFER TO THE ANGLE OF THE MOUTH

By the simple technique of muscle transfer from either the temporalis or masseter, elevation of the angle of the mouth can be achieved when the teeth are clenched. In an intelligent patient this technique can produce satisfactory reanimation with practice.

20

Upward extension of the preauricular incision and the three perioral incisions provide adequate access for tunnels to be developed.

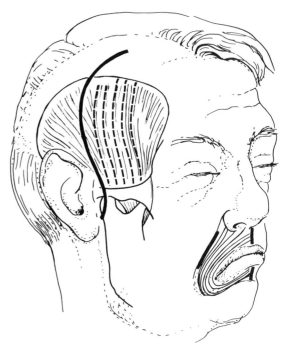

20

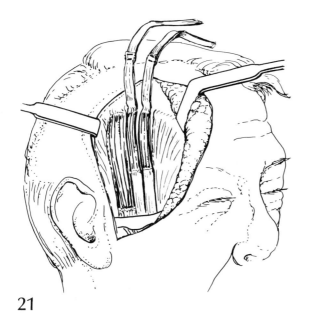

21

21

Two separate strips of temporalis fascia are raised to provide the additional length required to reach the midline of both lips. These strips are sutured to the fasciomuscular strips with non-absorbable stitches. Care must be taken not to divide the nerve fibres when developing the muscle strips; they must be teased apart.

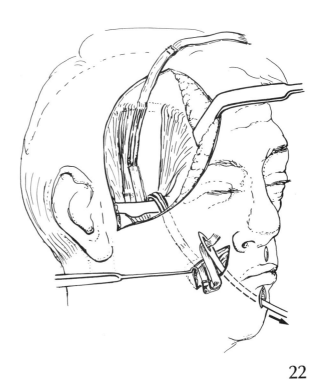

22

22 & 23

To achieve the cross-over at the angle of the mouth the anterior fasciomuscle strip is passed to the lower lip and the posterior strip to the upper lip. The strips are then stitched at the angle of the mouth. The tension developed when the strips are positioned must be adequate to raise the paralysed side to the normal level. Alternatively a loop of fascia lata can be used around the lips (*see* section on 'Static support for the angle of the mouth'); this provides additional support for the attachment of the temporalis muscle slips.

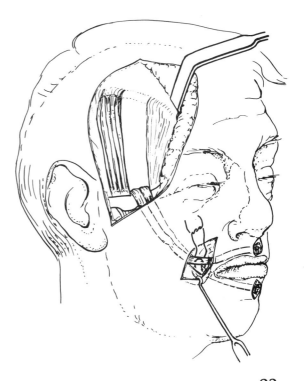

23

24

Detachment of slips from the insertion of the masseter muscle and their attachment to the angle of the mouth can also elevate the angle of the mouth when the jaws are occluded.

Nasolabial and submandibular incisions provide the access required. A separate fascia lata sling around the lips may be necessary to provide attachment for the muscle slips.

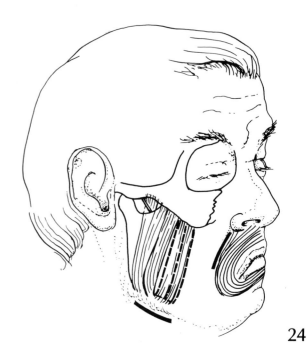

24

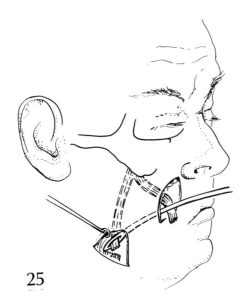

25

25

Two slips of the masseter muscle are carefully detached from the insertion of that muscle at the angle of the mandible. It is essential to retain the aponeurotic insertion with the muscle slips as this provides a satisfactory tissue to hold the stitches. The muscle slips must be teased apart in order to preserve the nerve fibres.

26

The two slips are brought out through the nasolabial incision and sewn to the modiolus of the oral angle or to a fascia lata loop. Excess skin can be removed by excision of a nasolabial ellipse or by a face lift approach.

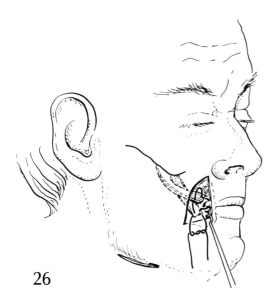

26

Conclusion

Muscle transfer can give a small range of movement of the angle of the mouth and provide tonic support for the flaccid paralysed face.

Facial palsy – nerve grafting and nerve anastomosis

H. Millesi MD
Head, Unit of Plastic and Reconstructive Surgery, 1. Chirurgische Universitätsklinik;
Director, Ludwig Boltzmann Institute of Experimental Plastic Surgery, Vienna, Austria

Introduction

Plastic surgery is concerned with the facial nerve in its extratemporal course. The plastic surgeon can be confronted with lesions of the facial nerve arising from a number of different causes.

Acute injury

When division of the facial nerve or some of its branches by an open injury occurs a decision has to be made whether continuity should be restored as a primary or as a secondary procedure.

If the lesion involves peripheral rami, it has to be considered whether a repair is indicated at all (see Section V).

Lesions of the facial nerve due to a fracture of the temporal bone are not a problem primarily for the plastic surgeon and are not discussed here.

Sequelae of injury

In the case of division of the facial nerve by past injury, restoration or continuity is attempted. It is surprising how, after long periods of denervation, the facial muscles can reassume function. The presence of contractile ability has to be proved by electrophysiological studies before such an attempt is undertaken.

Treatment of lesions of the facial nerve due to a fracture of the temporal bone by intratemporal operations is not dicussed here. However, if spontaneous recovery is not likely to occur and an intratemporal operation is not indicated, one of the techniques of nerve transfer (nerve anastomosis) or one of the palliative procedures can be considered.

Central lesions of the facial nerve

These lesions are recognized by the fact that the muscles of the face are usually not completely paralysed because they are supplied by nerves from both hemispheres. Restoration of continuity is impossible. Again, a nerve transfer (nerve anastomosis) or a palliative procedure is indicated.

Bell's palsy

In cases of Bell's palsy without spontaneous recovery, nerve transfer (nerve anastomosis) is considered if the time of denervation is not too long and contractile ability is present.

Tumours of the cerebellopontine angle

If the facial nerve has been destroyed by the tumour or during surgery, a nerve transfer (nerve anastomosis) is indicated.

Tumours of the parotid gland

If the facial nerve has to be resected for reasons of radicality, restoration of continuity or nerve transfer can be considered. Immediate restoration of continuity by nerve grafts is the logical treatment following resection of the facial nerve. The indications to do so are influenced by the general state of the patient, his or her age and the prognosis as far as the tumour is concerned. An alternative is an immediate nerve transfer (nerve anastomosis).

There are cases in which secondary repair after a waiting period is preferred.

In summary, whenever possible, the restoration of continuity is the treatment of choice. If this is out of the question, neuronization of the paralysed muscles by nerve transfer (nerve anastomosis) is considered. If this is contraindicated or has failed, one of the palliative techniques can improve the situation. For palliative procedures such as muscle grafting or muscle transposition with or without neuronization, see chapter on 'Static support for facial palsy', pp. 418–428.

Exposure of the facial nerve in its extratemporal course

This exposure can be performed at three different levels:

1. At the main trunk.
2. At the level of the intraparotid course when the main branches of the facial nerve are involved.
3. Beyond the parotid gland when the peripheral rami are involved.

Surgical exposure is indicated: if an acute traumatic lesion is suspected; in cases of secondary repair after trauma; in cases of parotid gland tumours to define the main trunk and the rami before the tumour is attacked; and if a nerve transfer is planned.

Skin incision

1

The skin incision is performed in one of the skin folds immediately anterior to the auricle; it curves round the lobe and turns downwards again, following the sterno-cleidomastoid muscle.

Alternatively an incision as for a facelift, with wide undermining of the skin, can be used or an incision beginning at the mastoid process and running obliquely along the body of the mandible.

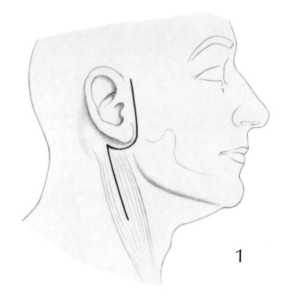

1

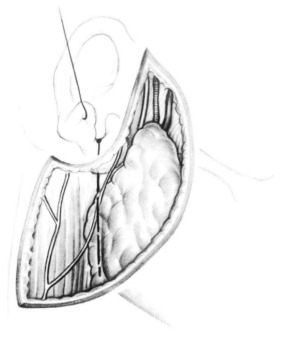

2

2

The skin is undermined in both directions. An anteriorly based skin flap is raised. Two structures are met at a superficial level, the external jugular vein and the great auricular nerve, both of which have a longitudinal course. Both structures are defined and retracted.

Dissection between the sternocleidomastoid muscle and the posterior border of the parotid gland

The anterior border of the sternocleidomastoid muscle and the lower and posterior border of the parotid gland are defined. In the superior border of the operative field the auricular cartilage is exposed. The tragal cartilage may have a small process pointing in the direction of the facial nerve. The anterior border of the sternocleidomastoid muscle is crossed by the posterior auricular artery and its concomitant vein, and by the posterior auricular nerve, which is a branch of the facial nerve. The facial nerve should be found parallel to a line between the external acoustic meatus and the angle of the mandible. The facial nerve is situated at a rather deep level.

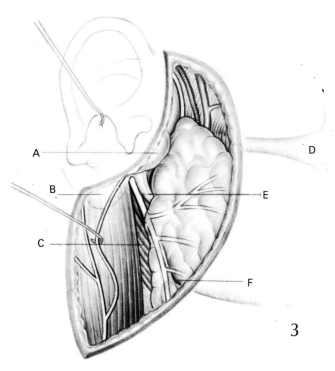

A = tragus; B = mastoid process; C = digastric muscle; D = zygomatic arch; E = styloid process; F = angle of mandible

3

3 & 4

Exposure of the main trunk of the facial nerve

The parotid gland is lifted and its posterior border is retracted anteriorly. The mastoid process is defined by palpation as is the styloid process. The tragal cartilage lies cranial to the posterior belly of the digastric muscle, which is defined. The posterior facial vein lies on top of this muscle. All the other important structures (internal carotid artery, internal jugular vein, external carotid artery and the accessory, hypoglossal, vagus and glossopharyngeal nerves) are deeper to this muscle.

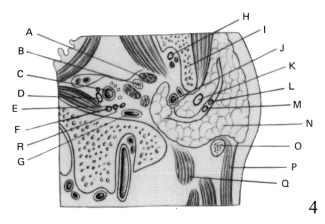

4

Horizontal section across the right parotid area – seen from above. A = styloglossus muscle; B = styloid process; C = internal carotid artery; D = vagus nerve; E = hypoglossal nerve; F = accessory nerve; G = jugular vein; H = inferior alveolar nerve; I = mandible, J = external carotid artery; K = retromandibular; L, M = branches of facial nerve; O = tip of mastoid process; P = sternocleidomastoid muscle; Q = digastric muscle; R = superior cervical ganglion

5

The facial nerve is situated cranial to the posterior belly of the digastric muscle. It has to be remembered that the stylomastoid foramen is situated quite a distance medial to the lateral contour of the bone. It is also medial to a line connecting the mastoid and the styloid process.

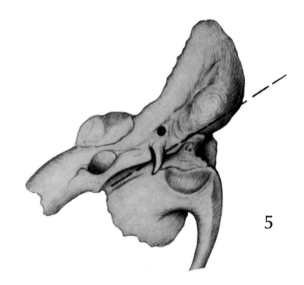

5

Exposure of the main branches of the facial nerve

After location of the main trunk of the facial nerve the branches are exposed by following the main trunk into the parotid gland. Within the parotid gland the nerve usually divides into two main branches. The upper one turns about 90° in an anterior direction. The lower branch continues to follow the line between the external acoustic meatus and the angle of the mandible.

Exposure of the proximal stump of the facial nerve in the stylomastoid foramen

In cases of very proximal damage, the proximal stump of the facial nerve can be defined only after opening of the stylomastoid foramen by careful chiselling and drilling.

Care must be taken not to damage the chorda tympani. This structure leaves the facial nerve on its lateral aspect in a retrograde direction. The course of the chorda tympani then turns anteriorly and runs lateral to the canal of the facial nerve.

Exposure of the branches of the facial nerve within the parotid gland (parotid plexus)

If after section of the facial nerve no distal stump is found, the fascia of the parotid gland is incised at its posterior border. Dissection proceeds between the major superficial part of the gland and the minor deep one. The superficial part is elevated. The branches of the facial nerve are located between the layers of the gland.

Exposure of the rami of the facial nerve peripheral to the parotid gland

6

If, in the case of a parotid gland tumour, the gland has to be removed radically or, if in the case of trauma, dissection within the parotid gland is difficult due to scar tissue formation, the peripheral rami are exposed at the level where they leave the gland. A larger skin flap is undermined and elevated as in a facelift procedure. The rami leave the parotid gland at its superior, anterior and inferior borders. There is great variation in the ramification of the facial nerve (see below) and, therefore, the terminology is not uniform. The following rami have been described: temporal, zygomatic, infraorbital, buccal, mandibular and cervical.

Other structures

The parotid duct is situated at the same depth running parallel and inferior to the infraorbital rami.

The superficial temporal artery is situated posterior to the temporal branches.

The transverse facial artery runs parallel and superior to the infraorbital branches.

The facial artery is crossed by the mandibular branch and by the labial and buccal branches of the facial nerve.

The anterior facial vein is situated lateral to the facial artery and follows the same course.

The buccinator fat-pad is deep to the branches of the facial nerve.

Other nerves

The auriculotemporal nerve (branch of the trigeminal nerve) is situated lateral to the superficial temporal artery.

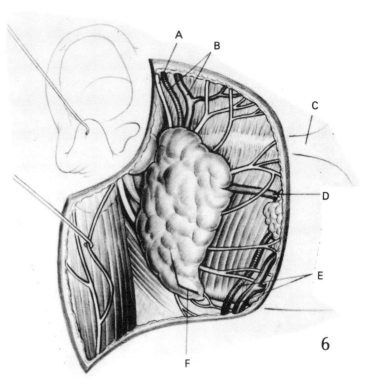

6

A = auriculotemporal nerve; B = temporal artery and vein; C = zygomatic arch; D = parotid duct; E = facial artery and vein; F = angle of mandible

The great auricular nerve (branch of the cervical plexus) has been mentioned already. Branches of this nerve are met in the pre-auricular area and superficial to the parotid gland.

The buccal nerve (branch of the trigeminal nerve). Branches of this nerve ascend in the area of the buccinator fat-pad from deeper layers and may form an anastomosis with the facial nerve rami in this area.

The infraorbital nerve (the second branch of the trigeminal nerve). Branches of this nerve emerge from the infraorbital foramen and ascend superficially to supply the skin of the cheek and the lower eyelid.

Variations in the ramification of the facial nerve

7a–f

After division of the main trunk of the facial nerve into the two first-order branches within the parotid gland, these branches divide again into second-order branches. Anastomoses occur between these branches forming the parotid plexus. More peripherally a further division into rami of third and fourth order occurs. The manner of ramification is subject to many variations. Six types of ramification are differentiated in the literature[1,2], as shown in the illustrations (with selective frequency). In the majority of cases (80 per cent) anastomoses are present between the zygomatic and buccal branches. Only in about 5–12 per cent do anastomoses occur between the buccal and the mandibular branches[3].

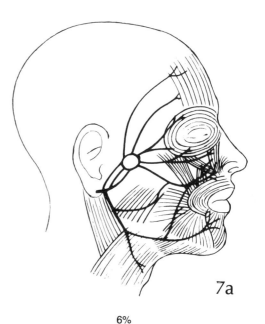

7a

6%

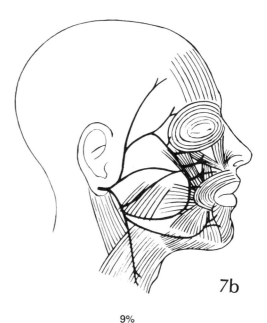

7b

9%

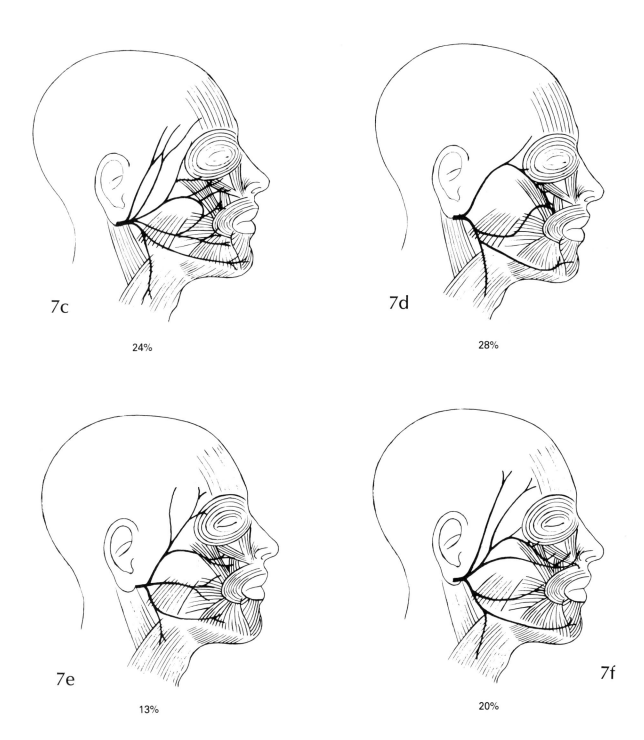

7c

24%

7d

28%

7e

13%

7f

20%

Intraneural topography

Information about intraneural topography is based on a study of 10 facial nerves in human cadavers, performed by G. Meissl[4,5].

At the stylomastoid foramen in all 10 specimens the facial nerve consists of three major fascicles and several smaller ones. After leaving the foramen the three fascicles fuse into the one large fascicle, divided by several perineural septa into compartments. One large fascicle is surrounded by several small ones, like satellites. In the middle third the large fascicle has divided into three fascicle groups. The cranial fascicle group joins the upper branch. In the final third of the main trunk the central fascicle group divides, the upper joining the upper branch, the lower the lower branch. The caudal fascicle groups join the lower branch.

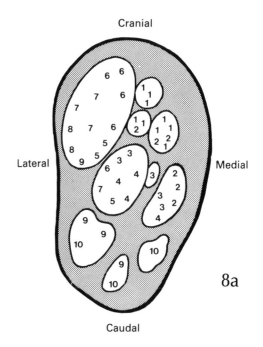

8a–d

The nerve fibres supplying individual muscles are not diffusely distributed over the cross-section but show distinct prevalences in certain areas as shown in the illustrations. Comparing (a) and (b) it can be seen that on leaving the stylomastoid foramen the main trunk turns about 90° anticlockwise.

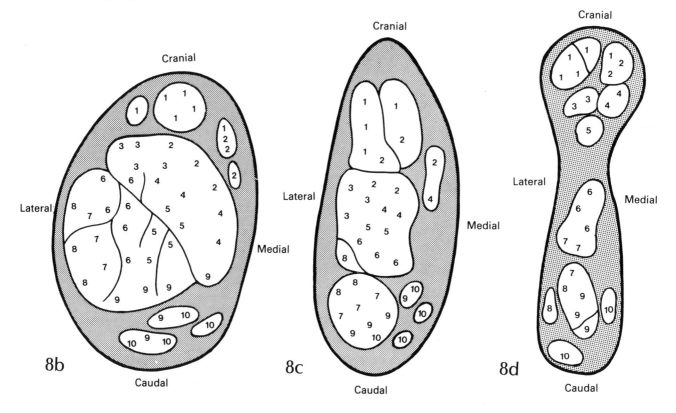

Restoration of continuity

BASIC CONSIDERATIONS

The technical approach for dealing with a facial nerve damaged in its extratemporal course is different in primary or secondary repair. It is influenced by the site of the lesion and by whether the nerve was cut cleanly without a defect, or whether there is a nerve deficiency.

After traumatic section of the facial nerve a primary repair has advantages. The anatomical situation is usually clearer than in secondary exposure and there is no retraction. However, very often the facial nerve lesion is part of a major injury and an immediate operation may be contraindicated. Secondary repair within several months has at least an equally good chance of producing a satisfactory result. It can be performed by an experienced surgical team under elective conditions.

The technique of exposure and repair will be different for a main trunk lesion and for lesions of the branches within the parotid or of the rami in the cheek and in the temporal area. Due to the plexiform structure, division of some of the peripheral rami does not produce a permanent functional loss. However, under certain conditions, repair is still indicated.

If there is a clean division, the two stumps are separated by elastic forces. These forces have to be overcome to unite the two stumps again if a primary repair is performed. In the case of secondary repair the retraction due to elastic recoil is very often fixed; in addition, a neuroma is present at the central and a glioma at the peripheral stump and these have to be resected. Therefore, even in the case of a clean cut, there will be some difficulties.

In blunt injury the nerve tissue of the two stumps has suffered some damage, but it is difficult to assess the amount at primary surgery. In secondary repair the damaged tissue can be recognized easily because it has become fibrotic. It has to be resected. In such a case one finally has to deal with a larger defect.

A small distance between the two stumps can be overcome by mobilization and by rerouting the nerve to a straight instead of a slightly curved course. If the deficiency extends beyond a certain limit a stump-to-stump coaptation can be achieved only by approximating the two stumps with tension. If there is tension proper coaptation is difficult to achieve and to maintain and much more surgical manipulation is necessary. Nerve grafts can be used to achieve an indirect coaptation between the two stumps. The great disadvantage of nerve grafting lies in the fact that the regenerating axons have to cross two sites of coaptation instead of one. For this reason in the past nerve grafts have been considered inferior to stump-to-stump coaptation. During the past few years sufficient material has been collected to prove that indirect coaptation by a nerve graft, in spite of the two sites of union, can produce better results than direct union under tension.

The classic technique of nerve repair since the 1870s has been epineural nerve suture. Attempts to repair the individual fascicles of a divided nerve by perineural stitches did not become popular because of the increased surgical trauma during such a procedure. Since the development of microsurgical techniques, optical magnification combined with very fine instruments has permitted intraneural manipulations with an acceptable amount of trauma, and much more attention can be paid to the intraneural structures[6].

In classifying the intraneural structures three main types of peripheral nerves can be differentiated:

1. Nerves which consist basically of one large fascicle (monofascicular nerves);
2. Nerves having a few large fascicles (oligofascicular nerves); and
3. Nerves consisting of many smaller fascicles (polyfascicular nerves).

The fascicles of a polyfascicular nerve may be arranged in fascicle groups or may be diffusely distributed over the cross-section.

TECHNICAL CONSIDERATIONS

The technique of nerve repair consists basically of four steps: preparation of the stumps; approximation; coaptation; maintaining the coaptation.

Preparation of stumps

The two stumps are prepared by resecting the damaged tissue in primary repairs and by resection of the neuroma and the glioma respectively, including the fibrotic parts, in secondary repairs.

9a, b & c

Lesions of the main trunk near the stylomastoid foramen

In this area the facial nerve consists of one large fascicle. There are only a few very small fascicles like satellites around this large fascicle. The central stump in this area is prepared by resection of slices from the periphery towards the centre, using a sharp instrument such as a razor blade or a No. 11 blade. The resection is repeated until normal tissue is encountered.

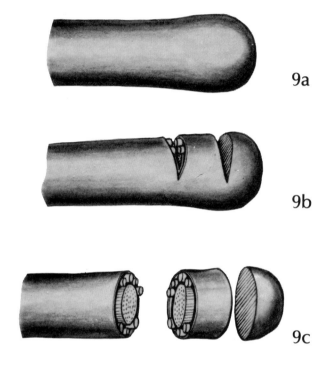

9a

9b

9c

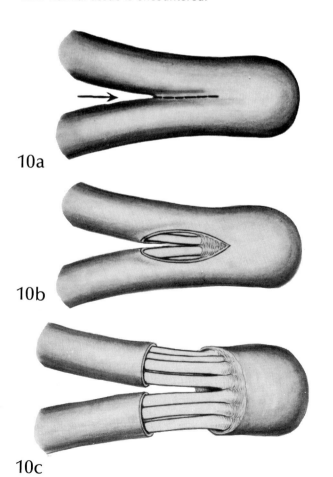

10a

10b

10c

10a, b & c

Lesions of the peripheral part of the main trunk

At this level the facial nerve has a polyfascicular structure with group arrangement. Therefore, the preparation of the stump is performed in a different way. The epineurium is incised in the normal tissue zone and separated from the underlying fascicles. Two to four fascicle groups can be isolated and the epifascicular epineurium is cut at the division. Under microscopic view the dissection proceeds from the normal tissue towards the neuroma and the glioma, respectively, and the resection is performed exactly at the level where the normal fascicles lose their normal appearance.

In peripheral lesions the branches and rami are treated like one fascicle group and no further intraneural dissection is performed.

Approximation

The prepared nerve stumps are approximated to achieve coaptation. This is done by using a 10/0 nylon stitch for manipulation. This stitch can be anchored in the epineurium, in the perineurium of a fascicle or in the interfascicular tissue.

Coaptation

The aim is to achieve a coaptation which is as close as possible to the normal anatomy. Whenever possible, that is if the two stumps have an identical fascicular pattern, the individual fascicles should be coapted exactly.

Fascicular coaptation is easily achieved in nerves consisting of a few large fascicles but very difficult in a polyfascicular part of a nerve. The fascicular coaptation is achieved under microscopic view by gentle manipulation. A compromise has to be established between maximum precision and minimum surgical trauma. It is sometimes necessary to improve the fascicular coaptation by one or two additional stitches at the most (10/0 nylon). There is a point beyond which the surgical trauma outweighs the advantage of increased accuracy.

If in a polyfascicular nerve the fascicular pattern of the two stumps does not correspond, the best that can be done is to identify the corresponding fascicle group and achieve a coaptation between these groups (interfascicular coaptation).

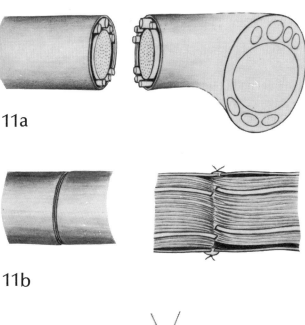

11a

11b

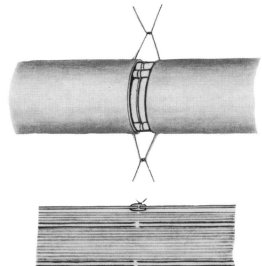

11c

11a–d

For a lesion of the main trunk without a gap fascicular coaptation of the large fascicle has to be established (a). It is of no importance whether epineural, perineural or interfascicular stitches are used.

In the case of a tight union with epineural stitches where the large fascicle is still in good shape, the small fascicles may be buckled and without contact (b). If the coaptation is performed loosely without tight contact of the circumferential margin of the epineurium, the fascicular coaptation of the smaller fascicles can be controlled in a much better way (c). Tight contact of the circumferential margins of the epineurium is not relevant to the result, nor is tight contact of the circumferential margins of the perineurium of the individual fascicles. A fibre film forms within a very short time between these margins and in a few days a collagen sheath is established. If the fascicular pattern does not correspond and an interfascicular coaptation is performed, due to the different fascicular pattern tight contact between the margins of the perineurium is *a priori* impossible. In spite of this, good results can be expected.

Coaptation in a malrotated position has to be avoided (d).

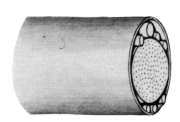

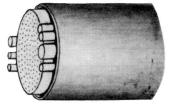

11d

12

In this case a central stump consisting basically of one large fascicle with some satellites has to be united with a peripheral stump containing a polyfascicular structure with group arrangements. Three or four nerve grafts can be used for individual coaptation. One graft is connected to the upper part of the central cross-section (1, 2) and the upper fascicle group in the peripheral stump (1, 2). The second graft connects the upper and medial aspect with the intermediate fascicle group (2, 3, 4). The third graft is united with the lateral aspect of the proximal stump and leads to the upper half of the lower fascicle group (5, 6, 7, 8). The fourth graft unites the lower medial aspect with the lower half of the lower fascicle group (7, 8, 9, 10). Some fibres (5, 6, 7) will go in the wrong direction because the fibres of different qualities are not well separated and there are no sharp boundaries between areas where fibres of a certain quality are predominant. Instead of the first and the second grafts, one larger graft can be used.

The example given here and those in all other figures are based on individual dissections and it should be kept in mind that there is a great variation between individual cases.

13

In deficiencies between the main trunk and the branches within the parotid, four nerve grafts of different sizes are again used for indirect coaptation. One graft unites the upper aspect of the central stump with the upper half of the upper branch (1, 2), the second graft the upper medial aspect with the lower half of the upper branch (3, 4, 5), the third graft the lower lateral aspect with the upper half of the lower branch (6, 7, 8), and the fourth graft the lower medial aspect with the lower half of the lower branch (7, 8, 9, 10, 5).

Some fibres (5, 6, 8) will go in the wrong direction.

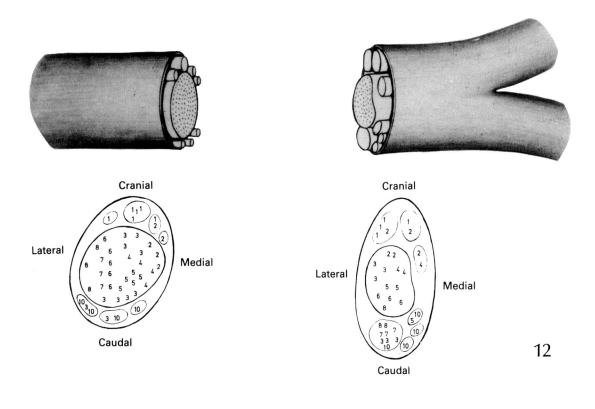

12

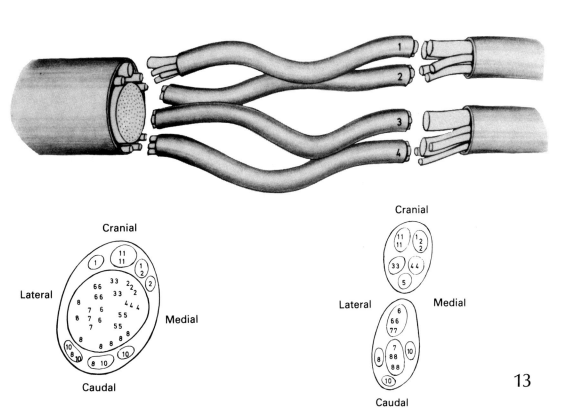

13

14

Deficiencies between the main trunk and the peripheral rami

Six to eight smaller nerve grafts are used. The first nerve graft is used to connect the upper aspect of the cross-section in the central stump with the temporal branch, the second is used to unite the upper medial aspect with the zygomatic branch, the third graft connects the centre of the central stump with the infraorbital branch, the fourth graft the central and lateral part of the central stump with the buccal branches, the fifth graft the lower aspect of the proximal stump with the inferior buccal branch and the sixth graft the lower aspect of the central stump with the mandibular branch. This procedure has to be modified according to the individual case.

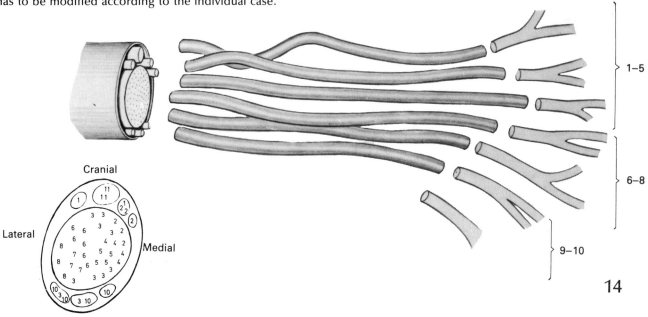

14

Maintaining the coaptation

The problem of maintaining the coaptation becomes more pronounced the greater the tension acting on the site of coaptation. If there is tension one stitch cannot produce contact between the two cross-sections; only contact at the site of the stitch is achieved and several other stitches have to be used to provide a better contact. If there is only very slight tension, an area of contact is established just by approximation using one stitch.

If there is no tension at all, natural fibrin clotting is sufficient to maintain the coaptation. Of course extreme care has to be taken to avoid shearing forces during wound closure, and immobilization for the early postoperative period is essential. If natural clotting is relied on, tension has to be wholly avoided.

The tensile strength of a sutureless coaptation can be increased considerably by application of a concentrated fibrinogen solution and induction of coagulation by adding thrombin, Ca^{++}ions and Factor XIII[7]. A similar procedure is advocated by Duspiva et al[8].

The use of artificial glues for peripheral nerve repair, as suggested by Heiss and Faul[9] did not prove very successful[10] in peripheral nerves. Extreme care has to be taken to avoid contact of the glue with the cross-section of the nerve stumps. Successful application of this technique to facial nerve repairs has been reported[11, 12] in combination with tubulization. In this case the glue is applied a certain distance from the site of coaptation, but still remains cytotoxic and produces marked tissue reaction. If tension is avoided these techniques can be disregarded.

Protection of the coaptation

To avoid adhesions between the site of nerve repair and the surrounding tissue, which may lead to an invasion of the site of coaptation by proliferating connective tissue, and to avoid the aberration of axon sprouts, wrapping up the site of coaptation has been recommended. Different materials have been used such as millipore, Silastic membranes and collagen membranes. Adhesions to the surrounding tissue can be prevented but the connective tissue proliferation originating from the margins of the epineurium remains inside the tube. This tissue proliferates between the nerve tissue itself and the walls of the tube. Axon sprouts can aberrate into this connective tissue layer. Collection of liquid in the space between tube and nerve has been observed. The material forming the tube may cause tissue reaction, especially if the site of repair is not completely immobile. Tubilization has been used to achieve and maintain a coaptation within a tube by application of the glues at the end of the tubes at a certain distances from the site of coaptation. The best technique for avoiding invasion of the site of coaptation by proliferating connective tissue and axon aberration is to establish a union without tension, leaving the axons an opportunity to proceed straight forwards as a result of reducing the gap and the tissue reaction between the stumps.

Repair of peripheral lesions

In the area anterior to the anterior border of the masseter muscle, anastomoses between the rami of the facial nerve form a plexifom structure as outlined above. Some of these rami can be divided without any visible loss of function. Therefore, a local injury in this area, even dividing some of the rami, may not lead to a circumscribed facial palsy. It is said that anterior to a vertical line passing through the lateral angle of the eye, a repair of facial nerve branches is not necessary. But there are cases in which the plexiform arrangement is less developed (see pp. 00–00) or severance of more branches has occurred. In these cases a circumscribed palsy results from such an injury. Primary or secondary repair of the peripheral rami is then indicated.

15a–e

An example is shown in the illustrations. A patient had suffered an injury which caused two deep wounds in his cheek. A permanent palsy of the major zygomatic muscle and the levator of the upper lip followed. There was no tendency towards spontaneous recovery. The site of the lesion and the original arrangement of the rami are shown (a). Exposure demonstrated that the nerve branch to the major zygomatic muscle and two other branches going to the upper lip had been divided (b). Two proximal stumps could be detected coming from the infraorbital rami. A third proximal stump arising from the buccal rami was encountered. After gentle mobilization repair by end-to-end coaptation of the two above-mentioned rami was performed (c). The third ramus was not restored. An alternative would have been the use of two small nerve grafts if approximation had been difficult (d).

Sometimes it may be impossible to locate all proximal stumps. In this case one would attempt to locate the proximal stump in the area of the buccal rami and transpose it to the peripheral stumps.

If no central stump had been detected, a local nerve transfer would have to be considered. After ensuring that enough rami to the angle of the mouth and the lower lip remain intact, one of these rami is divided, transposed to the peripheral stumps and united with them to activate the upper lip and the major zygomatic muscle (e).

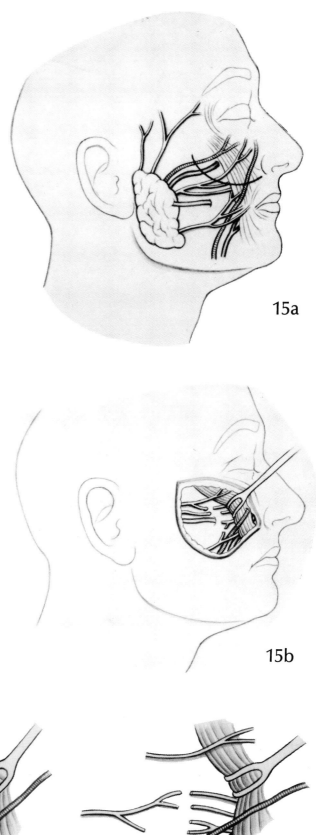

15a

15b

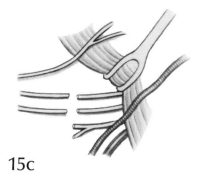

15c

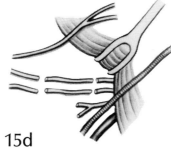

15d

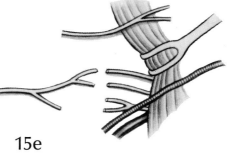

15e

Facial-facial-nerve transfer (anastomosis)

The idea is based on confidence in the value of long nerve grafts and on microsurgical technique, which can deal with such small nerve rami without too much traumatization.

The technique has been independently published[13, 14, 15].

The anatomical basis lies in the fact that the peripheral rami of the facial nerve are connected with each other by many anastomoses forming a plexiform structure. Some of these rami can be divided without loss of function. The central stump of such a divided ramus can be used to provide axons, which are transferred to the paralysed side via nerve grafts. These nerve grafts are connected with the peripheral stumps of facial nerves, nerve rami or branches on the paralysed side. It is of course extremely important to prove that there are at least two rami serving the same muscles before one of them is divided. This can be done by electric stimulation.

A facial-facial-nerve anastomosis is indicated if repair of continuity of the facial nerve is impossible. It is an alternative to the hypoglossal and accessory nerve transfer (anastomosis). It is not yet possible to give a final evaluation of this technique. The amount of motor recovery may be less pronounced than in the two other nerve transfers discussed. Better symmetry and better resting tonus may be achieved, and disturbing concomitant movements are avoided.

The operation can be performed in two stages:

1. The donor rami are exposed and identified. After procuring the nerve grafts the central ends of these grafts are coapted with the donor rami and the grafts placed into position via subcutaneous canals across the midline ('cross-face') to the paralysed side.

2. The peripheral ends of the grafts are exposed, the branches of the paralysed facial nerve are identified and transected, and the peripheral ends of the graft are coapted with the peripheral ends of the facial nerve branches. Usually a neuroma has formed at the peripheral end of the grafts, proving that the graft has been neuronized. Smith[14, 15], Millesi and Samii[16] and Samii[17] perform the operation in one stage, at least in young individuals with good chances of nerve regeneration. There are cases in whom a spontaneous innervation of paralysed facial muscles after the first stage of a two-stage procedure could be proved, from spontaneous contact of the peripheral ends of the graft and the paralysed muscles.

16

Smith[14, 15] uses an incision which parallels the nasolabial folds. The exact site of the incision is defined in the following way. A line is drawn to mark the inferior border of the maxilla. The summit of the malar prominence is noted and this establishes the site for drawing a vertical line. This vertical line usually lies about 2 cm lateral to the nasolabial fold. A transverse line about 1.5 cm or 1 fingerbreadth below the inferior margin of the zygoma is marked at the points where the vertical and the transverse line cross it, and it becomes the centre of a 5 cm incision that parallels the nasolabial fold. By dissection parallel to the expected course of the rami the nerve plexus can be identified in the depths of the wound. The nerves are usually deeper than expected. The rami of the facial nerve always enter the corresponding muscles on their deep surface. After identifying the facial artery at the level of the nasolabial fold, the rami crossing the facial artery can be identified. Some cross the artery superficially and others deeply. The rami of the facial nerve are superficial to the buccinator fat-pad. It has to be remembered that at this level branches of the buccal nerve, derived from the trigeminal nerve and carrying sensory fibres, ascend from deeper layers and may form anastomoses with the facial nerve. Other sensory fibres in this area come from the infraorbital nerve (second branch of the trigeminal nerve).

Smith uses one nerve graft, containing four to six fascicles, which are united with branches of the zygomatic and buccal rami.

A similar incision is made on the paralysed side. The plexus formed by the zygomatic and buccal rami is identified. The peripheral end of the graft is connected with branches proximal to the plexus. One graft 9–14 cm in length is necessary. It is suggested that the graft be placed in reverse direction (antidromal), connecting what was the peripheral end of the graft to the proximal stumps of the facial rami; thus, loss of axons by unsatisfied branches is prevented.

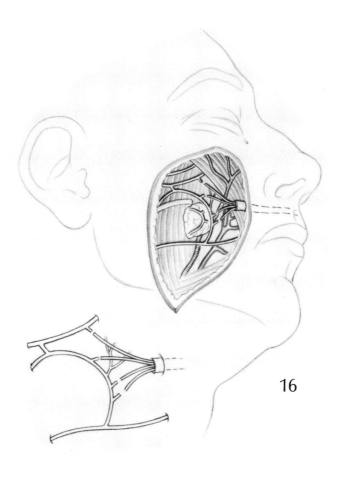

16

17

Anderl[18, 19] advocates a two-stage procedure. He uses three to four grafts. Three incisions are made on the non-paralysed side.

The *first incision* is placed 1.5 cm lateral to the orbit and is about 3 cm in length. This incision serves to identify the zygomatic rami. This plexus lies superficial to the orbicularis muscle. Anderl identifies the rami by electric stimulation. By application of local anaesthetic (0.5 per cent lignocaine + adrenaline) to the rami to be transected and electric stimulation of paralleling rami it can be proved that function is still preserved.

A *second incision*, 4 cm in length, is made about 1.5 cm behind the nasolabial fold. The rami of the facial nerves are identified deeply beneath the fat tissue in the layer of the deep muscle groups. Usually three rami of this plexus are selected for transection. In the lower part of the exposure branches leading to the buccinator and orbicularis oris muscle are identified. Three or four of them are selected for transection.

A *third incision* is made 1.5 cm anterior to the facial artery where it crosses the mandible. By this incision the terminal rami of the mandibular branch can be identified.

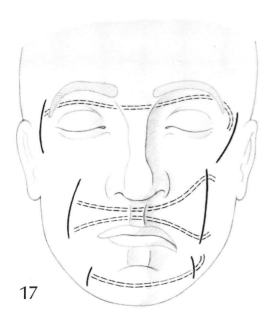

17

18

Three to four grafts are used. Therefore, it is necessary to utilize two sural nerves.

One graft (15–17 cm in length) is placed in a channel passing through the frontalis muscle and the superior part of the orbicularis muscle on both sides. The graft is put into place in an orthodromal direction, its proximal end being united with the central stumps of the facial nerve rami. The inset shows how the fascicles of the graft are coapted with different proximal stumps. If axons leave the nerve through small unsatisfied branches, they can grow into the paralysed frontal and orbicularis oculi muscles. An additional neuronization of these muscles is expected. The insertion of the graft is facilitated by a small incision in the area of the glabella. The peripheral end of the graft is brought to the paralysed side, using an incision 1 cm in length, just anterior to the hairline and superior to the zygomatic arch. Care is taken to ensure that this incision will not interfere with the site of the operation at the second stage.

One or two grafts, 13–15 cm in length, are passed across the upper lip to the paralysed side. This is facilitated by an incision in the philtrum. The peripheral ends of the grafts are brought to the paralysed side, using two additional short incisions in the paralysed cheek, anterior to the parotid gland. It is important that the peripheral ends of the grafts come into an area which is posterior to the site where the union with the peripheral stumps of the paralysed facial nerve will be performed in the second stage. Also, these grafts are inserted in normal proximal/distal orientation. Usually two grafts are used, except in cases where a sufficient number of rami cannot be utilized, when one graft only is inserted.

Another graft 6–8 cm in length may be inserted between the rami of the mandibular ramus. This graft is used especially if insufficient rami in the buccal area are available and only one graft has been used across the upper lip[19].

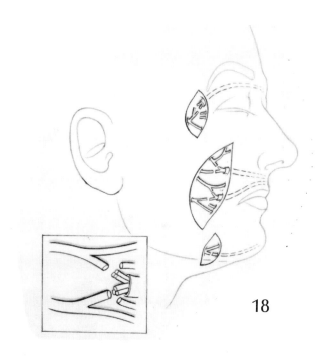

18

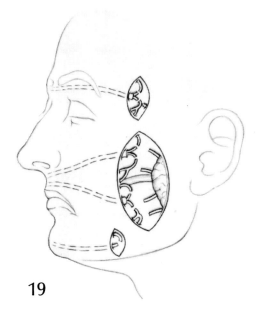

19

19

Usually the second stage is performed 5 months later. An incision is made over the zygomatic arch in the direction of and lateral to the lateral margin of the orbit. The second incision is 4 cm in length and made anterior to the parotid gland. If the graft across the chin is used, the third incision is made over the mandible near the facial artery. The peripheral ends of the grafts are identified and the neuroma at the peripheral ends resected. The fascicles of the sural nerve grafts are separated. The rami of the paralysed facial nerve are identified as they leave the parotid gland. After transection coaptation is performed between the peripheral ends of the grafts and the peripheral stumps of the facial nerve rami. The second stage can also be performed through a facelift incision.

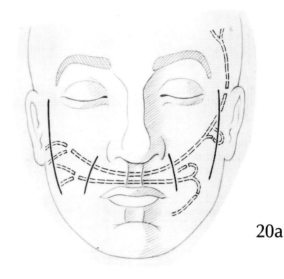

20a

20a–d

Samii[17] uses a one-stage procedure. He performs the exposure from an incision which is located 1.5 cm anterior to the tragus. By elevating an anterior flap the facial nerve rami are identified in the preparotid area. Some of the zygomatic and buccal branches are used for the transfer. Two nerve grafts are inserted across the upper lip, using additional incisions in the nasolabial fold. The peripheral anastomosis is performed using a similar incision 1.5 cm anterior to the tragus.

Based on fibre counts which revealed that the zygomatic branch of the facial nerve usually contains about 40 per cent of the nerve fibres of the whole facial nerve territory, Samii now restricts the procedure to connection of only the zygomatic branches of both sides.

The coaptation, regardless of which technique is used, follows the principles already outlined. Under magnification (×10–16) the fascicles of the sural nerves are separated and coapted with the fascicles of the facial nerve rami. One 10/0 nylon stitch is used to achieve approximation. As the coaptation is without any tension, no additional manipulations are necessary to maintain it.

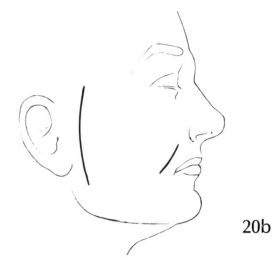

20b

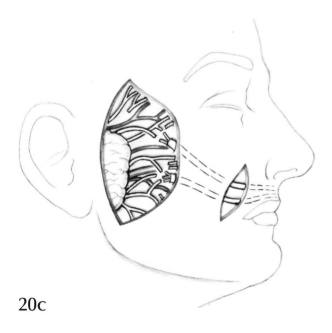

20c

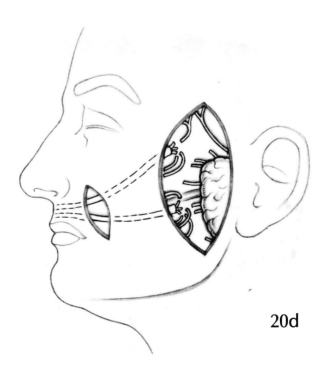

20d

Hypoglosso-facial-nerve transfer (anastomosis)

21a, b & c

An incision is made along the anterior border of the sternocleidomastoid muscle. Superficial to the muscle the external jugular vein and the branches of the great auricular nerve are encountered. The vein is ligated and transected, the branches of the postauricular nerve being retracted in a dorsal direction. By dissection between the anterior border of the sternocleidomastoid muscle, the posterior and lower border of the parotid gland and the cartilage of the external acoustic meatus, the main trunk of the facial nerve is exposed as described previously. The exposure is extended to the carotid triangle. The posterior belly of the digastric muscle is identified. Deep to this muscle the external jugular vein and the external carotid artery are seen. There are two arteries branching off the external carotid artery in this area: the occipital artery and the sternocleidomastoid branch.

The hypoglossal nerve descends between the internal carotid artery and the internal jugular vein. It is located superficial to the vagus nerve and the superior cervical ganglion (see *Illustration 4*). Inferior to the lower border of the digastric muscle the hypoglossal nerve lies between the external carotid artery and the jugular vein. It divides into the descending branch, which follows the artery to form the Ansa hypoglossi profunda. The main trunk turns anteriorly and crosses the external carotid artery on its outer aspect. However, there are cases in which the hypoglossal nerve turns not only around the artery but also around the internal jugular vein. The nerve is crossed by the common facial vein.

The main trunk of the hypoglossal nerve is transected (C, D) as far peripherally as possible; it is then turned upwards and laterally. The facial nerve is divided close to the stylomastoid foramen and turned downwards. A coaptation between the proximal stump (A) of the hypoglossal nerve and the peripheral stump (B) of the facial nerve is established. To avoid atrophy of the homolateral side of the tongue the descending branch of the hypoglossal nerve is transected (C) at a level sufficient to provide a long proximal stump. This is turned upwards and united with the peripheral stump (D) of the main trunk. Thus, re-innervation of the tongue is obtained.

Hypoglossal nerve transfer usually results in a powerful neuronization of the facial muscles. Some resting tonus is provided. Many patients are embarrassed by the concomitant movements of the facial muscles during speech and swallowing. For this reason, some patients insist on giving up an otherwise successful anastomosis.

Conley[19] reported on a large successful series of hypoglosso-facial-nerve-transfers. He performed this in selected cases simultaneously with a radical resection of the parotid gland with sacrifice of the facial nerve.

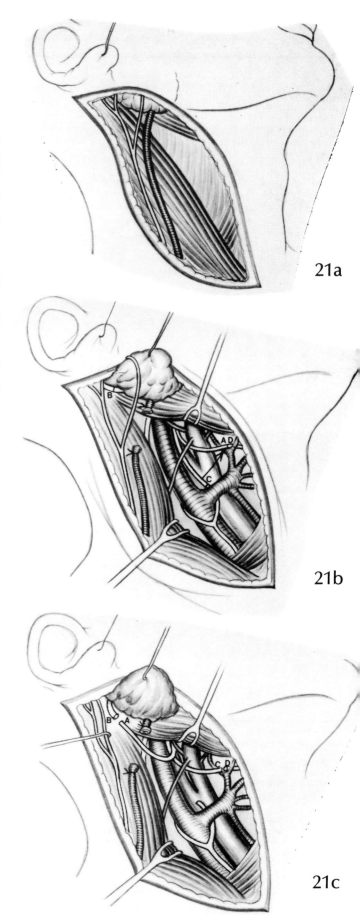

21a

21b

21c

Accessory-facial-nerve transfer (anastomosis)

22

An incision is used which runs parallel to the anterior border of the sternocleidomastoid muscle. The branches of the great auricular nerve are retracted posteriorly, and the external jugular vein is ligated. The main trunk of the facial nerve is exposed as described previously. The accessory nerve descends between the internal carotid artery and the internal jugular vein. It is deep to the hypoglossal nerve. It crosses the internal jugular vein posteriorly in two-thirds of the cases. In about one-third of the cases the nerve crosses the vein on its anterior and lateral surfaces. The nerve enters the sternocleidomastoid muscle on its medial side. At this level the nerve is divided into fascicles supplying the sternocleidomastoid and fascicles going on to supply the trapezius muscle. Only the part supplying the sternocleidomastoid muscle is used for the nerve transfer to avoid functional loss in the shoulder area[21]. Identification is facilitated by electrostimulation. The supply to the sternocleidomastoid muscle is separated from the remaining nerve and transposed in a cranial direction.

The main trunk of the facial nerve is transected close to the stylomastoid foramen and the peripheral stump swung down, to be approximated to the proximal stump of the transected part of the accessory nerve. Sometimes a direct coaptation is not possible and a small nerve graft has to be used for indirect union.

Accessory nerve transfer gives powerful innervation. Functional loss is acceptable if the part of the accessory

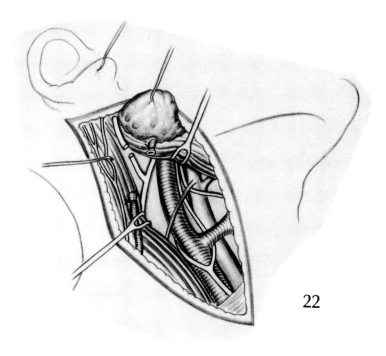

22

nerve going to the trapezius muscle is spared. The disadvantages are that symmetry at rest is poor if the patient does not innervate the facial muscles voluntarily and there are troublesome concomitant movements of the shoulder and head.

In cases of partial facial nerve paralysis, function can be restored by performing a selective nerve transfer of branches of the accessory nerve and the paralysed rami of the facial nerve via nerve grafts[22].

Providing the nerve graft

Sural nerve

23

The sural nerve is generally used if long nerve grafts are required. The sural nerve provides a nerve graft of 35–40 cm in length with a minimum of branching. The intraneural structure of the sural nerve differs depending on the level. At very proximal levels it can be a monofascicular nerve, more peripherally the number of fascicles increases, and in its peripheral part it is a polyfascicular nerve, showing some group arrangement. For this reason sections of the sural nerve can be selected according to the fascicular pattern required.

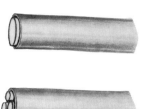
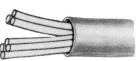
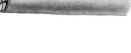

23

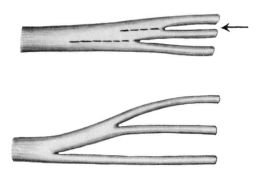

24

24

Proximal to the external malleolus the sural nerve divides into two or four branches. These are already preformed at higher levels and, by intraneural dissection, the peripheral portion of the sural nerve can be dissected into a graft with a main trunk centrally and several branches of the length desired at its peripheral end.

25a–e

The sural nerve is exposed through a small oblique incision behind the external malleolus. It is deep and lateral to the small saphenous vein. At this level there are at least two branches which are very small and difficult to define. Another incision is made 4–5 cm proximally; here the sural nerve is again very close to the small saphenous vein in the subcutaneous compartment. The nerve is fixed by a rubber band and is divided at a level behind the external malleolus. By gentle traction at the proximal incision the smaller branches are put under tension, can be identified now easily by palpation and are divided. After division of these branches the sural nerve can be easily extracted through the proximal incision.

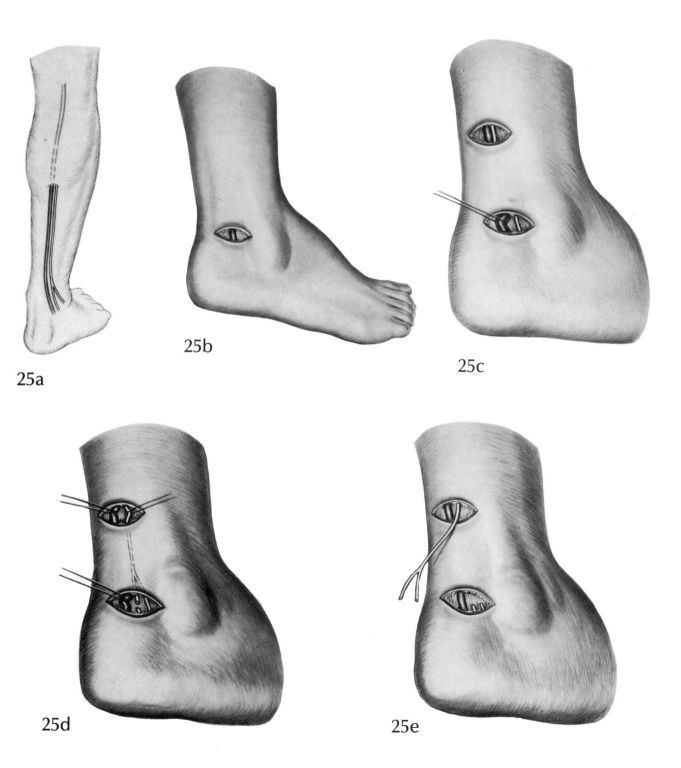

25a

25b

25c

25d

25e

26

By gentle traction the course of the sural nerve is identified proximally. Just below the popliteal fossa the sural nerve can be palpated. Again a transverse incision is used; the fascia has to be incised, and the sural nerve is identified lying between the two heads of the gastrocnemius muscle. A stripper could be used to liberate the sural nerve for extraction, but in about 15 per cent of cases the sural nerve receives another branch, usually from the lateral side.

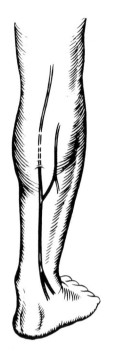

26

This additional branch would be destroyed by the use of a stripper. It is therefore preferable to make another incision in the mid-calf and identify the sural nerve there, which can be done easily by palpation with gentle traction on the peripheral stump. Here the nerve usually is immediately underneath the fascia. The presence of an additional branch can be detected by palpation when pulling. If it is certain that there is no additional branch or the additional branch has been identified and liberated by one or two additional incisions, the whole sural nerve can be extracted from the proximal incision. At the level of division a neuroma is formed. To minimize the risk of the development of neuroma pain it is always wise to perform the division at the level where the sural nerve is subfascial. Even if quite a small length of the nerve is needed, it is preferable to excise the whole sural nerve in order to leave the level of division deep between the muscles. Another advantage of excising the whole sural nerve is that the right portion of the nerve can be selected according to the desired intrafascicular structure. After preparation according to its fascicular pattern, the nerve is cut to give a graft of the desired length. The sections are carried out with scissors with undulated blades, using several gentle bites. With each bite the epineurium is shifted away from the site of the division to prevent overlapping of the cross-section by epineural tissue. A resection of the epineural tissue at the ends of the graft is not necessary, because the connective tissue proliferation from this free-grafted epineurium will be retarded and will not be able to interfere with the fascicular coaptation.

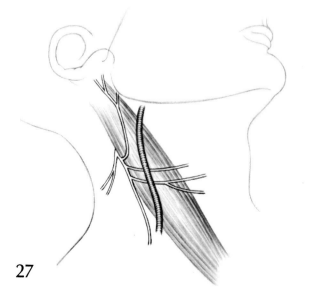

27

27

Cervical plexus

Nerves originating from the cervical plexus may be used as donors for nerve grafts. The branches of the auricular nerve are usually identified when the main trunk of the facial nerve is exposed. In the same way the anterior cutaneous nerve of the neck can be used. It has also been suggested that the main trunk of the C3 root could be united with the main trunk of the facial nerve and the great anterior auricular nerve of the neck connected with the branches. Thus, a nerve graft may be provided which corresponds to the basic features of the facial nerve. Due to the change of the interfascicular pattern it is uncertain whether with the use of such a compound graft the corresponding axons of the proximal and the distal stumps will be connected. Therefore, it is much better to reconstruct the pattern of the facial nerve by the use of individual nerve grafts instead of a compound unit.

References

1. Davis, R. A., Anson, B. J., Budinger, J. M., Kurth, L. Surgical anatomy of the facial nerve and parotid gland based upon a study of 350 cervicofacial halves. Surgery, Gynaecology and Obstetrics 1956; 102: 384–412

2. Shapiro, H. H. Maxillofacial anatomy. Philadelphia: Lippincott, 1974

3. Dingman, R. O., Grabb, W. C. Surgical anatomy of the mandibular ramus of the facial nerve based on the dissection of 100 facial halves. Plastic and Reconstructive Surgery 1962; 29: 266–272

4. Meissl, G. Facial nerve suture. In: Facial Nerve Surgery. U. Fisch. Ed. Amstelveen: Kugler Medical Publication BV; Birmingham, Ala.: Aesculapius Publishing Co., 1977

5. Meissl, G. Die intraneurale Topographie des extraniellen Nervus facialis. Acta Chirurgica Austriaca 1979; Suppl., 25

6. Millesi, H. Zum Problem der Überbrückung von Defekten peripherer Nerven. Wiener Medizinische Wochenschritt 1968; 118: 182–187

7. Matras, Helen, Dinges, H. P., Lassmann, H., Mamoli, B. Zur nahtlosen interfaszikulären Nerventransplantation im Tierexperiment. Wient. med. Wschr. 1972; 122 Jhrg.: 37, 517

8. Duspiva, W., Blümel, G., Haas-Denk, Sylvia, Wriedt-Lübbe, Ingrid. Eine neue Methode der Anastomosierung durchtrennter peripherer Nerven. Chirugisch Forum, Suppl., 100, 1977

9. Heiss, W. H., Faul, P. 'Nervennaht' mit Klebstoff. Langenbecks Archivfur Klinische Chirurgie 1965; 313: 710–713

10. Berger, A., Ganglberger, J., Millesi, H. Experimentelle Untersuchungen zur Nervennaht mit Klebestoffen. Symp. Klebestoffe i.d. Chirurgie, Verl. d. Wr. Med. Akademie 1968; 269

11. Miehlke, A. Surgery of the Facial Nerve, 2nd Edn. Philadelphia: W. B. Saunders, 1973

12. Conley, J. Salivary Glands and the Facial Nerve. Stuttgart: Georg Thieme, 1975

13. Scaramella, L. L'anastomosi tra i due nerve facciali. Archs ital. Otol. 1971; 82: 209

14. Smith, J. W. 'A new technique of facial animation.' In: Transactions of the Fifth International Congress of Plastic and Reconstructive Surgery (1971), pp. 83–84. Sydney: Butterworths, 1971

15. Smith, J. W. Facial nerve paralysis and microsurgery. In: Daniller, A. I., Stauch, B. Eds. Symposium on Microsurgery; New York City, 1974, pp. 172–176. St. Louis: C. V. Mosby, 1976

16. Millesi, H., Samii, M. Erfahrungen mit verschiedenen Wiederherstellungsoperationen am Nervus facialis. In: Plastische und Wiederherstellungschirurgie, pp. 111–127. Stuttgart, New York: H. Höhler, 1975

17. Samii, M. Modern aspects of peripheral and cranial nerve surgery. In: Advances and Technical Standards in Neurosurgery, Vol. 2. Ed. H. Krayenbühl. Vienna: Springer Verlag, 1975

18. Anderl, H. 'Reconstruction of the face through cross-face nerve transplantation in facial paralysis.' Chirurgia Plastica 1973; 2: 17–46

19. Anderl, H. 'Cross-face nerve grafting – up to 12 months of seventh nerve disruption.' In: Reanimation of the paralysed face: new approaches, Ed. L. R. Rubin, 241–277. Saint Louis: C. V. Mosby, 1977

20. Conley, J. Management of facial nerve paresis in malignant tumours of the parotid gland. In: Reanimation of the paralyzed face: new approaches. Ed. L. R. Rubin, 224–234. Saint Louis: C. V. Mosby, 1977

21. Bragdon, F. H., Gray, G. H. Differential spinal accessory-facial anastomosis with preservation of function of trapezius. Journal of Neurosurgery 1962; 19: 981

22. Yanagihara, N. In panel discussion, 'Classification and standardized documentation of surgical results.' In Facial Nerve Surgery, pp. 527–554, Ed. U. Fisch. Amstelveen: Kugler Medical Publication BV; Birmingham, Ala.: Aesculapius Publishing Co., 1977

Superficial musculoaponeurotic system platysma facelift

John Q. Owsley Jr MD, FACS
Clinical Professor of Surgery, Department of Plastic Surgery
University of California Medical Center, San Francisco, California;
Chairman, Department of Plastic Surgery, R. K. Davies Medical Center, San Francisco, California, USA

Introduction

The facelift operation is performed to improve the appearance of facial ageing by correcting laxity of the skin of the face and the neck. The operation starts with incisions made in the temporal and occipital scalp that are connected to incisions partially encircling the ear in the pre- and postauricular region. Through these incisions, undermining of the skin of the face and neck is initiated in the superficial subcutaneous plane. The undermining is carried forward in the neck near, or to, the midline, and in the cheek approaches the area of the nasolabial fold. After undermining, the redundant skin is lifted superiorly and the overlapping skin is trimmed, and the incisions sutured under moderate tension. In the classic facelift operation, the undermining is entirely at the subcutaneous level[1].

In recent years, plastic surgeons have recognized that the skin of the cheeks and anterior neck is an interconnected three-layer unit. This facial skin unit is comprised of the superficial epidermal-dermal layer, the underlying subcutaneous fat, and beneath that a gliding fascial membrane composed in part of smooth fibrous connective tissue and in part muscle. The gliding fascial membrane is called the superficial musculoaponeurotic system (SMAS). The SMAS has multiple fibrous extensions that attach through the subcutaneous fat to the superficial epidermal-dermal portion of the skin which allow the three layers to move together as a unit.

In the neck, the SMAS membrane incorporates the platysma muscle which extends from the lower jaw area to the clavicle. The platysma is involved in certain facial expressions involving the lower face and neck, such as extreme grimacing. The chronic spastic contraction of the platysma muscle produces neck cords, which with ageing can gradually create persistent vertical folds beneath the chin and on the upper anterior neck.

As the facial skin ages, there is gradual loss of elasticity in the epidermal-dermal layer of the skin as well as in the SMAS membrane. Gravity produces sagging of the cheek skin unit along the jaw creating fleshy 'jowls' and often a 'double chin' appears. This is due to the drooping of the fatty portion of the lax skin unit along the anterior and lateral jaw area. At the nasolabial fold, the cheek skin unit sags forward with ageing to increase the prominence of the fold which ultimately extends downward below the mouth, lateral to the chin, to become continuous with the jowl. Sagging of the subcutaneous fat and the gliding SMAS membrane contributes as much to the appearance of facial ageing as does the loss of elasticity in the superficial epidermal-dermal layer.

1a & b

In the SMAS facelift, the three-layer unit of facial and neck skin is freed by undermining at the level of the natural gliding plane just beneath the SMAS layer. After undermining, all three layers are lifted together, with the tension being placed on the underlying SMAS layer. The lift placed on the SMAS layer also corrects sagging of the overlying fat and brings the interconnected epidermal-dermal layer to an improved lifted position as well. Placing the tension of the lift on the deeper supporting SMAS layer produces a snug lasting lift in the chin and jawline that is not pulled in appearance. Since it is not necessary to place excessive tension on the superficial epidermal-dermal cheek layer in front of the ear, the skin incision can be placed behind the tragus, making that incision invisible.

Because the undermining performed with the SMAS facelift is at a natural gliding plane where few blood vessels cross, less bleeding occurs than with the classic skin facelift where many blood vessels are cut during the undermining in the subcutaneous plane. Consequently, less bruising occurs with the SMAS facelift than is typically encountered with the standard facelift and healing time is accelerated. The important nerves that are present in the layers beneath the SMAS plane can be protected by careful technique. In more than 600 patients operated upon with the SMAS technique during a period of 6 years at the University of California Medical Center, there have been no occurrences of injury to the facial nerve.

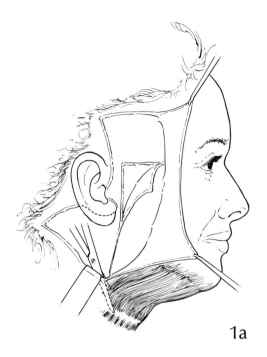

1a

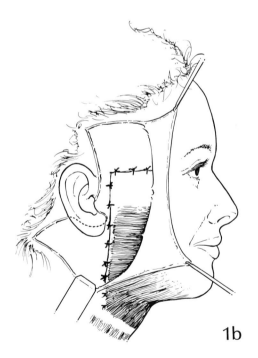

1b

The operation

Anaesthesia

The operation may be performed under either local or general anaesthesia. The author's preference in most instances is to combine local anaesthesia with intravenous sedative medication consisting of diazepam and small incremental doses of a selected narcotic such as fentanyl or pethidine. The patient is positioned supine preferably in a slight reversed Trendelenburg position.

Marking the incisions

2

The hair is trimmed in preparation for the incisions in the temple and postauricular occipital scalp, and the hair is controlled with tape and sterile towels. The line of the skin incision is marked including a post-tragal incision which outlines a small ellipse of skin to be removed first from over the tragus to facilitate skin flap elevation.

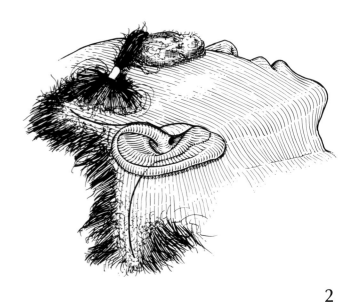

2

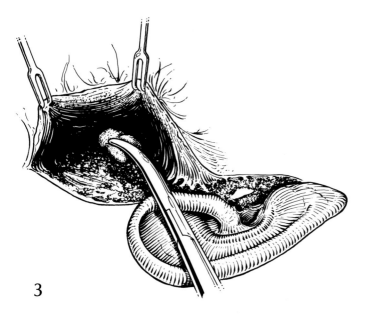

3

Temple and preauricular incisions

3

After infiltration with 0.5 per cent and 0.25 per cent bupivacaine (Marcain; Marcoine) the temple and preauricular incisions are made, with the ellipse of skin being removed first to expose the tragal cartilage. Dissection is started in the temple area, elevating the skin flap at a subcutaneous plane. Blunt dissection with a peanut sponge is recommended to avoid injury to the hair follicles and the underlying frontalis branch of the facial nerve which runs just beneath the superficial frontalis fascia on a line about midway between the ear and the lateral orbit.

4

Postauricular and occipital incisions

The postauricular and occipital incisions are begun after undermining the temple and cheek flap for a short distance in front of the ear. The postauricular skin flap is elevated over the mastoid region using sharp scalpel dissection.

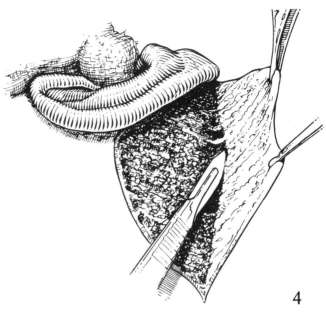

4

5

Undermining in subcutaneous plane

The undermining of the skin flaps in the subcutaneous plane in the lateral neck is extended for 8–10 cm below the earlobe. The subcutaneous dissection in the cheek is limited to only 3–4 cm anterior to the preauricular incision. In the classic skin facelift, the dissection at a subcutaneous plane would be extended anteriorly toward the nasolabial fold in the cheek and the midline in the neck area.

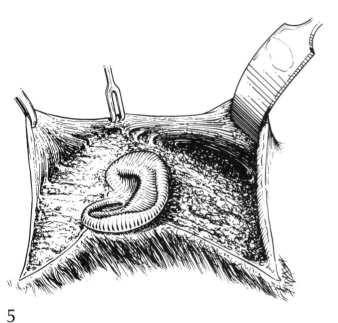

5

SMAS dissection

6

In the SMAS platysma facelift, the anterior undermining will be extended at this point beneath the SMAS in the cheek and mandibular area. In the preauricular region this plane of dissection is superficial to the true parotid fascia. An incision is begun at the level of the zygomatic arch, parallel and about 1 cm anterior to the skin incision in the preauricular area, and is deepened to expose the parotid gland with its thin investing fascia. Tensing the cheek skin with countertraction facilitates identification of the proper depth of the SMAS incision.

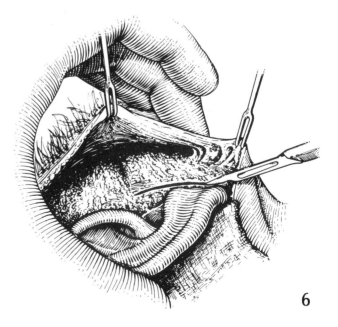

6

7

The incision in the preauricular SMAS extends downward through the platysma to the lower limit of the undermining of the skin flap in the lateral neck. Care in this area must be exercised to avoid injury to the external jugular vein which can be located by external observation.

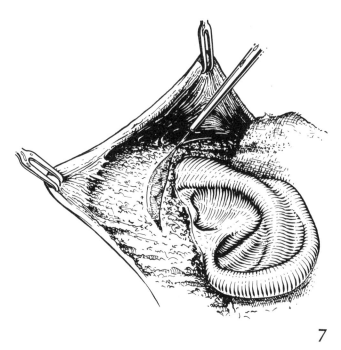

7

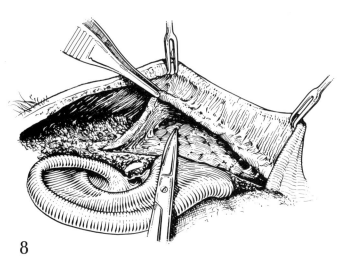

8

8

Small sharp pointed scissors are used to elevate an SMAS flap from the underlying parotid fascia. Leaving the SMAS attached to the skin during this dissection decreases the likelihood of accidental perforation of the SMAS flap which in some patients, is quite thin in the upper cheek area. The sharp scissor dissection can be extended forward for 2–3 cm over the parotid gland which covers and protects the underlying branches of the facial nerve.

9

The dissection is then extended down the lateral neck beneath the platysma muscle. In the lateral neck the dissection is carried out by spreading with blunt tipped scissors to avoid injury to the large veins encountered. After the entire flap is developed laterally, the incision is extended anteriorly in the lower neck. Spreading scissor dissection elevates the platysma overlying the thyroid cartilage up to the cervicomental angle. At the mandibular angle the marginal mandibular branch of the facial nerve must be protected. The fibrous attachments from the parotid and masseteric fascia to the undersurface of the SMAS and platysma can be easily dissected in blunt fashion with a gauze sponge. It is not necessary to sever completely these attachments but merely to create sufficient mobility of the SMAS platysma skin flap for satisfactory upward advancement.

In the cheek, anterior to the parotid gland, the SMAS is freed by blunt dissection with the scissor blades in the region of the buccal fat pad, carrying the spreading dissection as far forward as the nasolabial fold. Carefully avoiding any cutting motions of the scissors in the area of the buccal fat pad prevents injury to the facial nerve branches.

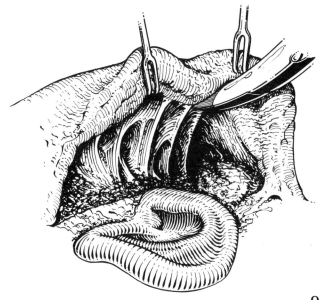

9

10

Development of SMAS flap

After undermining, the SMAS flap is incised along its attachment at the zygomatic arch and is lifted upward to tighten the submental and anterior mandibular region. The attachments of the overlying skin of the flap must be dissected superficially to allow resection of the redundant SMAS platysma tissue and suture fixation of the deep flap.

When indicated to correct hypertrophic platysma bands, the platysma muscle is split transversely from its deep aspect at the midneck level prior to elevation and fixation of the SMAS platysma flap[3].

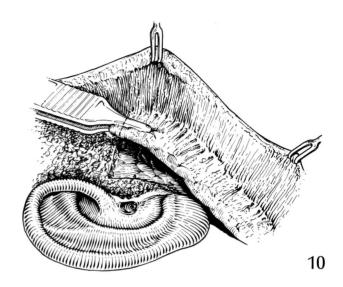

10

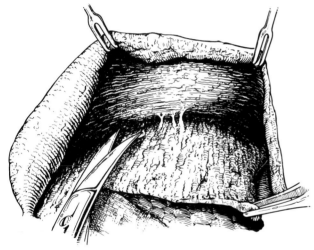

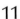

11

The skin of the cheek and the lateral neck is undermined sharply to separate it from the SMAS platysma flap. This dissection is carried only as far forward as necessary to allow resection of the redundant SMAS platysma tissue while eliminating any obvious tethering point between the two layers as they are advanced separately.

Fixation of SMAS flap

12

The SMAS platysma flap has been trimmed and sutured under tension along the zygomatic arch. This upward advancement and fixation creates a sling effect in the submental area of maximum correction of laxity in that region. The remaining portion of the redundant SMAS platysma flap is pulled laterally and the excess trimmed and sutured to the lateral side of the SMAS platysma incision.

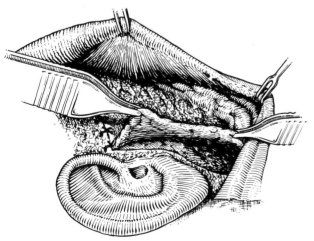

12

13

The SMAS platysma incision is approximated with interrupted absorbable sutures of 4/0 Vicryl, which extends down to the lateral neck well below the angle of the mandible (*see Illustration 16*).

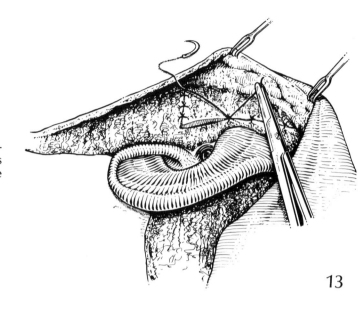

13

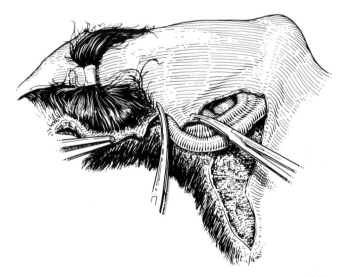

14

Lifting and suturing the skin flaps

14

After the SMAS platysma layer has been sutured, undermining in the upper and central cheek is extended in the superficial subcutaneous plane over the malar eminence and midcheek area. This frees the skin sufficiently for maximum lifting in the area of the nasolabial fold.

15

Traction on the temporal and cheek skin flap is exerted laterally to effect maximum lifting of the nasolabial fold. The skin flap is incised through the overlapping excess and an initial fixation suture is placed at the level of the insertion of the superior helix of the ear. Excessive tension is avoided to prevent necrosis at the suture line and possible temporal hair loss due to ischaemia of the skin flap.

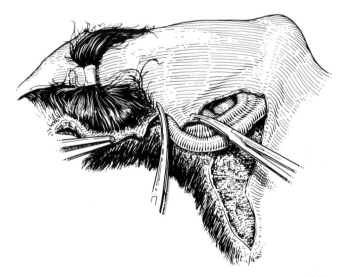

15

16

The postauricular skin flap is pulled upwards to avoid a dog-ear at the posterior extremity of the incision. The overlapping flap is split to the level of the superior edge of the incision and the second fixation suture placed. Excessive tension must be avoided to prevent ischaemia of this thin skin flap which would result in necrosis at or below the suture line.

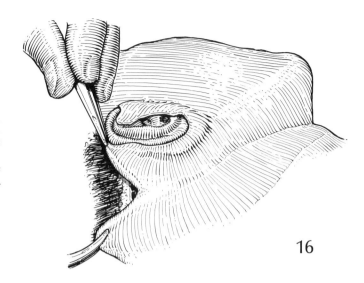

16

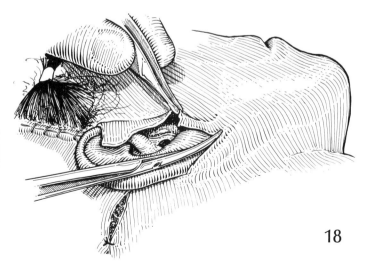

17

17

The overlapping flap is trimmed forward to the postauricular sulcus and the third tension suture is placed.

18

The skin flap overlying the ear is split down to the level of the incision which encircles the earlobe so that the flap will fit around the ear without tension at the insertion of the earlobe.

18

19

The overlapping redundant skin in front of and behind the ear is trimmed so that the edges of the skin incision meet without tension. In the tragal area, a skin flap is fashioned to suture over the tragus to the post-tragal incision without deforming tension.

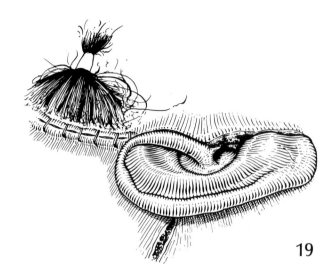

19

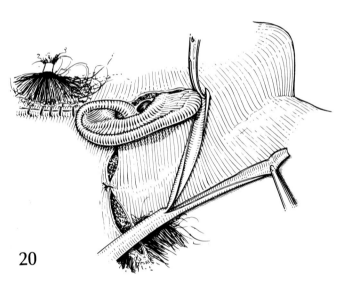

20

20

Insertion of drain

A Penrose drain is split, one portion being placed in the lower extreme of the lateral neck at the SMAS platysma incision and the other just behind the earlobe. The drain exits at the posterior end of the occipital skin incision.

21

Closure

The incision in the hairbearing areas is closed with stainless steel staples and a few nylon sutures. Staples are preferred because of their ease and speed. Alternatively, a combination of interrupted and running 4/0 nylon sutures may be used in the scalp areas. The post-tragal and postauricular incision is closed with interrupted sutures of 4/0 plain catgut. Only one buried 4/0 catgut suture is placed at the insertion of the earlobe to the skin flap. The preauricular incisions are closed with running 5/0 nylon sutures.

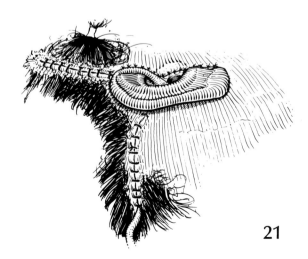

21

22

A padded compression dressing with an Ace bandage is placed to reduce swelling and serum collections. The dressing is left in place for 24 hours and then replaced with a lighter bandage.

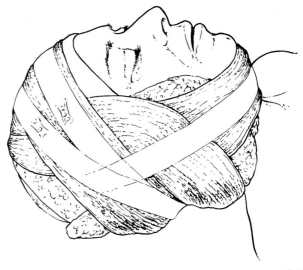

22

References

1. Rees, T. D. Aesthetic plastic surgery, Vol. 2. Philadelphia, London, Toronto: W. B. Saunders, Co., 1980

2. Owsley, J. Q. Jr. Platysma fascial rhytidectomy: a preliminary report. Plastic and Reconstructive Surgery 1977; 66: 843–850

3. Owsley, J. Q. Jr. SMAS platysma facelift. Plastic and Reconstructive Surgery 1983; 71: 573–576

Illustrations by Angela Christie

Dermoid cysts

David M. Evans FRCS
Consultant Plastic Surgeon, Wexham Park Hospital, Slough,
and Ashford Hospital, Middlesex, UK

Introduction

Congenital dermoid cysts arise from ectodermal cells that have settled or become trapped in a subcutaneous or deep position. Their occurrence in characteristic sites, mainly in the head and neck, and either in the midline or near the eye, led to the idea that ectoderm was buried as the various migrating processes met and fused, but as it is now accepted that these processes are mesodermal structures migrating beneath intact ectoderm, such a theory is untenable. Littlewood[1] has advanced evidence to suggest that at least some midline nasal dermoids are derived from neuroectoderm. This is based on embryological and clinical studies. A condensation of dural tissue is found at an early stage between the two cartilagenous laminae that form the septum; deep extensions of midline nasal dermoids may also be found in this site. Familial occurrence has been reported[2].

Most congenital dermoid cysts are present at birth or appear within 5 years, although some are not apparent until adult life. As noted by New and Erich[3], they are found in the head and neck in four areas: around the eyes, on the nose, in the floor of the mouth and in miscellaneous other midline sites (occiput, forehead, lip, neck and soft palate). They are soft cystic structures, often deeply placed and adherent to underlying fixed tissues. This distinguishes them from sebaceous cysts which are attached to the skin, as are implantation dermoid cysts. Confusion with other lesions is unlikely, but lipomas and angiolipomas may occur in some of the sites frequented by dermoid cysts, and meningoceles and gliomas are found in the nose.

There may be a sinus overlying a dermoid cyst from which sebaceous material is discharged and hairs emerge; if there is a history of recurrent infection the cyst will be adherent to surrounding structures.

EXTERNAL ANGULAR DERMOID

The **outer** end of the eyebrow is the commonest location for **a dermoid** cyst on the face. The cyst is usually about 2 cm **in diameter** and more frequently occurs on the left than **the right**. The presence of a fistula at this site is uncommon. Larger cysts have a doughy consistency and **may extend** into the temporal region or upper eyelid. The **treatment** is by surgical excision under general anaesthetic. Infiltration with 1:200000 adrenaline solution aids a clean dissection.

The operation

1

The incision follows the upper or lower edge of the eyebrow at its outer end, if necessary curving laterally away from the eyebrow to the limit of the cyst. A mobile cyst may be manipulated to lie beneath an elected incision, but removal through too small an incision is unwise.

2

The wound is deepened until the outermost fibres of orbicularis oculi are encountered. These are split by scissor dissection, taking care to avoid injury to the frontal branch of the facial nerve, which is not far above the line of dissection. As the tissues are further separated the thin white wall of the cyst appears. It should not be handled with forceps at this stage or it will tear easily because of the fixity of its deep surface.

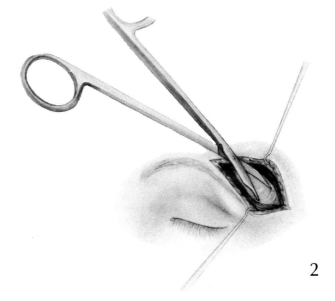

3

With small blunt retractors holding the muscle layer apart, the plane on the surface of the cyst is carefully opened in all directions; this can be done without handling the cyst at all. It may be necessary to cut numerous fine connections between the cyst wall and its surroundings. These can then be held with forceps to apply gentle traction to the cyst.

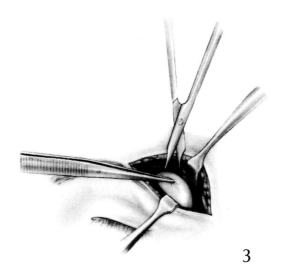

4

At this stage the cyst is frequently found to be adherent to periosteum and may be resting in a crater at the root of the zygomatic process of the frontal bone. The periosteum should be incised around the perimeter of its attachment to the cyst and elevated from the bone surface. Occasionally a cord-like structure runs from the cyst wall into surrounding soft tissue or bone and this should be traced and excised with the cyst. Rarely the cyst lies in a defect in the skull and its deep surface has to be dissected off the dura.

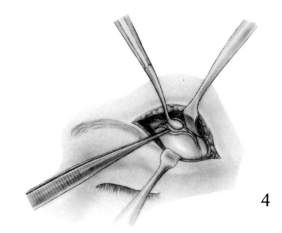

4

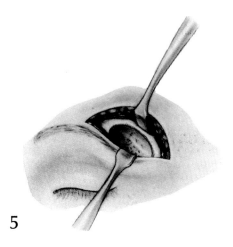

5

5

Rupture of the cyst should be avoided, but if it does happen no effort should be spared to remove the entire wall and its contents, and the wound should be irrigated copiously with normal saline. Failure to remove debris may result in a recurrent cyst, and subsequent surgery will be more difficult than on the first occasion.

6

When bleeding has been stopped the wound is closed in layers without drainage, using fine interrupted stitches or subcuticular nylon and adherent skin tapes. No dressing is required.

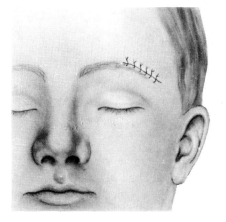

6

Postoperative care

Some oedema of the upper eyelid is to be expected. The skin sutures are removed after 5 days.

NASAL DERMOID

These are rare but troublesome lesions. They may be true cysts, or there may be one or more fistulae emerging on the bridge of the nose, with hairs sprouting from them.

They usually present in early childhood, but may do so later, or even in adulthood. The need for and timing of treatment must be considered in relation to each individual patient, bearing in mind the fact that these lesions may not give rise to serious complications. Incomplete removal will lead to recurrent swelling and discharge, and radical complete removal may lead to an extensive deformity requiring reconstruction. If symptoms or deformity warrant it treatment is by surgical excision which must be complete, with consideration given to the fate of the cavity left behind and reconstruction of the nasal support if necessary.

Preoperative

Nasal dermoid cysts may be extensive. The first exploration gives the best opportunity for complete excision. It is therefore important to know the extent of the lesion beforehand if possible. Widening of the nasal bridge with or without hypertelorism suggests that the cyst extends into the nasal septum. A plain anteroposterior X-ray will reveal any widening of the septum, and the limits of such swelling can be determined by tomography. Other skeletal defects of the nasal bones or base of the skull will also be demonstrated. Lipiodol inserted into a fistula shows its extent on a lateral film.

Excision of a nasal dermoid should be performed under general anaesthesia, with adequate preparation and time allotted for an extensive operation; it is wise to have blood available.

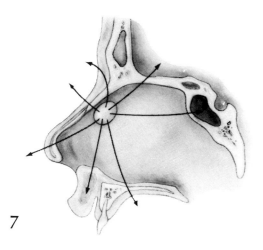

7

7

The fistulous track may be present anywhere along the arrows. More than one of these areas may be occupied.

8

Pre- or intraoperative X-ray studies may give prior warning of intracranial extension, in which case neurosurgical considerations take priority. A probe passed gently into the track will give some indication of its depth, and a lateral X-ray of the probe in place may provide sufficient grounds for intracranial exploration.

8

9

The neurosurgeon may require other investigations. A CT scan is valuable if possible, but tomography of the anterior cranial fossa should reveal a defect. The track usually extends upwards between the leaves of the dura forming the falx cerebri.

The craniotomy and excision of the intracranial part of the cyst are usually better carried out before excision of the nasal lesion. A synchronous approach is inappropriate because of the risk of ascending infection, and the turned-down frontal flap obstructs access to the nose. When the patient has fully recovered the nasal dermoid may be removed in complete safety.

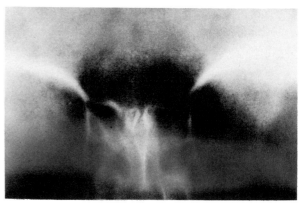

9

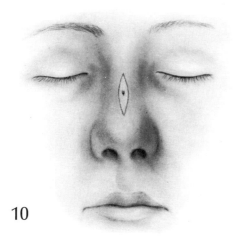

10

The operation

10

If there is no reason to suspect an intracranial extension, or it has already been dealt with, the cyst or sinus is explored through a vertical incision, including an ellipse of skin if necessary. Keeping close to the surface of the lesion, dissection is continued until hampered by the small incision which is then extended upwards or downwards.

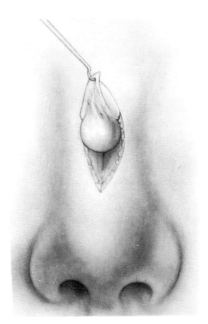

11

11

A small cyst may lie in a shallow depression in the edge of the septum and will be dissected out without difficulty. This may be all there is of the lesion.

12

At any point a track may be encountered extending deep to the nasal bones or further back into the septum. If this is divided and remains unnoticed the cyst will recur.

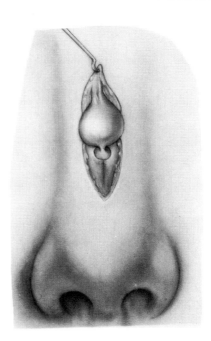

12

13

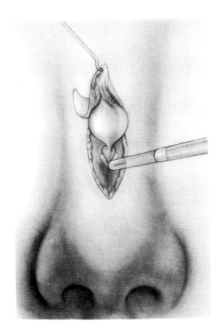

13

Initially the cartilagenous bed to the superfical cyst is incised, and if the underlying lesion demands it the bony nasal bridge is split in the midline with a sharp osteotome. If there is a large underlying cyst, that part of the vertical plate of the ethmoid will be missing.

The emphasis during excision must be on a flexible approach, following the cyst or its tracks wherever they go.

14

In small children the nasal bones may be pliable enough to spread apart. If not, an upper horizontal cut in the nasal bones will help, and a lateral osteotomy may also be needed; this is best made by a separate approach through a small incision in the upper buccal sulcus as in *Illustration 15*.

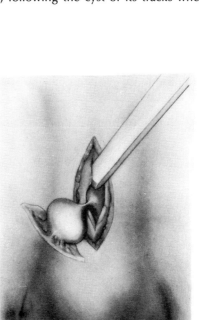

14

15

In adults, or when a large deep component of the cyst is expected, the anterior shell of the nasal bone complex may have to be lifted to give deep access and be replaced at the end of the operation.

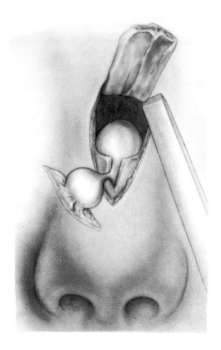

15

16

If the size of the lesion requires a longer skin incision a staggered lateral extension towards the eyebrow on one or both sides gives wide exposure and leaves an excellent scar. This also gives good access to the rare internal angular dermoid.

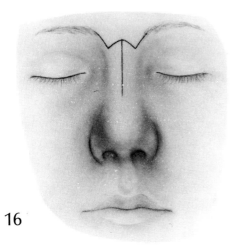

16

17

When the preoperative studies have given enough information to know that there is a large intraseptal cyst or track which is not extending too high, external scarring can be avoided by lifting the entire nasal soft tissue off the skeleton as described for removal of nasal glioma[4] and replacing it afterwards. The incision runs around the alar groove, along the intercartilagenous line and across the columella. Weisman and Johnson[5] lifted the nasal bones with the soft tissues.

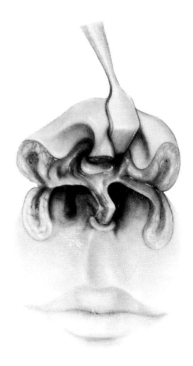

17

18

When the cyst lining or track has been completely excised, the cavity is temporarily packed, then checked for bleeding. Kazanjian[6] proposed that an opening should be established into the nasal cavity, and it is very likely that such a communication will have occurred accidentally during dissection. A final inspection is made for any lining remnants within the cavity. If a very friable cyst wall has been removed piecemeal the cavity should be curetted and any suspicious areas diathermied to destroy residual lining.

In spite of the precautions mentioned on pages 467 and 468 a sinus may unexpectedly connect with a process of dura mater through a defect in the cribriform plate area or behind it. With caution a serious dural tear should be avoided, but a cerebrospinal fluid leak may occur and subsequent management should be in collaboration with a neurosurgeon. A small tear may be sealed with a gelatin foam pack held firmly in place for 30 minutes[5]. A larger dural tear may require a fascia lata repair. Penicillin and sulphadiazine should be given.

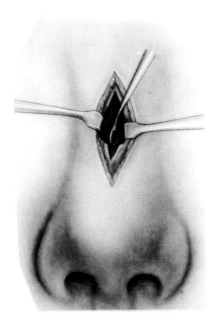

18

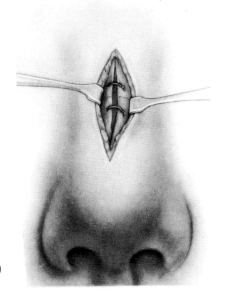

19

19

Closure commences with skeletal reconstruction. Displaced or removed skeletal components are wired in place. Occasionally previous nasal deformity requires simultaneous correction, in which case a hump removed for access need not be replaced, and an infracture will help to collapse the underlying cavity.

If the nasal bridge support is missing a bone graft is used to reconstruct the bridge line, but in the presence of a large cavity it may be wiser to defer this to a second operation.

20

Subcutaneous sutures will avoid adherence of the scar to underlying structures, and the skin wound is closed with 6/0 silk to avoid the cutting effect of nylon in nasal skin.

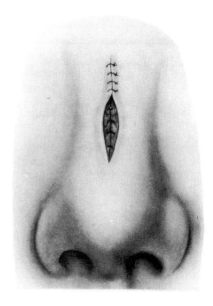

20

21

A plaster of Paris splint holds the nasal bones in place and immobilizes soft tissues.

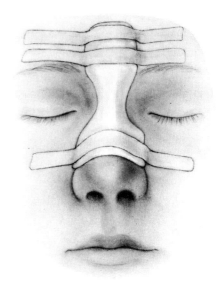

21

Postoperative care

If there has been extensive bone work the splint is left on for 14 days and the sutures removed at this time. Otherwise the sutures may be removed at 5–7 days.

Acknowledgements

The X-rays were provided by Mr D. M. Auger, Senior Medical Photographer, Stoke Mandeville Hospital. The author thanks Mr B. N. Bailey for permission to publish the X-rays and Mr C. B. T. Adams for advice on the neurosurgical aspects of this chapter.

References

1. Littlewood, A. H. M. Congenital nasal dermoid cysts and fistulae. Plastic and Reconstructive Surgery 1961; 27: 471–488

2. Muhlbauer, W. D., Dittmar, W. Hereditary median dermoid cysts of the nose. British Journal of Plastic Surgery 1976; 29: 334–340

3. New, G. B., Erich, J. B. Dermatoid cysts of head and neck. Surgery, Gynecology and Obstetrics 1937; 65: 48–55

4. O'Brien, P. The surgical approach to nasal glioma. British Journal of Plastic Surgery 1970; 23: 30–35

5. Weisman, P. A., Johnson, G. F. S. Concealed extensions of dermoid cysts of the nose; how can the surgeon be forewarned? Plastic and Reconstructive Surgery 1964; 34: 373–381

6. Kazanjian, V. H. Treatment of dermoid cysts of the nose. Plastic and Reconstructive Surgery 1958; 21: 169–176

Illustrations by Gillian Oliver

Parotidectomy

Michael Hobsley TD, MA, M.Chir, PhD, FRCS
Professor of Surgery, Head of the Department of Surgical Studies, The Middlesex Hospital Medical School, and
Consultant Surgeon, The Middlesex and University College Hospitals, London, UK

History

The commonest indication for the removal of parotid tissue is the presence in the salivary gland of a lump that might be a neoplasm. The facial nerve runs through the gland and is clearly at risk. Moreover, around many salivary tumours there appears to exist a good surgical plane. Surgical endeavour was therefore initially concentrated on limited resection, cutting down on the lump via a small incision, entering the plane and enucleating the tumour with blunt (or even digital) dissection.

Such limited operations are not free of the risk of damage to the facial nerve[1] – after all, about 15% of lumps turn out to be deep to the nerve – but at least at first there appeared to be an acceptably low recurrence rate. However, it gradually became apparent with sufficiently long follow-up that the recurrence rate of the commonest lesion, a slowly growing pleomorphic salivary adenoma, was 1% per annum[2]. The addition of radiotherapy has not been shown to reduce this recurrence rate[3], and further surgical interventions are even more hazardous to the facial nerve and even less likely to cure the patient[4].

The alternative approach of formal parotidectomy with exposure of the facial nerve was pioneered by Janes in Canada[5], Bailey[6] in the United Kingdom and Redon[7] in France, and its increasing use in the English-speaking world owes much to the powerful advocacy of Patey and Thackray[8], who demonstrated the basic pathological reasons why enucleation was bound to entail a high risk of recurrence.

Principles of formal parotidectomy

The trunk of the facial nerve is found as it plunges into the posterior border of the parotid a few millimetres below its point of exit from the skull, the stylomastoid foramen. The trunk and its branches are then dissected forwards through the gland to remove that part of the gland superficial to the nerve – thus the term superficial parotidectomy. If the lump lies in this part of the parotid, this completes the excision and the wound is closed. If the lump lies deep to the nerve, the latter must be elevated from its bed to permit the mobilization and removal of the deep part of the gland. The external carotid artery runs through the deep part, and must be tied and divided at the lower and upper poles. Throughout the dissection great care must be taken not to breach the surface of the lump; a margin of normal tissue must be left at the periphery of the lesion. Removal of both the deep and the superficial part with preservation of the facial nerve constitutes total conservative parotidectomy.

The operation of total conservative parotidectomy is described. Modifications depending on unusual operative findings or different clinical situations are discussed afterwards.

Preoperative

The patient is informed that a degree of paresis of the facial muscles is usual after conservative parotidectomy but that this always recovers, provided that the nerve and all its named branches are anatomically intact at the end of the operation. Moreover, his informed consent must be obtained to the sacrifice of one or more branches of the nerve, or even of the trunk itself, if it becomes apparent during the dissection that the tumour is invading the nerve. Such consent is rarely withheld when the patient realizes that the chance of this eventuality is small, that techniques for reinnervation exist, and that neoplastic invasion of the facial nerve itself inevitably produces facial palsy so that the nerve might just as well be sacrificed in the hope of achieving a cure.

Shaving of the face and neck is carried out from the front of the pinna to a line joining the lateral margins of eye and mouth, and also over an area extending 3 cm above and behind the pinna and 6 cm below it (see Illustration 2).

Anaesthesia

After induction, the trachea is intubated with a pernasal or peroral tube to guarantee patency of the airway. Induced hypotension is an invaluable, but not essential, adjunct.

Position of patient

1

The patient lies supine, with the head turned 20–30° towards the side opposite to the lesion and its position stabilized with a head ring. To minimize venous congestion the head end of the table is tilted head up, sufficiently to make the external jugular vein collapse. If necessary, the foot end of the table can also be tilted downwards, with a foot piece in position to prevent the patient slipping.

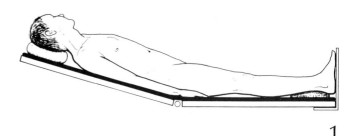

2

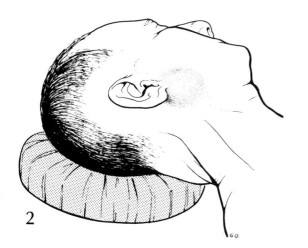

The area of shaving is shown in the detail of the head.

3

Drapes

The towels are arranged to leave exposed the pinna, and the face and neck from the zygoma above to the supraclavicular region below, and from behind the mastoid process behind to the lateral corner of the eye and the mouth in front.

I prefer to sew the towels on, but the use of a skin-adhesive is equally satisfactory.

Before skin cleansing and towelling is commenced the anaesthetist must protect the eye by inserting an ointment and taping the lids shut. Once the skin has been prepared and towelled, the surgeon inserts a twist of wool into the external auditory meatus to protect the drum.

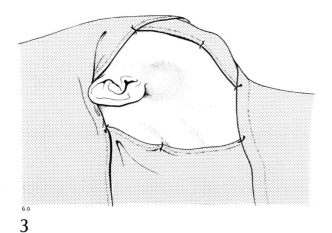

The operation

The complete skin incision is S-shaped and at least 22 cm long (see *Illustration 21*). It has a cervical, a mastoid and a facial component. If such a long incision is made all at once, control of bleeding can be time-consuming and tedious. The author therefore makes the three components separately, starting from below.

Cervical phase

The incision

4

The cervical skin incision is made in the upper skin crease of the neck. With the patient in the illustrated position, the landmark for the posterior end is vertically below the point where the lower border of the pinna meets the face. The incision is carried forwards to end a few millimetres in front of the external jugular vein. The incision is deepened carefully, and only just through the platysma.

It is important to note how low in the neck this incision lies. The interrupted and dotted lines indicate the outline of the parotid and of the posterior border of the mandible, and the incision lies well below these.

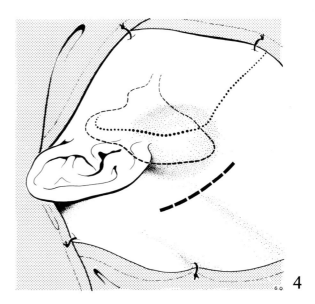

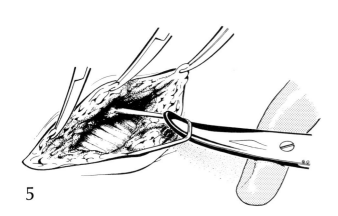

Great auricular nerve

5

Blunt dissection in the zone midway between the anterior and posterior ends of the incision reveals the great auricular nerve. In this orientation it runs almost vertically upwards and slightly backwards towards the pinna, often as a larger, more posterior and a smaller, more anterior branch. Adequate clearance of the lower pole of the parotid requires that at least the posterior branch is divided, and it is therefore as well to make a virtue of necessity and excise a conveniently long (at least 4 cm) segment of the nerve. This is kept in a bowl of physiological saline until the end of the operation, since it could prove useful as a cable graft to repair an excised defect in the facial nerve. The dissection of the nerve is pursued mainly downwards, not upwards where it might impinge on the lesion.

Deepening the cervical incision

6

Artery forceps are placed on the subcutaneous tissues of the upper flap, which is retracted upwards. The incision is then deepened along the lower flap, i.e. as far as possible from the lump, to expose first the anterior border of the sternomastoid muscle and then the posterior belly of the digastric. The latter is found most easily in the posterior angle of the wound, where it still lies in a superficial position. Below this region it trends away from the surgeon and deeply into the neck towards the midline. If the patient's head is turned more than 30° towards the opposite side, this tendency is enhanced and finding the muscle is more difficult.

The external jugular vein is preserved at this stage since tying it might increase venous stasis in the region and accentuate bleeding. The posteriorly running tributary of the vein is not a constant feature, but fairly common.

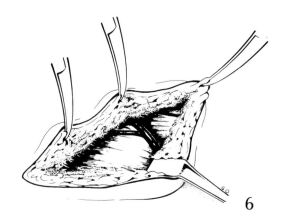

6

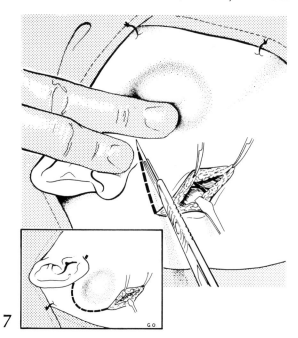

7

Mastoid phase

The incision

7

The mastoid part of the incision extends from the point at which the lower pole of the pinna meets the face to the posterior end of the cervical incision. During the incision the lump is pushed forwards by the surgeon's left index finger to ensure that it is kept away from the blade of the scalpel.

If the lesion happens to be at the postero-inferior extremity of the parotid, overlying the mastoid process, the incision can be modified by curving it well backwards. It is essential not to cut inadvertently into the lump.

Deepening the mastoid incision

8

First the anterior border of the sternomastoid and then, more deeply, the anterior border of the digastric muscle are followed upwards to the mastoid process. At all stages the lump is pushed gently away from the instruments if the margin seems to be narrowing.

When this part of the dissection has been completed, further blunt dissection in front of the posterior belly of the digastric reveals the third muscular landmark, the stylohyoid muscle. It runs in front of and roughly parallel to the posterior belly of the digastric muscle, and its anterior border is also cleared up towards the mastoid process.

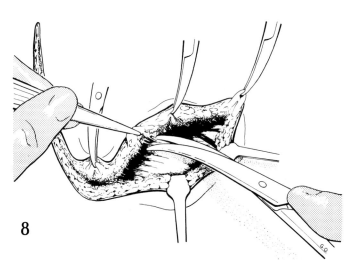

8

Facial phase

The incision

9

The facial incision lies vertically in the skin crease between the front of the pinna and the face. It extends from the zygoma above to the upper end of the mastoid incision below.

Again, the lump must be pushed forwards, away from the knife.

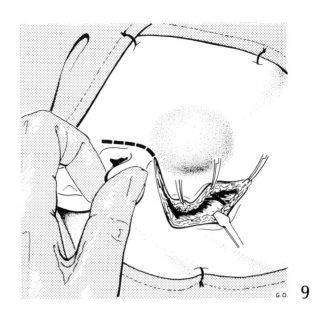

9

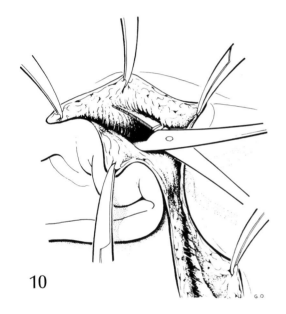

10

Deepening the facial incision

10

The facial incision is deepened cautiously, keeping strictly to the surface of the cartilage of the external auditory meatus. Curved scissors are particularly convenient for this manoeuvre, as their blades fit snugly to the contour of the cartilage. At a depth of 3–4 mm a beautiful surgical plane of cleavage is entered between the cartilage behind and the gland with its contained tumour in front. This plane is readily (and usually fairly bloodlessly) opened up with a pair of artery forceps as shown, and the cleft is then deepened until the surgeon can feel, in the depths of the wound, where the cartilage is joined to the bone of the external auditory meatus.

Facial nerve

11

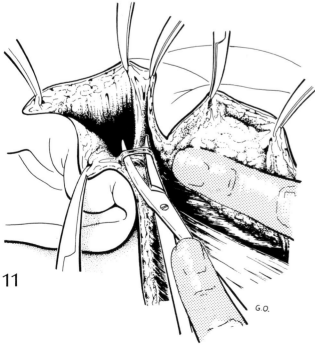

11

There is now one cavity in front of the ear, another in front of the three muscles in the neck and, between these two cavities, in front and just above the mastoid process, a bridge of tough tissue consisting of parotid fascia together with some underlying parotid glandular tissue. This bridge is now whittled away piecemeal by combined blunt and sharp dissection. The blades of the artery forceps are thrust through a 2 mm thickness of tissue as shown and the strip is then divided with a pair of scissors. The lump, covered with intact parotid tissue, is again pushed gently forwards, away from the dissection.

12

The process of whittling away the bridge continues until (inset) the final stroke displays the trunk of the facial nerve. If the trunk is very short, the bifurcation becomes immediately visible. Often, however, the trunk is much longer, and it is then necessary to dissect forwards to display the bifurcation, therefore confirming that the whole nerve has been found and not just a branch.

The uppermost branch of the upper main division of the nerve and the lowermost branch of the lower division are then traced towards the anterior skin margin of the wound. The same combination of blunt and sharp dissection is used as for the bridge of tissue overlying the trunk of the facial nerve.

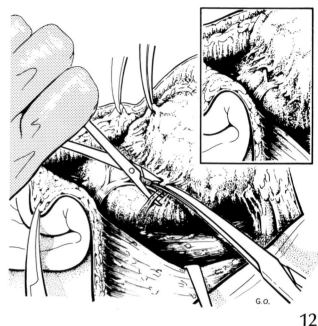

12

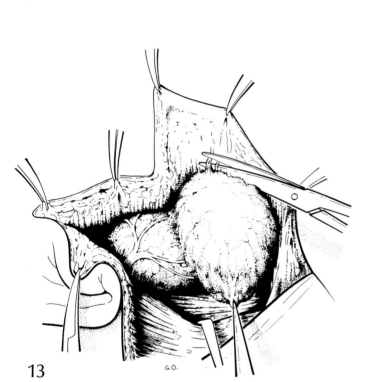

13

Reflection of skin

13

Exposure of the uppermost branch is now complete and that of the lowermost branch nearly so. Since the lump in this case is clearly superficial to the branches of the facial nerve, it is now safe to raise the anterior skin flap. Sometimes with a large deep tumour the superficial parotid undergoes pressure atrophy, leaving the facial nerve dangerously near the skin so that the unwary surgeon might divide it if he reflects the skin flap at an early stage of the operation.

Great care must be taken not to breach the capsule of the tumour during the reflection of the skin. This is not always easy. Useful aids are vertical upward traction applied to the skin flap, and backward pull on the gland behind the lump.

The beginnings of the zygomatic and upper buccal branches from the upper division, and the lower buccal branch from the lower division of the facial nerve, can be seen.

Removal of superficial parotid

14

The various facial nerve branches are now dissected forwards, elevating the superficial parotid with its contained lump. The arrangement of the branches is by no means constant, but it is common, as shown here, for the upper and lower buccal branches each to give rise to a branch which unites with its opposite number to encircle the parotid duct. This is why it is dangerous to cut down on the duct in the cheek, for example, in order to try and find a stone in the duct.

At the stage shown in this illustration, cutting across the duct frees the superficial part of the gland and completes the superficial parotidectomy. It is not necessary to tie the duct remnant. Closure is as after total parotidectomy (see *Illustration 21*).

The author's practice is to divide the duct as far forwards as possible, i.e. after the dissection has reached the intrabuccal fat pad, since this step seems to minimize the possibility of a postoperative parotid fistula.

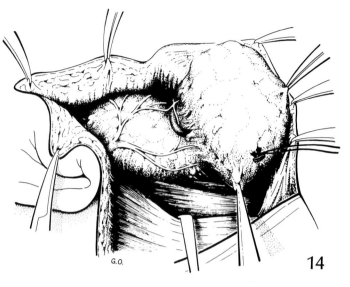

Removing the deep parotid

15

When mobilizing the deep part of the parotid, it has to be taken into account that the external carotid artery plunges into the lower pole of the deep part, runs through the gland and emerges at its upper pole, shortly to divide into the superficial temporal artery and the maxillary artery. The three vessels (and any companion veins, an inconstant feature) must therefore be divided before the deep part can be freed.

In this illustration the external carotid artery has been identified rising from deep to the stylohyoid muscle, a segment has been cleared by blunt dissection, and an aneurysm needle is being used to place the first of three ligatures around the vessel. The artery is divided between the uppermost and the lower two ligatures.

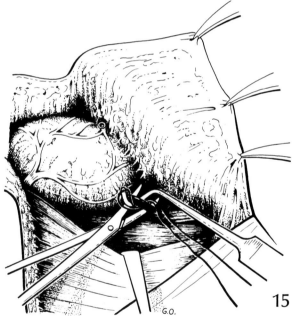

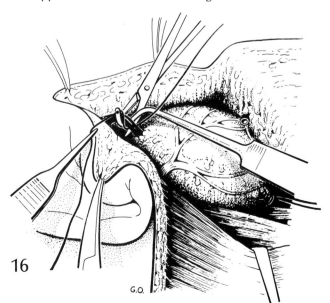

16

If there is a high division of the external carotid artery, well above the upper pole of the deep parotid, a ligature is placed with an aneurysm needle around the termination of the external carotid. Frequently the subdivision of the artery is at the upper pole, and it is then necessary to tie and divide the two terminal branches individually.

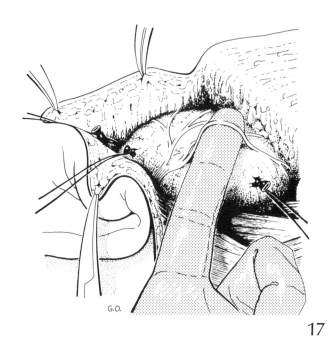

17

17 & 18

The next step is to free the facial nerve and its branches on their deep aspect from the underlying deep parotid tissue. This manoeuvre should be performed very gently, using a finger to elevate the nerve and sharp, delicate scissors to snip the connective tissue anchoring the nerve to the parotid. Each branch in turn is attacked until all lie freely across the surface of the deep parotid.

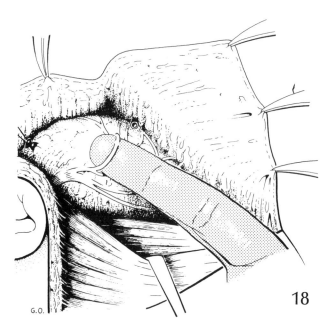

18

19

Attention is then paid to freeing the deep surface of the gland from its bed. Much of this dissection has to be done blind, by gentle use of a finger. Also at this stage considerable areolar tissue binding the anterior margin of the parotid to the posterior border of the mandible has to be divided. There is a similar collection of fibrous and areolar tissue at the posterior border of the gland, deep to the trunk of the facial nerve, binding the gland to the base of the skull in the region of the styloid process. Ultimately, the gland is sufficiently free that the surgeon's two index fingers can meet deep to the gland, having been passed behind upper and lower poles respectively.

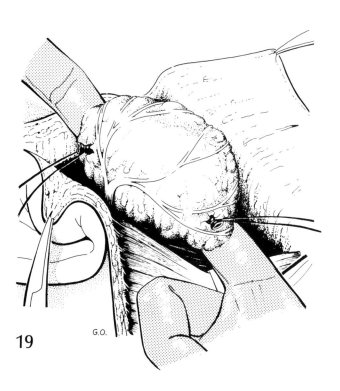

19

20

The final manoeuvre in removing the deep part is to extricate it gently from its position deep to the facial nerve and its branches. The illustration shows this being done in a downward direction, and this is usually the easier way, but sometimes it is easier to dislocate the gland upwards or even through the central gap between the branches of the upper divisions and those of the lower divisions of the facial nerve.

The tilted head end of the table is returned to the horizontal, the anaesthetist is asked to bring the controlled hypotension to an end, and any renewed bleeding due to the effect of the return of the blood pressure towards normal is stopped. Swabs and instruments are checked.

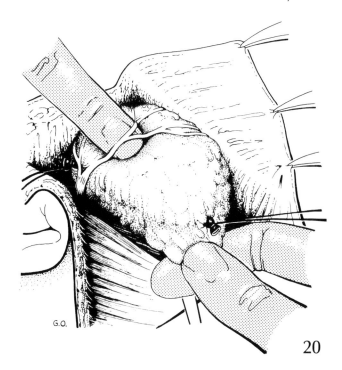

20

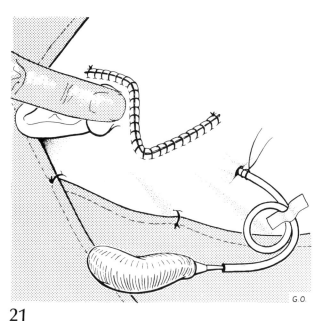

21

Closure

21

Suction drainage is instituted via a separate stab incision, the firm plastic drainage tube being anchored to the skin with a stitch tied with a clove-hitch. The skin is closed with a non-absorbable (the author uses silk) continuous blanket suture which provides side-to-side apposition along the whole wound instead of only at cross-over points. Quite apart from providing ideal wound healing conditions, this stitch is a useful aid in producing an airtight wound, an essential requisite for efficient suction drainage.

During the suturing of the skin, continuous suction is applied to the drainage tube to prevent its being blocked by clotted blood. After the wound has been closed, a light occlusive dressing is applied and the tube is connected to any convenient form of mobile suction apparatus such as the rubber bulb which is favoured by the author.

Postoperative care and complications

Reactionary haemorrhage

This is an important complication in that it has occurred in about 5% of the author's cases. Important precautions are to make sure (especially after hypotensive anaesthesia) that the patient's blood pressure has reached at least 110 mmHg (or 20 mmHg below his normal pressure) for at least 5 minutes before closing the wound, and to try to prevent the drainage tube blocking (see under 'Closure' above).

Small haematomas can be left to absorb, but those of any significant size threaten the integrity of the skin flap. The patients should therefore be returned to the operating theatre and the haematoma evacuated, bearing in mind the superficial and vulnerable position of the facial nerve. Any bleeding points found are dealt with and the wound is closed in the same way.

Fistula

The author has seen fistula develop after formal conservative parotidectomy in three patients. In two the fistula persisted for only a few days or weeks but in the third patient it seems to be permanent. However, in over 100 operations since the institution of the manoeuvre of always finding the main parotid duct and excising it right up to a few millimetres from the oral orifice, there has been no instance of even a temporary fistula.

Facial nerve paresis

After conservative parotidectomy, i.e. with the trunk and all named branches of the facial nerve anatomically intact at the end of the operation, the author has not seen any patient with a permanent loss of power in the facial muscles. Temporary paresis, however, is the rule rather than the exception. The median time to full recovery as assessed by a trained observer is 9 months, although from the point of view of the patient and his friends and relatives it is shorter than that. Very occasionally, recovery can take as long as 2 years.

After semi-conservative parotidectomy, if only one named branch has been sacrificed, the pattern of facial paresis differs not at all from that after a conservative operation. If more than one named branch is sacrificed, there is an incidence of permanent disability, but grafifyingly less often and to a less severe degree than one might expect from the anatomical lesion. The necessity to sacrifice named branches is, of course, only likely to arise if the lesion is infiltrating nerves, i.e. if it is malignant.

References

1. Ward, C. M. Injury of the facial nerve during surgery of the parotid gland. British Journal of Surgery 1975; 62: 401–403

2. McFarland, J. Three hundred mixed tumors of salivary glands of which sixty-nine recurred. Surgery, Gynecology and Obstetrics 1936; 63: 457–468

3. Armistead, P. R., Smiddy, F. G., Frank, H. G. Simple enucleation and radiotherapy in the treatment of the pleomorphic salivary adenoma of the parotid gland. British Journal of Surgery 1979; 66: 716–717

4. Watkin, G. T., Hobsley, M. Influence of local surgery and radiotherapy on the natural history of pleomorphic adenomas. British Journal of Surgery 1986 (in press)

5. Janes, R. M. Treatment of tumours of salivary glands by radical excision. Canadian Medical Association Journal 1940; 43: 554–559

6. Bailey, H. Treatment of tumours of parotid gland, with special reference to total parotidectomy. British Journal of Surgery 1941; 28: 337–346

7. Redon, H. Remarques sur le traitement des tumeurs dites mixtes de la parotide. Mémoires d'Académie de Chirurgie 1942; 68: 338–342

8. Patey, D. H., Thackray, A. C. The treatment of parotid tumours in the light of a pathological study of parotidectomy material. British Journal of Surgery 1958; 45: 477–487

Further reading

Patey, D. H. Tumours and other diseases of the salivary glands in relation to general physiology and pathology. Journal of Laryngology and Otology 1968; 82: 853–866

Hobsley, M. Sir Gordon Gordon-Taylor: two themes illustrated by the surgery of the parotid salivary gland. Annals of the Royal College of Surgeons of England 1981; 63: 264–269

Illustrations by Robert N. Lane

Carcinoma of the tongue

G. Westbury FRCS, FRCP
Professor of Surgery, Institute of Cancer Research and Royal Marsden Hospital, London, UK

General considerations

Carcinoma of the tongue is best managed by a combined radiation–surgical approach and calls for close team work between the specialties. The author generally prefers radiotherapy as the primary treatment for small and intermediate-sized carcinomas of the anterior two-thirds and for all carcinomas of the base of the tongue; in these circumstances surgery is reserved for radiation failure. Surgery forms the primary management of carcinomas involving bone and/or cervical lymph nodes. These more advanced lesions usually receive planned preoperative radiotherapy and sometimes chemotherapy. The surgical procedures to be described therefore, when necessary, take into account the influence of prior irradiation on healing. In this respect, interstitial irradiation, with its predominantly localized effect, produces fewer problems than external beam therapy which involves normal tissues over a wider field. Regional flap reconstruction, which brings in a healthy blood supply from outside the irradiation field, allows safe primary repair of major resections, planned or for salvage, following external radiotherapy.

The operations

Local excision

Local excision may be used for small carcinomas of the anterior two-thirds of the tongue, and especially of the tip where interstitial irradiation is impracticable. In the non-irradiated tongue repair is usually by layered closure. The irradiated tongue is best and safest left unsutured: postoperative complications are minimized and epithelialization is complete within 3–4 weeks. Limited areas of premalignant change may be excised and closed by suture. Extensive sacrifice, especially of dorsal mucosa, requires resurfacing with split skin.

The operation is performed under general anaesthesia with nasotracheal intubation. Moderate hypotension is helpful. Full exposure of the oral cavity is obtained by using a mouth gag and cheek retractors; perfect lighting and effective suction are essential.

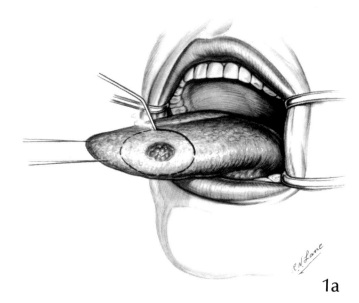

1a

1a & b

The line of excision is marked with Bonney's blue dye. A minimum clearance of 1 cm, and preferably 2 cm, in all three dimensions is required. Frozen-section monitoring is mandatory. Excision is performed either with the knife or the cutting diathermy. Larger arteries are controlled by transfixation-ligation and smaller vessels by diathermy coagulation.

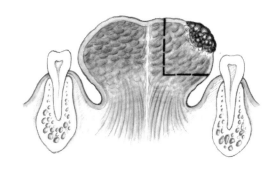

1b

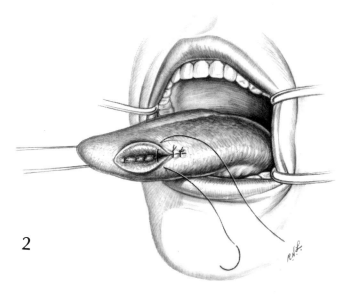

2

2

Muscle is repaired when necessary with 2/0 or 3/0 chromic catgut, taking care to obliterate dead space. The mucosa is repaired with 3/0 silk.

Postoperative care

Most patients can take a fluid diet by mouth from the first day. A few require nasogastric tube feeding for 48 to 72 hours.

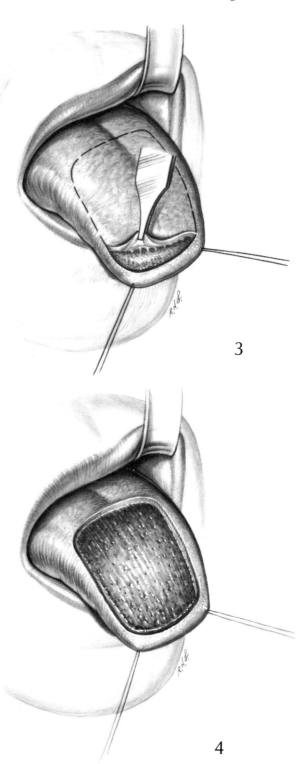

3

EXCISION OF MUCOSA OF DORSUM AND RESURFACING

This procedure is indicated for extensive premalignant change of the dorsal mucosa and may be combined with local excision of a small carcinoma of the anterior two-thirds of the tongue.

3 & 4

The mucosa is excised with a thin layer of subjacent muscle.

4

5

A split skin graft is cut to size and first sutured in place to the edges of the defect. Apposition of graft to the raw surface is obtained by a series of quilting stitches which anchor the split skin and provide sufficient immobility of each square so produced to ensure take.

Postoperative care

The patient is fed by nasogastric tube for one week.

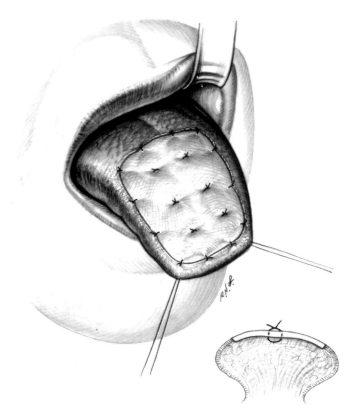

5

Composite operations

Excision of the tongue, partial or total, in continuity with neck dissection, is indicated for more extensive carcinomas, especially when disease extends to the floor of the mouth. The mandible may be spared, provided there is a margin of 1 cm or more of healthy tissue between it and the tumour. In such a case a pull-through procedure or median mandibulotomy with mandibular swing is preferred to jaw resection. When the tumour lies closer to the mandible, provided there is no radiographic evidence of gross bone destruction, clearance can be achieved by splitting the mandible sagittally so that the adjacent inner table forms part of the specimen while the remaining outer table maintains continuity of the mandibular arch. This, in effect, is an extended pull-through procedure. If the strength of the outer table is in question or in the presence of gross bone invasion, full thickness sacrifice is required. In elderly patients the entire hemimandible is sacrificed so far forward as to include the mental foramen. In younger patients part of the ascending ramus may be preserved and the defect bridged either with a temporary spacing prosthesis with a view to later bone grafting or, in selected circumstances, by an immediate vascularized compound graft, pedicled or transferred as a free flap with microvascular anastomosis. Full radical neck dissection is preferred on the side of the tumour. When simultaneous contralateral dissection is indicated, modifications such as complete dissection with preservation of the internal jugular vein, supra-omohyoid or suprahyoid dissection are used as appropriate.

Regional flap repair is almost always required. A variety of techniques are available and the choice will depend on the nature of the defect and the experience of the surgeon. The pectoralis major and latissimus dorsi pedicled myocutaneous flaps supply lining and bulk as well as protecting the exposed carotid arterial tree. Where less bulk and greater flexibility are required the radial forearm flap is ideal. The deltopectoral flap is now seldom used but the narrow pedicled forehead flap (see *Illustrations 12–15* and *19*) remains a useful alternative. It is reliable, versatile and restores an acceptable jaw contour after complete hemimandibulectomy.

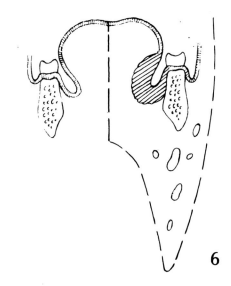

6

PARTIAL GLOSSECTOMY, HEMIMANDIBULECTOMY AND NECK DISSECTION

The incision

6 & 7

For anteriorly placed lesions adequate exposure can usually be obtained without splitting the lip. For extensive and more posteriorly placed tumours the lip split provides superior access. Tattoo points are made on the muco-cutaneous junction and chin. The skin incision divides the vermilion of the lip obliquely and descends vertically in the midline to join the incision for the neck dissection. Especially in the irradiated neck, this should avoid any junction points over the carotid artery, and the U-shaped flap illustrated, which usually includes the platysma, is preferred. The blunt apex of the flap lies two fingers' breadths above the clavicle. The lower part of the posterior triangle is readily exposed by retraction. The base of the flap is made as broad as possible by taking the posterior limb well behind the mastoid process.

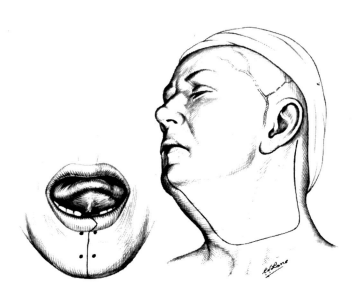

7

Neck dissection and approach to oral cavity

8

The neck dissection proceeds from below upwards as far as the lower border of the submandibular gland. The lingual and facial arteries are divided, and the trunk of the external carotid, which continues as the superficial temporal artery, is carefully preserved to nourish the forehead flap. The cheek flap is reflected off the mandible as far back as the anterior border of the masseter muscle, where the facial artery and the vein are divided. The mandible is sectioned with a Gigli saw anterior to the mental foramen.

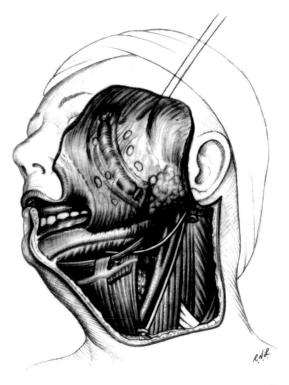

8

Intraoral dissection

9 & 10

The line of section of the tongue is drawn with Bonney's blue. The plane of section is determined by the extent of the tumour and, if necessary, may transgress the midline or extend to the adjacent faucial pillar. The tip of the tongue is preserved complete, provided it is clear of disease. This produces a better functional and aesthetic result than the sharp point which is left after formal hemiglossectomy. Dissection is deepened vertically through the tongue and this plane determines the correct plane of further dissection upwards in the submandibular triangle so that the two fields now meet. Lateral retraction of the mandible with the divided tongue and floor of mouth allows progressive exposure and resection of the posterior extent of the tumour.

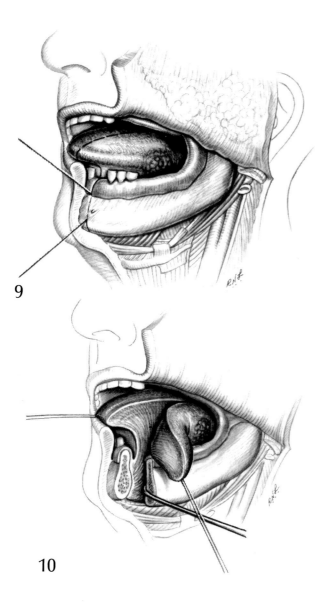

9

10

Section of coronoid and disarticulation of the mandible

11

The masseter muscle is divided down to bone and the lateral surface of the ascending ramus bared with a periosteal elevator. The coronoid process is divided at its base with bone-cutting forceps and left attached to the temporalis muscle insertion to facilitate formation of the tunnel for the forehead flap. The mandibular head is disarticulated, taking care to avoid damage to the maxillary artery running deep to its neck, and especially to the superficial temporal artery. Division of the lateral and medial pterygoid muscles finally frees the specimen.

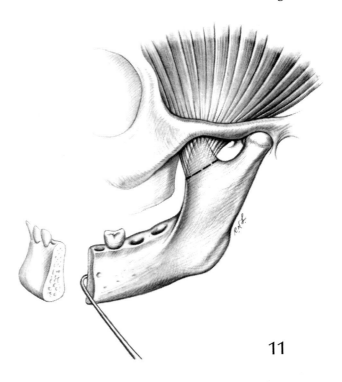

11

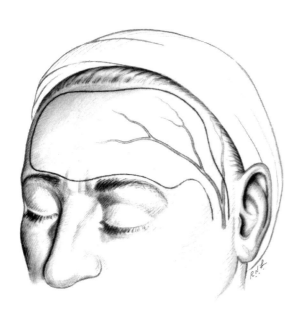

Reconstruction

12

The narrow pedicled forehead flap is planned and raised as a complete cosmetic unit.

12

13

A Kocher's forceps is used to push the coronoid fragment upwards and carry the temporalis insertion deep to the zygomatic arch so that the greater part of the muscle can be resected.

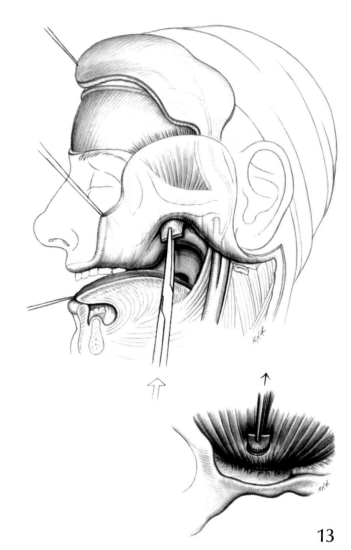

13

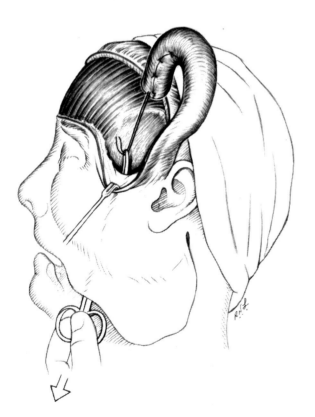

14

14

The incision in the temporal fascia is enlarged sufficiently to allow free passage of the flap and its pedicle deep to the arch and into the mouth.

15a & b

The tip and anterior part of the tongue are closed as far as possible with minimum tension and the flap is then set in to provide a mobile tongue, reconstitute the floor of the mouth and reform the jaw line. The neck is closed after insertion of two wide-bore suction drains.

Tracheostomy is performed using a cuffed tube. A fine nasogastric feeding tube is introduced.

Postoperative care

The cuffed tracheostomy is replaced by a silver tube when oral exudate and secretion subside, usually within 72 hours. The silver tube is removed as soon as the normal airway is clear. Oral fluids are commenced on the 7th day and the nasogastric tube is removed when adequate intake is established.

The pedicle is divided and returned in 3 weeks.

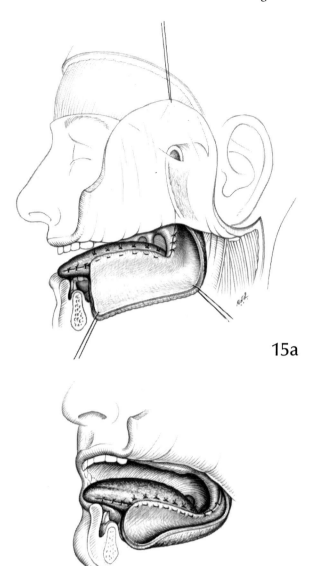

15a

15b

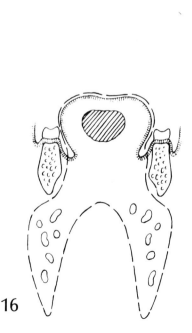

16

PULL-THROUGH SUBTOTAL GLOSSECTOMY

16

This is indicated for carcinoma which has extensively infiltrated the oral tongue but is free of the mandible on both sides. As already mentioned, it may be extended to include part of the inner table of the mandible in selected instances.

The resection

17 & 18

Bilateral neck dissections are completed as indicated above. The upper edge of each dissection reaches the lower border of the mandible, whose periosteum is incised and elevated from the inner table as far as the mucosal reflection. The mucous membrane of the floor of the mouth is incised anteriorly and laterally as far back on each side as dictated by the extent of disease. A fringe of mucoperiosteum is left, sufficient to take sutures for the repair. Incision of the already elevated periosteum throws the oral and cervical components into continuity. The tip of the tongue is grasped firmly from below with a tongue clip or stay sutures and delivered behind the mandibular arch into the neck. The tongue is finally transected through its pharyngeal portion in the plane of the body of the hyoid bone.

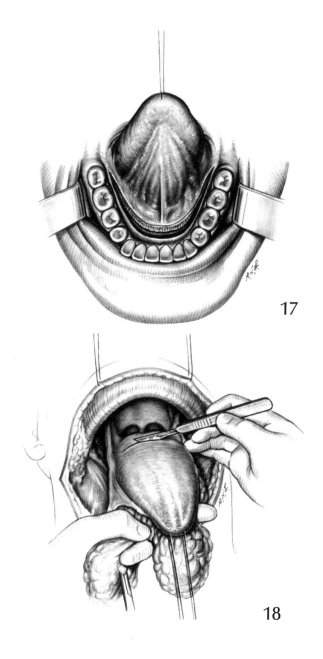

17

18

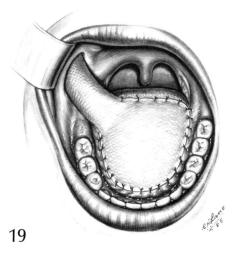

19

The repair

19

A variety of flaps are available. The pectoralis major and latissimus dorsi pedicled or free myocutaneous flaps supply bulk to the reconstructed floor of mouth. The patient illustrated shows the use of the narrow pedicled forehead flap. The flap is planned and raised, and then tunnelled superficial to the zygomatic arch and into the mouth via an incision in the buccal mucosa. If necessary, the coronoid process may be resected to accommodate the pedicle more comfortably. The flap is sutured to the alveolar mucoperiosteum and pharyngeal remnant of the tongue.

The pedicle is divided and returned in 3 weeks.

Median mandibulotomy and mandibular 'swing'

For larger and more posteriorly placed carcinomas, generous access can be provided by division of the mandible at the symphysis so that the jaw can be swung laterally. An alternative line of section lies just posterior to the canine tooth.

20

The lip and chin are split and a stepped cut is made through the symphysis. Extraction of a central incisor tooth may be necessary.

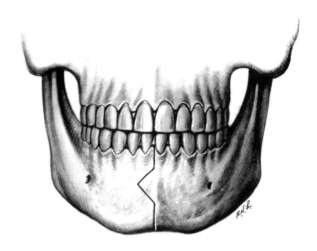

20

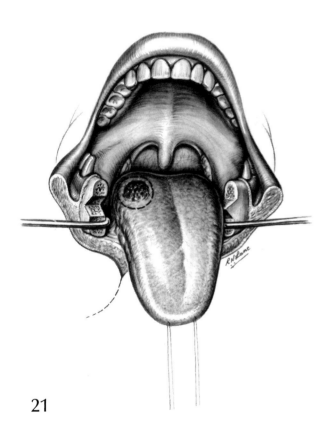

21

21

Division of the floor of the mouth on the affected side allows half of the mandible to be retracted widely laterally. Partial glossectomy can be done in continuity with neck dissection and an appropriate flap introduced for repair.

22

The mandibulotomy is stabilized by two stainless steel wires.

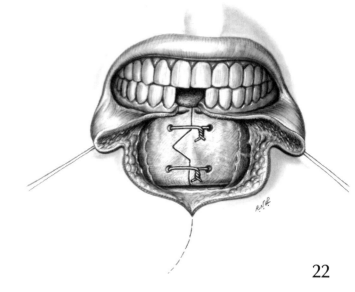

22

CARCINOMA OF THE BASE OF THE TONGUE

Carcinoma of the base of the tongue usually presents with the primary lesion locally advanced, and the cervical nodes are involved clinically or histologically, often bilaterally, in a high proportion of cases. These facts dictate a major role for radiotherapy in management and, where surgery is required, call for wide resection and radical lymphadenectomy.

Excellent exposure for radical excision of the tongue base is obtained by the standard commando approach with preliminary lymph node dissection and division of the mandible just in front of the ascending ramus. Full mobilization of the carotid trunk allows safe resection of involved lateral pharyngeal wall, and posteriorly dissection may extend as far as the mucosa of the epiglottis. The specimen is resected *en bloc* with the posterior part of the hemimandible. Extension of disease to the vallecula may require the addition of laryngectomy, not only for clearance but also to obviate aspiration of saliva and food, which is especially dangerous in the elderly.

Illustrations by Robert N. Lane

Tongue flaps

Vahram Y. Bakamjian MD
Chief Reconstructive Surgeon, Roswell Park Memorial Institute, New York, USA

The tongue has always played an elemental role in the repair of excisional oral defects because of its relatively large size and central location in the cavity of the mouth, and its free mobility, marked stretchability and rich vascularity. Thus, before the development in the last three decades of a variety of external flap techniques for undelayed transfer into the oral cavity, all immediate oral repairs depended almost exclusively on pulling *en masse* the salvaged portion of the tongue for direct suturing into the area of an adjoining defect. Often the result was more costly than even unavoidable tethering and functional impairment of the residual tongue; and in many cases closure had to be effected by sacrificing a segment of mandible, not because of invasion by the cancer, but in order to allow the cheek to collapse and thus facilitate closure by direct suture.

1

Somewhat different in approach to closure by direct suture is the concept of redistributing the mucosa more equitably by borrowing a pedicle flap from an area of relative abundance on the tongue for transfer into a deficit in its vicinity.

The idea may be said to have originated as early as 1909 with Lexer, who reported two cases in which he repaired a defect in the mucosa of the cheek by advancing into it mucosa from the lateral floor of the mouth on a pedicle based on the lateral border of the tongue. The idea, however, seems not to have taken root, and did not re-emerge until half a century later when it evolved into a variety of better forms.

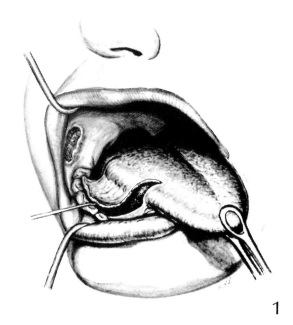

1

Anatomy

2

Two symmetrical halves of the tongue are separated longitudinally by a fibrous raphe, each half comprising two sets of muscles: the extrinsic, whose muscle fibres originate from outside before entering and terminating in the organ; and the intrinsic, whose fibres are contained entirely within it.

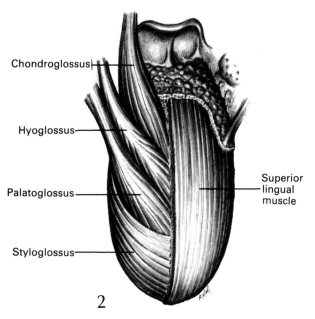

Chondroglossus

Hyoglossus

Palatoglossus

Styloglossus

Superior lingual muscle

2

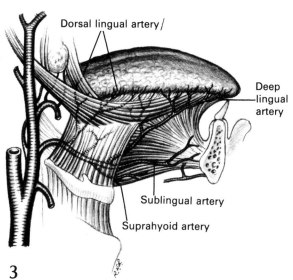

Dorsal lingual artery

Deep lingual artery

Sublingual artery

Suprahyoid artery

3

3

Each half receives its own lingual artery: a dorsal lingual branch ascends posteriorly to supply the base of the tongue, the epiglottis, tonsil and soft palate; and a large terminal branch, the deep lingual or ranine artery, proceeds forwards and upwards along the undersurface of the body of the tongue, at intervals giving off vertical branches into the lingual substance before reaching the tip of the organ. There are no significant cross-communications between the vessels of the two sides, except at the very tip and some at the base.

Smooth on the ventral surface, the investing mucous membrane becomes papillary on the dorsal surface. It adheres closely to the corium, which is a submucous feltwork of connective tissue with elastic fibres and numerous penetrating vessels and nerves which supply the papillae. The corium in its turn adheres closely to the superior lingual muscle, which is the outermost stratum of intrinsic musculature of the tongue.

The flaps

POSTERIORLY BASED DORSAL TONGUE FLAP

4

Taken lengthwise from either side of the midline on the upper surface of the oral portion of the tongue, a flap can be based posteriorly at the crest of the lingual base and extended to the tip. Raised in a thickness of approximately 7 mm, it includes along with mucosa the intimately adhering underlying submucous corium and the stratum of intrinsic superior lingual musculature. Slightly angular in outline at its end, the donor wound can be closed by direct suturing in a straight line. This narrows the lingual body somewhat but does not shorten it sufficiently to interfere appreciably with normal function. The closure must be effected with scrupulous attention to haemostasis and obliteration of all potential dead space in the wound by using two or more rows of buried sutures, lest a haematoma form and infiltrate the loose stroma of the tongue, causing a massive swelling which would endanger not only the flap but also the airway.

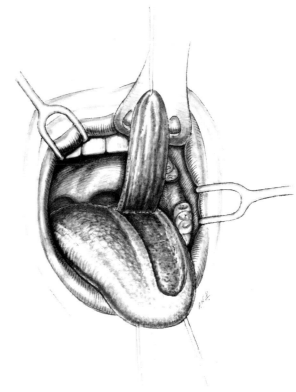

4

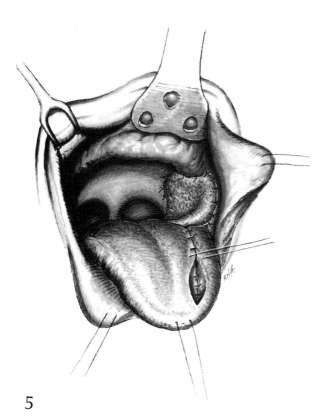

5

Repair of defects in the faucial or retromolar region

5

With lateral and backward rotation the posteriorly based dorsal tongue flap may be used to cover moderately sized defects in the faucial or retromolar area. (The size of the defect so managed can, of course, be larger, if a cancerous segment of the mandible is also included in the resection.)

6

A wide posteriorly based flap from the ipsilateral dorsum of the tongue can be used to close a defect left by resection of a tumour in the retromolar or faucial region.

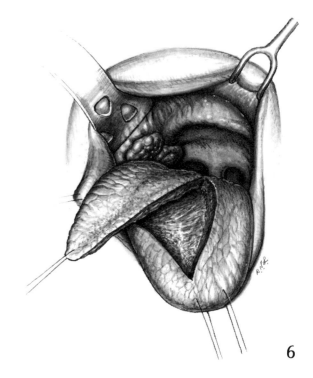

6

7

The donor site on the dorsum of the tongue is easily closed by direct approximation.

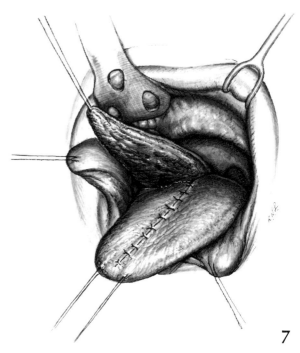

7

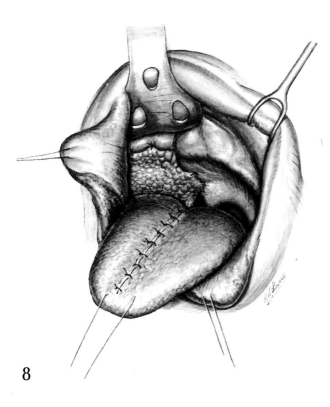

8

8

The flap is then transported and sutured into the defect in the tonsillar area.

Provision of cheek mucosal lining

9

With lateral transposition and a lesser degree of backward rotation the posteriorly based dorsal tongue flap may be used to replace mucosa in the cheek of edentulous patients or those with an edentulous space in the molar area through which the flap can pass to its buccal destination.

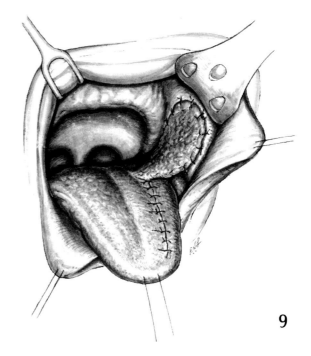

9

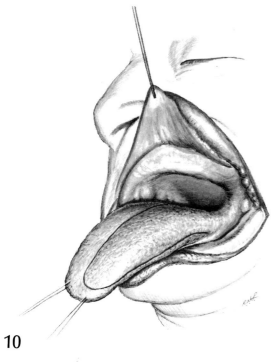

10

10

The posteriorly based tongue flap can also be used to provide lining for the repair of a full thickness cheek defect.

11

The donor defect on the dorsum of the tongue is closed by direct approximation.

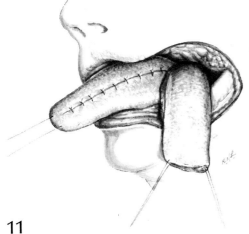

11

12

The flap is then sutured into position to line the oral side of defect. Cover will be provided by the outlined sternomastoid musculocutaneous flap.

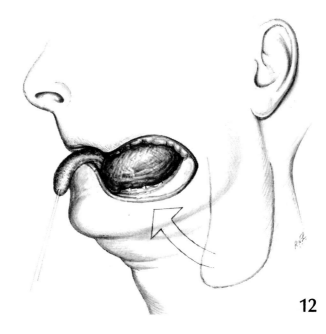

12

ANTERIORLY BASED DORSAL TONGUE FLAP

13

Similar in all respects except for its anterior base, this flap enjoys greater mobility and a wider range of application than the posteriorly based flap. It can be used in the anterior environs of the mouth to cover defects in the cheek, lip, floor of mouth or oral roof. When it has to cross the teeth in order to reach its destination, as, for example, in a cheek or lip reconstruction, a bite block, specially prepared for each patient, has to be worn in the early days after operation to protect the pedicle. Also, unlike with posteriorly based flaps, the pedicle of anteriorly based flaps needs to be divided from the donor tongue after a period of about 3 weeks. It is interesting to note how little speech and swallowing are inconvenienced in most cases during this interval.

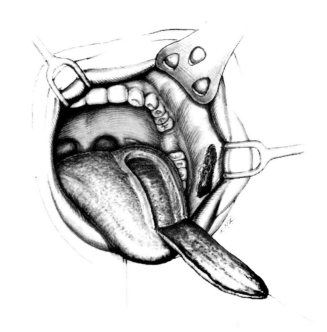

13

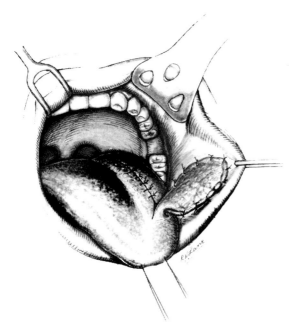

14

14

With lateral and forward rotation the anteriorly based flap may be used for repair in the anterior areas of the cheek and the lip commissure.

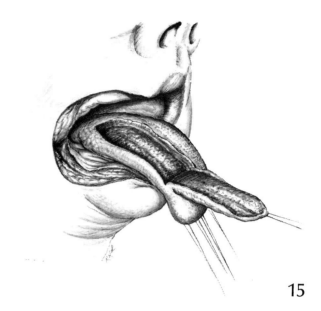

15

Provision of cheek lining after full thickness resection of carcinoma

15 & 16

The anteriorly based tongue flap is raised and sutured into position to provide lining for the reconstruction. The donor area is closed by direct approximation. A submental random flap is marked out.

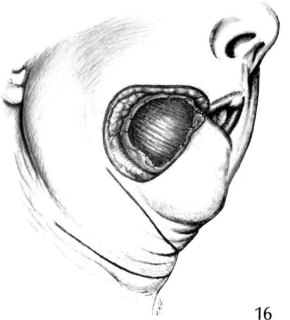

16

17

The submental random flap is then raised and transposed into the cheek defect to provide cover over the lining tongue flap. The pedicle of the anteriorly based tongue flap will require subsequent division and inset to fill the tip of the tongue.

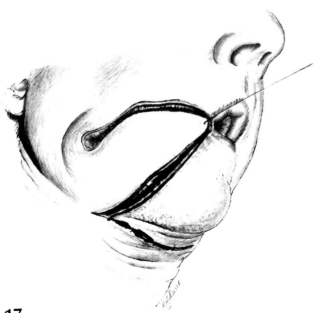

17

Provision of lining for lower lip

18

With a full forward rotation and a twist to face the raw surface of the flap outward, the anteriorly based tongue flap can be used for lining in a reconstruction of the lower lip.

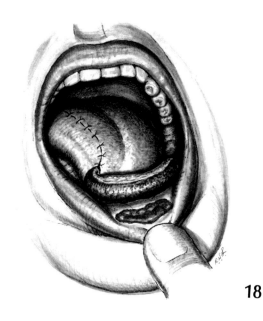

18

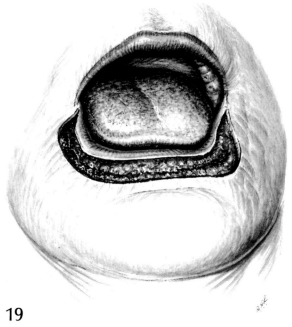

19

19–21

For a full thickness defect of the entire width of the lower lip (e.g. after full thickness resection of a carcinoma) the flap is rotated into the lip defect with the mucosal surface facing inwards, and sutured into position to provide lining for the lip reconstruction.

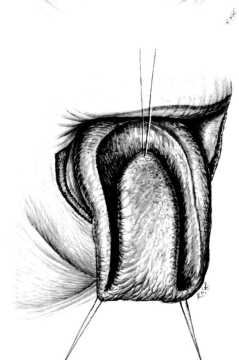

20

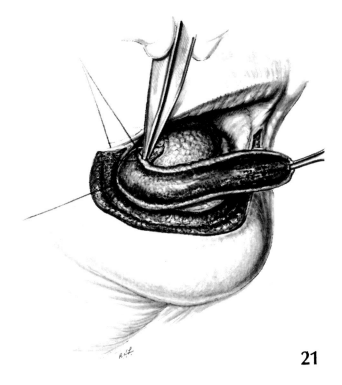

21

22

Reconstruction of the external aspect of the lip is accomplished by a bipedicled random flap of neck skin. The reconstructed lip is being retracted to show the lining tongue flap.

The pedicles of both the tongue flap and the bipedicled neck flap are later divided and inset. Division of the pedicle of the tongue flap is needed to preserve mobility of the tongue.

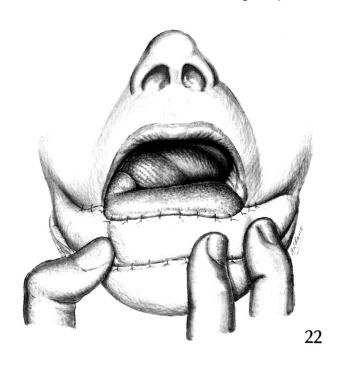

22

Repair of defects in the floor of the mouth

With similar rotation, but a twist that faces its raw side downward, the anteriorly based flap may by used to replace mucosa in the anterior floor of the mouth.

23

The flap should be raised on the **contralateral** side to the defect.

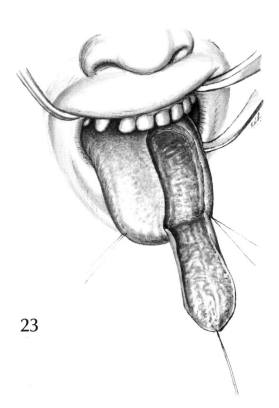

23

24

It is then rotated and sutured into place to reconstruct the defect in the floor of the mouth. (A catheter is placed around the pedicle of the flap to retract the tongue for demonstration).

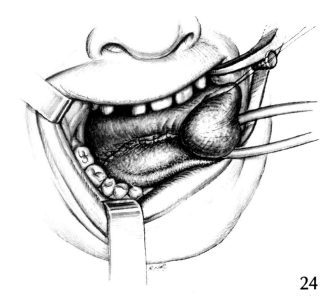

24

25

For some defects of the floor of the mouth, passing the anteriorly based flap through a midline incision through the full thickness of the tongue may be preferable.

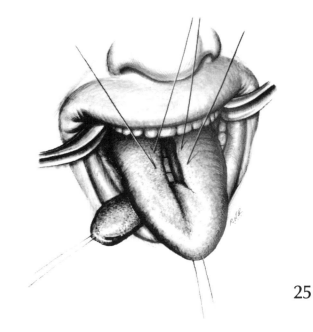

25

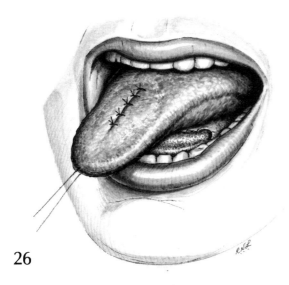

26

26

Ten days later the pedicle of the flap is divided and inset into the donor site, preserving the form and function of the tongue.

Repair of defects in oral roof

27

Forward reflection of tongue flap for closure of an anterior palatal fistula.

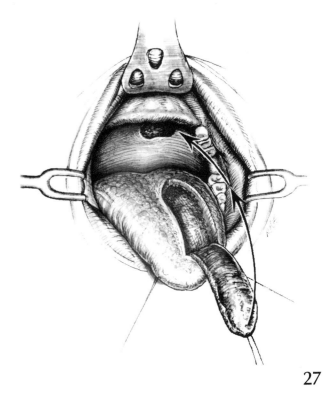

27

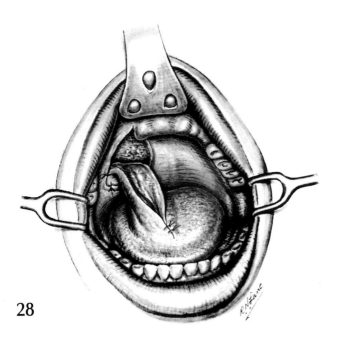

28

28

180° twist of the pedicle in using the flap to repair an excisional defect of the ipsilateral half of the hard palate.

BIPEDICLED TRANSVERSE TONGUE FLAP

29

A transverse flap developed across the dorsum of the anterior third of the lingual body may be applied to the anterior floor of the mouth, or to the lower lip when the front teeth are missing. It must have two pedicles, based laterally, as a single one cannot support any portion that extends beyond the median raphe to the opposite side. Because closure of the donor wound by direct suture causes undue shortening and blunting of the lingual tip, indiscriminate use of this flap is not recommended.

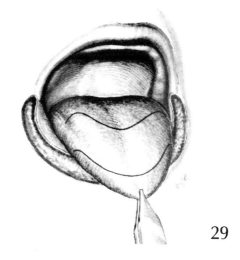

29

30

For reconstruction of a full thickness defect of the lower lip the flap is raised near the tip of the tongue and the donor defect closed by direct approximation.

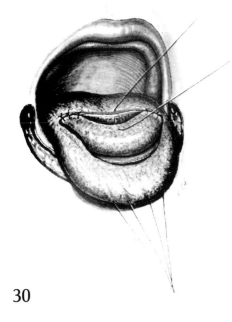

30

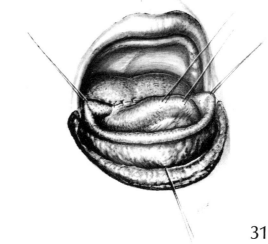

31

31

The flap is then rotated on its pedicles so that the raw surface faces forwards. The upper margin of the flap is rolled outwards to form the vermilion border of the reconstructed lip.

32

The reconstruction of the external surface of the lip is completed with two nasolabial flaps.

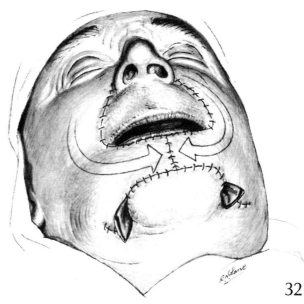

32

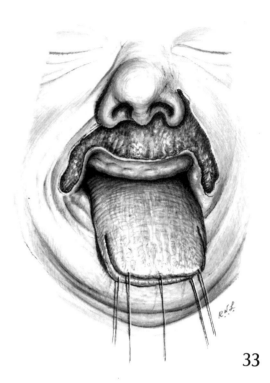

FLAPS FROM TIP OF THE TONGUE

A variety of these flaps, reflected either dorsally or ventrally, can be designed to be used principally in the reconstruction of the lips. They are much shorter than they are broad, and extremely viable. Discretion is important, however, to avoid undue functional impairment of the lingual tip.

Reconstruction of the upper lip

33 & 34

A short, broad flap, based posteriorly across the dorsal surface of lingual tip, may be reflected dorsally to line an upper lip, for example after resection of a carcinoma.

33

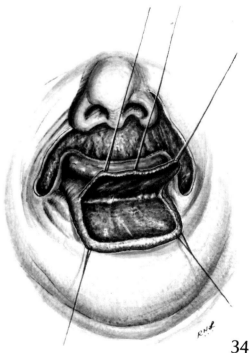

34

35

The outer side of the reconstructed upper lip is fashioned from a transposition flap from the submental area. The smooth margin of the tip of the tongue will form the vermilion border of the reconstructed lip.

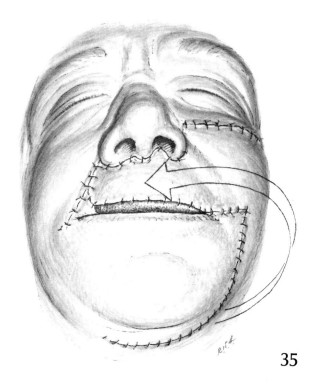

35

36

The tongue is later detached from the reconstructed upper lip and the defect on the tip closed by direct approximation. The portion of the tip of the tongue forming the vermilion border of the lip will be sutured to the underlying lining flap previously raised from the dorsum of the tongue.

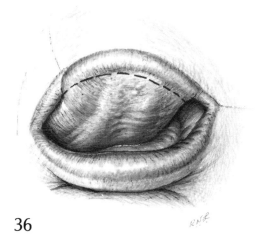

36

37

The repair is completed by division and inset of the flaps. Good protrusion of the remaining tongue is demonstrated.

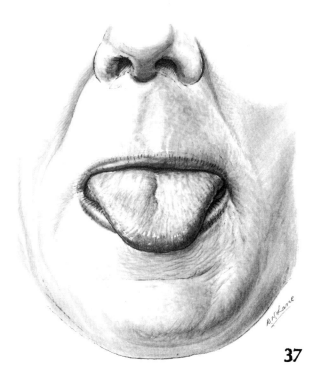

37

Provision of new vermilion

38

Through an incision along the front ventral edge to unroll the smooth tip of the tongue dorsally, a flap is formed which can provide the new vermillion for the lower lip total vermilionectomy. (The reverse, with incision along the dorsal front edge and a ventrally unrolled tip, can be used for upper vermilion.)

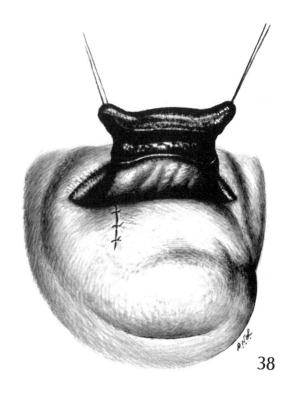

38

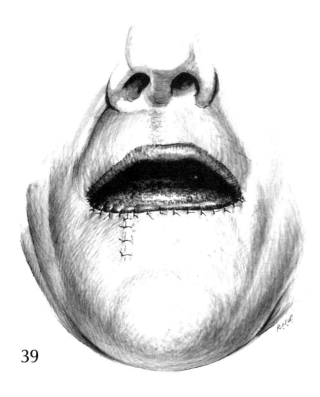

39

39

The flap is unrolled and sutured to the lower lip to reconstruct the vermilion border.

40

The flap is later divided and inset, and the donor defect on the tongue closed. Good postoperative protrusion of the tongue is demonstrated.

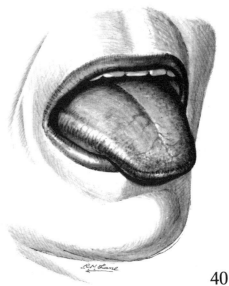

40

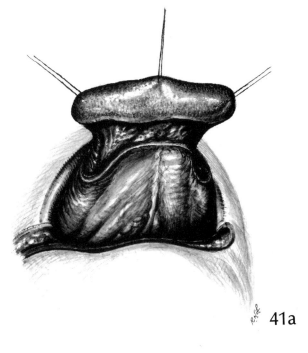

41a

Reconstruction of the lower lip

41a & b

Similarly, through a transverse incision across the ventral side, carried around on each side dorsally towards a central base, a two-winged flap (reminiscent of the hammerhead shark) is formed which can provide both lining and vermilion in a reconstruction of the lower lip.

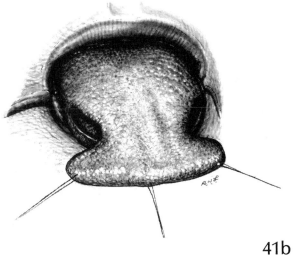

41b

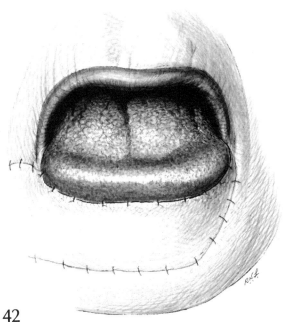

42

The flap is unrolled dorsally and sutured to the reconstructed lower lip.

42

43

The base of the flap is later divided and inset to complete the repair. The donor defect on the tongue is closed by direct approximation.

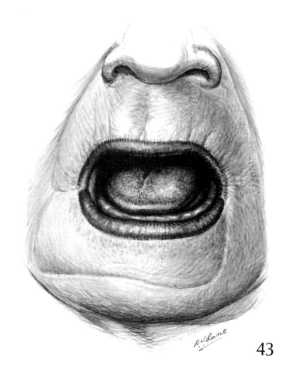

43

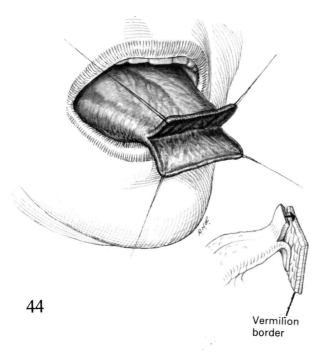

Vermilion border

44

44

A variation of the two previously described flaps, with the incision a little on the dorsal side of the lingual tip and the tongue tip split in fish-mouth fashion, can give two flaps, one reflected dorsally to supply vermilion, and a slightly longer one reflected ventrally to supply lining in a reconstruction of the lower lip. The vermilion so provided may not be as smooth as desired but will improve in time with atrophy of its papillae.

VENTRAL TONGUE FLAPS

The flaps so far described are all formed totally or largely from the dorsum of the tongue, although the smoother ventral mucosa would look better in labial reconstructions, particularly of the vermilion. Ventral mucosa is, of course, in much shorter supply. It is also much thinner and does not lend itself as easily to the formation of sizeable flaps and direct closure of the donor wound without undue tethering and impairment of important functions of the tongue.

45

A defect of the anterior floor of the mouth after resection of a carcinoma can be closed by two posteriorly based flaps from the lateral underside of the tongue.

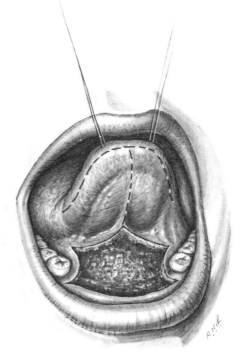

45

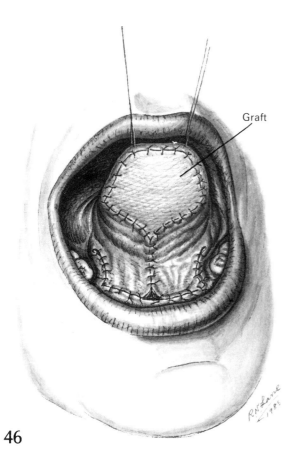

46

46

The flaps are rotated forward and medially to cover the surgical defect. A skin graft is used to close the donor defect in order to avoid tethering of the tongue.

Excision of carcinoma of floor of mouth

Michael F. Green FRCS, FRCS(Ed)
Consultant Plastic Surgeon, Welsh Centre for Burns, Plastic and Reconstructive Surgery, St Lawrence Hospital, Chepstow, Wales

Introduction

Excisional surgery for carcinoma of the floor of the mouth depends not only on the tumour type, size and site, but also on the surgical capability and experience of the surgeon. Total excision with a surround of normal tissue is required, and no elegant reconstruction, however complex, overshadows this need. The outcome of inadequate primary excision is local recurrence and either further operative procedures or failure, for both the surgeon and, more importantly, the patient. The surgeon should assess whether he can complete the procedure, both excision and reconstruction, before embarking upon it. If not, he should limit himself to a diagnostic biopsy or surgical excision alone and refer the patient to a specialist unit for secondary reconstruction. The extent of the excision depends on histological tumour type and degree of involvement of adjacent tissues and structures. The excision needs to be wider along the preferential lines of metastases, e.g. around the periosteal margin of the mandible, along the course of the mental nerve and towards the cervical neck glands. The tumour, usually a squamous cell carcinoma, is slow-growing and may prevent an adequate diet being ingested. It is worth while, in spite of any delay involved, to improve the nutritional state by vitamin and food supplements before surgery. Ideally this should be started at the time of initial diagnosis so that the patient will have gained weight by the time of operation.

The operations

BIOPSY

1

A thorough examination and the biopsy are ideally performed under general anaesthesia. If a local anaesthetic is used the patient may be more comfortable in the sitting position. Cheek retractors are positioned around the mouth to provide the optimal view, and good lighting and suction should be available. An ellipse of tissue of adequate size to include tumour and adjacent normal mucosa and deep tissues is excised. In cases with widespread mucosal changes particular care should be taken to biopsy areas of 'red' leucoplakia. Care should be taken to observe which tissue planes are transgressed, for subsequent surgical excision must extend past these planes. A little thought at this stage may prevent unnecessary damage making the excision and subsequent repair more difficult. Bleeding may be profuse and suturing difficult. Haemostasis by direct pressure may be necessary. Non-absorbable sutures allow easy subsequent recognition of the biopsy site. Complete excision biopsy of small lesions may be carried out but must be followed by careful histological and clinical surveillance.

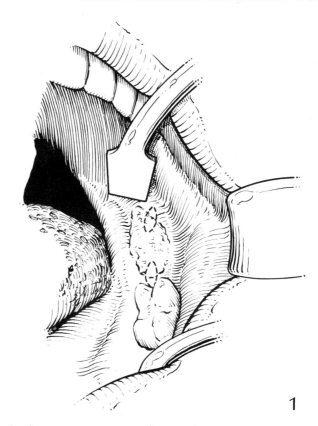

1

MAJOR RESECTIONS OF INTRAORAL STRUCTURES

A general anaesthetic is given by nasotracheal intubation or elective tracheostomy. The tracheostomy incision should be placed so as not to impair the vertical blood supply to the neck skin flaps. The patient is prepared for a long operative procedure, and facilities for vital sign monitoring, temperature regulation and fluid replacement should be available. Immediately before the resection a final examination is carried out under general anaesthesia to confirm that the apparent limits of the lesion agree with those of the earlier, pre-anaesthetic examination, which may have been hampered by pain or gagging.

The skin of the head and neck is cleaned with povidone iodine solution and draped with head towels sutured into place. Other areas of the patient are prepared as required. The donor areas for split skin grafts should be shaved, but not potentially hairy donor flap sites.

The incisions

2

The skin incisions should be marked with the head in the normal position so that they follow the natural skin creases. This may be carried out preoperatively. Accurate repositioning on suturing is facilitated by making the incisions slightly cross each other.

Starting at the midpoint of the neck, a transverse line is drawn across the neck in a skin crease to a point 1 cm posterior to the anterior border of the trapezius muscle. The posterior vertical incision is marked just behind the anterior border of the trapezius along its length. The midline incision extends from the midpoint of the neck to beneath the chin, just above the hyoid. It then continues around the natural chin prominence on the contralateral side to the proposed mandibular section, thus separating the skin from the bone and mucosal incisions.

The lip is marked, preferably in the midline, but always ensuring clearance by intra-oral inspection of the tumour.

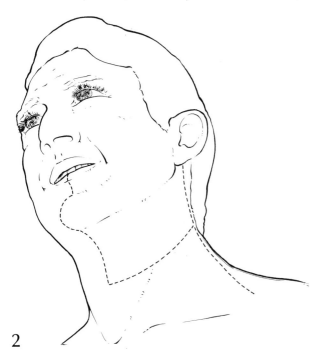

2

Elevation of skin flaps

3

The head is rotated to one side in order to improve access and to tighten and delineate the neck muscles, thus making elevation of the flaps easier. However, as this obstructs the superficial veins, it is important to rotate the neck back and recheck haemostasis before replacing the skin flaps at the end of the operation. The transverse incision is made first, taking care to identify and avoid the external jugular and anterior cervical veins. The platysma muscle retracts (it is deficient anteriorly) and the numerous vertical veins and arterioles present in the flap require haemostasis. The flap is then elevated in relatively avascular fascial planes. Skin-only flaps can be raised when the platysma is considered close to the tumour.

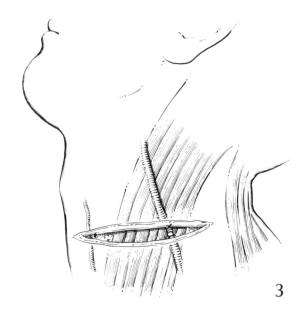

3

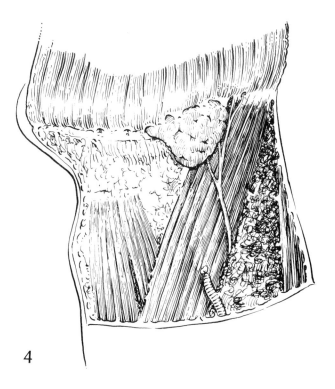

4

4

The upper flap is elevated until the lower border of the mandible is palpable from symphysis to mandibular angle, and the lower pole of the parotid and insertion of the sternocleidomastoid muscle from the mastoid process are visible. The latter's insertion into the skin may produce profuse superficial bleeding which can be controlled by pressure. This exposure may be sufficient for intermediate excisions where continuity of the mandible is being maintained, and in experienced hands for more major excisions. Elevation of the lip flap should be delayed until the *en bloc* dissection is almost completed, as this shortens the time the flap is malpositioned.

Elevation of lip flap

5

The lip is split while maintaining haemostasis by digital compression until the labial vessels are ligated. The incision around the contralateral chin is made through skin and muscle, and the flap is then elevated carefully, keeping close to the periosteum without broaching it. The muscular elements of the chin are attached to the bone and their muscle bellies normally keep the skin from draping directly on to the hard bone. Their removal reduces this effect and, on resuturing, the flap may be at risk because of the loss of uniform flap thickness and therefore possible vascular impairment.

6

The lesion and the extent of labial mucosal excision required for adequate tumour clearance can now be seen. The labial mucosa and the platysma insertion into the mandible are incised under direct vision as the skin flap is turned back from the mandible, the masseter muscle and the lower parotid fascia. The mental nerve is sectioned clear of the mental foramen. The mandibular branch of the facial nerve may occasionally be preserved if the lower pole of the parotid is not being included in the excision. The elevated flaps are retracted and secured with sutures through the subcutaneous tissue, taking care to maintain flap viability.

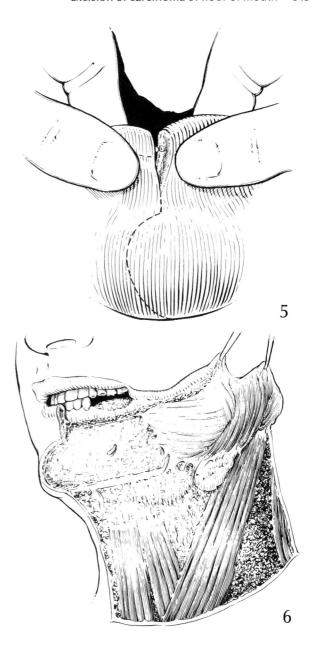

5

6

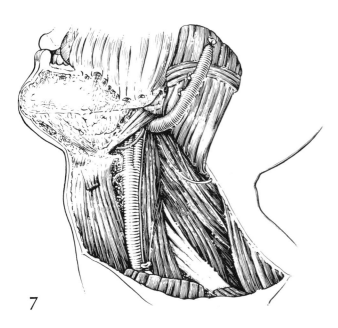

7

7

The elevated flaps reveal the sternomastoid muscle dividing the anterior and posterior triangles of the neck, and the anterior digastric muscle dividing the submental and digastric triangles. The hyoid, its greater cornu and the lower border of the mandible can be palpated.

The block dissection of the neck (*see* chapter on 'Radical neck dissection', pp. 523–537) at this level includes the sternomastoid muscle, the ligated lower end of the internal jugular vein, and the cervical fascia and glands. Division of the cutaneous cervical branches allows upward elevation of the block to expose the posterior belly of the digastric and the stylohyoid insertion into the hyoid. The lingual veins and artery, the hypoglossal nerve and the carotid bifurcation lie deep to these muscles.

Anterior dissection

8

The submandibular fascia enclosing the submandibular gland is elevated and then incised with scissors along the line of the hyoid. Small vessels along the border are a guide, but may produce troublesome bleeding anteriorly where they coalesce to form the anterior facial vein.

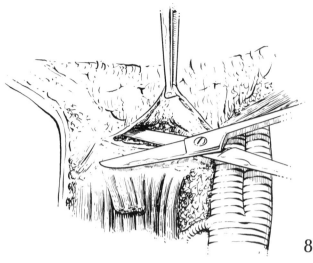

8

9

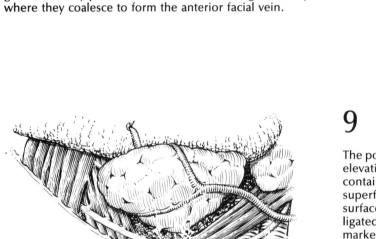

9

The posterior edge of the mylohyoid muscle is exposed by elevation of the mental and digastric triangles which contain the submandibular gland with the facial vein superficial and the facial artery passing into the deep surface of the gland. This should be exposed and either ligated or, if required for later microvascular anastomosis, marked and preserved along with suitable veins, e.g. the superior thyroid. The mylohyoid muscle is elevated and divided with scissors from the hyoid bone to the midline, exposing the hyoglossus and genioglossus muscles. This should be continued across to the contralateral side in anterior tumours. The mylohyoid muscle and the deep submandibular gland and duct are then elevated from the side of the tongue. The lingual nerve, if it is to be preserved, must be dissected free at this stage.

10

The surface of the hyoglossus is followed deep to the mandible while checking the required medial excision by intraoral examination. The digastric muscle is preserved as a landmark until the final excision. The contents of the mental triangle are freed from the midline towards the mental foramen. The anterior belly of the digastric and the geniohyoid muscle may occasionally be preserved in bilateral cases to act as support for the hyoid and thus the base of the tongue and larynx.

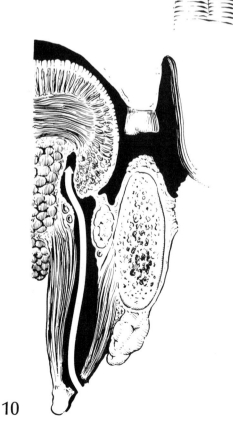

10

Posterior dissection

11

The posterior belly of the digastric muscle is followed to its origin from the mastoid notch, where it lies under the sternomastoid. The deep surfaces of sternomastoid and digastric muscles are freed by blunt dissection from behind and divided by sharp dissection from the skull. Bleeding from multiple small vessels is common and moist swab packing aids haemostasis while the surgeon continues with the anterior dissection. The contents of the posterior triangle, including the group of glands at the apex, are dissected from the muscles of its floor (the splenius capitus, levator scapulae and scalenus muscles). The upper end of the internal jugular vein, found at the level of the palpable transverse process of the atlas vertebrae, can be dissected safely on its deep surface where there are no branches and doubly ligated with non-absorbable sutures. It is important, however, not to damage the small emissary veins joining the upper end of the jugular vein just beneath the skull.

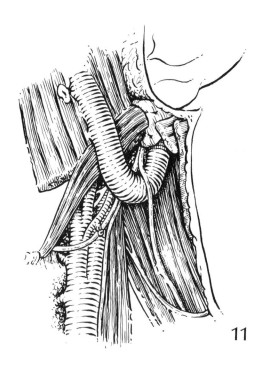

11

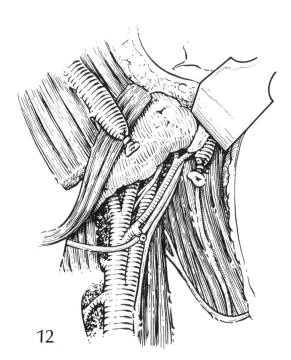

12

12

Anterior displacement of the muscles and block brings the deep surface of the parotid into view. The facial nerve trunk lies adjacent and deep to the palpable styloid process. If there is any involvement of the facial nerve and parotid duct, either by tumour or surgical excision, appropriate remedial surgery, e.g. tarsorrhaphy, is included in the reconstruction. The parotid edge is elevated below the ear to expose the external carotid trunk entering its deep surface and the postauricular artery branch.

A plane of section that ensures tumour clearance, including the expected lymphatic drainage from the tumour site, is now decided upon. This may entail:

1. no parotid excision in anterior lesions;
2. lower pole excision in lateral lesions; and
3. major resection in posterior and ascending lesions.

Removal of the lower pole below the superficial temporal and maxillary arteries, with preservation of the main facial nerve trunk, is sufficient in the majority of lateral and anterior floor lesions. The superficial temporal artery must be preserved if a forehead flap reconstruction is envisaged.

Posterior mandibular transection

13 & 14

The bone is sectioned using a Gigli saw, dental burrs or a mechanical saw. The mechanized methods allow greater accuracy, especially in horizontal cuts and in the formation of the bone ends to aid reconstruction. It is an advantage to carry out both osteotomies partially while the jaw is still stable, before completing either. The posterior line of transection is made by direct incision down to bone. Incision of the parotid results in venous bleeding and care should be taken in haemostasis not to inflict unnecessary damage to branches of the facial nerve. Bipolar diathermy may be preferred. The masseter muscle is divided at the same level and causes bleeding from the maxillary artery branches. The periosteum at the posterior border of the mandible is incised and elevated only enough to allow section. The remaining periosteum maintains the viability of the bone. The periosteum can be easily elevated from the sides but a sharp-edged elevator is required for the anterior edge. Care must be taken on the deep surface to stay in the subperiosteal plane, as the maxillary artery passes close behind the mandibular neck.

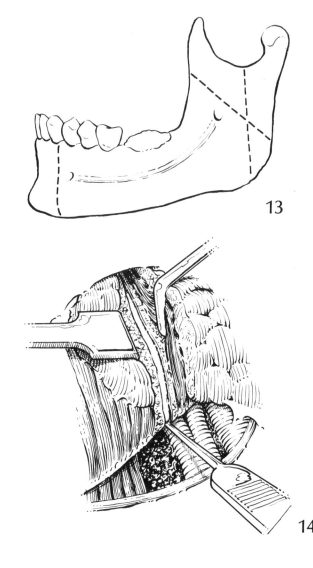

13

14

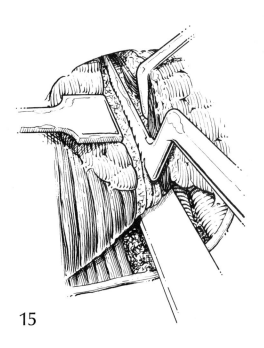

15

15

A protective guide is placed within the deep periosteum and the mandible is cut along the line of transection. It is essential to remove all of the inferior dental canal. The medial pterygoid muscle insertion is elevated with the periosteum. For posterior lesions requiring dislocation of the mandible for tumour clearance, the temporalis insertion must be released from the coronoid process. This is more easily carried out after the anterior mandibular resection. In cases where metastasis to the parotid nodes is unlikely, the parotid fascia and masseter may be incised at a lower level and a subperiosteal reflection carried out, preserving the parotid gland and facial nerve but allowing a higher transection of the mandible.

Anterior mandibular transection

16

The line of anterior mandibular transection is marked clear of the tumour, but always includes the mental canal. The periosteum is elevated from the line of excision without undermining the adjacent bone. The periosteum strips easily from the lower border and sides of the mandible from below but is strongly adherent on the upper edge, and incision and elevation from the oral surface is easier. Any teeth in the transection line should be extracted. Retractors and guards are placed to prevent inadvertent damage to surrounding tissues. A curved clip is passed behind the mandible and one end of the Gigli saw is drawn through. Holding the saw at an oblique angle, the handles are fitted and the bone is cut, taking care that the saw does not jump out on completing the osteotomy.

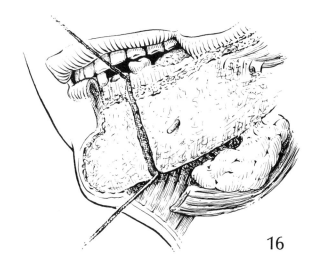

16

Tumour excision

17

The tumour mass and the block dissection are now suspended on the medial mucosal lining. A review of the planned excision should now be made to ensure that there are no soft tissue attachments containing structures that will prevent removal of the tumour once the medial incisions have been made. It is important that no structures due to be preserved, e.g. the lingual artery or nerve, are damaged inadvertently at this stage if sudden bleeding obscures the view. The divided mandible is retracted at the anterior end to improve the view of the tumour. The labial mucosal incision made when raising the lip flap is extended towards the posterior line of transection, taking care to avoid the parotid duct. Deeper removal of the cheek, including the buccinator muscle, allows the buccal pad of fat to intrude into the wound and this may need temporary suture to control. A medial incision, well clear of the tumour, is made through the mucosa and adjacent tongue into the space already developed on the hyoglossus and continued to the posterior margin of the excision. The submandibular duct and submental gland are included in the excision. The posterior incision is deepened through the divided mandible, the deep mandibular periosteum and medial pterygoid muscle insertion to the posterior plane of dissection, freeing the tumour and block dissection in continuity.

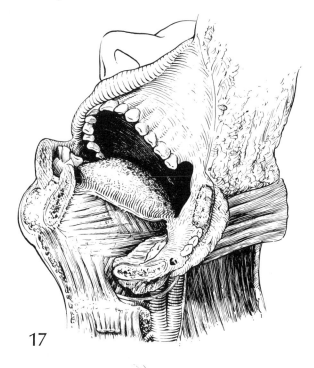

17

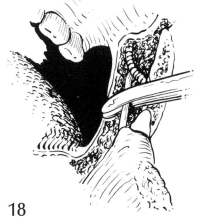

18

18

The proximal end of the mental nerve should be isolated and excised as high as possible. If frozen sections of the nerve demonstrate tumour involvement, further excision of the nerve is indicated. Haemostasis is obtained and a moist pack applied to the area.

MAJOR RESECTIONS INVOLVING SKIN

19

The incisional markings for the neck dissection and tumour removal are adjusted to the circumstances. The deep approach to the mandible is performed as described. The area of skin involved in the tumour is marked with a wide uninvolved margin. The actual skin incision should be placed to match functional and aesthetic facial contours outside this margin. The incisions in the skin should be wider than in the deeper muscular layers, decreasing in a stepped fashion. This aids flap replacement by providing underlying support to the suture lines. The soft tissue incision is deepened through the muscles of the face to join the intra-oral incisions. The combined radical block dissection (mandible with attached tumour) and the involved skin are then removed *en bloc*. The excisional defect is assessed and a reconstructive plan decided upon.

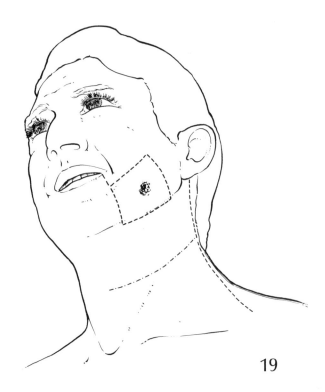

19

CONSERVATIVE RESECTION OF THE MANDIBLE

The major procedure has been described first, as lesser procedures should only be carried out for specific reasons in suitable cases and tumours. The upper cervical skin flap is raised to the lower border of the mandible. The contents of the submental and anterior triangles are dissected from the hyoglossus and genioglossus and the side of the tongue. The jugulo-digastric group of glands are dissected with the proposed excision. The lingual mandibular periosteum is elevated from the lower border to the level of the mental canal and from the mental foramen to the coronoid notch. Externally the attachment of the masseter and labial depressors is delineated and left in contact with the mandible and overlying soft tissue. This maintains the blood supply to the mandibular strut. The labial periosteum superior to this is freed by passing a narrow elevator above the muscle insertion via an anterior incision in the gum made clear of the tumour at the level of bone excision.

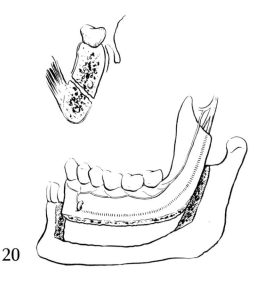

20

20

Using a reciprocating mechanical saw, a horizontal cut is made in the horizontal mandible, holding the saw at an angle to preserve the lower border and outer rim (with muscular attachments). A vertical cut behind the mental canal is made to join this near the mandibular angle. The whole course of the mental nerve should be excised in every case. Internal or external fixation may be necessary, depending on the depth of strut remaining, to prevent early fracture in the postoperative period.

The mucosa from the lingual side is cut with scissors passed into the plane developed beside the tongue. The lateral mucosa is incised clear of the tumour, and both incisions are joined to the posterior incision. The tumour and attached mandible segment may then be removed.

RECONSTRUCTION

Reconstruction of the intra-oral defect needs to provide a competent oral sphincter; a functioning jaw allowing mastication; and a normal facial appearance, as similar as possible to the original. It is also important that defects from the donor flap sites are as unobtrusive as possible.

To the patient, appearance is critical for a successful return to normal life. Nevertheless, the paramount primary aim of treatment is removal of the tumour and not the repair. The variety of new musculocutaneous and microvascular free flaps has added greatly to the reconstructive armamentarium of the surgeon. Vascularized bone grafts produce rapid ossification of the bone junctions and improved functional repair. However, no single repair is perfect and the choice of operation must depend on the extent and limits of the excisional defect. Reconstruction should always be kept in mind during the excision to ensure that possible repair options are kept open while not compromising the excision. I prefer the following two main repairs.

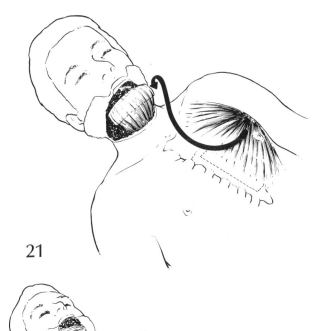

21

21

The sternal pectoralis major musculocutaneous flap provides bone, muscular cover and oral lining, and if necessary also external skin cover. The sternal outer table is malleable and can be curved to the shape required, but this needs temporary fixation until stable. It can be divided between the muscle interdigitations and angled to produce an ascending strut. This flap may also be used to carry a rib. The pectoralis muscle replaces the excised sternocleidomastoid muscle and fills the flat neck dissection defect. If possible, the pedicle should be reduced to the vessels only as the flap passes over the clavicle. Dividing the motor nerve supply allows the muscle bulk to degenerate while still providing cover to the carotid vessels.

22

Recently developed microvascular techniques allow single-stage transfer of vascularized bone and lining. A skin and radius bone segment based on the radial artery and linked into the branches of the external carotid artery, with drainage into the jugular vein or veins around the thyroid, provides bone of matching diameter capable of osteotomy for contouring. It is particularly useful as skin only in rim preserving excisions and in conjunction with functional neck dissections.

The donor area is the surgeon's responsibility and should be chosen and repaired with the greatest care. The skin defects should be contoured. Defects requiring grafting should have their free edges sutured down to the underlying tissue in order to lessen the potential contour deformity.

22

Wound drainage and closure

23

The wound is drained through two suction drains, one lying horizontally, avoiding the carotid artery, and the other lying vertically along trapezius. One is therefore always dependent whether the patient is lying down or sitting. The suction drains produce a concave surface on the neck and any tendency towards flattening or, worse, convexity signifies the formation of haematoma, which must be investigated. Large haematomas may develop even though the drains appear to be functioning, and must be evacuated promptly. The drains are removed when only small amounts of fluid are collected. Large volumes of fluid, particularly if milky in appearance, indicate a chylous fistula.

Before wound closure the head is placed in the normal position, the skin flaps are replaced and their viability is checked. The oral mucosal edges are sutured to the reconstructed lining with absorbable sutures. The small cross-hatch extensions and square angles enable the skin to be accurately reapproximated. The subcutaneous/platysma layer is closed with absorbable sutures, e.g. polyglycolic acid sutures, to provide complete skin apposition. The horizontal skin incision is repaired using a subcuticular suture with occasional interrupted external skin sutures. The vertical incisions are repaired with a combination of subcuticular and external skin sutures. The lip flap must be replaced on the chin by suturing the muscles to those remaining on the mandible and matching in the lip. The lip mucosa is repaired with fine absorbable sutures. The muscles of the lip, especially in the vermilion border, where muscle retraction occurs, should be sutured in their original positions to facilitate rapid return of functional mobility.

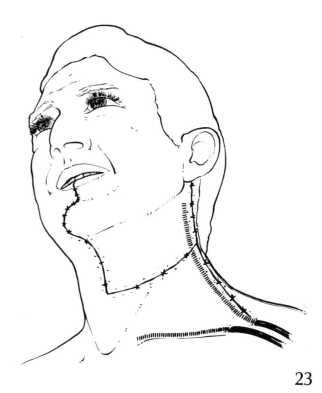

23

Antibiotic cover

The division of the mucosal barrier and the lymphatic drainage of the neck increase the risk of infection, and consideration should be given to the use of antibiotics against β-haemolytic streptococcal, Bacteroides species, and staphylococcal infections.

Postoperative care

A fine-bore nasogastric tube is passed into the stomach at the end of the procedure. The presence of swallowed blood may lead to a short period of gastric atony but as soon as the alimentary canal is functioning (usually within 12 hours) the total fluid and food requirement can be given via this route. No oral fluids are given. Once adequate fluid input is achieved, salivation will recommence, obviating the patient's need for sips, etc. The withholding of oral fluids limits swallowing movements of the tongue against the repair edges, which may still be insensitive and therefore liable to disruption. Oral fluids are commenced at approximately 4–5 days. Postoperative observation and care must be meticulous, both immediately after operation and subsequently. The reconstruction will require particular observation and may necessitate systemic, postural or surgical revision. The position of the intraoral suture lines may not be obvious from the external appearance.

Suture removal

The interrupted skin sutures are removed at 5 days, while the subcuticular sutures are left *in situ* or, if nylon, removed at 14–21 days. The intra-oral sutures are left in situ unless producing discomfort.

The patient's morale can be maintained by planning a sequence of steps: removal of drains, removal of catheters, start of oral fluids, removal of sutures, start of feeding, planning of discharge.

Illustrations by Robert N. Lane

Radical neck dissection

P. M. Stell ChM, FRCS
Professor of Otorhinolaryngology, University of Liverpool, UK

Introduction

The lymphatic drainage from almost all the sites in the head and neck where carcinomas may arise is into the lymph nodes of the neck, which form an interconnecting system with virtually only one outlet, at the inferior end of the internal jugular chain. The lymph nodes of the neck thus form an efficient barrier to the spread of cancer of the head and neck, and even if the tumour has metastasized to these nodes, distant metastasis does not occur for many months, so that treatment is still worthwhile at this stage.

Although the primary tumour often responds to radiotherapy, lymph nodes invaded by squamous carcinoma seldom do so and must be treated surgically. Operation may therefore be needed on the nodes alone or for removal of the nodes in continuity with the primary tumour. In this chapter the operation for removal of the nodes alone will be described.

Types of neck dissection

Several operations have been described for removing the lymph nodes of the neck and they must be described briefly first. A radical neck dissection is the classic operation, first described by Crile in 1906, in which the entire lymph-bearing area between the clavicle and the mandible, the midline and the trapezius is removed; with rare exceptions, this is the operation which should be adhered to. A block dissection consists of removal of the primary tumour in continuity with an enlarged mass of nodes; this operation will often leave behind smaller involved nodes and should not be done. An elective or prophylactic neck dissection has in the past been recommended when there are no palpable nodes but the primary tumour is known to metastasize frequently. It is thus hoped that nodes which may be involved histologically will be removed before they become palpable. There is no evidence that this procedure improves the cure rate compared with a policy of 'wait and see', and it is in general unjustifiable to carry out this operation, with its attendant increase in morbidity and mortality, until acceptable evidence is produced that it confers benefit on the patient.

Several partial neck dissections have been described, among them a functional neck dissection, preserving the sternomastoid muscle and the accessory nerve, and suprahyoid dissection in which only the tissues above the hyoid are cleared. Neither of these appear to be safe procedures and are not recommended. Indeed the only place for a local removal of palpable nodes appears to be in the treatment of papillary carcinoma of the thyroid, a tumour with a long natural history, which never breaks out of the capsule of the thyroid gland and does not follow the usual lymphatic channels taken by other head and neck carcinomas.

Preoperative

The patient is shaved between the level of the angle of the mouth and the nipple, including the hair over the mastoid process.

A general endotracheal anaesthetic is used. If a bilateral neck dissection is being performed a tracheostomy should be made to protect the patient from oedema of the airway, and the anaesthetic can be delivered through this.

The towels should be applied as for any other head and neck operation, and should be stitched in place to prevent them slipping.

The patient's neck is extended, and the head turned towards the opposite side by a pillow under the shoulder on the same side as the operation.

The operation

The incisions

1a, b & c

Two basic types of incision are in use for a radical neck dissection: the Y-type (a) and the double horizontal incision (b).

If the patient has not been irradiated, a Y incision is used. If the patient has been irradiated, a double horizontal incision protects against the danger of wound breakdown and is preferred. In either case the upper incision extends from the point of the chin down to the hyoid bone and ends over the mastoid process.

If a Y incision is used, the vertical limb starts about the middle of and at a right angle to the horizontal limb. The limb then continues down in an S-shape; when the scar contracts this becomes a straight line, but if a straight line were used in the first place a web might result. This incision must not cross the clavicle as this would compromise any future chest flaps.

In a double horizontal incision the second incision lies about 2 cm above the clavicle, starting laterally at the anterior border of the trapezius and ending medially at the midline. The lateral end of this lower incision can be turned up if necessary to improve access.

A bridge flap is lifted between the two incisions. The entire lower part of the dissection must be done first and the specimen passed under this flap to allow completion of the upper part of the dissection.

A further incision which can be used for either irradiated or unirradiated patients, and which can easily be modified for all major operations on the neck, is the half-H incision (c). This incision respects the two areas of vascular territory in the neck: the one supplied inferomedially from branches of the subclavian system and the other superolaterally from branches of the external carotid system.

Raising the flaps

Applied anatomy

During dissection of the upper flap, two branches of the facial nerve must be preserved, the cervical and mandibular.

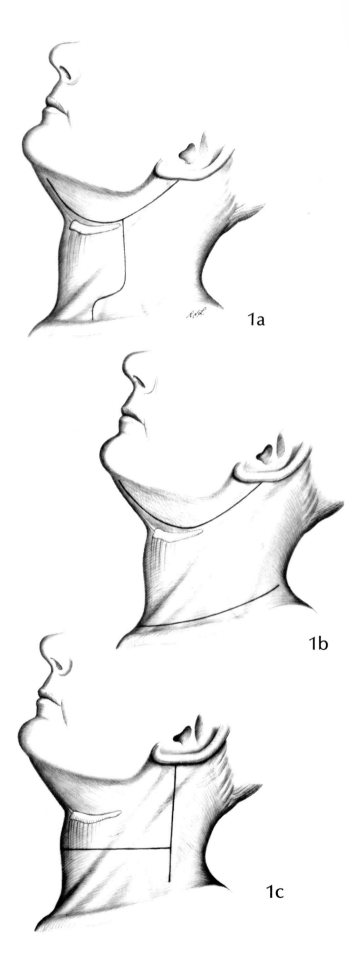

1a

1b

1c

2

The cervical branch supplies the part of the platysma which crosses the mandible and is inserted into the corner of the mouth, and the mandibular branch supplies the muscles around the mouth. Division of either nerve, therefore, leads to drooping of the lower lip. Both nerves curve downwards, below and in front of the angle of the mandible, across the facial vessels about one finger's breadth below the mandible. The mandibular branch then runs immediately superior to the submandibular gland, while the cervical branch runs lateral to this gland. Both nerves then curve upwards again to reach their destination.

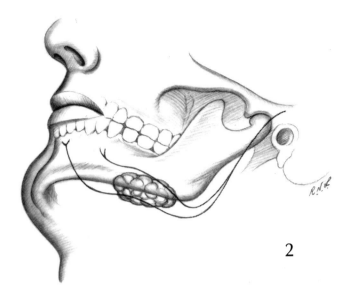

2

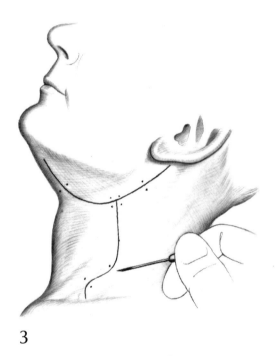

3

3

The incision is marked out with methylene blue using either a mapping pen or a sharpened orange stick. The skin should not be scratched with a needle to indicate suture marks; it is better to dip the tip of an intramuscular needle in methylene blue and make dots on the skin in three or four places for critical sutures.

4

The skin is incised in one movement down to and through platysma muscle. In the posterior part of the neck the platysma is very thin and the fibres of the sternomastoid are inserted directly into the skin, resulting in a little bleeding in this area. The platysma should be kept on the skin flaps as it increases the strength of the wound and increases the blood supply to the skin flaps.

The skin is retracted by double skin hooks placed underneath the platysma. These are pulled directly upwards while applying counter-traction to the specimen to expose the subplatysmal plane. Dissection here causes no bleeding provided the branches of the external and anterior jugular veins are tied. Bleeding usually signifies that a new and wrong plane has been entered.

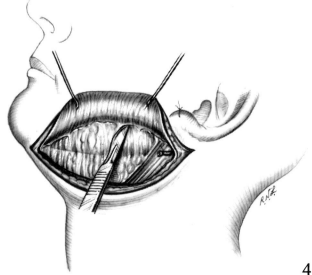

4

5 a & b

In a double horizontal incision the lower flap and the lower half of the middle flap are raised from below and the upper flap and the upper half of the middle flap from above. Access is gained by retracting the middle bridging flap with tapes.

When raising the upper flap the branches of the facial nerve must be preserved. The usual method of protecting these nerves, by ligating and dividing the facial vessels on the submandibular gland and lifting them over the mandible, is dangerous when the nerve's course is lower than usual; this manoeuvre also compromises removal of the pre- and postfacial nodes which are often affected in oral tumours. It is also difficult to preserve these branches if the platysma is left on the specimen.

The easiest way to preserve the branches of the facial nerve is to cut right through the fascia at the level of the hyoid bone, down to the capsule of the submandibular gland, and elevate the resulting flap in continuity with the skin flap.

When the flaps have been elevated they are stitched back to the towels, care being taken not to pass the needle through the epidermis. This excludes the skin surface from the wound.

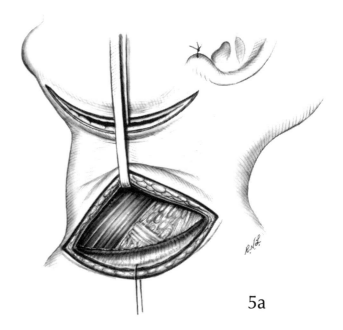

5a

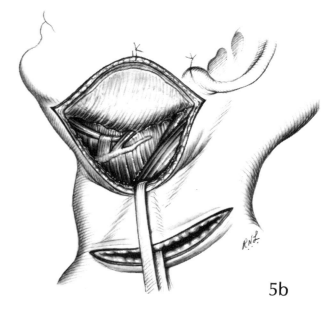

5b

Lower end of the internal jugular vein

6

Applied anatomy

The lower end of the internal jugular vein lies posterior to the lower end of the sternomastoid muscle, within the carotid sheath. The common carotid artery lies posteromedially, with the vagus nerve between the two structures, so that the nerve is in danger. A small unnamed tributary often joins the internal jugular vein about 2.5 cm above the end of the clavicle and can be the cause of troublesome bleeding.

Immediately lateral to the lower end of the carotid sheath lies the scalenus anterior muscle, with the phrenic nerve running from lateral to medial across it.

On the left side the thoracic duct ascends medial to the internal jugular vein, passes laterally, posterior to the vein, and then descends to enter the junction of the internal jugular and subclavian veins. Its size, position, tributaries and ending are very variable, and it should be looked for carefully in the root of the neck on the left side.

Posterolateral to the lower end of the common carotid artery, next to the medial border of the scalenus anterior, lies the thyrocervical trunk, which is short and immediately divides into the inferior thyroid, suprascapular and transverse cervical arteries. The latter two pass across the field of dissection. At the point where the inferior thyroid artery turns medially, there arises the ascending cervical artery, which is closely applied to the posterior wall of the carotid sheath, so that traction on this vessel can tear the thyrocervical trunk and indeed the subclavian artery.

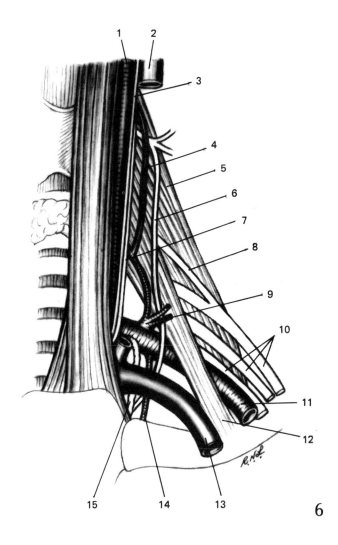

6

1 = Common carotid artery; 2 = internal jugular vein; 3 = vagus nerve; 4 = ascending cervical artery; 5 = scalenus medius muscle; 6 = phrenic nerve; 7 = inferior thyroid artery; 8 = C5 nerve; 9 = thyrocervical trunk; 10 = brachial plexus; 11 = subclavian artery; 12 = scalenus anterior muscle; 13 = subclavian vein; 14 = internal thoracic artery; 15 = thoracic duct

7

Technique

It is a basic principle of cancer surgery that the main vein draining the area being operated upon must be divided first, to reduce the number of systemic metastases caused by tumour emboli released by manipulating the tumour. The lower end of the internal jugular vein must, therefore, be divided first after exposing it by dividing the sternomastoid muscle, the assistant applying traction to the lower end while the surgeon does the same to the upper end. The muscle is then divided with a knife until the blueness of the vein is seen. Usually one vessel needs to be tied in the lower part of the sternomastoid. The lower, divided end of the sternomastoid muscle should not be transfixed. This produces a large mass of necrotic muscle which will almost certainly form an abscess leading to breakdown of the wound.

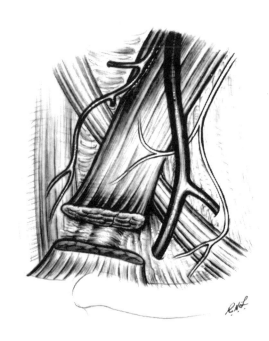

7

8

The carotid sheath is opened right down to the vein wall and the vein is freed using right-angled forceps at right angles to the vein. When the vein is free, it is retracted laterally with a small vein retractor. Only when the vagus nerve has been identified on the wall of the common carotid artery should ligatures of 2/0 silk be passed round the vein wall; three ligatures, two at the lower end and one at the upper end, are used. Each end is then transfixed with 3/0 silk. The vein is then held up by the long ends of the suture and divided with a knife between the transfixion stitches.

8

Supraclavicular dissection

9

Applied anatomy

The posterior triangle of the neck is divided by the omohyoid muscle into the occipital triangle and the supraclavicular triangle; the latter will be considered in this section, the former in the next. The supraclavicular triangle is filled by fat, and its floor is formed by the prevertebral fascia overlying the phrenic nerve and brachial plexus. Its important contents are the omohyoid muscle which forms its upper boundary, the subclavian vein in the very lowest part of the triangle behind the clavicle, the external jugular vein crossing its roof, and the transverse cervical artery passing laterally over the fascia of its floor.

Technique

The omohyoid muscle occasionally overlies the internal jugular vein but it is usually found immediately lateral to it; it can be divided without clamping as it will not bleed if cut through its tendon. The fascia over the fat pad lateral to the internal jugular vein is incised and this fat pad is elevated to identify the phrenic nerve passing over the scalenus anterior muscle from lateral to medial. The nerve lies behind the prevertebral fascia, which must not be incised as it protects the phrenic nerve and also the brachial plexus, which is encountered next. Diathermy must not be used over the fascia as this can also damage these nerves.

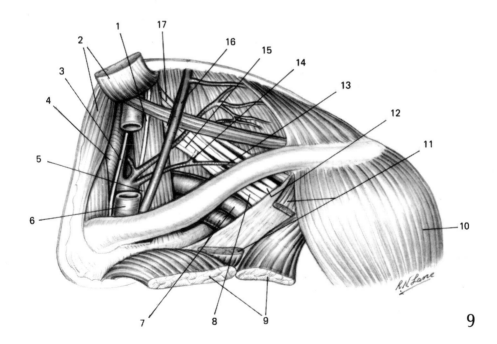

9

1 = Phrenic nerve; 2 = sternomastoid muscle; 3 = vagus nerve;
4 = common carotid artery; 5 = scalenus anterior muscle;
6 = internal jugular vein; 7 = subclavian artery and vein;
8 = posterior cord of brachial plexus; 9 = pectoralis major
muscle; 10 = deltoid muscle; 11 = pectoralis minor muscle;
12 = lateral cord; 13 = suprascapular artery; 14 = descending
scapular artery; 15 = lower trunk; 16 = external jugular vein;
17 = upper trunk of the brachial plexus

10

Dissection of this area can be greatly facilitated by using the plane between the fat pad and the prevertebral fascia. A finger is passed laterally, anterior to the prevertebral fascia, as far as the anterior border of the trapezius; the transverse cervical artery and vein in this area are ligated and divided if necessary. The external jugular vein is also divided and tied. The fat in the supraclavicular fossa can now be divided without bleeding by cutting down onto the finger, taking care not to cut the subclavian vein as it is pulled out of the thorax by the upward finger retraction.

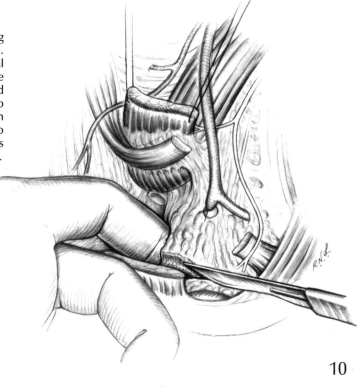

10

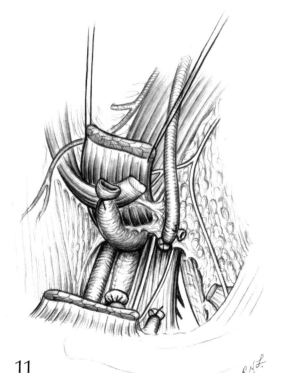

11

11

Now turning to the anterior part of the specimen, the internal jugular vein is elevated out of the carotid sheath.

Great care is needed so as not to tear a high thoracic duct on the left side, and a plane is established on the wall of the common carotid artery. The specimen must not be pulled up too hard at this point as it is possible to tear off the thyrocervical trunk because of traction on its inferior thyroid branch.

The occipital triangle

12

Applied anatomy

The other half of the posterior triangle is the occipital triangle, formed by the sternomastoid, the trapezius and the omohyoid muscles. Its floor is formed by the levator scapulae, which will be seen later to be of importance. The triangle is filled by fat, and contains only two items of interest to the surgeon: the accessory nerve coursing laterally to end in the trapezius muscle, 5 cm above the clavicle, and the branches of the transverse cervical artery. The latter artery divides at the anterior margin of the levator scapulae into a superficial and a deep branch; the superficial branch ascends deep to the anterior edge of the trapezius muscle and is accompanied by a vein.

The third and fourth cervical nerves give off a number of small branches, usually three or four, that pass posteriorly across the floor of the posterior triangle. The branches from the third cervical nerve may joint the accessory nerve just proximal to its insertion into the trapezius, or may enter the muscle directly. The branches from the fourth cervical nerve pass directly to the deep surface of the trapezius. On the deep surface of the trapezius muscle the spinal accessory and the cervical nerve branches form a plexus to supply the muscle. Contrary to previous opinions, these branches from the cervical plexus are motor nerves to the trapezius muscle.

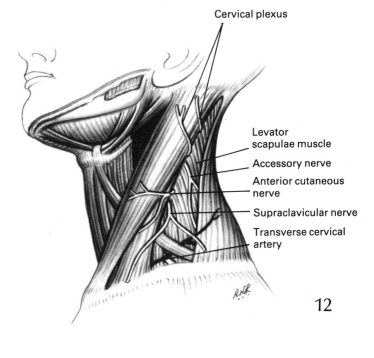

Cervical plexus

Levator scapulae muscle

Accessory nerve

Anterior cutaneous nerve

Supraclavicular nerve

Transverse cervical artery

12

Ascending branches of the transverse cervical artery run along the anterior border of the trapezius muscle, making dissection along this part of the muscle bloody and tedious.

Technique

13

The easiest method is to develop a tunnel with the finger over the prevertebral fascia immediately anterior to the border of trapezius. The fat is divided between two large artery forceps until the sternomastoid is reached. During this part of the dissection the accessory nerve is cut, causing the shoulder to jump.

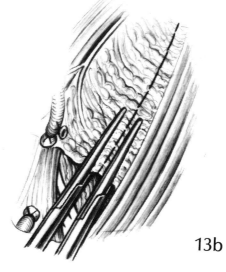

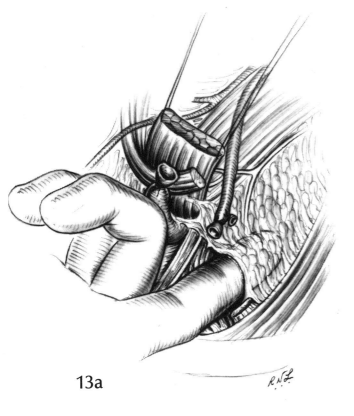

13a

13b

14

With the specimen now free inferiorly and posteriorly, it is pulled medially and the fat pad is elevated off the prevertebral fascia. This is best accomplished by the assistant taking the specimen in a swab and pulling it upwards very hard. The specimen is freed by sharp dissection with a knife, together with countertraction. It is tacked down in three places, however, by the three cutaneous branches of the cervical plexus; these neurovascular bundles consist of a vein, an artery and a nerve and should be clamped, divided and tied high on the specimen to avoid damage to the phrenic nerve and to the branches arising from C3 and C4 which course across the floor of the posterior triangle to supply the trapezius muscle. It is important to preserve these nerves, as this step preserves movement of the shoulder girdle in about 80 per cent of cases.

Dissection is continued along the common carotid artery on the adventitial plane up to the bifurcation, taking care to preserve the vagus nerve.

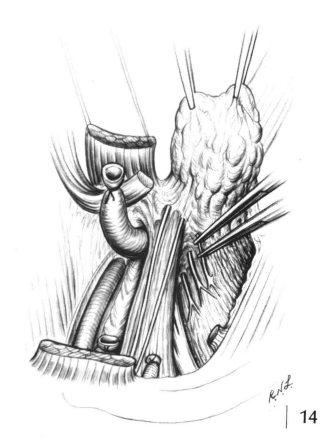

14

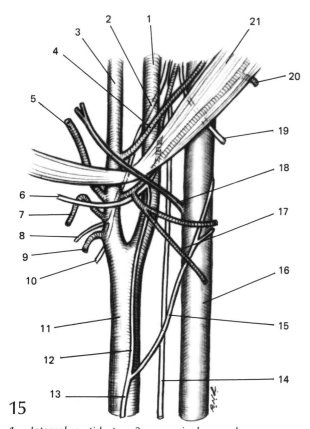

15

1 = Internal carotid artery; 2 = superior laryngeal nerve;
3 = external carotid artery; 4 = posterior auricular artery;
5 = facial artery; 6 = hypoglossal nerve; 7 = lingual artery;
8 = internal laryngeal nerve; 9 = superior thyroid artery;
10 = external laryngeal nerve; 11 = common carotid artery;
12 = descendens hypoglossal nerve; 13 = hypoglossal nerve;
14 = vagus nerve; 15 = descendens cervicalis nerve;
16 = internal jugular vein; 17 = lower sternomastoid branch of occipital artery; 18 = facial vein; 19 = accessory nerve;
20 = upper sternomastoid branch of occipital artery;
21 = digastric muscle (posterior belly)

The upper end of the internal jugular vein

15

Applied anatomy

It is customary to divide the upper end of the internal jugular vein at the level of the easily palpable transverse process of the first cervical vertebra. At this point the vein is covered by the posterior belly of the digastric muscle, which is the key to dissection in this area. This muscle has few superficial relations except for the tail of the parotid gland and the common facial vein. Once the upper end of the sternomastoid muscle, with the overlying external jugular vein, has been divided, it is easy and safe to expose the posterior belly of the digastric. The internal jugular vein will be found issuing from beneath the muscle, with the accessory nerve lying over the vein. The internal and external carotid arteries are posteromedial to it at this point, and the hypoglossal nerve emerges between the vein and the internal carotid artery, lying medially in the carotid sheath. The occipital artery runs laterally along the inferior border of the digastric muscle and can be a troublesome source of haemorrhage. At the level of the transverse process of the atlas (CI), the internal jugular vein is often joined by the occipital vein.

echnique

6

ie sternomastoid muscle is divided from the mastoid
ocess and the internal jugular vein is followed upwards
the transverse process of the first cervical vertebra from
:low, dividing the fascia of the carotid sheath with
issors. This frees the jugular vein on three sides and by
:eping close to the wall it is an easy matter to pass
;ht-angled forceps round it anteriorly and put on the
ree 2/0 silk ties – two above and one below the point of
vision.

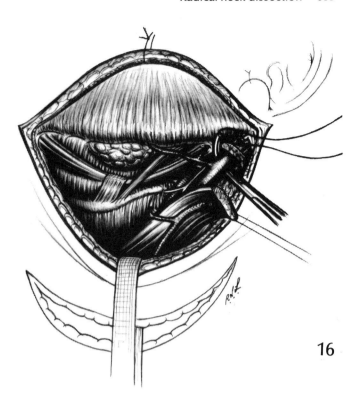

16

17

An alternative way of identifying the internal jugular vein
is to cut down onto the posterior belly of the digastric
muscle – there are no vital structures superficial to it at this
point except the common facial vein. The muscle is
retracted upwards, and the vein will be seen emerging
from beneath it with the accessory nerve overlying it.

It is not necessary to remove the posterior belly of the
digastric muscle since it is so helpful in covering closure
lines and for carotid artery protection. However, in order
to remove as much jugular vein as possible the posterior
belly of the digastric is retracted upwards to allow the
ligatures to be slid up as high as possible, but before tying
the ligature the vagus and hypoglossal nerves must be
identified. The occipital artery crosses the posterior part
of the vein; it is ligated and divided, as is the occipital vein
if present, before dividing the main vein. After transfixion
with 3/0 silk, the upper end of the internal jugular vein is
divided.
Dissection then proceeds anteriorly. The posterior
branch of the posterior facial vein is found 13 mm anterior
to the internal jugular vein; it is ligated and divided. The
tail of the parotid gland is then divided in a line between
the mastoid tip and the angle of the jaw. If at this point the
knife is angled upwards the facial nerve may be cut, so
that the knife must be angled slightly downwards to the
transverse process of the first cervical vertebra, thus
cutting the parotid gland obliquely.

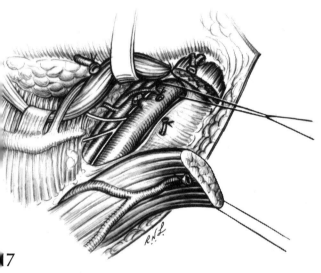

7

18

The hypoglossal nerve is then identified and traced to the bifurcation of the common carotid artery. Bleeding may occur from veins accompanying the hypoglossal nerve – these veins generally run medial to the nerve but send three or four anastomotic branches anterior to it. These anastomotic vessels are freed by dissection along the hypoglossal nerve on the perineural sheath, clamped, divided and tied; diathermy must never be used in this area. If bleeding occurs from these veins it is important to realize that the bleeding point will retract medial to the hypoglossal nerve. The only way to stop this bleeding without damaging the hypoglossal nerve is to lift the nerve, either up or down, with a blunt hook, find the bleeding point, apply a small artery forceps and tie the bleeding point.

Finally the hypoglossal nerve is traced forwards into the submandibular triangle.

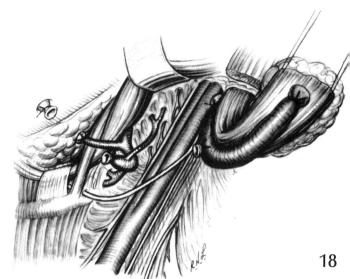

18

The submandibular triangle

19

Applied anatomy

The important anatomical feature of the submandibular area is its floor, from which the gland must be separated safely. The floor is formed by the mylohyoid and hyoglossus muscles, with the lingual and hypoglossal nerves passing laterally across them. The hypoglossal nerve is seldom in danger, however, since it is protected by the anterior belly of the digastric muscle. The lingual nerve describes a curve, U-shaped downwards, being tethered by its branch to the submandibular ganglion. Anteriorly the nerve disappears medial to the mylohyoid muscles accompanied by the submandibular duct, around which it does its well-known swerve, medial to the mylohyoid muscle, and not in the area of dissection. The facial artery enters the triangle between the submandibular gland and the posterior belly of the digastric muscle.

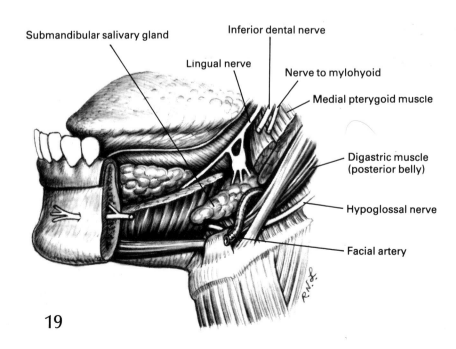

Submandibular salivary gland

Lingual nerve

Inferior dental nerve

Nerve to mylohyoid

Medial pterygoid muscle

Digastric muscle (posterior belly)

Hypoglossal nerve

Facial artery

19

Technique

The upper border of the submandibular gland is freed by dividing and tying the vessels, including the facial artery, which cross the lower border of the mandible.

The fat in the submental area is separated from the chin and the anterior belly of the digastric muscle displayed. The anterior part of the submandibular gland is then identified and freed in a posterior direction to the posterior border of the mylohyoid.

20

The mylohyoid muscle can now be pulled forwards to show the submandibular duct and the lingual nerve pulled down in a curve. The latter is freed by dividing the fascia around the submandibular ganglion with a knife, whereupon the lingual nerve springs upwards behind the body of the mandible. The submandibular duct is tied and divided.

The neck specimen is removed after transfixion and division of the facial artery at the posteroinferior border of the gland, and division of the fascia over the strap muscles in the region of the hyoid bone.

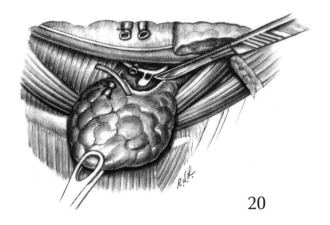

20

Protection of the carotid artery

The carotid artery must be protected in any patient whose skin wound is likely to break down, or who is likely to develop a fistula; this includes patients who have been irradiated, poorly nourished patients and diabetics. Several methods of carotid artery protection have been described, but the only absolutely reliable method is that of using the levator scapulae muscle.

21

The levator scapulae is identified and its posterior border freed. The lower border is also freed as near to the scapula as is possible and divided. It is then easy to swing the muscle forwards, pedicled on its anterior border like a page of a book; this preserves its blood supply entering from its anterior border. The brachial plexus must not be injured during division of the lower end.

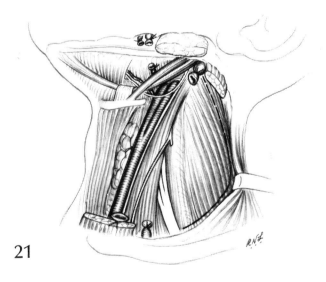

21

22

The muscle is stitched over the carotid arteries using interrupted 3/0 chromic catgut sutures, usually to the sternohyoid muscle anteriorly, to the posterior belly of the digastric superiorly, and to the stump of the sternomastoid inferiorly.

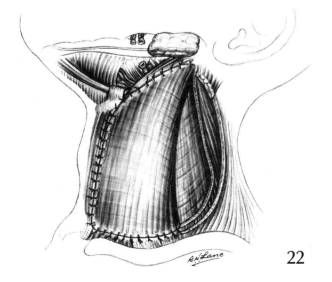

22

Closure

The wound is washed, dirty instruments are discarded and the entire operating team change their gowns and gloves. Haemostasis is completed with coagulation diathermy. Blood always pools at the insertion of the trapezius muscle to the clavicle because any bleeding that occurs in the neck will run down to this point. Continuous suction-drainage should be used, preferably of the Haemovac type.

Two Haemovac drains are introduced, from the under-surface of the lower flap to the outside. It is safer to put them in from within out since, if they are inserted in the opposite direction, the sharp introducer may damage the carotid artery if it slips. The drains are held with 3/0 chromic sutures, one along the anterior border of the trapezius and the other in front of the carotid artery curving upwards into the submandibular region. Drains should never cross the carotid sheath, and they should be cut to the correct length so that there are no holes outside the skin, otherwise an airtight closure will not be possible. The drains are secured to the skin with a Roman garter stitch of 3/0 silk. A final check is now made for: bleeding from the veins accompanying the hypoglossal nerve; bleeding on the undersurface of the middle flap, if a double horizontal incision has been used; a chylous leak. These are the three commonest causes of trouble in the postoperative period.

Division of the thoracic duct on the left side is often necessary and the duct is often injured. This is of no importance, but it must be recognized during the operation. Since the patient is starving, the chyle will be clear and scanty. It is therefore important to look carefully for it at this stage in the groove posterolateral to the lower end of the common carotid artery. If there is a slight collection of chyle, the surrounding fascia should be oversewn until the area is dry.

Buried sutures of 3/0 chromic catgut are placed at the skin marks and further similar interrupted sutures are placed until the flap is airtight. In order to check for this, suction is applied to the Haemovac drains. If any air leaks, further sutures are inserted.

The skin is closed with a blanket stitch of 5/0 Dermalene and air tightness is again checked.

No dressing is needed if all bleeding has been stopped and the wound closed so that it is airtight. Nobecutane should not be used on the wound as this sticks to the skin and stitches, so that when the stitches are removed, removal of the film of Nobecutane may drag the wound edges apart.

Radical neck dissection as part of a combined procedure

When a primary tumour is removed in continuity with a neck dissection, it is important to keep a band of continuity between the neck dissection and the primary growth.

Laryngeal cancer

In a total laryngectomy, the neck dissection should be left attached along the whole length of the larynx to include the superior and inferior lymphatic pedicles.

Pharyngeal cancer

When a laryngopharyngectomy is performed the pedicle must be as broad as possible and is best left along the whole length of the pharynx.

Oral cancer

Oral cancers drain to the submandibular, submental and upper deep cervical nodes. Therefore, the specimen should be left attached along the lower border of the mandible and should include the inner layer of the periosteum, to preserve continuity.

Oropharyngeal cancer

Tumours of the oropharynx drain by a pedicle to the upper deep cervical nodes. The specimen should be left attached, therefore, near the tail of the parotid gland.

Postoperative care

1. Continuous suction to the drains.
2. Intravenous fluids until the next day.
3. Feeding by mouth can begin the next day.
4. Antibiotics should never be needed unless basic surgical principles have been contravened.
5. The drains are not removed until drainage is less than 10 ml per day – usually about the fourth day.
6. Stitches are removed on about the fifth day.

Complications

(1) *Haemorrhage* Possible sites include either end of the jugular vein, the subclavian vein, pharyngeal veins, superior and inferior thyroid pedicles and the posterior surface of the bridge flap.

(2) *Chyle leak* If the thoracic duct has been damaged and this has not been recognized, when feeding begins, abundant white milky fluid will issue from the suction drain. The neck must be re-explored immediately and the end of the duct found and oversewn.

(3) *Nerve lesions* It is possible to damage the following nerves – phrenic, sympathetic trunk, brachial plexus, vagus, accessory, facial nerve and its lower branch, hypoglossal and lingual.

(4) *Facial oedema*

(5) *Cerebral oedema* This may come on after a bilateral neck dissection; after a second, staged neck dissection; or after the first neck dissection, if a large dominant internal jugular vein has been removed. The symptoms are restlessness and a bursting headache, with a falling pulse rate and a rising blood pressure; the face is swollen and cyanosed, whereas the extremities remain pink and warm. It should be treated by sitting the patient up, releasing all constricting dressings round the neck and giving an intravenous infusion of 200 ml of 25 per cent mannitol.

(6) *Infection and wound breakdown* These are usually due, apart from lapses in surgical technique, to the injudicious use of a Y-type of incision in a patient who has been irradiated. If the flaps become non-viable, necrotic material must be excised if present, and local soaks, such as eusol, used. A culture of the infected material often reveals opportunist Gram-negative bacilli, so that antibiotics are not often indicated. The pyocyaneus, which secretes pyocyanin, a toxin that dissolves skin, can often be eliminated by 1 per cent acetic acid soaks.

(7) *Rupture of the carotid arteries* This may be a sequel to wound breakdown in an irradiated patient if the arteries have not been protected by a levator scapulae graft. If this complication occurs, the artery must be tied off, ensuring as far as possible that the cerebral blood flow is maintained, by replacing lost blood, keeping the head low and not allowing CO_2 retention. At least half the patients who suffer this complication will die, and many of the survivors suffer a hemiplegia.

(8) *Frozen shoulder* In the classical procedure all the innervation of the trapezius muscle is divided. The muscles that abduct the shoulder are still innervated but the patient cannot fix his shoulder girdle, which therefore falls forwards, making abduction of the arm mechanically impossible. He is therefore given exercises to brace the shoulder girdle backwards and to maintain mobility of the shoulder joint to prevent a frozen shoulder. In the technique described above of preservation of the branches from C3 and C4 of the cervical plexus, normal shoulder movement is retained in 80 per cent of patients.

(9) *Recurrence in the skin or glands*

Illustrations by Sandra Neophytu

Malignant melanoma of the head and neck

T. P. F. O'Connor FRCS, FRCSI
Consultant Plastic Surgeon, Southern Health Board, The Regional Hospital, Cork, Ireland

D. C. Bodenham FRCS, FRCS(Ed)
Consultant Plastic Surgeon, Frenchay Hospital and United Bristol Hospitals, Bristol, UK

1

Malignant melanoma of the head and neck accounts for approximately one-third of all malignant melanomas. Treatment is based on an understanding of three types: the flat type of lentigo maligna, the plateau type or superficial spreading, and the polypoidal type or nodular lesion.

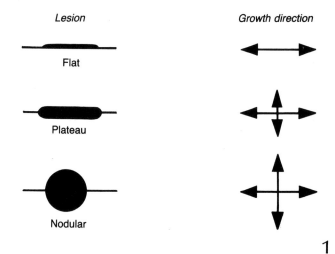

The vertical growth component of the tumour has the greatest significance because as the tumour invades the dermis the chances of metastases via the lymphatics or blood vessels in the dermis increase. The height of the tumour above the surface of the skin is also helpful in determining prognosis. Early treatment is essential, as flat lesions, which are eminently curable, will progress and eventually develop a vertical growth component. This lessens the chances of curative treatment. Prognosis for females is 10 per cent better than for males, but this is not sufficient difference to justify special treatment.

The face is the commonest site for malignant melanoma. It is also an area of great cosmetic and functional importance. Mutilation should therefore be avoided and function preserved by reconstructive procedures commonly practised by the plastic surgeon. The incidence of melanoma on the scalp and neck is relatively low and more easily dealt with.

Diagnosis

Early diagnosis is of utmost importance. Suspicion should be aroused if a mole becomes itchy, changes colour (either darkening or becoming lighter), increases in size (area or volume) or bleeds. Approximately 80 per cent of lesions can be diagnosed by naked eye examination. The remaining 20 per cent will require microscopic examination by a pathologist experienced in the pattern and behaviour of melanoma cells. Excision biopsy, and not incision biopsy, is carried out. The specimen is sent for frozen section or urgent paraffin section examination to confirm the diagnosis. Further excision is carried out as soon as possible if the diagnosis of malignant melanoma is confirmed.

Although lentigo maligna is radiosensitive, other forms of malignant melanoma are radioresistant. Painful bony and some other metastases may respond favourably. Surgery is quicker, more positive and without the risk of local irradiation effects on the skin, which can be troublesome. Chemotherapy has no place in the primary management of malignant melanoma at present. Immunotherapy has not yet been shown to improve the recurrence-free interval or survival of the patient[1].

Success of treatment is related to the margin of surgical excision (*Table 1*). As this increases from zero there will be a rise in cure rate for the first few millimetres, but the law of diminishing returns applies to more radical treatment. Surgery can only deal with purely local disease and, to a very limited extent, with locally spreading disease. Elsewhere on the body there is not the cosmetic or functional penalty of an equivalent excision on the face – for example close to an eyelid.

The lax skin of elderly patients allows a relatively simple surgical procedure which can often be carried out under local anaesthesia. The lesion should be excised down to deep structures, preserving, for example, the VIIth cranial nerve.

Table 1 Guidelines for determining margin of excision

Type of tumour	Size of tumour (mm)	Margin of excision (mm)
Flat lesion	up to 10	3
	10–25	5–10
Plateau	up to 5	10
	5–10	20
Nodular	up to 5	20
	5–10	20–30

Lymph nodes

Opinion no longer favours prophylactic lymph node dissection, which may be harmful by diminishing the host's immune defence mechanism. If the regional lymph nodes are enlarged or suspected of harbouring malignant disease they should be removed. If the primary lesion is nodular and overlies the draining lymph nodes then excision of the lesion in continuity with the lymph nodes may be indicated.

Methods of repair

Surgical defects may be repaired by any of the following methods: direct closure, free skin graft, local flap, or pedicle flap.

Examples of the above reconstructive procedures are described in subsequent paragraphs.

Preoperative

Anaesthesia

General anaesthesia via an endotracheal tube with a pharyngeal pack in position is the anaesthetic of choice when operating for malignant melanoma of the head and neck. For small lesions where a simple repair is possible and/or general anaesthesia is contraindicated, local anaesthesia with adrenaline, e.g. 2 per cent lignocaine in 1:250 000 adrenaline, is preferable.

Position of patient

The patient is placed in the supine position with the head resting on a rubber ring. Some degree of head-up tilt helps to reduce bleeding during the operation.

Preparation

The skin is cleaned with an aqueous antiseptic solution of choice. Head towels are applied, exposing the whole face.

General postoperative management

Sutures

Fine silk or monofilament nylon sutures such as 6/0 or 5 are used on the face. The stitches are tied securely but n so that they are tight, and are removed in 5–7 days whe possible to avoid stitch marks. When sutures are remove the wound may be supported with Steristrips or th equivalent.

Postoperative wound toilet

The wounds receive daily toilet, removing any crust exudate.

Complications

Loss of skin flaps or skin grafts, or wound breakdow results from faulty technique, infection or haematom formation. Meticulous technique and haemostasis a essential. At the first sign of infection a wound swab taken for culture and sensitivity determination, and th appropriate antibiotic prescribed. Any accumulation pus or haematoma is released.

The operations

Malignant melanoma of the cheek

EXCISION AND DIRECT CLOSURE

The lax skin of the cheek in elderly patients allows relatively simple surgical excision with direct closure of the wound, but the repair should be planned to avoid pull on the lower eyelid and undue tension on the skin edges. Defects of up to 2 cm in the elderly will usually close. Where possible, scars are placed in the natural crease lines.

2

The lesion with surrounding margin of healthy skin is outlined with pen and ink (Bonney's blue) and then excised.

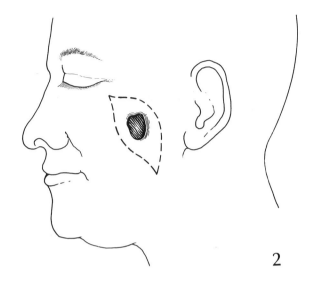

2

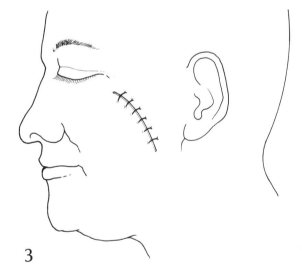

3

3

The wound edges are easily sutured together when margins have been adequately undermined and the excision has been properly planned.

EXCISION AND FREE SKIN GRAFT

4

When the wound, following excision of a malignant melanoma, cannot be closed directly, a skin graft may be used. A split thickness skin graft (Thiersch graft) gives a poor cosmetic result on the face because of its different quality and tendency to contract. When using a skin graft the maximum amount of graft should be inserted into the defect to allow for shrinkage.

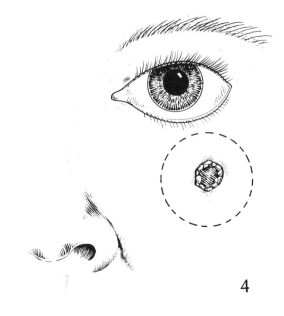

4

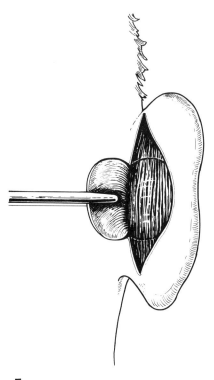

5

5

A full thickness skin graft from the sulcus behind the ear, cut to correct size and shape, gives a good cosmetic result. The colour and texture of the skin graft match well with that of the face. Any fat or subcutaneous tissue is removed from the graft. The repaired donor wound is well concealed behind the ear, where most defects can be closed by simple suture.

6

Having been cut to the correct pattern for accurate fit, the graft is sutured edge to edge along its margin. Some of the sutures on all sides are left long.

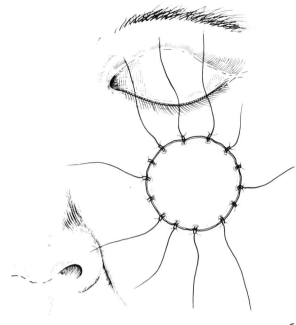

6

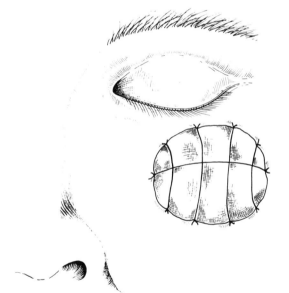

7

7

A piece of polyurethane foam or flavine wool pack is used to exert pressure on and to immobilize the graft. The long sutures are tied over the foam or wool pack. The pack and sutures are removed in 5–7 days.

EXCISION AND LOCAL FLAP REPAIR

The primary defect is repaired by moving adjoining tissue into it. The secondary defect is then closed by direct approximation, free skin graft or use of a further local flap. If possible the secondary defect is placed in a position where it can be more readily concealed.

8

The margins of excision of the lesion at A are marked. Flaps B and C are outlined for the repair. The principle is to transfer the defect from the cheek to the postauricular area.

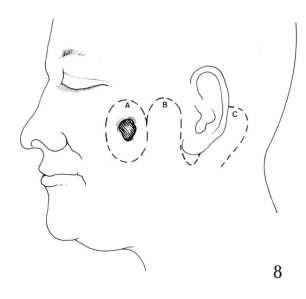

8

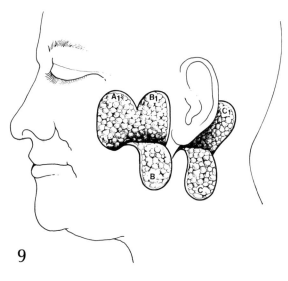

9

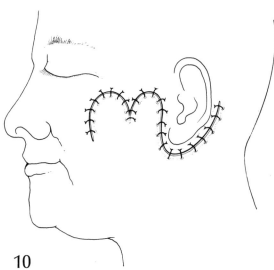

10

9 & 10

The lesion is excised, creating the defect A_1. The pre-auricular flap B is elevated for its repair, creating a secondary defect B_1. A second local flap C is then elevated from the postauricular area and used to fill the defect B_1. The defect C_1 is in an inconspicuous area and can be repaired by direct closure or a free graft.

Melanoma of the nose

LATERAL NASAL FLAP

Melanomas of the nose are extremely rare. Lesions of the nasal mucosa often present late and carry a bad prognosis. Simple excisional defects of the nose may be repaired by conventional methods using free grafts or flaps.

11

The excision is planned to create a triangular skin defect at the site of the lesion. A lateral nasal flap which does not transgress the midline and extends upwards into the glabellar region is outlined to transpose into the primary defect. A secondary defect will be created in the glabellar region.

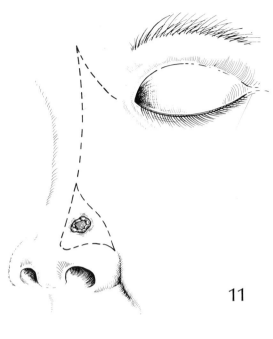

11

12

The flap is incised and elevated. Careful undermining of the flap is required to allow adequate transposition.

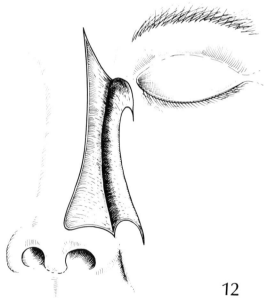

12

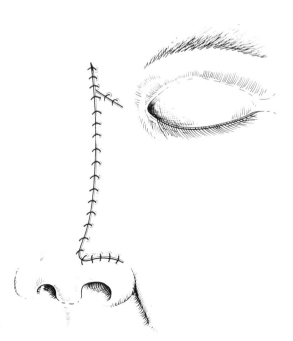

13

Suturing commences at the tip of the nose. The lax skin of the glabellar region is easily approximated to allow closure of the secondary defect. A slight temporary distortion of the nose often occurs but this corrects itself.

13

AMPUTATION OF THE NOSE

14

Amputation of the nose may be required to eradicate an infiltrating tumour of the nose which arises from the skin or the nasal mucosa.

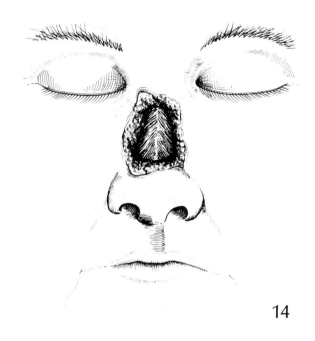

14

15

The nose is excised with an appropriate margin of skin and mucosa.

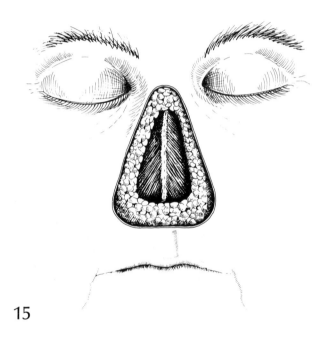

15

Closure by skin-to-mucosa approximation

16

With adequate undermining and resection of the bony margins the skin and mucosa at the margins of excision can be sutured together.

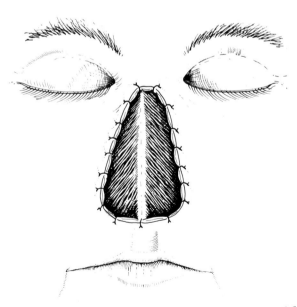

16

Closure by skin grafting

17

If direct closure is not possible a split skin graft is required to cover the raw surface between the skin and mucosa. The graft is secured in place with flavine wool and tie-over sutures.

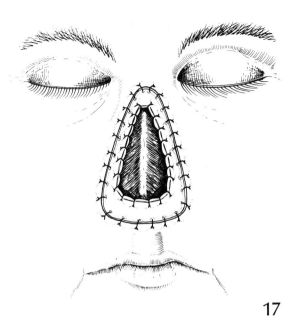

17

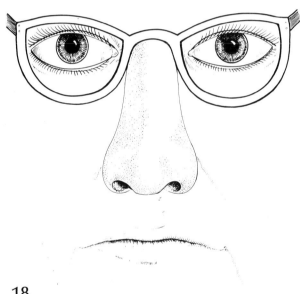

18

External nasal prosthesis

18

If there is any doubt as to the advisability of flap reconstruction because of the age or infirmity of the patient, or in the case of an aggressive tumour such as melanoma, a spectacle-frame nasal prosthesis provides a satisfactory alternative and does not prejudice reconstruction at a later date. Time may be saved and a better prosthesis manufactured if the technician sees the patient before operation.

Melanoma of the eyelids

Melanoma of the eyelids is rare and can be diagnosed early. Fortunately the lesion is more commonly of the flat (lentigo maligna) variety and nearly always involves the skin of the lower eyelid. When the lesion is near the margin of the lid a full thickness wedge of up to one-third of the eyelid is excised and the resultant defect may be closed directly after freeing the lateral canthal ligament while preserving full function and appearance. Defects of more than one-third of the eyelid require some form of flap reconstruction. A full thickness flap from the lower eyelid, based on the marginal vessels, may be used to repair defects of the upper eyelid. The vessels are preserved in a pedicle of 5–6 mm width which is divided after 2 weeks. In the author's experience subtotal defects

of the lower eyelid can be easily and satisfactorily repaired using a conjunctival flap from the upper fornix, which is covered by a free skin graft.

Total reconstruction of the lower lid is satisfactory, but the upper eyelid, with its necessary range of movement, is more difficult to repair. The result is usually unsatisfactory, but part of the lower eyelid may be used to reconstruct an upper eyelid to protect the cornea.

In the case of advanced disease, exenteration of the orbit is necessary. A split thickness skin graft is used to resurface the bony orbital cavity. The skin graft is applied immediately and carefully secured in place with a pack of flavine wool or foam sponge.

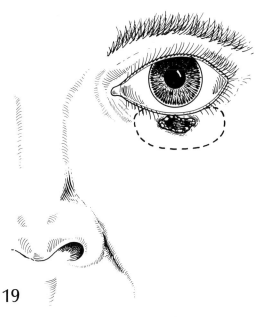

19

EXCISION AND FREE SKIN GRAFT

19

The lesion on the lower eyelid is outlined with a 3–5 mm margin of normal skin. The lesion is excised down to muscle with the surrounding margin of normal skin. The skin defect is measured.

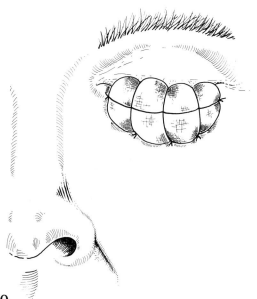

20

20

A full thickness graft of adequate size to fill the defect is taken from behind an ear as previously described. The graft is sutured accurately to the wound edges and secured in place with a tie-over dressing. A split thickness graft is less bulky and is preferred for the repair of skin defects of the more mobile upper lid.

WEDGE EXCISION OF THE LOWER EYELID WITH LATERAL CANTHOTOMY

21

The eye is protected with a plastic shield. The wedge of eyelid including the lesion is outlined for excision.

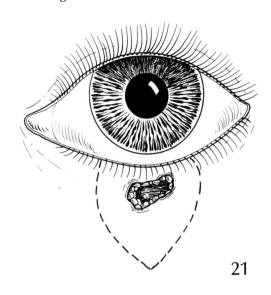

21

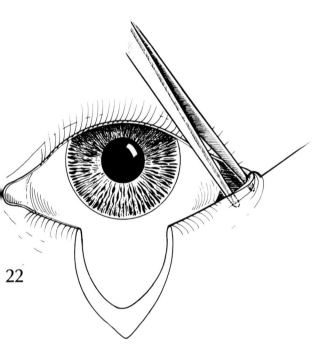

22

22

Having excised the lesion, that part of the canthal ligament attached to the lower commissure is divided by inserting the points of fine scissors through the conjunctiva and cutting the fibres until the commissure is free.

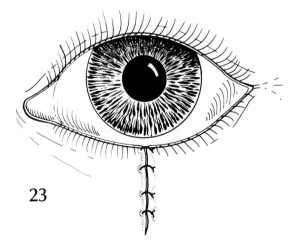

23

23

The lid is closed in two layers. The tarsal plate and conjunctiva are approximated with interrupted catgut sutures, taking care not to penetrate the inner surface of the conjunctiva so that the sutures do not rub on the cornea. The skin is repaired with interrupted 6/0 silk sutures. A single suture unites the grey line at the lid margin. The eye shield is removed when the repair is complete.

LARGE DEFECTS OF THE LOWER EYELID

Large defects of the lower eyelid are repaired by transposition of a conjunctival flap to provide lining and a free skin graft for external cover. The procedure is carried out in two stages.

Stage I

24

The area of excision is outlined with pen and ink.

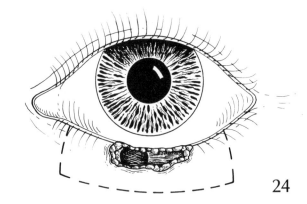

24

25

The lesion is excised with a knife and the width of the defect is measured.

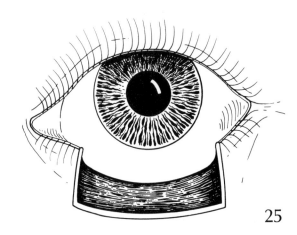

25

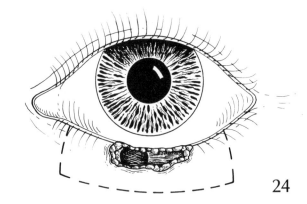

26

26

Using a knife, a horizontal incision is made in the conjunctiva parallel to and about 4–5 mm from the margin of the upper lid. With scissors the conjunctival flap is dissected from the upper border of the tarsal plate along the full width and then superiorly from the levator muscle. A piece of tarsal plate may be taken with the flap. The lateral margins of the flap are incised with scissors. The flap is advanced and sutured to the conjunctiva at the margins of the defect with interrupted 4/0 or 6/0 chromic catgut sutures. The knots are tied on the external surface so that they do not rub on the globe.

27

The size of the skin defect is measured. A free skin graft, preferably a full thickness graft, is taken from the sulcus behind the ear. This graft is applied accurately to the raw surface of the conjunctiva which is now lining the defect and sutured carefully to the skin margins with 6/0 silk. The upper lid margin is placed over the conjunctival flap in the position it normally occupies.

A paraffin gauze dressing and eye pad are applied and secured with adhesive tape.

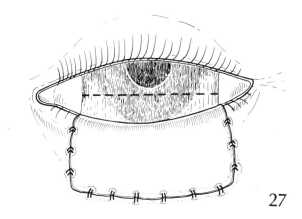

27

Postoperative care

The dressings are changed daily and the skin sutures removed in 1 week.

Stage II

Three weeks after the lid reconstruction a probe is passed under the conjunctival flap, which is divided high up at the upper level of the tarsal plate with blunt scissors. The divided flap should be slightly too large in a vertical direction to allow for shrinkage. No sutures are necessary.

28

Within a few weeks the lower lid has a good cosmetic appearance and functions well. Restoration of eyelashes is not necessary.

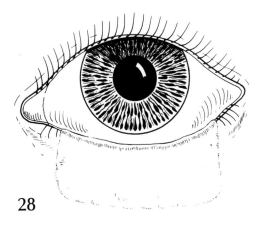

28

Melanoma of oral cavity

Melanomas of the oral mucosa are uncommon and are very aggressive tumours. The roof of the mouth is the commonest site. Local recurrence is frequent and there is lymphatic spread to the regional cervical lymph nodes. Treatment is similar to that for lesions of the skin but a compromise is necessary when determining the margin of surrounding mucosa to be excised. A free split skin graft is applied to the defect. Involved lymph nodes in the neck are excised *en bloc*.

LESION OF THE CHEEK MUCOSA

29

The lesion with a 1–2 cm margin of surrounding mucosa is outlined with pen and ink and excised down to the healthy tissue beneath. Bleeding points are controlled by diathermy coagulation.

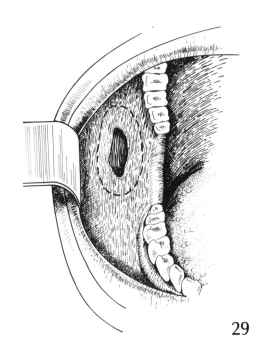

29

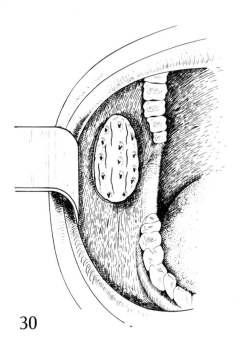

30

30

A split thickness skin graft taken from the arm or thigh is applied to the defect and secured in place with multiple anchoring catgut sutures, giving a quilted appearance, as described by McGregor[2]. Multiple small slits are then made in the graft[3] to prevent haematoma from accumulating under the graft.

Postoperative care

The diet is kept soft, and frequent gentle mouthwashes are given, especially after meals. The graft usually takes in 5–7 days, at which time the surplus graft around the margins of the defect may be trimmed off.

Dissection of pre-auricular lymph nodes

The pre-auricular lymph nodes lie on and within the parotid gland; one or two are subcutaneous, lying superficial to the parotid fascia. They may become diseased secondarily to melanomas of the temple, vertex, eyelids and orbit, and from lesions of the pre-auricular region. To remove the diseased glands a superficial parotidectomy is carried out, taking care to preserve the facial nerve and its branches unless it is involved by tumour.

aesthesia and position of patient

neral anaesthesia is given by endotracheal tube, as this
ives the operative field clear for the surgeon. Anaes-
etic measures to reduce bleeding facilitate the dissec-
n. Use of the faradic nerve stimulator is of great help in
ating the VIIth nerve and its branches if no muscle
axant is used. The patient is placed supine with a slight
ad-up tilt, the neck slightly extended and the head
rned away from the surgeon.

eoperative preparation

1

e operative field is cleaned with an aqueous germicidal
lution. Drapes are applied from the midline of the
rehead to the mastoid and hyoid, and from the hyoid to
e mastoid, leaving exposed the homolateral eye and
rner of the mouth so that any stimulation of the facial
rve may be observed.
A cotton wool plug is placed in the external auditory
eatus for the duration of the operation to prevent blood
cumulating in the meatus. The surgeon must remember
remove this at the end of the procedure.

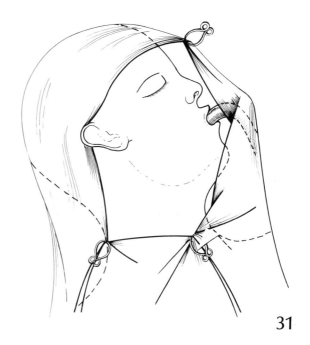

31

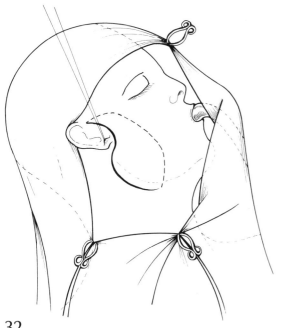

32

The incision

32

The approach is the same as for parotidectomy. The skin
incision begins at the level of the zygomatic arch and
continues down in a skin crease immediately in front of
the pinna, curving below the root of the lobule to the
mastoid. It is then extended downwards and forwards in a
skin crease two fingerbreadths below and parallel to the
mandible over the sternocleidomastoid to the level of the
horn of the hyoid. The shape of the incision is that of a
reversed lazy S.

Flap elevation

33

Keeping close to the undersurface of the skin, a skin flap with platysma in the lower part is raised using a knife or blunt-tipped curved scissors. The flap is freed as far as the anterior border of the parotid. The elevated flap is reflected forwards and secured to the skin of the cheek with one or two sutures.

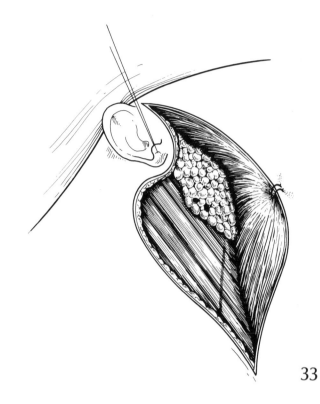

33

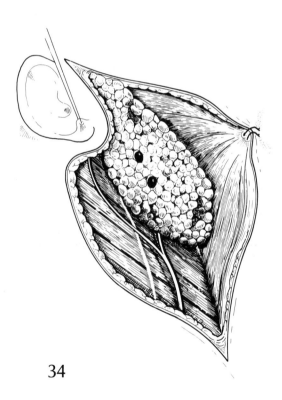

34

Deepening of cervical part of incision

34

The parotid fascia and glandular tissue overlying the upper end of the sternomastoid are stripped forwards, and the anterior border of the muscle is defined up to the mastoid process. During the dissection the external jugular vein is freed and preserved. The posterior facial vein is traced upwards to the lower pole of the superficial lobe of the parotid. Care is taken not to divide the mandibular branch of the facial nerve which crosses over the posterior facial vein near the lower margin of the gland. Because of the proximity of diseased lymph nodes the great auricular nerve is sacrificed where it crosses on to the parotid gland.

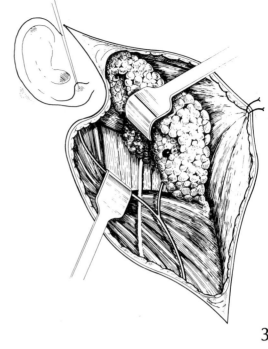

35

Deepening of facial part of incision

35

The ensheathing fascia of the parotid gland is now incised with the knife immediately below and in front of the external auditory meatus, and a plane of cleavage is opened up between the meatus and the gland, securing any small vessels which are divided. The dissection is deepened in this situation close to the cartilaginous meatus until the sharp bony ridge of the anteroinferior margin of the bony meatus is reached.

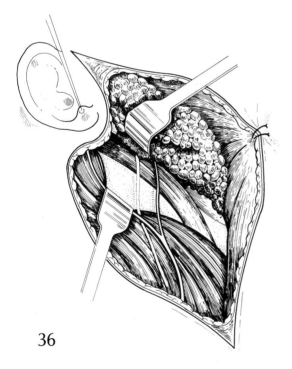

36

Exposure of posterior belly of digastric muscle

36

The posterior belly of the digastric muscle and the stylohyoid muscle are located by blunt dissection deep to the anterior border of the sternocleidomastoid muscle. The posterior belly of the digastric muscle is exposed from the intermediate tendon anteriorly to the point where it disappears beneath the mastoid process posteriorly.

   If the jugulodigastric group of lymph nodes is found it is worth removing it for biopsy.

Exposure of facial nerve

37

The trunk of the facial nerve is found after it has emerged from the stylomastoid foramen beneath the sharp ridge of the anteroinferior margin of the bony meatus, crossing the upper border of the posterior belly of the digastric muscle and lying superficial to the styloid process.

The stylomastoid branch of the posterior auricular artery runs below and parallel to the trunk of the nerve. This should be ligated and divided. The face should be observed constantly during the dissection of the facial nerve and its branches, and any facial twitching noted. The nerve stimulator is useful in identifying the nerve trunk and its subsequent branches.

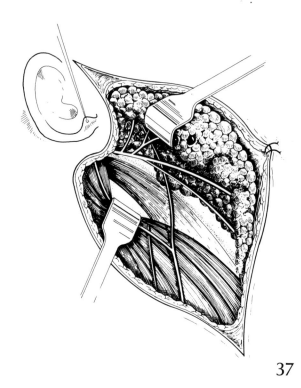

37

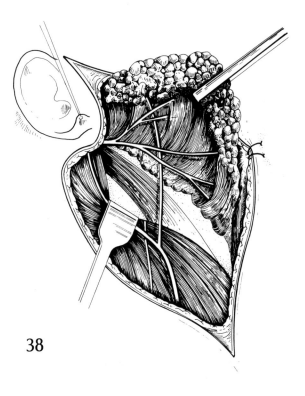

38

Dissection of facial nerve branches

38

The assistant retracts the gland forward. The surgeon, by careful blunt dissection, displays the two main divisions of the facial nerve and their branches before cutting free the superficial lobe of the gland with the lymph nodes, using a knife or scissors. Care must be taken not to inadvertently divide the branches of the nerve, which may be distorted by the tumour, during retraction of the gland. The branches of the nerve lie immediately superficial to the posterior facial vein and its plexus in the gland. Careful haemostasis with diathermy and/or ligatures is essential during this meticulous procedure. If the nerve or major branch is accidentally divided it is repaired by direct suture or by nerve grafting, using a segment of the great auricular nerve.

Completion of freeing and removal of superficial parotid with lymph nodes

39

Once the nerve and its branches have been displayed and preserved, the remaining attachments of the superficial lobe of the gland to the deep lobe are divided. The parotid duct is ligated at the anterior border of the gland and divided. To free the upper pole of the gland it is necessary to divide the superficial temporal vessels between ligatures.

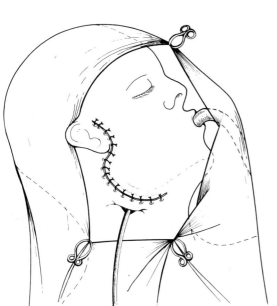

39

Closure

40

A suction drain is inserted and brought out through a stab wound near the inferior end of the wound. The lower half of the wound is repaired in two layers: platysma and skin. The upper half of the wound requires skin sutures only.

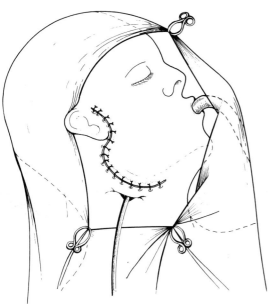

40

Postoperative care

The suction drain is removed as soon as the aspirate ceases, usually within 2–4 days. The sutures are removed at 5–7 days.

Complications

Haemorrhage The wound must be reopened and haemorrhage arrested. Blood transfusion is given if required.

Haematoma All haematomas should be evacuated, as they absorb slowly and leave a swelling which can persist for several months.

Facial weakness Temporary weakness due to stretching of facial nerve fibres is occasionally seen, but this usually recovers spontaneously within 2–3 weeks. Owing to cross-anastomosis minor nerve filaments may be divided without loss of function, but division of a major trunk leaves a permanent paralysis.

Anaesthesia Anaesthesia of the pre-auricular region and outer aspect of the lower half of the pinna results from division of the great auricular nerve.

Gustatory sweating In this condition there is sweating in the pre-auricular skin and sometimes flushing (Frey's syndrome[4]) whenever salivation is stimulated. The problem is rarely severe enough to require treatment.

References

1. O'Connor, T. P. F., Labandter, H. P., Hiles, R. W., Bodenham, D. C. A clinical trial of BCG immunotherapy as an adjunct to surgery in the treatment of primary malignant melanoma. British Journal of Plastic Surgery 1978; 31: 317–322

2. McGregor, I. A. In: Gaisford, J. C. ed. Symposium on cancer of the head and neck. St. Louis: C. V. Mosby, 1969

3. McGregor, I. A. 'Quilted' skin grafting in the mouth. British Journal of Plastic Surgery 1975; 28: 100–102

4. Frey, L. Le syndrome du nerf auriculo-temporale. Revue Neurologique 1923; 2: 97–104

Illustrations by Peter Cox

Surgery of malignant disease of the maxilla and orbit

R. T. Routledge FRCS
Senior Consultant Plastic Surgeon, Frenchay Hospital, Bristol, UK

Introduction

Tumours of the orbitomaxillary complex pose particular problems both as regards surgical ablation of the disease and also in the reconstruction of the attendant tissue defects. The long-term results of individual conventional therapy are not good and it may well be that advances in treatment will be along the line of therapy combination – for example preoperative chemotherapy, surgical excision and postoperative radiotherapy. However, as things stand at the moment, at some point in the treatment regimen, radical surgical ablation is mandatory.

The poor prognosis for malignant disease in this area is probably directly related to the paucity of definitive symptoms produced by the disease. For this reason patients report late, at a time when considerable progression of the tumour has occurred. The disease arises in an area separated only by thin bony walls from the ethmoid air cells, the nasal and orbital cavities and even the anterior cranial fossa. Spread into the pharyngopalatine fossa with its rich lymph network is common. It is therefore not unusual to find that a tumour is, by reason of its extension to the skull base, irresectable or certainly surgically incurable at a time when the patient first reports with vague symptoms suggesting chronic sinusitis.

A complete preoperative assessment is of the utmost importance. The majority of these patients will be over 60 group, many will undergo surgical procedures of considerable magnitude, and every effort must be made to protect them. Preoperatively, tumour assessment may be difficult and inadequate despite modern radiographic techniques which include stereotomography and EMI scan, and one must always be prepared to accept that accurate assessment may have to await surgical exploration. Forward planning must be so detailed that one is able to deal satisfactorily with the exigencies of the moment.

Tumours of the orbit

ENUCLEATION OF THE EYE

Indications

Malignant melanoma confined within the globe and retinoblastoma are indications for enucleation. More commonly the surgeon will find himself carrying out this procedure because of extensive secondary involvement of the conjunctiva in basal cell or squamous cell lesions of the eyelid.

Method

1

The conjunctiva at the limbus is lifted and incised with sharp pointed scissors around the circumference of the limbus and undermined widely to bare the globe. In succession, and facilitated by traction-rotation of the globe, a blunt hook is passed around each extrinsic muscle close to its insertion before it is then divided.

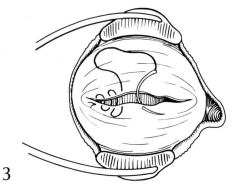

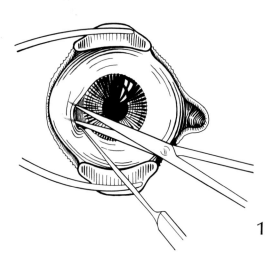

2

The optic nerve is divided by blunt curved scissors passed around behind the posterior surface of the globe. The fairly brisk haemorrhage which ensues from the ophthalmic artery is easily controlled by pressure and, when bleeding abates, the severed artery can be tied.

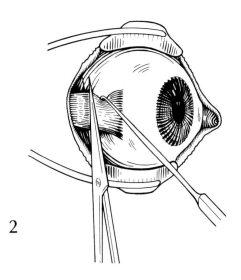

3

The conjunctival incision is closed with 4/0 catgut and the socket lightly packed with Vaseline gauze.

It is possible to secure the stumps of the recti to a Silastic implant to which a suitably adapted prosthetic eye may be fitted later, in order to provide some movement of the prosthesis.

EXENTERATION OF THE EYE

Indications

Exenteration is indicated for squamous carcinoma or basal cell carcinoma of the eyelid secondarily involving the eye or periocular structures. The procedure is also indicated in the treatment of certain neoplasms arising within the orbit, including melanosis of the conjunctiva and malignant melanoma of the choroid.

Method

4

A circumorbital skin incision is deepened in its full length through periosteum to the bony orbital margin.

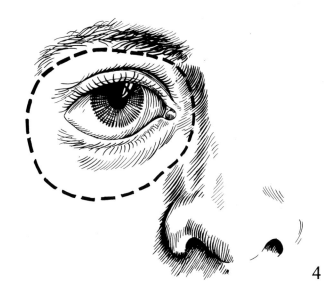

4

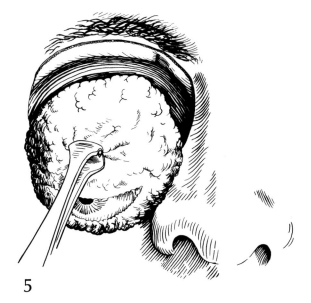

5

5

Using a small rongeur the entire periosteal sheath of the orbit is elevated back towards the superior orbital fissure and the optic foramen. This is completed cleanly and easily though some resistance will be evident at the peripheral attachments of the medial and lateral canthal ligaments.

Curved scissors cleanly divide the optic nerve and ophthalmic vessels and the entire contents of the orbit are delivered. Haemostasis is secured once the brisk haemorrhage has been controlled largely by pressure.

6, 7 & 8

It is perfectly possible to resurface the entire area using a split-skin graft removed from the medial aspect of the upper arm. This usually takes satisfactorily even on a bony bed but the resultant appearance is unattractively cadaveric. A more elegant result is achieved using a forehead flap, even though this will give rise to a secondary cosmetic defect and is usually a two-stage procedure demand the return after 2–3 weeks of the carrying portion of the flap. It is important to design the flap wide enough so that it will sink into the deep concavity of the defect and obliterate all dead space.

An island flap of forehead skin based on the transverse branch of the superficial temporal artery is also applicable and has the advantage of being a one-stage procedure, although it is somewhat more hazardous than the conventional forehead flap.

Alternatively the temporalis muscle can be detached from its origin from the skull and transposed into the empty orbit, skin cover being achieved by applying a split skin graft onto the muscle bed.

It is customary to provide the patient with a cosmetic complex of eyelids and eye which can be conveniently mounted behind the lens of a standard pair of spectacles, thus providing very effective camouflage.

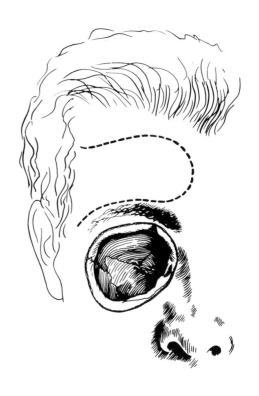

6

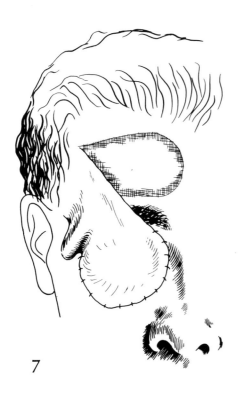

7

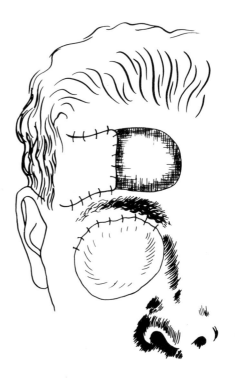

8

ORBITECTOMY

Indications

Adenocarcinoma of the lacrymal gland demands a radical approach. It is commonly diagnosed late and simple exenteration of the eye fails to ablate this typically aggressive tumour. Malignant involvement of any kind of the periocular structures with penetration of bone and dural involvement will similarly demand this extended excision.

Method

9

The skin excision, which follows the line of the orbital rim, is deepened in its full length through periosteum.

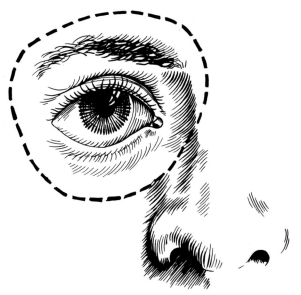

9

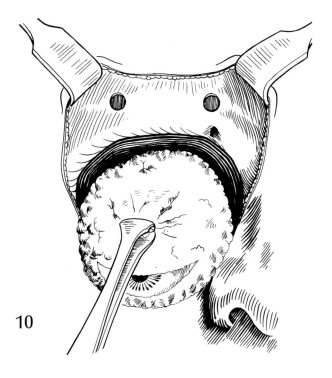

10

10

Superiorly periosteum is stripped from the face of the frontal bone and two burr holes are made above the supraorbital ridge.

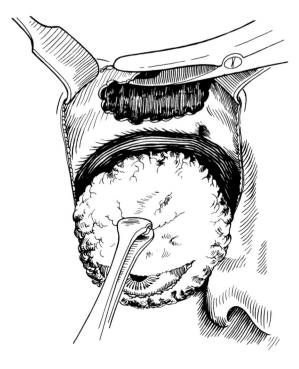

11

These are deepened to dura and the intervening bone removed by nibblers to produce an elliptical bony defect.

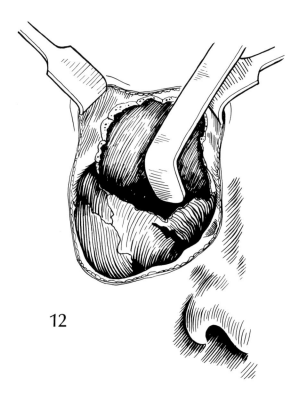

12

This is extended medially to remove the anterior wall of the frontal sinus, the lining of which is then curetted. Dura investing the inferior surface of the frontal lobe is then carefully elevated until the area of dural involvement by growth is clearly visualized. Involved dura and brain are widely excised and the whole of the orbital roof is nibbled away back to the superior orbital fissure. This usually completes the bony excision but if the medial and lateral walls are involved they may be totally removed as well. The entire orbital contents enclosed within their periosteal sac are delivered.

The dural defect is repaired by carefully suturing into place a patch of fascia lata removed from the outer aspect of the thigh and a forehead flap completes the repair. Such a layered repair provides a totally watertight seal and leak of cerebrospinal fluid postoperatively will not be encountered. In the immediate postoperative days the patient is covered by a sulphonamide regimen.

Malignant tumours of the maxilla

By far the commonest tumour is squamous cell carcinoma arising from the pseudostratified columnar epithelium of the antral lining. Less commonly an adenocarcinoma arises from the mucus-secreting glands within the mucous membrane. On occasions the maxilla may be secondarily invaded by malignant tumours arising in the palate, the nose or other paranasal sinuses. Spread to glands in the cervical chain occurs in less than 20 per cent of cases, so excision of the upper jaw is not combined with a radical neck dissection unless involved nodes are palpable.

Prognosis is best for those tumours arising from the floor of the antrum or wholly contained within the maxillary sinus. The wider the area of involvement the more radical must be the ablative procedure. It is possible therefore to classify a range of upper jaw excisions, segmental, partial, total or extended.

For all these procedures hypotensive anaesthesia is of assistance, but if the patient's poor general condition rules this out satisfactory operation conditions are provided by a combination of free unobstructed airway and a fairly steep head-up tilt. An oroendotracheal tube is preferable. In any excisional operation on the upper jaw where doubt may exist, as it so often does, concerning the extent of spread, permission must be obtained preoperatively for removal of the eye should it become necessary.

13

SEGMENTAL MAXILLARY RESECTION (PALATOALVEOLAR RESECTION)

Indications

This type of resection is used for growths limited to the anterior part of the floor of the antrum or the alveolus of the upper jaw.

Method

An upper central incisor is extracted. A mucosal incision extends from the socket vertically up to the upper buccal sulcus and then horizontally around the sulcus to the maxillary tuberosity. An incision through mucoperiosteum of the palate extends from the incisor socket back in the midline to the junction of hard and soft palate where it turns at a right angle to separate soft from hard palate, and link up with the incision in the tuberosity region.

The thin bone of the anterior antral wall is conveniently divided by fissure burr from the piriform fossa back to the tuberosity as it tends to shatter easily with an osteotome or chisel. The anterior bony alveolar cut and hemisection of the palate are completed with an osteotome and, after similarly cutting through the tuberosity and separating muscle attachments posteriorly, the entire inferior maxillary segment is lifted out. Healing of the raw edges is rapid without a graft and the defect is then conveniently closed by means of an acrylic obturator.

PARTIAL MAXILLECTOMY

Indications

Partial maxillectomy is indicated for tumours of the maxilla contained within the antrum and not transgressing the upper quarter of the cavity, so that the eye may be spared safely.

Method

13

An upper central incisor on the side of the lesion is extracted. The upper lip is divided in the midline. Pinch pressure on the two halves of the lip adequately control bleeding at this stage so that the severed labial artery can be picked up and ligated. The skin incision continues in the midline between the two philtrum columns, turns out at the base of the columella to skirt the base of the ala of the nose and continues up the side of the nose to the inner canthus. The incision may be extended horizontally to the outer canthus by dividing the skin in a horizontal direction 2 mm from the lash line.

14

Within the mouth the mucosal incision extends from the lip-split horizontally along the upper buccal sulcus and around the maxillary tuberosity into the soft palate where it runs along the posterior margin of the hard palate and joins a midline incision through the mucoperiosteum of the hard palate.

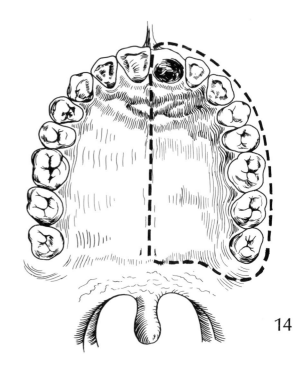

14

15

With a rougine the periosteum is stripped from the whole anterior surface of the maxilla as far laterally as its junction with the body of the zygoma which can then be divided with an osteotome. The upper end of this osteotome cut is continued through the front face of the maxilla just below the inferior orbital rim as far medially as the medial canthus. In most instances this horizontal cut will open into the infra-orbital foramen and the nerve can be carefully dissected free and preserved as it runs on to the soft tissue cheek flap.

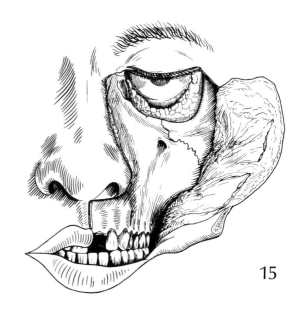

15

An osteotome frees the nasal bone from the maxilla and a scissor cut detaches the side wall of the nose down to the piriform fossa. Here an osteotome is introduced and the upper alveolus is divided in the midline. This osteotome cut continues posteriorly in the midline to divide the hard palate.

The soft palate is divided from the hard palate by deepening the mucosal incision, which has already been made, and the maxilla is now held only by the pterygoid plates and the posterior muscle attachments. A 2 cm wide curved osteotome slips conveniently behind the body of the maxilla and the pterygoid plates are divided. When the few remaining muscle attachments are cut the maxilla can be delivered. Brisk bleeding is encountered from the maxillary artery which retracts into the pterygoid muscle bellies. If the cavity is packed with gauze for a minute or two haemorrhage is controlled to the point where the arterial stump can be seen, picked up in haemostats and tied.

16

Any bony irregularities around the edges of the defect and within its depth are trimmed and a block of polyethylene foam is cut in pyramidal form to fit the defect snugly. A split-skin graft cut from the thigh is wrapped around this foam shape, and tacking sutures through foam and skin graft and the mucosal edges of the defect anchor it firmly in position.

After one week the sutures and foam are removed and the grafted areas trimmed. Primary healing of the cavity has been achieved within a few days so that scarring and contracture will be at a minimum.

A temporary acrylic obturator may be inserted, the definitive obturator being fitted when the cavity achieves its final shape and size after 2–3 months.

This procedure can be modified considerably to suit individual circumstances. If tumour is found to involve the upper portion of the antral cavity the upper bony cut is replanned to run from the zygoma at one end and the medial canthal region at the other, backwards and inwards into the inferior orbital fissure so that the bony orbital floor is removed with the specimen. Some prolapse of the eye should be anticipated after this, although subsequent scar contracture and support from an obturator largely corrects the deformity. Persistent visual disturbance is uncommon.

There are, of course, other methods of providing suitable graft fixation. If convenient teeth are present in the upper jaw a dental splint capable of carrying a suitable tray may be fitted before operation, and, after excision of the jaw, gutta percha is moulded into the defect and kept in place by attaching the tray to the splint.

Alternatively, the gutta percha mould with its supporting tray may be retained by means of stainless steel bars and universal joints attached to supraorbital screws. This method has superseded the now outdated head cap method of providing an anchor for stainless steel bars.

TOTAL MAXILLECTOMY

Indications

All maxillary tumours which have breached the bony antral wall require total maxillectomy.

Extra-antral spread occurs posteriorly into the pterygopalatine fossa or superiorly into the orbit and supramedial group of paranasal sinuses. Less commonly spread is in a downward direction into the mouth.

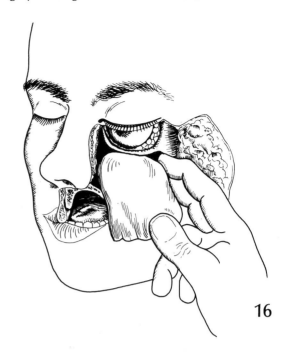

16

Method

The skin and mucosal incisions remain as described for partial maxillectomy. The incision at the outer canthus can be extended out on to the cheek to facilitate division of the masseter from its attachment, if section of the zygoma through its arch is indicated.

Retraction of the upper skin flap at the medial canthal region will permit ablation of the ethmoid group of sinuses by removal of the medial wall and ablation of the frontal sinus by removal of the anteroinferior wall.

The orbital floor is removed with the main maxillary block in the manner already described and the orbit is exenterated. The lash-margin is trimmed from the upper lid as is the conjunctival lining. The orbital defect can then be closed by suturing together the skin edges and packing the skin diaphragm into the socket. The large maxillary defect is lined by a split-skin graft retained by one of the methods already detailed.

This procedure deals adequately with tumour which has spread superiorly or inferiorly, but may prove less than adequate if spread has occurred widely into the pterygopalatine fossa. To open up this space in its entirety and improve exposure, it is recommended that a formal excision of the ascending ramus, the neck and condyle of the mandible be carried out through a conventional submandibular approach. Once this section of mandible is out of the way the surgical attack can be efficiently directed into a widely opened cavity which, until now, has been but poorly visualized in the depths of the maxillary cavity.

EXTENDED MAXILLECTOMY

Even so radical a procedure as that described under 'Total maxillectomy' may be insufficient to deal with tumour which has spread widely to involve either the soft tissue of the cheek or the bone of the skull base with the underlying, closely applied dura mater. In both these instances the maxillectomy must be extended so that an entire block of diseased tissue may be ablated, and suitable reconstructive procedures devised to achieve primary wound healing and minimize, as far as possible, the mutilation which inevitably accompanies so destructive a procedure.

Extended maxillectomy with removal of soft tissue of cheek

In a case where tumour has erupted through the skin of the cheek, total maxillectomy with wide removal of all involved skin is mandatory. In such cases surgical exposure poses no problems and a through-the-cheek

removal of the upper mandibular segment is possible if tumour spread renders this additional, bony removal necessary.

There are several ways of reconstructing the complex defect. Basically the essential components of any successful repair are skin cover and mucosal lining, but bone and muscle may also be provided in order to effect a more physiological reconstruction.

Repair using forehead and deltopectoral flap

In its simplest form cover can be provided by a forehead or deltopectoral flap, lining being substituted by a split-skin graft sutured to the raw surface of the flap and supported by a foam block sewn into the cavity in the manner already described.

Alternatively, combined use may be made of two full-thickness skin flaps, taking a deltopectoral flap to replace lining and a forehead flap to provide cover.

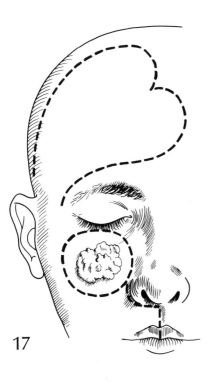

17

17–21

Repair using bilobed scalp-forehead flap

In suitable cases, and usually in patients with little scalp hair, an elegant repair is provided by a bilobed scalp-forehead flap based on the transverse and ascending branches of the superficial temporal artery. A preoperative arteriogram will demonstrate the arterial pattern so that a suitable flap may be safely designed.

The large flap is raised back to the main trunk of the superficial temporal artery, and the donor area is resurfaced with a split-skin graft. The bilobed flap is folded on itself to provide an inner and outer skin surface and is sutured into the defect along its medial and superolateral edges, leaving a temporary slit fistula along the inferior edge. After 3 weeks the flap is divided, and the carrying portion is replaced onto the forehead. The bilobed flap is divided along the full length of its fold and the two cut edges sutured into the freshened inferior edge of the defect, thereby closing the fistula and reconstituting the cheek.

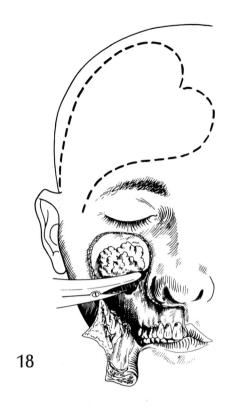

18

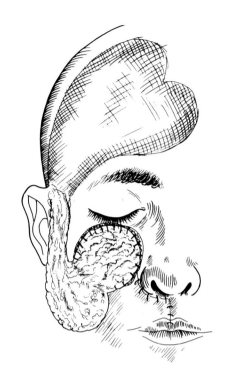

19

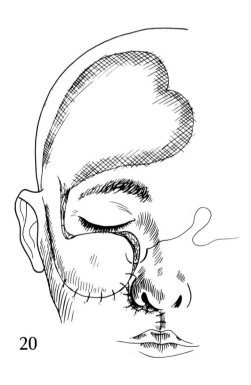

20

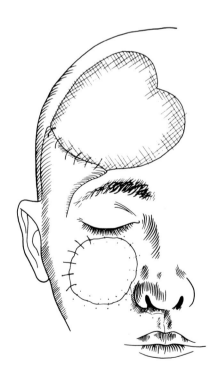

21

Repair using myocutaneous and free flaps

With the rise in popularity of the myocutaneous flap and the free flap even more sophisticated methods of reconstruction are now available.

A pectoralis major myocutaneous flap will provide two skin paddles, one for cover and one for lining, with a large bulk of muscle filler to recreate cheek contour. It has been claimed that portions of ribs may be carried on this flap into the defect but considerable doubt must exist as to whether such bone is truly vascularized or acts merely as a free graft.

Trapezius myocutaneous flaps may similarly be used to provide skin for cover and lining with a muscle filler.

In some cases, although certain specific indications must exist, a suitable free flap containing skin, muscle and bone can be transferred into the defect using standard microvascular anastomoses between the vessels of the flap and suitable vessels in or close to the defect, e.g. the superficial temporal or facial arteries. Convenient donor sites for the free flap are the groin, using a composite flap based on the deep circumflex iliac artery, or the back, employing a latissimus dorsi free flap based on the subscapular artery.

Extended maxillectomy with excision of skull base

For several years an extended resection with removal of part of the base of the skull has been practised for cases of ethmoid carcinoma at a late stage. In the region of the cribriform plate the thin perforated bone is readily penetrated by a biologically aggressive tumour with involvement of meninges and brain. So long as reconstruction is as vigorously pursued as the excision the procedure is safe and a percentage of otherwise hopeless cases may be rescued or at the least very significantly palliated.

If preliminary investigative studies suggest that the anterior skull base is involved by tumour which does not, however, occupy the cavernous sinus, an extended maxillectomy is planned with neurosurgical assistance. All incisions should be planned and executed at the outset by the reconstructive surgeon, bearing in mind that the widest exposure possible is desirable. Subsequent reconstructive procedures should not be jeopardized by misplaced skin incisions.

The standard maxillectomy incisions in the face and within the mouth are applicable with an extension passing medially from the inner canthus across the nose bridge. An offset midline forehead flap is raised on the side opposite to the lesion, based on the supra-orbital-supratrochlear arterial complex. A conventional forehead flap is raised based on the superficial temporal artery on the same side as the lesion. With all incisions deepened and skin flaps developed, the maxilla is removed and the orbit exenterated with sacrifice of periorbital soft tissues. Through the upper medial extension of the facial incision the nasal bone is divided by osteotome at the frontonasal suture. The nose can then be rotated laterally away from the defect to expose the entire nasal septum. Most cases will demand excision of the entire upper half of the septum, following which a surgical attack can be launched on the cribriform plate from below. The entire ethmoid group together with the frontal and sphenoid sinuses is ablated and all involved bone of the skull base can be removed back to the foramen lacerum. Through the large bony hiatus, involved dura and brain are excised from below. The dural defect is patched using a free fascia lata graft cut oversize so that it may be tucked under the edges of the bone defect. A watertight seal is achieved by rotating the median forehead flap to cover the fascial patch, anchoring it in place by sutures passed through drill holes at the edges of the bony defect. The laterally based forehead flap is sutured into place to close the orbital defect. The maxillectomy incisions are closed in layers and the cavity grafted and foam-packed in a conventional manner.

After 3 weeks both forehead flaps are divided and finally inset, and the carrying portions are returned.

Such a procedure, although necessarily mutilating, provides an excellent functional reconstruction and cerebrospinal leaks will not be encountered. A very reasonable cosmetic result can be achieved by fitting an overall Silastic or acrylic prosthesis.

Illustrations by Gillian Oliver

Resection of tumours involving the anterior and middle cranial fossa

Ian T. Jackson MD, FRCS, FACS
Professor of Plastic Surgery, Head of Plastic Surgery, Mayo Foundation, Mayo Clinic, Rochester, Minnesota, USA

Introduction

Tumour involvement of the anterior cranial fossa may result from malignant lesions in any area of the upper face. The principal regions are the orbit, the nose, the nasopharynx, the ethmoid and frontal sinuses, and the forehead. Fibrous dysplasia can occur in the orbit and frontal bones. This often requires total resection and reconstruction with bone grafts because of deformity and/or visual problems. When the nasopharynx is entered, this area must be carefully closed off from the extradural space, otherwise fatal infection may occur.

Middle cranial fossa tumours can be meningiomas or neurofibromas that escape through the foramina in the base of the middle fossa to invade the infratemporal fossa. From here they may enter the orbit through the inferior orbital fissure, infiltrate down the wall of the pharynx, or escape from behind the ascending ramus of the mandible to appear as tumours of the deep lobe of the parotid. Tumours arising in or invading the pterygoid area may enter the middle cranial fossa in a similar way. It is also possible for malignant tumours to enter the middle cranial fossa anteriorly from the orbit or the maxilla. The main problem in resection of these tumours is surgical exposure. The most useful methods to achieve this will be presented in this chapter.

The operations

Anterior cranial fossa tumours

PENETRATING MEDIAL CANTHAL CARCINOMAS

These are usually basal cell carcinomas that invade the ethmoid sinuses and then involve the cribriform plate.

1

The excision is outlined around the tumour.

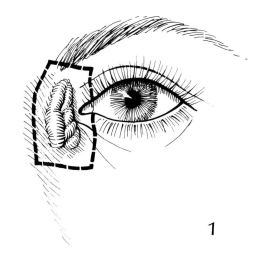

1

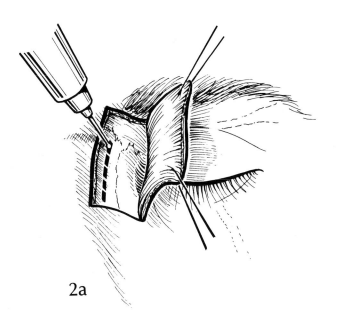

2a

2a & b

After incision through the skin down to periosteum, the underlying bone is cut with an air drill medially, inferiorly and laterally.

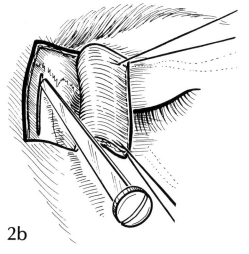

2b

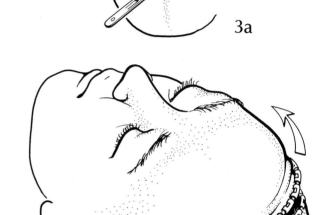

3a

3b

3 & 4

The anterior cranial fossa is approached by raising a coronal flap.

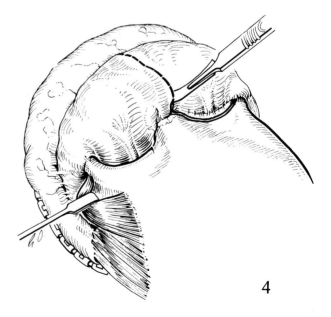

4

5

A frontal bone flap is removed and the frontal lobes are retracted; the dura is left on the cribriform plate if necessary for complete resection. A cut is made around the roof of the ethmoids with an air drill.

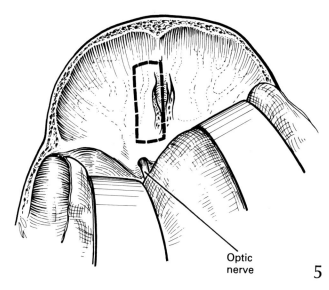

Optic nerve

5

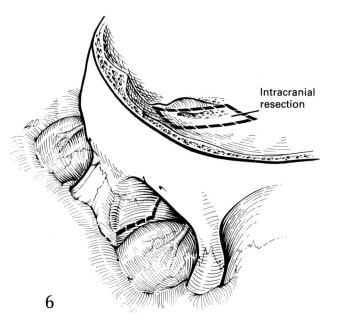

Intracranial resection

6

6

The orbits are exposed and the block of tumour is left attached to the nasal area. The bone cuts are continued posteriorly.

7

The total block is now resected.

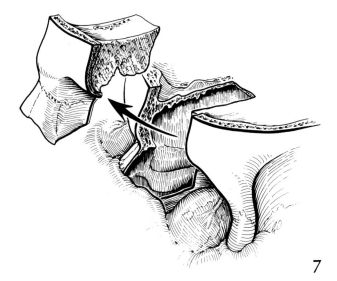

7

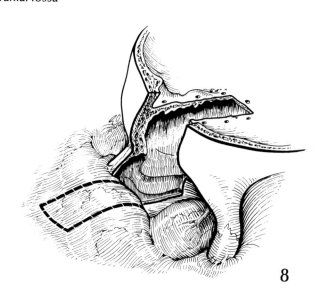

8

8 & 9

The anterior fossa defect in continuity with the nasopharynx is closed with a galeal frontalis flap, and the frontal bone flap and coronal flap are replaced in position with suction drainage.

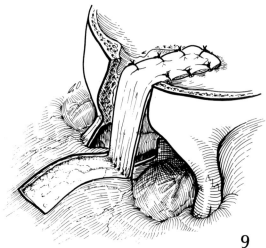

9

PENETRATING MIDFACE CANCERS

These are usually basal cell or squamous cell carcinomas that have recurred after incomplete resection of medial canthal tumours. Radical resection is mandatory for cure. Failure to completely isolate the cranial cavity from the nasopharynx may result in meningitis. Often a portion or all of the nose has been previously resected.

10

There may be multiple recurrences in the area of previous resection. Computerized tomographic (CT) scanning will reveal the extent of orbital and intracranial involvement. The line of resection is then drawn out.

10

11

The skin and subcutaneous tissues are incised down to the maxilla, orbits and nasal bones. The bone cuts are made with an air drill.

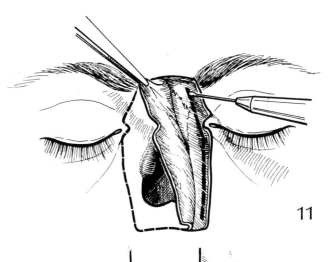

11

12

A coronal scalp flap is turned down. A localized frontal craniotomy is performed and the central face is resected, including medial orbital walls, cribriform plates, dura and nasal septum.

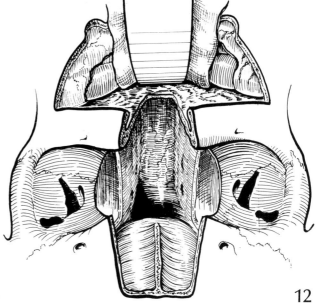

12

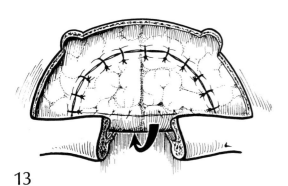

13

A meticulous dural repair is performed with careful closure under the frontal lobes.

13

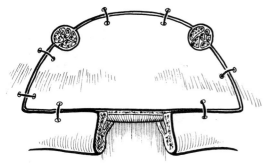

14

The bone flap is replaced and wired. The burr holes are grafted with chip bone grafts from the skull (see Illustration 39). The coronal flap is returned and sutured.

14

15

A glabellar flap is outlined based on the medial eyebrow/upper eyelid region.

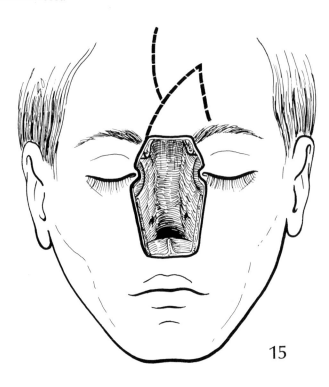

15

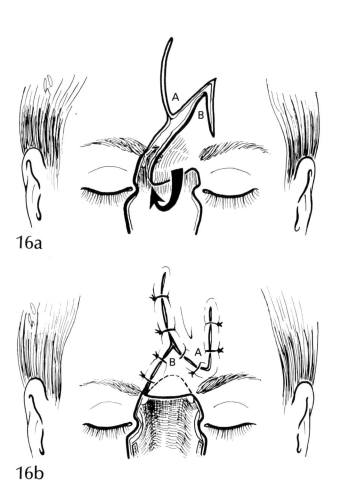

16a

16b

16a & b

In order to close the donor site, an unequal Z-plasty is designed on the forehead. The glabellar flap is turned in and its leading edge taken back to the posterior part of the resection – the posterior wall of the sphenoid sinus. Holes are drilled in the base where convenient, and the flap is stabilized by sutures.

17

The cavity is now completely lined with a split skin graft, and packing is inserted to hold this in place.

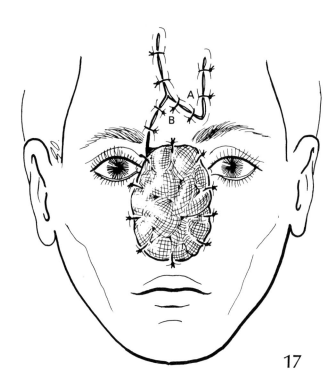

17

NASAL SEPTAL TUMOURS

The commonest tumour of the nasal septum is squamous carcinoma, but occasionally chondrosarcoma may occur. When this is far back in the septum and involves the cribriform plate, the approach is somewhat different from that described above.

18

A coronal flap and face-splitting incision are used. The latter is an extended Weber-Ferguson approach.

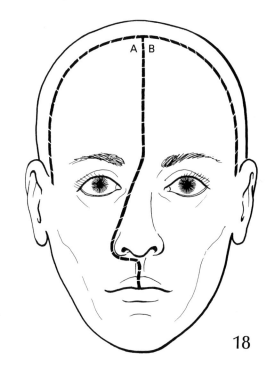

18

19

The flaps are elevated to expose the frontal area, orbits, nose and maxilla. One or both flaps may be folded back completely. The frontal bone flap is removed, as are the glabellar area, nose, medial portions of both orbits and the central part of the maxilla, but sparing the teeth.

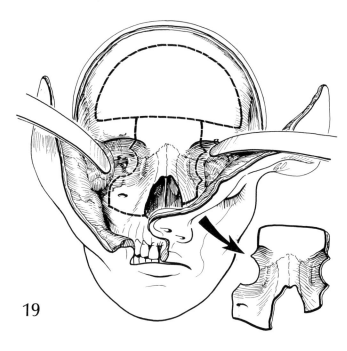

19

20

The tumour is resected with neighbouring dura, cribriform plates, medial walls of orbits and nasal septum.

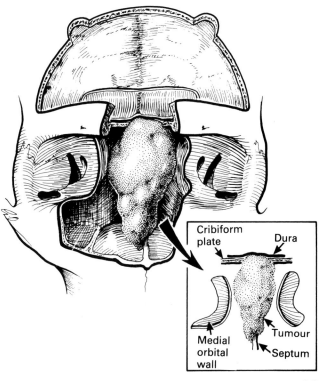

Cribiform plate
Dura
Medial orbital wall
Tumour
Septum

20

21

Holes are made in the anterior cranial fossa floor and posterior wall of sphenoid, and a galeal frontalis flap is sutured in position to close the nasopharynx from the extradural space (see *Illustration 9*).

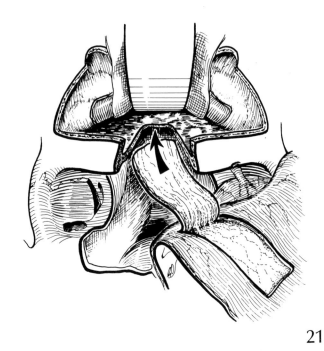

21

22

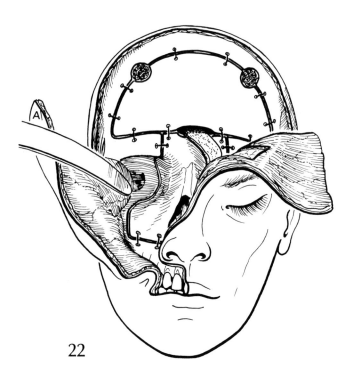

22

The remainder of the cavity is filled with a split skin graft, and this is packed in position. The frontal bone flap and the removed midface skeleton are wired back in position. A defect is left in the glabellar area for the pedicle of the galeal frontalis flap.

23

The end of the packing for the skin graft is brought out through the nostril for later removal. The skin incisions are sutured.

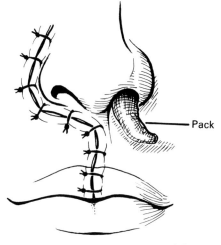

Pack

23

LATERAL ORBITAL TUMOURS

These may be penetrating squamous or basal cell carcinomas or malignant tumours of the lacrimal gland. Intracranial and orbital involvement is assessed by CT scanning.

24

The skin area to be resected is outlined, and an incision is made down to orbital and frontal bone.

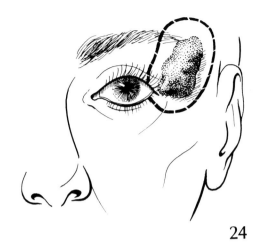

24

25

The frontotemporal area is exposed using a coronal flap. The temporalis muscle is elevated medially and a bone flap is removed. The frontal lobe is retracted, as are the orbital contents.

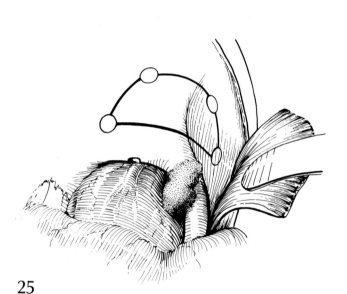

25

26

The tumour is resected by making bone cuts through the supraorbital rim, roof, lateral orbital margin and lateral orbital wall.

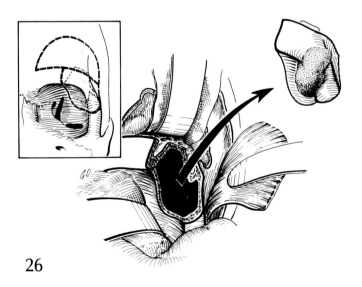

26

27

The frontal bone flap is wired back into position. The excisional defect is left without reconstruction.

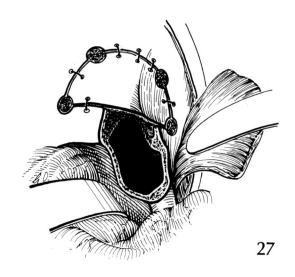

27

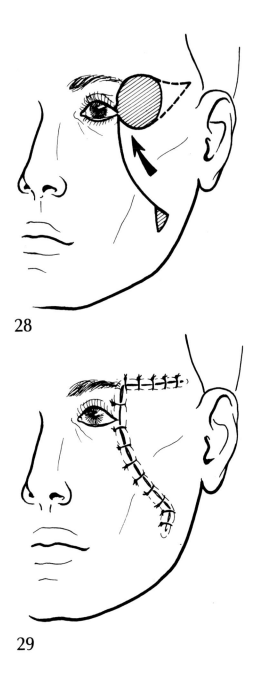

28

28 & 29

There are many methods of skin closure. The inferior rotation flap causes least distortion of hairline, eyebrow and, in the male, hair-bearing facial skin.

29

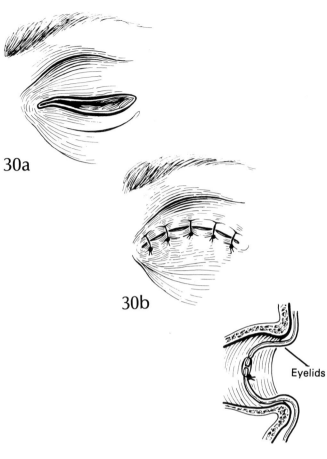

30a

30b

Eyelids

30c

30

If the orbital contents are exenterated, two methods of reconstruction are possible. When the eyelids are preserved, the skin of the lids can be used to resurface the socket after removal of the eyelash-bearing rim.

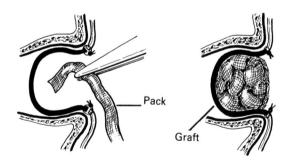

Pack

Graft

31

31

If the lids are sacrificed, the cavity is lined by a split thickness skin graft and packed. The orbit is unusual in that a skin graft will take on the bone denuded of periosteum.

TUMOURS REQUIRING TOTAL ORBITAL RESECTION

Total orbital resection is performed for malignant tumours involving the orbital contents, the skin and the bone, e.g. melanoma, advanced maxillary carcinoma, sarcoma.

32

The external area to be excised is outlined and an incision made down to the bone on all sides.

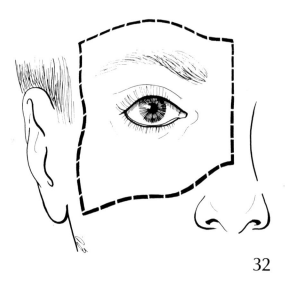

32

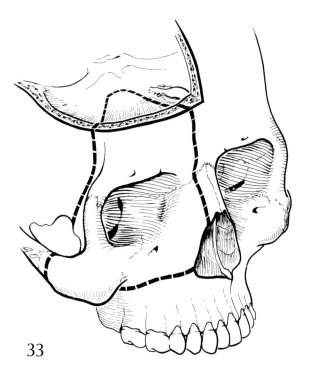

33

33

A coronal flap is turned down and a frontal bone flap removed. The frontal lobe is retracted to expose the floor of the anterior cranial fossa. A cut is then made with the air drill through the floor along the edge of the cribriform plate and laterally to the lateral orbital wall. The anterior cuts can be made through the resection incisions medially, laterally and transversely along the anterior surface of the maxilla.

From the anterior cranial fossa floor, the apex of the orbit can be exposed, and the ophthalmic vessels and optic nerve clamped, divided and ligated.

The removal of the specimen leaves a large defect opening into the nasopharynx. If the dura has been resected, careful repair and closure with a galeal frontalis flap (see *Illustration 9*) is advocated.

The simplest reconstruction at this point is a split skin graft with a pack on top. Failing this, a pectoralis major myocutaneous flap may be used as cover (see *Illustrations 59 and 60*). The pedicle is divided in three weeks. As with any missing facial area, rehabilitation is achieved by an external prosthesis made of silicone or acrylic.

FIBROUS DYSPLASIA INVOLVING THE ANTERIOR CRANIAL FOSSA

This strange disease of bone may occur in the orbital roof, supraorbital rim or frontal bone. It may be recurrent or progressive and may cause visual problems such as diplopia and reduction of visual acuity. There may also be considerable aesthetic disturbance due to the increase in bone bulk. Cure necessitates complete resection and reconstruction with bone grafts.

34

Through the standard coronal approach, the involved fronto-orbital area is exposed. The condition usually affects the lateral and medial orbital walls, and the nasal skeleton may also be extensively involved.

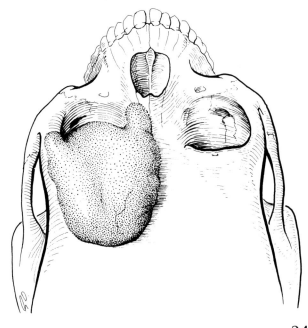

34

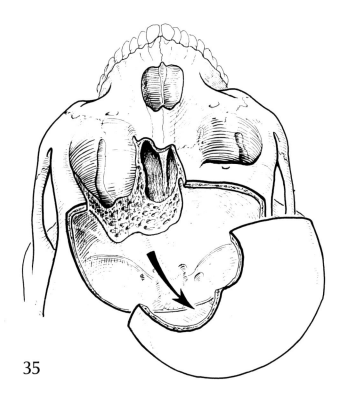

35

35

All affected areas are resected: the frontal area, roof of orbit, medial and lateral nasal walls, cribriform plate and nasal skeleton.

36

If there is failing visual acuity, the optic canal is unroofed to decompress the optic nerve. Dural repair may be required as a result of dural thinning or previous surgery.

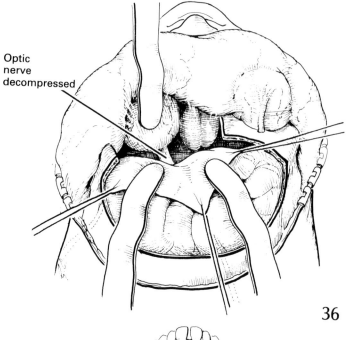

Optic
nerve
decompressed

36

37

The dural defect is repaired with lyophilized dura. This is carefully sutured with fine nylon. The orbit and supra-orbital ridges are reconstructed with split rib bone grafts. These are wired together and to any adjacent stable bone.

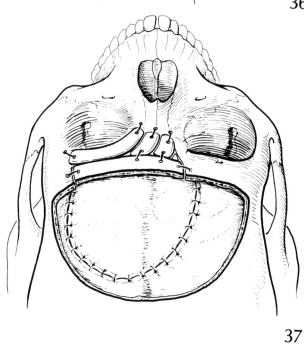

37

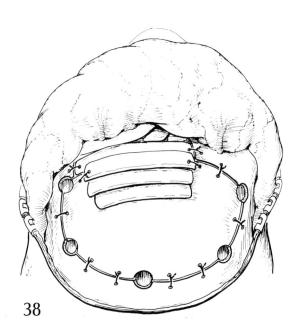

38

38

The skull is reconstituted by frontal bone flap replacement and split rib grafts to close the post-excisional defect. The scalp is closed with suction drainage.

SKULL BONE GRAFTS

In skull and orbital reconstruction split skull is used increasingly as a graft. These membranous bone grafts seem to survive better than grafts from enchondral bone.

39

The outer table of the skull is frequently taken as a bone graft. A contouring burr is used to drill a trough around the area to be taken. It is then removed after splitting with an osteotome as illustrated. Small shavings of bone can be taken for grafting of small areas, using a hammer and chisel as a sculptor or a wood carver would.

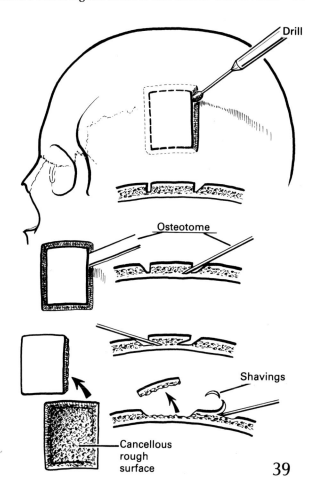

39

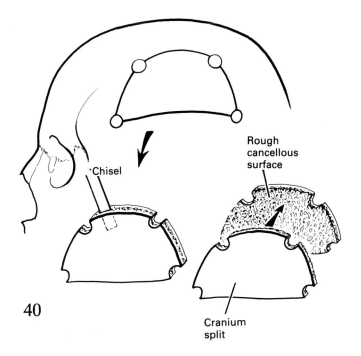

40

40

Alternatively, a bone flap is removed and then split using a hammer and chisel. In this way larger plates of bone may be obtained for grafting. This does, however, necessitate a craniotomy.

Middle cranial fossa tumours

As stated earlier, these tumours may originate in the middle cranial fossa and escape into the pterygoid area through foramina in the base of the skull, or the fossa may be invaded from the orbit or the skull base area. Surgery for tumours involving the petrous temporal bone will be included in this section.

Resection is precluded if the cavernous sinus is invaded and must be carefully considered if the internal carotid is infiltrated. In the latter situation, cross-cerebral blood flow should be assessed.

41

The position of a middle cranial fossa skull base tumour is shown in relation to the facial bones. The arrows indicate the potential routes of spread – to the orbit, pharynx and retromandibular area.

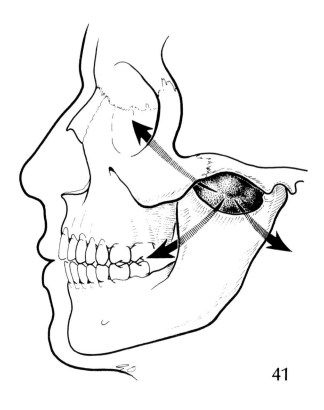

41

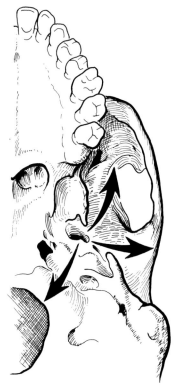

42

42

These tumours escape from inside the skull by way of basal foramina.

The lateral approach has been found to be the most satisfactory method of performing these extremely difficult resections.

43

The skin incision is curvilinear, commencing in the sagittal area of the scalp, running posteriorly in the temporal region and sweeping forward to the preauricular area. From here it is taken down into the neck to the clavicle in a lazy-S fashion.

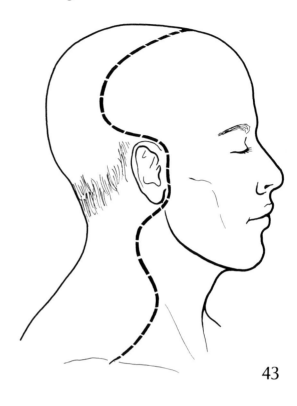

43

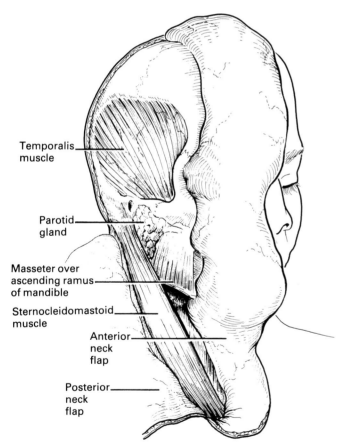

Temporalis muscle

Parotid gland

Masseter over ascending ramus of mandible

Sternocleidomastoid muscle

Anterior neck flap

Posterior neck flap

44

44

The large scalp/anterior neck flap is elevated to expose the temporal skull, temporalis muscle, zygomatic arch, parotid, masseter and anterior neck contents. The posterior neck flap is elevated and retracted to reveal the posterior neck anatomy.

45

A temporal craniotomy is performed and the temporal lobe elevated from the base of the middle cranial fossa. The tumour is visualized and the feasibility of resection assessed.

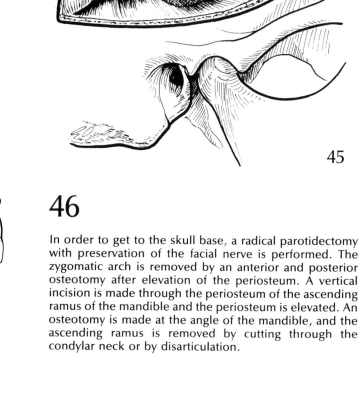

45

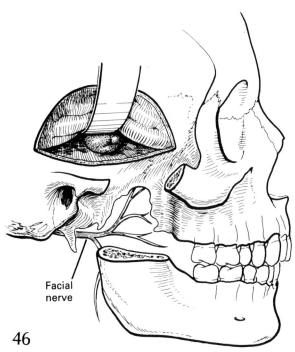

Facial nerve

46

46

In order to get to the skull base, a radical parotidectomy with preservation of the facial nerve is performed. The zygomatic arch is removed by an anterior and posterior osteotomy after elevation of the periosteum. A vertical incision is made through the periosteum of the ascending ramus of the mandible and the periosteum is elevated. An osteotomy is made at the angle of the mandible, and the ascending ramus is removed by cutting through the condylar neck or by disarticulation.

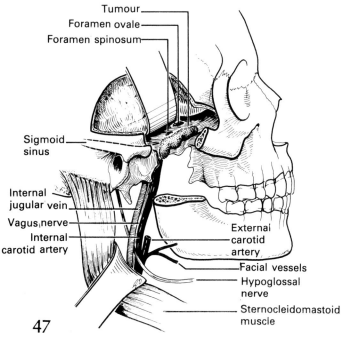

Tumour
Foramen ovale
Foramen spinosum

Sigmoid sinus

Internal jugular vein
Vagus nerve
Internal carotid artery

External carotid artery
Facial vessels
Hypoglossal nerve
Sternocleidomastoid muscle

47

47

In the neck, an upper dissection is performed to identify and isolate the internal jugular vein and internal carotid artery. The sternomastoid muscle is preserved. The tumour is visualized at this point as the pterygoid fossa is exposed. The vessels are followed to the skull base, and their relation to the tumour mass is noted; this makes for safer tumour resection.

48

Beginning at the inferior margin of the craniotomy, a subperiosteal dissection is performed until the involved foramen is reached. All skull base lateral to this point is removed. The skull base and the tumour can be removed *en bloc* without damage to the vessels.

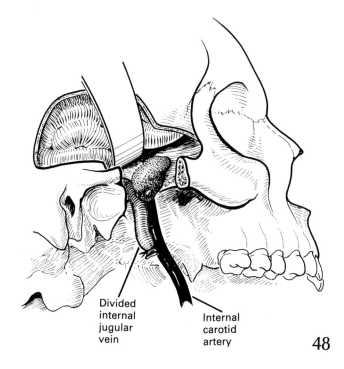

Divided internal jugular vein

Internal carotid artery

48

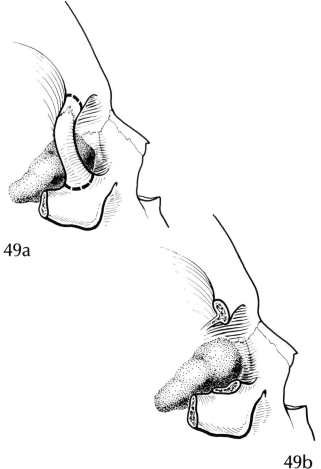

49a

49b

49a & b

If the orbit is involved, an orbital osteotomy is performed to effect tumour removal.

50

The sternomastoid muscle is divided inferiorly and elevated, preserving its superior blood supply.

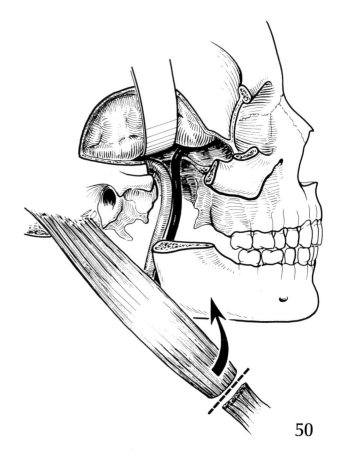

50

51

The bone flap, orbit and zygomatic arch are wired back in position, and the sternomastoid is taken up to protect the defect in the base of the skull. Frequently there has been a dural repair in this area. The ascending ramus of the mandible is replaced if indicated, and the incision is closed with drainage.

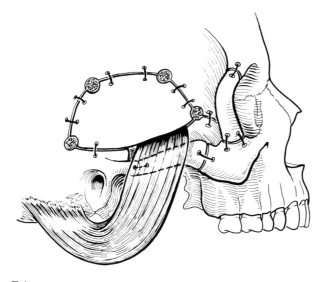

51

Ear and parotid tumours

PETROSECTOMY

This is perfomed for penetrating tumours – basal cell or squamous cell carcinoma of the external ear, malignant parotid tumours, and middle ear carcinomas. It may be partial or complete. Only the latter will be considered.

52

In most cases the approach is similar to that shown in *Illustration 43*. Frequently the external ear is removed. When the cancer arises in the middle ear, it may be preserved on either the anterior or the posterior flap.

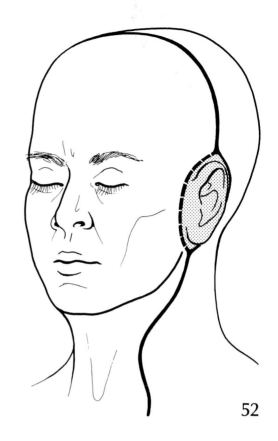

52

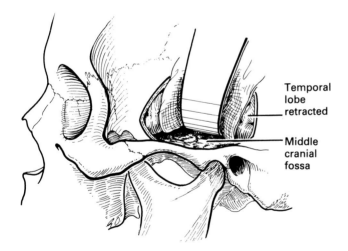

Temporal lobe retracted

Middle cranial fossa

53

53

A temporal craniotomy is performed to assess the feasibility of surgery. If there is extension through the dura or into the cavernous sinus resection may be hazardous or impossible.

54

In these tumours a neck dissection is advised, since there may be occult metastases and also in order to allow accurate identification of the carotid artery and the jugular vein. More and more, the sternomastoid muscle is preserved if possible.

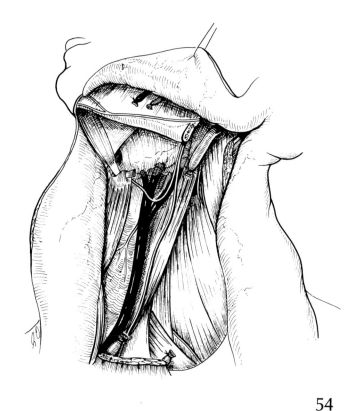

54

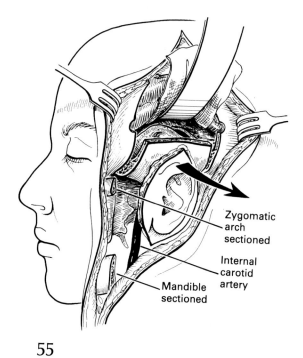

Zygomatic arch sectioned

Internal carotid artery

Mandible sectioned

55

55

The zygomatic arch is exposed and resected, as is the ascending ramus of the mandible. Bone cuts are made downwards from the inferior margin of the craniotomy.

56

The course of the internal carotid artery in the petrous bone should be understood. It enters the bone inferiorly, deep to the styloid process (a); runs posteriorly in its canal (b); and exits from the foramen lacerum in the middle cranial fossa (c).

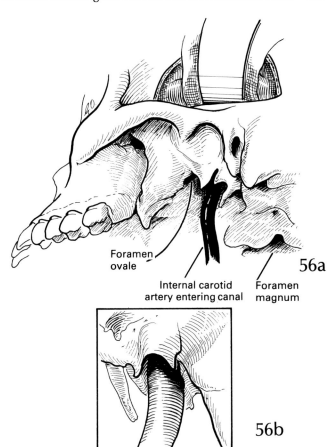

Foramen ovale

Internal carotid artery entering canal

Foramen magnum

56a

56b

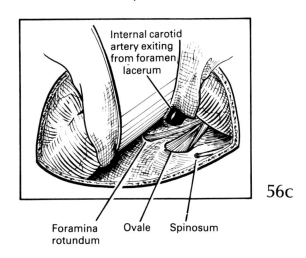

Internal carotid artery exiting from foramen lacerum

Foramina rotundum   Ovale   Spinosum

56c

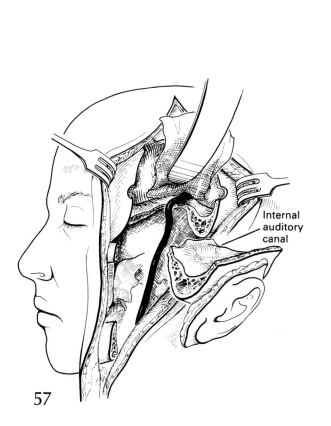

Internal auditory canal

57

57

The neurosurgeon exposes the artery from above, and the plastic surgeon unroofs it from below.

58a–d

Osteotomies are then made to give complete tumour resection, and the ear, petrous bone and neck dissection are removed.

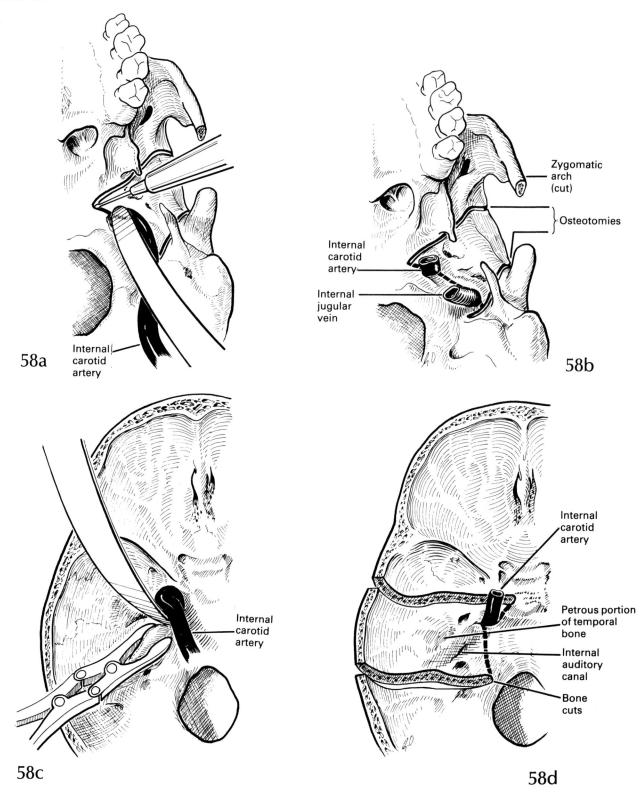

Internal carotid artery

58a

Zygomatic arch (cut)

Osteotomies

Internal carotid artery

Internal jugular vein

58b

Internal carotid artery

58c

Internal carotid artery

Petrous portion of temporal bone

Internal auditory canal

Bone cuts

58d

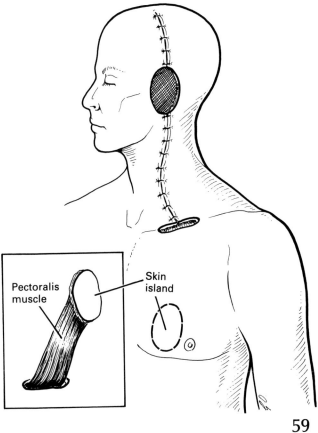

59 & 60

Following this the incisions are closed. If the ear has been sacrificed and there is a large defect on the side of the head, a pectoralis major myocutaneous flap is used to close this area.

59

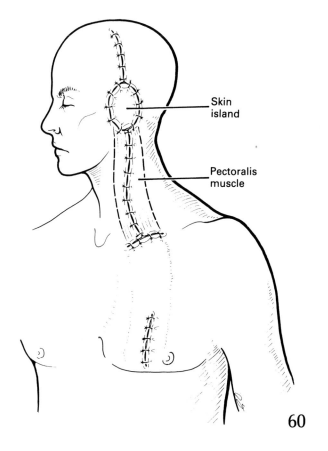

60

Further reading

Jackson, I. T. Treatment of cranio-orbital fibrous dysplasia. In: Proceedings of Seventh International Congress of Plastic Surgery (Rio de Janeiro, 1979)

Jackson, I. T., Hide, T. A. H. Further extensions of craniofacial surgery. In: Jackson, I. T. ed. Recent Advances in Plastic Surgery, 2, pp. 241–259. Edinburgh: Churchill Livingstone, 1981

Jackson, I. T., Hide, T. A. H. A systematic approach to tumours of the base of the skull. Journal of Maxillofacial Surgery 1982; 10: 92–98

Jackson, I. T., Hide, T. A. H., Gomuwka, P. K., Laws, E. R. Jr, Langford, K. Treatment of cranio-orbital fibrous dysplasia. Journal of Maxillofacial Surgery 1982; 10: 138–141

Jackson, I. T., Laws, E. R. Jr, Martin, R. D. A craniofacial approach to advanced recurrent cancer of the central face. Head and Neck Surgery, 1983; 5: 474–488

Jackson, I. T., Marsh, W. R. Anterior cranial fossa tumors. Annals of Plastic Surgery 1983; 11: 479–489

Jackson, I. T., Munro, I. R., Salyer, K. E., Whitaker, L. A. Atlas of Craniomaxillofacial surgery. St Louis: C. V. Mosby, 1982

Illustrated by Gillian Oliver

Osteotomies in the craniofacial area and orthognathic procedures

Ian T. Jackson MD, FRCS, FACS
Professor of Plastic Surgery, Head of Plastic Surgery, Mayo Foundation, Mayo Clinic, Rochester, Minnesota, USA

The main osteotomies for major craniofacial anomalies will be presented, although obviously a detailed description of the correction of these complex, multifaceted deformities is beyond the scope of this chapter. The orthognathic procedures will be explained in some detail.

Patients with major facial deformity require team assessment. The team should include a plastic surgeon, neurosurgeon, oral surgeon, otorhinolaryngologist, orthodontist, paediatrician, ophthalmologist, geneticist, speech therapist and social worker.

Various preoperative investigations such as computerized tomography (CT), special facial X-rays, cephalography, orthopantomogram and dental model studies are necessary for detailed evaluation of these difficult problems.

There are many potential complications, and these must be carefully explained to the parents or the patient. Failure to do this can lead to much grief in the postoperative period. It should also be appreciated that several procedures may be necessary to achieve the maximum improvement possible.

OSTEOTOMIES

Hypertelorism

In this condition the orbits are pushed apart by enlargement of the ethmoid sinuses, by a frontonasal encephalocoele, or by some variety of midface cleft. The deformity may be symmetrical or asymmetrical. Surgery is delayed until the tooth buds have descended enough in the maxilla to allow a transverse infraorbital osteotomy to be performed without damaging these essential structures.

1–7

The approach is by the coronal flap. This is turned down to expose the supraorbital rims. The orbital contents are dissected free at the subperiorbital level, and the dissection is taken down the nose and medial orbital walls. It then proceeds down the lateral orbital walls and across the floor of the orbit and the front of the maxilla. The zygomatic arches are exposed subperiosteally, and the temporalis muscles are elevated.

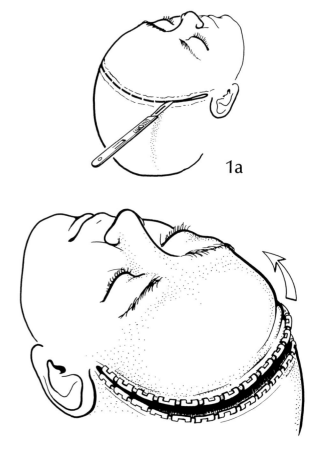

1a

1b

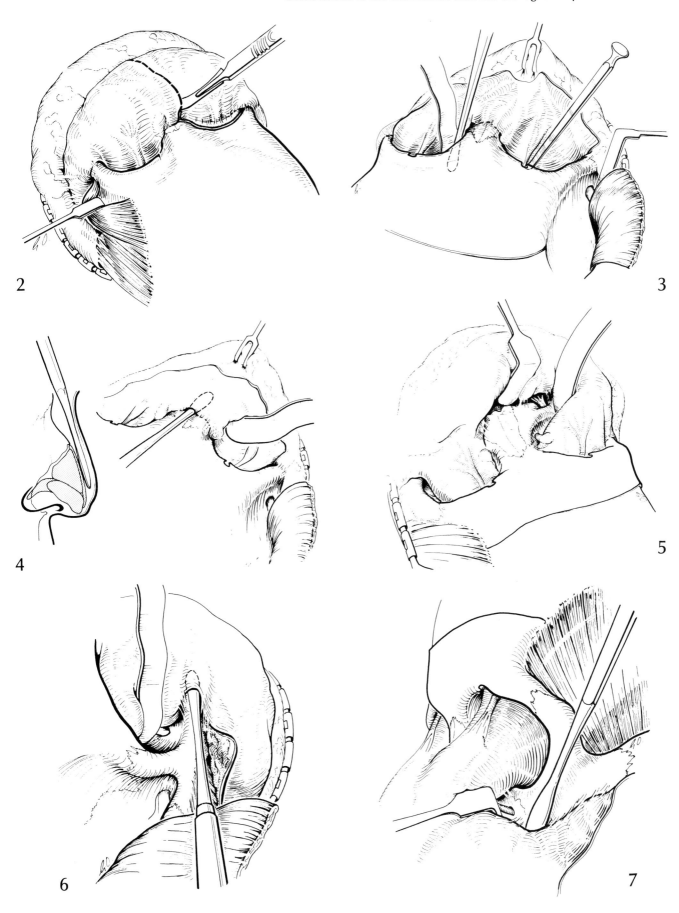

2

3

4

5

6

7

8

At this point, the medial canthal ligaments are identified using an external incision.

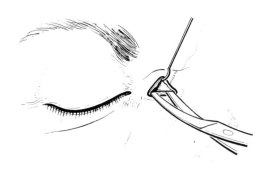

8

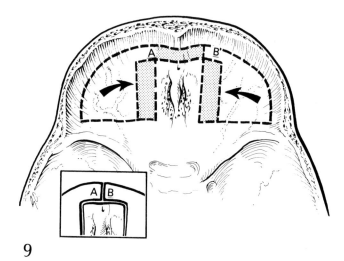

9

9 & 10

A frontal bone flap is removed and the frontal lobes are elevated. The shaded areas of bone are removed by cutting around them with a high-speed drill or saw.

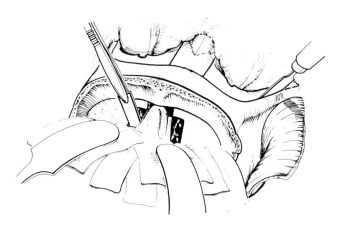

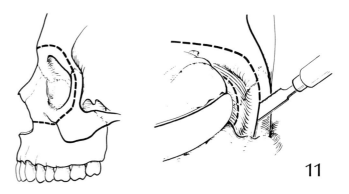

11

11, 12 & 13

In the orbital and nasal areas bone cuts are made around the orbits, across the maxilla and circumferentially around the orbital walls. The transverse maxillary cut is made by tunnelling from lateral to medial.

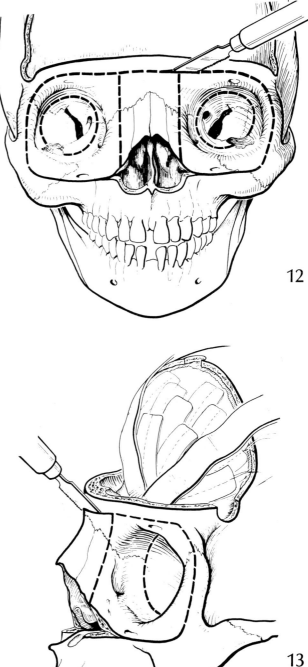

12

13

14

The central segment of bone is removed from the nasoglabellar area, leaving the cribriform plate intact. This can be done gently with a chisel. The ethmoid sinuses are removed with bone rongeurs.

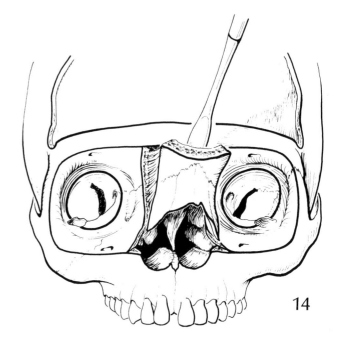

14

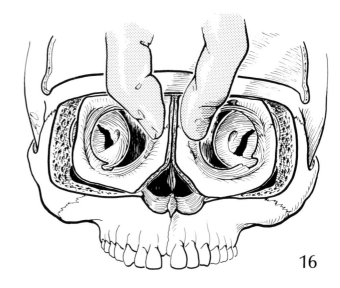

15

15

The orbits are now mobilized and are free to move in any direction required for correction of the deformity.

16

The orbits are brought together and wired in position. The lower medial portion is trimmed to give an adequate nasal airway. This is done with bone rongeurs.

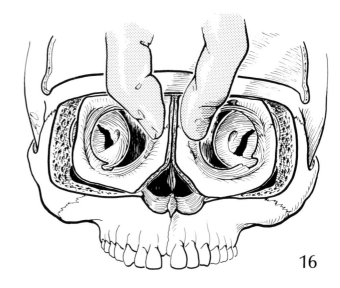

16

17

The medial canthi are wired in position using the method illustrated. It is important to choose a stout portion of bone over which to tighten the wires.

All bony defects are bone grafted using skull grafts (see *Illustrations 39* and *40* in the chapter on 'Resection of tumours involving the anterior and middle cranial fossa', pp. 572–598). The nasal skeleton is recreated in a similar fashion.

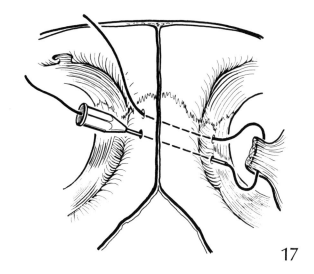

17

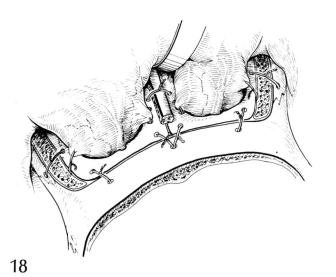

18

18

The frontal bone is replaced and the scalp closed with suction drainage. The method illustrated shows a sagittal split technique for the lateral orbital walls. As an alternative, the total lateral orbital wall may be shifted.

Subcranial deformity

In cases in which the lateral walls are in satisfactory position and there is only a bony telecanthus, the medial orbital walls may be moved in a subcranial fashion. The approach is, again, by a coronal flap.

19

The osteotomies are as shown. The paracentral segments are removed and the medial orbital walls are slid together.

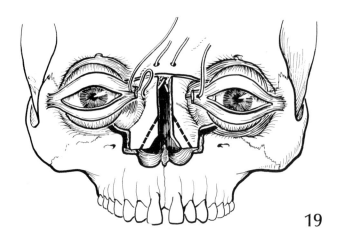

19

20

The medial orbital walls are wired in position, as are the medial canthi. The nasal airway is enlarged by removing bone inferiorly. The retained central strut gives a good nasal profile. Care must be taken not to enter the anterior cranial fossa superiorly.

In all these patients extensive soft tissue nasal surgery may be necessary and the lower lateral cartilages may have to be rearranged.

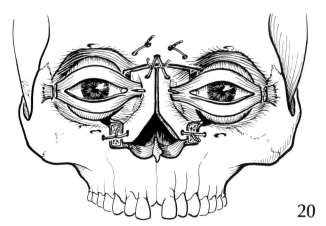

20

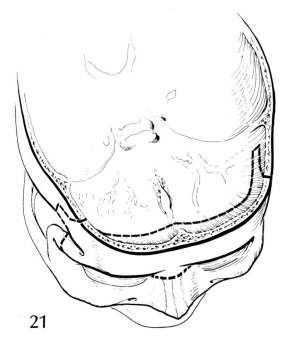

21

Retrusion of forehead and supraorbital ridges

This may be seen as an isolated problem, as in Carpenter's syndrome, or in conjunction with midface retrusion, as in Apert's and Crouzon's syndromes. The significant clinical features are a continually surprised look because of the elevated eyebrows, and the cornea lying in advance of the supraorbital rim. This deformity requires an intracranial procedure and may be corrected at any age. The approach is by the coronal flap.

21

The frontal lobes are elevated and bone cuts are made across the roof of the orbit. The cuts come forward medially and cross anterior to the crista galli.

22

Osteotomies are then made from the base of the frontal bone flap posteriorly out into the temporal area as a 'tongue'. This is continued down the lateral wall of the orbit, with the orbital contents protected, and then across the malar-lateral orbital wall junction to enter the orbit. The temporal tongue must be long enough to maintain contact on advancement (*see inset*). The nasal area is cut as an inverted V, taking care not to injure the medial dura.

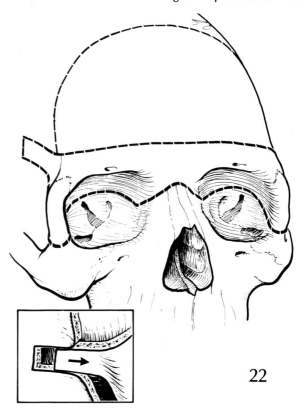

22

23

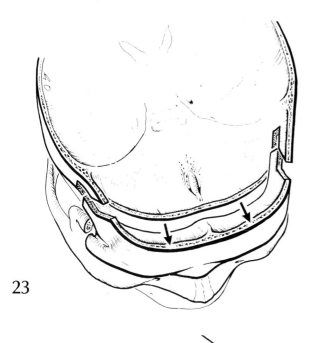

23

The supraorbital/nasal/orbital complex is mobilized and advanced to the required position. Laterally, at the junction of the orbit and temporal area, this may have to be mobilized with an osteotome.

24

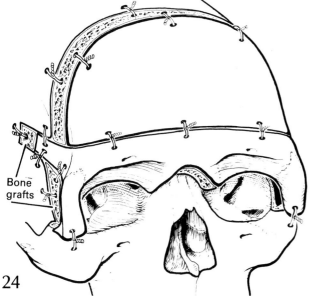

Bone grafts

24

All defects are bone grafted with skull bone, and the frontal bone is replaced and wired to the supraorbital rim. The coronal incision is closed with suction drainage.

Plagiocephaly

This is caused by unilateral coronal craniosynostosis, and results in retrusion of the supraorbital area with flattening of the frontal bone on that side.

25

A frontal bone flap is removed and an orbitonasal osteotomy is fashioned that is approximately half of that described in *Illustration 22*.

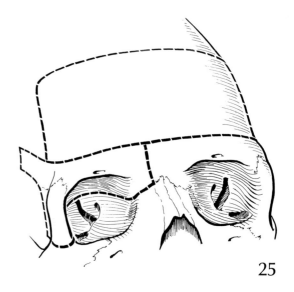

25

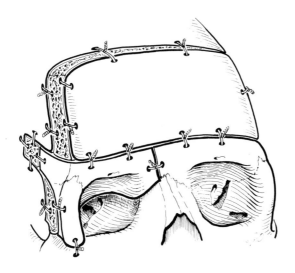

26

26

This orbital segment is advanced more laterally than medially, and is fixed in position with bone grafts and wiring. The skull segment is turned 180° so that the asymmetrical bone is under the hair; the symmetrical bone then forms the new frontal area. The coronal flap is sutured in position with suction drainage.

Midface advancement

This may be performed at different levels, depending on the clinical, cephalometric and dental model studies. It may be performed in isolation or simultaneously with a frontal advancement or a mandibular procedure. Maxillary advancement is employed to correct the craniofacial dysostoses, e.g. Crouzon's and Binder's syndromes, and the sequelae of cleft lip or trauma.

SUBCRANIAL LEFORT III

The approach is by the coronal flap (see *Illustration 1*) with extensive degloving of the orbits, temporal fossae and zygomatic arches.

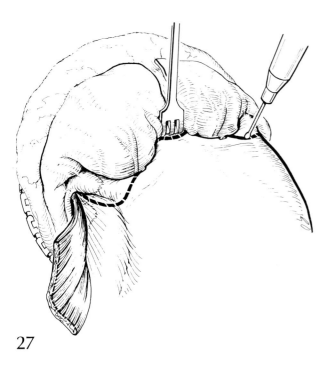

27

27

Osteotomies are made vertically in the lateral orbital walls, across the nasal bridge line and vertically down the medial orbital walls. The vertical osteotomies are joined across the orbital floor.

28

A finger is inserted down into the pterygoid area in order to identify the groove between the pterygoid plates posteriorly and the maxillary tuberosity anteriorly. An osteotome is inserted vertically from above, and the tuberosities are separated from the plates.

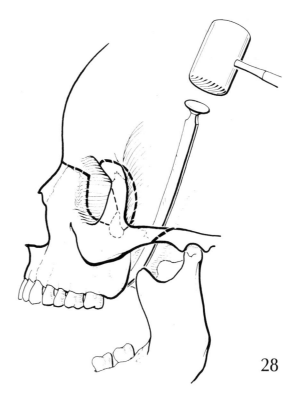

28

29

The zygomatic arch is divided at an angle.

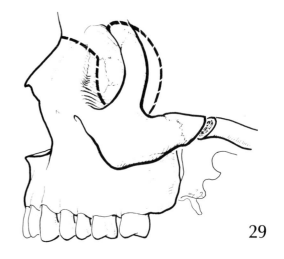

29

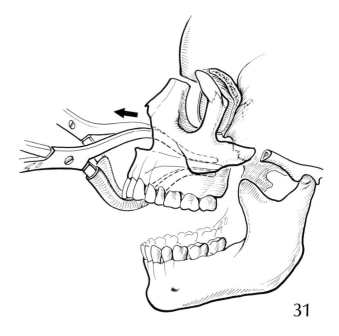

Cribriform plate

30

An osteotome is driven backwards and downwards through the nasal osteotomy to separate the vomer from the skull base. Care must be taken not to enter the anterior cranial fossa or to divide the endotracheal tube.

30

31

Using Rowe disimpaction forceps, the maxilla is mobilized and pulled forward so that the teeth will meet in correct occlusion.

31

32

The teeth are fixed in position, and the zygomatic arches are bone grafted with a full thickness and a split thickness rib graft as shown.

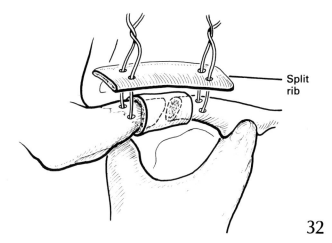

Split rib

32

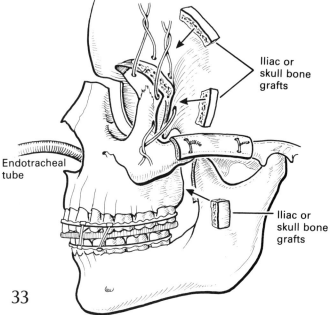

Iliac or skull bone grafts

Endotracheal tube

Iliac or skull bone grafts

33

33

Bone grafts are now inserted into all the bony defects resulting from the maxillary advancement.

34

The nasal gap is bone grafted, the lateral canthi are wired in position, and the temporalis muscles are advanced and sutured through drill holes in the lateral orbital rims. The coronal flap is returned and sutured, and suction drainage is established.

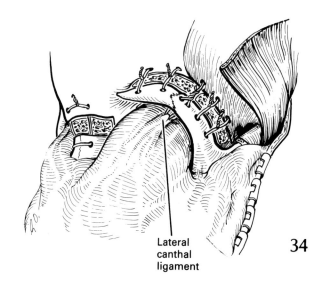

Lateral canthal ligament

34

VARIATIONS OF LEFORT III

Intracranial/extracranial

35

Part of the procedure may be performed intracranially to allow more of the supraorbital rim to be moved. A burr hole is made in the anterior portion of the temporal fossa over the anterior cranial fossa through which the frontal lobe can be retracted while the osteotomy is performed. The remainder of the operation is as described above.

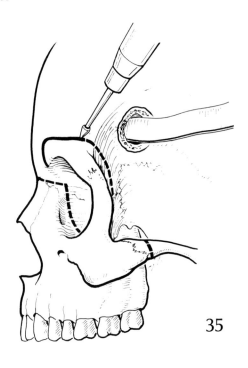

35

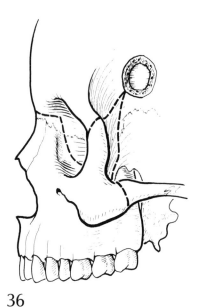

36

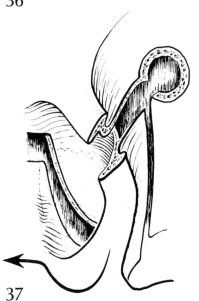

37

Self-stabilizing

36 & 37

Again, a burr hole is made in the temporal fossa. The osteotomy is such that a downward spike of lateral orbital wall is fashioned. The maxilla is then mobilized downwards, forwards and upwards so that it locks in front of this spike and is self-stabilized.

38

Further modification by introducing a long bone graft from the base of the skull down the lateral orbital wall to the maxillary tuberosity greatly enhances the stability.

The remainder of the operation is as described previously.

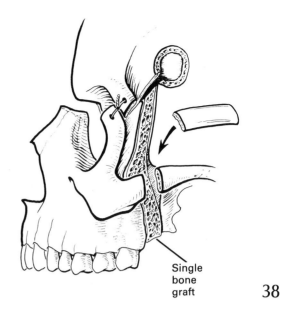

Single bone graft

38

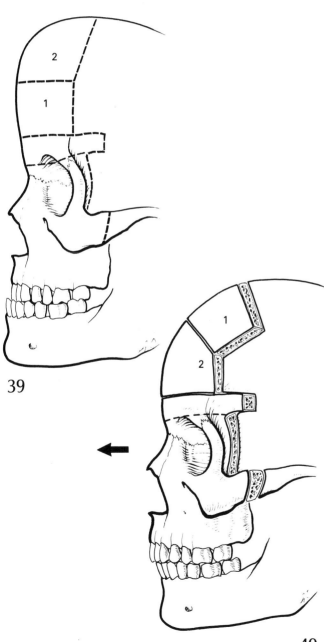

39

40

Step osteotomy

39 & 40

In addition to anterior movement of the maxilla, the supraorbital rims may be selectively advanced and the skull rearranged by transposition flaps.

LeFort IV (monobloc)

41 & 42

The supraorbital rims and maxilla may also be advanced as one block and the resulting defects bone grafted. The frontal bone is advanced by a similar amount and again stabilized by grafts.

All of these and the subsequent maxillary osteotomies are kept in intermaxillary fixation for 6 weeks. This is then removed and the patient is watched carefully. Should there be any tendency for relapse, the fixation is re-applied.

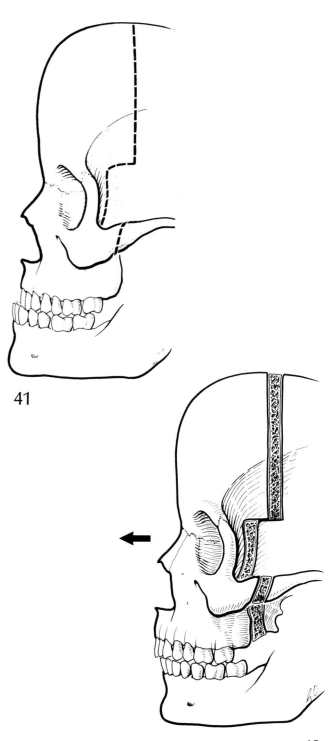

41

42

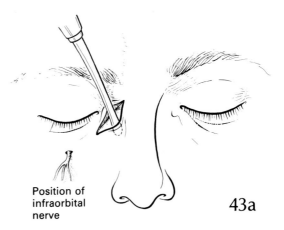

Position of
infraorbital
nerve

43a

LeFort II osteotomy

This is designed to deal with central midface retrusion, as in Binder's syndrome and some cleft syndromes. It advances the nose, the medial portions of the orbits and the upper teeth. The approach may be by a coronal flap or through limited paranasal incisions. Either method is acceptable.

43a–d

Through a paranasal incision the periosteum over the anterior aspect of the nose, the floor of the orbit and the nasal bones is raised (a). The lacrimal duct, which lies behind the infraorbital rim, is carefully dissected out from the lacrimal fossa with a small periosteal elevator (b). An osteotomy is then made with the drill, behind the duct across the infraorbital rim and down the anterior surface of the maxilla medial to the infraorbital nerve (c). Superiorly, this continues across the nasal bridge line so that the same procedure can be carried out on the opposite side (d).

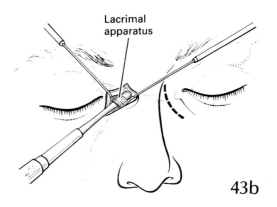

Lacrimal
apparatus

43b

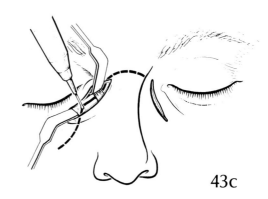

43c

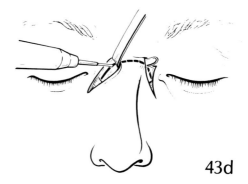

43d

44

An incision is then made in the upper buccal sulcus and the periosteum is elevated, revealing the osteotomy. This is continued downwards and then transversely to the pterygomaxillary groove. The septum is separated from the skull base with an osteotome.

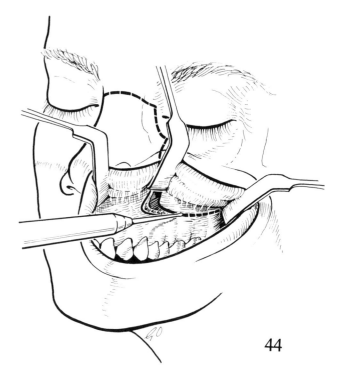

44

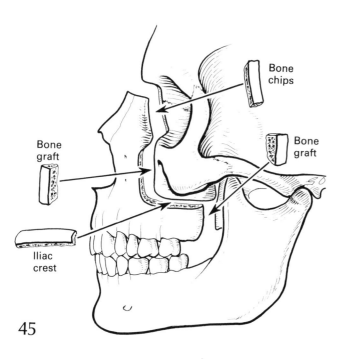

Bone chips

Bone graft

Bone graft

Bone graft

Iliac crest

45

45 & 46

The maxilla is mobilized with Rowe's disimpaction forceps, as described previously. Intermaxillary fixation is established, and the nasal bridge line is wired to the frontal area. Bone grafts are inserted and wired into all the gaps. If necessary, a nasal bone graft is inserted. All incisions are closed.

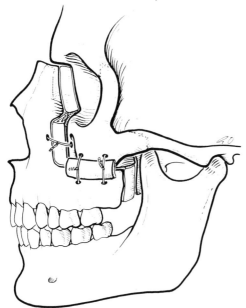

46

ORTHOGNATHIC SURGERY

Although the LeFort II osteotomy may be used to correct profile deformities, the workhorses are the LeFort I and mandibular procedures. These can be used to correct profile deformities as well as discrepancies in facial height. Again, careful cephalometric assessment, dental model studies and model surgery are necessary to ensure the correct choice of procedure and a satisfactory result. A course of orthodontic treatment is usually necessary to align the dental arches in order to ensure perfect occlusion at the end of the procedure. When only one jaw is being moved, an acrylic bite wafer is made, based on the correct occlusion established by model surgery. When both jaws are being moved, the maxilla is mobilized and fixed using an intermediate bite wafer, again fashioned as a result of the model surgery. The mandible is then operated on and the final occlusion established with the definitive bite wafer.

LeFort I osteotomy

The maxilla is most frequently advanced by the LeFort I osteotomy but it can also be shortened or impacted. Rarely, it may be retruded. In addition to pure orthognathic deformities, malocclusion in patients with secondary cleft lip and palate can also be corrected by this procedure.

47

A 'horse shoe' incision is made in the upper buccal sulcus, down through the periosteum, from tuberosity to tuberosity. A generous fringe of mucosa is left on the alveolus for final suture closure.

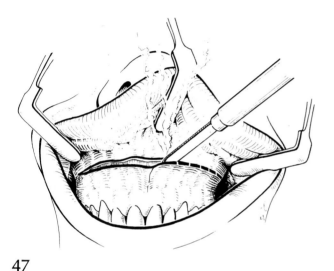

47

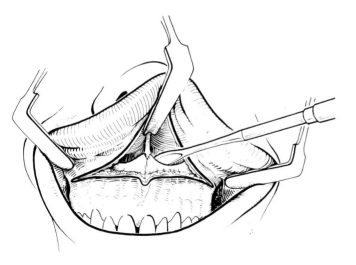

48

48

The periosteum is elevated to the pterygomaxillary fissure posteriorly and up to the infraorbital nerve superiorly. It is freed from the lateral pyriform aperture walls and the nasal floor. The lower part of the septum is freed of mucoperiosteum and mucoperichondrium.

49

A saw or drill is used to perform the transverse osteotomy from the pyriform aperture to the pterygomaxillary groove.

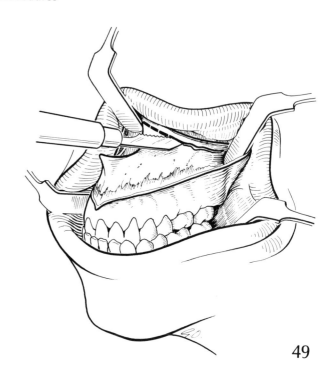

49

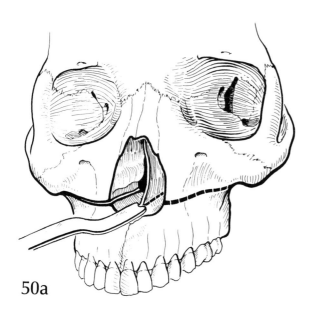

50a

50a & b

With a grooved septal osteotome, the septum and the lateral orbital walls are cut through to their full antero-posterior extent.

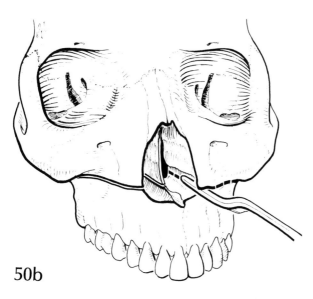

50b

51

A curved chisel is slipped behind the maxillary tuberosity, which is then separated from the pterygoid plates.

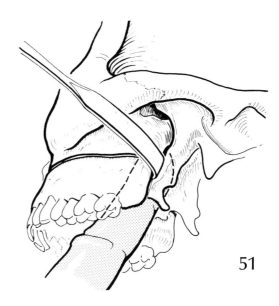

51

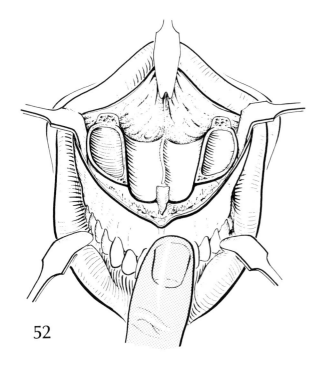

52

52

The maxilla can now be downfractured with finger pressure. Following this, it is completely mobile.

When the maxilla is to be impacted, the vomer is trimmed with rongeurs to ensure that the airway is not compromised by its bulk.

53

The maxillary segment is then advanced and/or impacted. In the latter case, a pre-calculated amount of maxillary bone is removed as a slice, an acrylic wafer is inserted between the teeth, and the maxilla and mandible are wired into intermaxillary fixation. Drill holes are made in the thickest portion of the maxilla and wires are inserted for osteosynthesis.

The subperiosteal dissection is continued up to the infraorbital rim and into the orbital floor. A drill hole is made through the rim and a wire passed; this is brought over the rim and on to the intermaxillary fixation. This inferior orbital suspension ensures absolute vertical fixation of the maxillary segment.

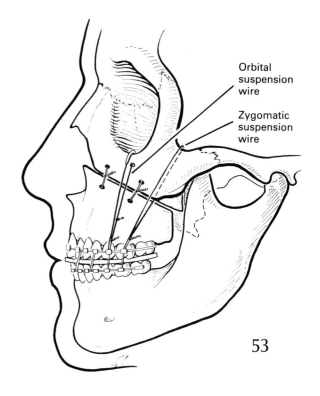

Orbital suspension wire

Zygomatic suspension wire

53

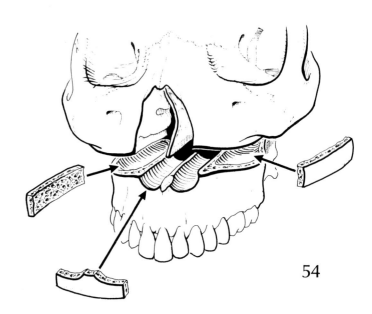

54

54 & 55

If the face is to be lengthened, the maxilla is extruded and bone grafts are placed and wired into the anterior maxillary defects. Small retrotuberosity grafts may be placed if there is a gap in this region. These are not absolutely necessary. The buccal sulcus incision is closed.

As in all maxillary osteotomies these patients are fed with a soft and fluid diet. The fixation is removed in 6 weeks.

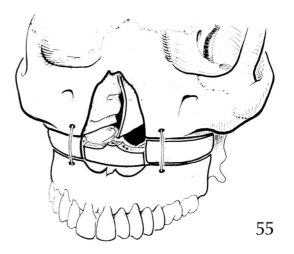

55

Mandibular osteotomy – sagittal split

By splitting the ascending ramus of the mandible it is possible to move the anterior segment in all directions. In this way, prognathism, retrognathism and laterognathism may be corrected. The large split areas allow good bone-to-bone contact. It is a quick and simple procedure. Permanent inferior alveolar nerve damage has been overemphasized; this should occur in less than 10 per cent of patients.

56

The procedure is performed intra-orally. The cheek is retracted and an incision is made posteriorly in the inferior buccal sulcus. Again, a generous cuff of buccal mucosa is left on the alveolus for later suturing.

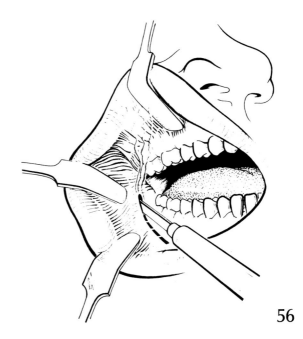

56

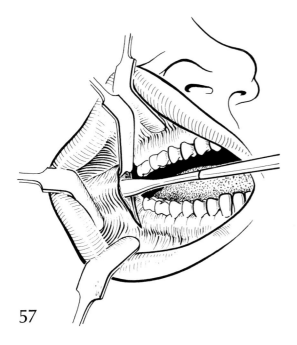

57

57

The periosteum is incised and elevated over the ascending ramus to the superior notch laterally. The posterior edge is then freed, as are the angle and the body to the second molar tooth. The pterygomasseteric sling is dissected free.

58

The medial subperiosteal dissection is performed by placing the special notched retractor on the pterygoid process and working down from the mandibular notch. In this way the inferior alveolar nerve and lingula can be exposed.

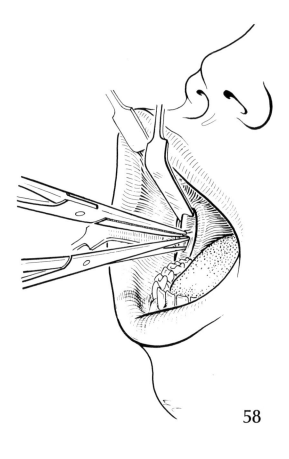

58

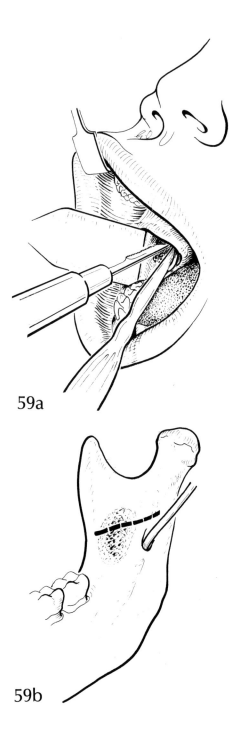

59a

59a & b

The periosteum is retracted laterally and the inferior alveolar nerve and periosteum are retracted medially. A horizontal cut is made above the nerve using a reciprocating saw or a drill. This cut goes part of the way through the ramus.

59b

60

The cut on the anterior surface of the ascending ramus is made as far laterally as possible, using a drill. This cut swings forward to the second molar tooth and then turns vertically downwards to the inferior edge of the mandible. The greater the advancement, the further forward this cut comes to ensure bone-to-bone contact.

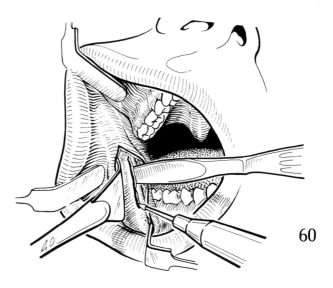

61

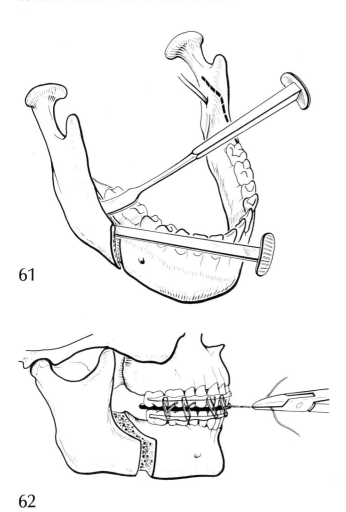

A fine Dautrey osteotome is now driven down between the lateral cortex and the cancellous bone. The split is achieved by a twisting movement, leaving the inferior alveolar nerve in the medial segment.

62

The jaw is moved into the correct pre-planned occlusion on the acrylic splint, which has been wired to the mandible. Intermaxillary fixation is applied.

63

The lateral segment is pushed firmly posteriorly and superiorly to ensure that the condyles are in the glenoid fossa. Drill holes are made on the superior part of the lateral segment and on a similar area on the medial segment behind the molars. These drill holes are used to wire the bony plates of the osteotomy securely in the correct position. The incisions are sutured.

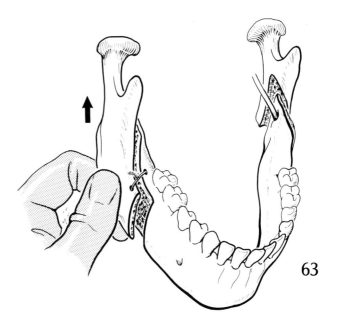

Genioplasty

This procedure can be used to advance the chin point, shorten it, lengthen it or retrude it. It may be performed in isolation or in conjuction with a mandibular procedure.

64

The chin is degloved subperiosteally through an inferior buccal sulcus incision. A good cuff of mucosa is left for later suturing. As much muscle attachment as possible is left on its posterior surface.

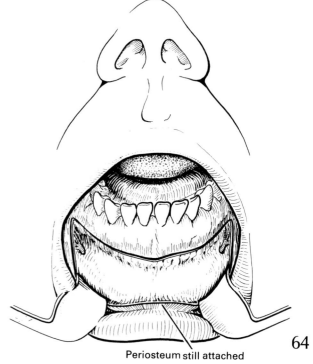

Periosteum still attached

64

65

The mandible is cut horizontally with a reciprocating saw or a drill. This cut is made below the level of the mental foramen.

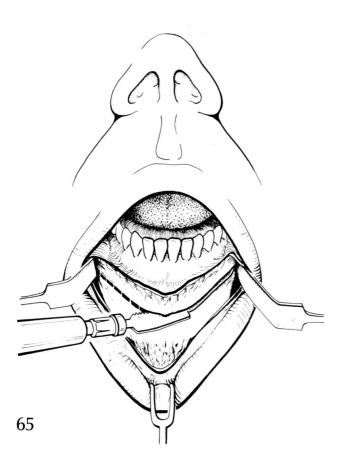

65

66

The segment is mobilized until it can be freely moved.

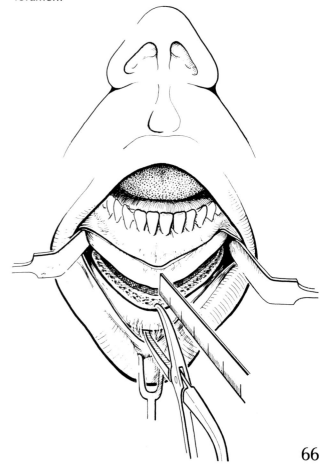

66

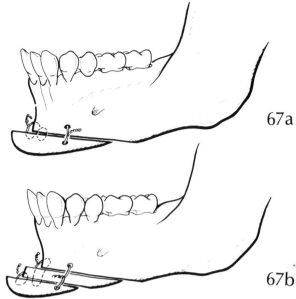

67a

67b

67a–d

The segment is moved and wired in position. This may be a one-step advancement (*a*), a two-step advancement (*b*), or correction of asymmetry (*c* and *d*). The incision is sutured. No intermaxillary fixation is necessary if only a genioplasty has been performed.

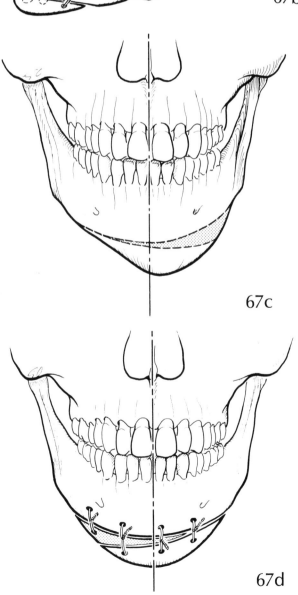

67c

67d

Bimaxillary procedures

68 & 69

In the long face syndrome with an open bite, a bimaxillary procedure may be necessary. The maxilla is impacted and the mandible split sagittally to close the bite. Frequently an advancement genioplasty will give an ideal profile.

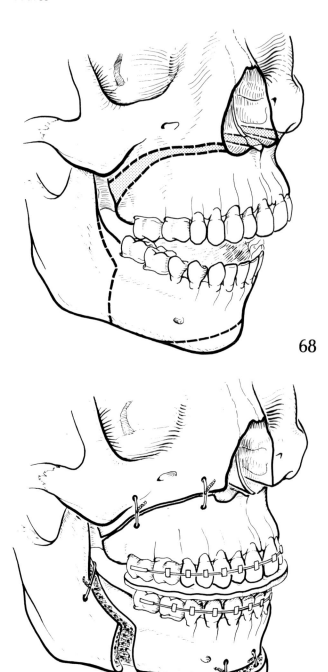

68

69

Further reading

Converse, J. M., Ransohoff, J., Mathews, E. S., Smith, B., Molenaar, A. Oculo hypertelorism and pseudohypertelorism: advances in surgical treatment. Plastic and Reconstructive Surgery 1970; 45: 1–13

Epker, B. N., Wolford, L. M. Middle third osteotomies: their use in the correction of congenital dentofacial and craniofacial deformities. Journal of Oral Surgery 1976; 34: 324–342

Freihofer, H. P. Jr. Correction of mandibular retrusion. In: Whitaker, L. A., Randall, P., eds. Symposium on reconstruction of jaw deformity, pp. 232–239. St Louis: C. V. Mosby, 1978

Henderson, D. The assessment and management of bony deformities of the middle and lower face. British Journal of Plastic Surgery 1974; 27: 287–296

Henderson, D., Jackson, I. T. Naso-maxillary hypoplasia: the LeFort II osteotomy. British Journal of Oral Surgery 1973; 11: 77–93

Jackson, I. T. Midface retrusion. In: Whitaker, L. A., Randall, P., eds. Symposium on reconstruction of jaw deformity, pp. 276–310. St Louis: C. V. Mosby, 1978

Jackson, I. T., Moos, K. F., Sharpe, D. T. Total surgical management of Binder's syndrome. Annals of Plastic Surgery 1981; 7: 25–34

Jackson, I. T., Reid, C. D. Nasal reconstruction and lengthening with local flaps. British Journal of Plastic Surgery 1978; 31: 341

Kufner, J. Four-year experience with major maxillary osteotomy for retrusion. Journal of Oral Surgery 1971; 29: 549–553

Munro, I. R. Combined maxillary and mandibular osteotomies. In: Whitaker, L. A., Randall, P., eds. Symposium on reconstruction of jaw deformity, pp. 311–326. St Louis: C. V. Mosby, 1978

Obwegeser, H. L. Surgical correction of small or retrodisplaced maxillae. Plastic and Reconstructive Surgery 1969; 43: 351–365

Tessier, P. Relationship of craniostenosis to craniofacial dysostoses and faciostenoses: a study with therapeutic implications. Plastic and Reconstructive Surgery 1971; 48: 224–237

Tessier, P. The definitive plastic surgical treatment of the severe facial deformities of craniofacial dysostosis, Crouzon's and Apert's disease. Plastic and Reconstructive Surgery 1971; 48: 419–442

Tessier, P. Anatomical classification of facial, craniofacial, and laterofacial clefts. Journal of Maxillofacial Surgery 1976; 4: 69–92

Trauner, R., Obwegeser, H. The surgical correction of mandibular prognathism and retrognathia with consideration of genioplasty. Oral Surgery 1957; 10: 677–689

Illustrations by Kevin Marks

Malignant melanoma of the skin

Ronald W. Hiles   FRCS, FRCS(Ed)
Consultant Plastic Surgeon, Frenchay Hospital, Bristol, Avon, UK

Introduction

Malignant melanoma is a tumour with a sinister reputation for early metastasis, although the overall prognosis is no worse than that for breast carcinoma. The most significant advances in surgical treatment have been a greater understanding of prognostic features in the primary tumour and earlier diagnosis.

Prognosis

It is now possible to predict the outcome with fair accuracy according to the morphological classification of the primary tumour.

Table 1 Malignant melanoma of the skin

Type	Clinical features	Prognosis (5-year survival)
Lentigo maligna	Flat, impalpable	Almost 100 per cent
Superficial spreading	Flat but palpable with mainly lateral growth	70 per cent
Nodular	Palpably and visibly raised with mainly vertical growth	44 per cent
Acral lentiginous	Occurs only in non-hairy skin	As low as 35 per cent

Clarke[1] first described the prognostic importance of the depth of penetration of the tumour into the dermis and classified the relative thickness of tumours according to five levels. There is increasingly poor prognosis the deeper the tumour extends.

Breslow[2] suggested a simpler classification depending on the absolute maximal thickness (depth of the fixed specimen measured histologically) of the tumour: tumours thinner than 0.75 mm rarely metastasize; those between 0.75 and 1.25 mm give a 5-year survival of 80 per cent; and of those patients with tumours thicker than 1.25 mm only 50 per cent survive 5 years.

The most recently described acral lentiginous type[3] accounts for some 30 per cent of melanomas occurring on the hairless volar skin of the feet and hands. This type can also arise in the sub- and paraungual positions and on or near mucosal surfaces. It often carries a poorer prognosis than its thickness would suggest.

The site of the primary tumour also carries prognostic significance – for example, for trunk and subungual melanomas the prognosis is bad but for facial and leg primaries it is better. There are also sex-related differences in the behaviour of melanomas in that females with melanomas survive longer than males overall.

Aims of surgery

The primary purpose of surgery is to establish or confirm a diagnosis and at the same time, if possible, to remove all detectable tumour. Secondarily, in the case of the wide excision, the aim is to remove undetectable localized tumour. As yet there are no recognized features in the primary which indicate which tumours make up the relatively small group of some 10–15 per cent of all tumours which subsequently develop local micrometastases. At present no other form of primary ablation is as effective in cure as surgery and none other leads to simultaneous histological confirmation of malignancy, so that it is still the primary treatment of choice. In addition there is probably no treatment that is less immunosuppressant than surgery. Surgery seems to help those cases in which micrometastases have already been produced by reducing total body tumour load; perhaps this releases immunological defence mechanisms to act on the smaller residuum of micrometastases.

The classic description of serial progression of malignant melanoma – at first by dermal lymphatic spread to form dermal satellite metastases, then by larger lymphatic pathways to regional nodes and subsequently, via the major lymphatics, onwards by haematogenous spread to distant organs – is by no means the rule. A very small primary tumour can often spread by the bloodstream at a very early stage and be lethal without any evidence of lymphatic spread. Hence the dilemma facing surgeons when deciding how wide a margin to take around the tumour at the first operation.

Lentigo maligna (carcinoma *in situ*) clearly needs no more than a simple complete excision with a 5 mm margin for certainty of clearance to effect a permanent cure. It can also be treated by cryotherapy or radiotherapy with good results. But what of the more aggressive types of tumour with a potential for metastasis? A wider clear margin of excision might well remove undetectable but already established local micrometastases which would eventually emerge as the classic satellite lesions if left or as recurrences in the scar of any inadequate excisions. Furthermore, each of these satellites would be a potential source of systemic metastases if the tumour had not already travelled further afield. There is still uncertainty and controversy about the optimum width of the margin of excision, but in the past 10 years there has been a growing awareness that the thin lesions metastasize either locally or systemically so infrequently as to make a margin of excision wider than 2 cm unjustified. It is frankly not known if wider initial excision in those cases in which local recurrences subsequently develop would have been wide enough to prevent them or early enough to prevent systemic spread. With our present methods of tumour detection and histological evaluation we are unlikely to get much nearer the truth than we are now. Controlled clinical trials involving various margins of excision are helping to clarify the position and are enabling us to

reduce the degree of mutilation that has accompanied surgery in the past.

Now that macroscopic and histological features can be more accurately related to prognosis, resection margins can be smaller for 'good' tumours but wider for the not so good. A wider clear margin of excision is still advised for the more aggressive grades of malignant melanoma as contemporary studies seem to indicate that if the margin drops below 2–3 cm the rate of local recurrence increases. With the present level of understanding of the pathology of malignant melanoma and with the limitations of our present means of tumour detection some working rules are possible, but each case is different and must be treated on its own merits and with some flexibility.

1. Always excise the tumour with a small but clear margin laterally and deep, even if the diagnosis is in doubt. This ensures that no primary tumour cells are left and that a comprehensive specimen is obtained for histological examination. Incision biopsy may give unrepresentative areas of the primary to the histologist, may make histological classification and thickness estimation either difficult or impossible and may theoretically also bring a risk of surgically induced metastases, although there is scant evidence for the latter. For lentigo maligna and for very thin lesions or lesions confirmed as benign by the histologist no further treatment is necessary.

2. If there is clinically no doubt that the diagnosis is malignant melanoma or if invasive malignancy has been shown histologically in previously doubtful lesions the excision is carried laterally 5–50 mm in all directions. The width of the margin of the excision should be dependent on the site and the grade of malignancy. For example, a greater margin is taken for a nodular than for a superficial spreading melanoma. When the primary is so situated that severe mutilation or disability would follow wide excision the benefits of the main effect of wide excision (which are the reduction in the rate of local recurrence and probably only slightly that of distant metastases) should be weighed against the undesirable effects, for example, of loss of function and mutilation by amputation of a thumb or the encroachment on to important facial features. There are diminishing returns of prognostic advantage as the radial margin of excision increases beyond the optimum, which may be as small as 30 mm but which has yet to be determined accurately and scientifically as opposed to empirically.

The operations

PRIMARY TUMOUR

Where diagnosis is in doubt

1

Excision biopsy should be carried out with a clear margin of at least 5 mm. Frozen section examination will usually distinguish between melanomatous lesions and those masquerading as melanoma, but only pathologists with great experience of melanoma are able to distinguish between malignant and benign melanoma without a full (and delayed) paraffin section. The long axis of the elliptical incision should be orientated in the direction of the local skin creases – that is, parallel to the lines of least tension.

If local analgesia is used it should be introduced in a ring around the tumour so as to reduce increases in tissue pressures within the tumour to a minimum.

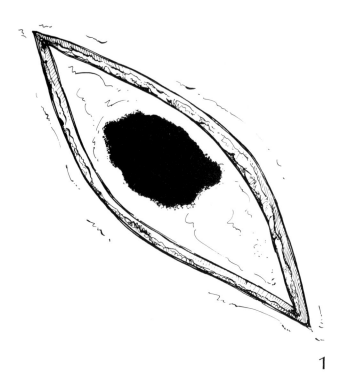

1

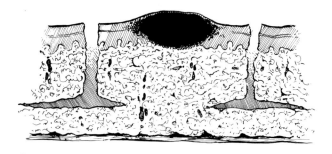

2

2

The excision is carried deep to clear the tumour well but not so deep as to extend right through the fat to the deep fascial plane. Tissue should be handled gently to reduce the risk of peroperative metastases and so as not to damage the specimen, which might make subsequent histological diagnosis difficult.

3a & b

The wound is closed by simple and accurate edge-to-edge suture in two layers.

Where diagnosis is not in doubt

Flat impalpable tumours (lentigo maligna and early superficial spreading melanoma)

The lesion is excised with a 5–10 mm margin of surrounding uninvolved skin. At some sites such defects can often be closed by direct apposition of the wound margins after conversion of the defect into an ellipse orientated in such a way as to allow ease of closure and minimal distortion to nearby features. A free split skin graft should be used when skin tension is too great to permit comfortable closure.

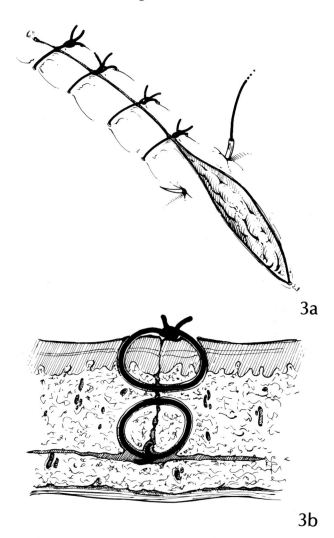

3a

3b

Palpable tumours

4

Starting proximally, excision is carried out with a wide margin of surrounding clear skin measuring 20–50 mm in all directions and extending to a depth which reaches but does not include the deep fascia. Olsen[4] has shown that the fascia acts as a lymphatic barrier and extension of the tumour to involve or pass deep to it is extremely rare. It is also an excellent base on which to place a split skin graft, but it is not always a very distinct layer – for example, on the posterior trunk, where there is little more than perimysium in most areas. The margin of excision is decided upon after consideration of the absolute thickness of the tumour, its site and whether or not there is either clinical evidence of local micrometastases or histological evidence of involvement of the intradermal lymphatics. The absolute indication for the maximum width of excision is evidence of local micrometastases and a site which allows wide excision without loss of function or inordinate mutilation. In many sites even a wide excision defect can be closed directly after conversion to an ellipse, undermining and advancing the wound edges.

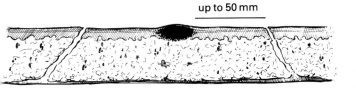

up to 50 mm

4

5

Where the defect left after an appropriate margin of excision cannot be closed directly the scalpel should be angled at approximately 45° so as to undercut the wound edges and clear them of fat.

The surgeon who is inexperienced in the diagnosis of melanoma should always carry out an excision biopsy of the whole lesion first, including a small clear margin, so as to establish the diagnosis and to measure tumour thickness histologically before extending the resection.

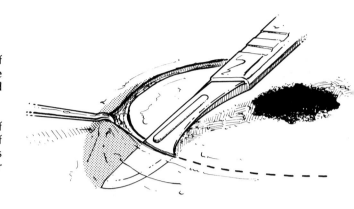

5

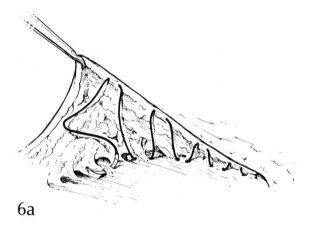

6a

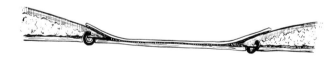

6b

6a & b

After wide excision with a view to skin graft repair the thin skin margins can then be sutured to the deep fascia with a continuous subcuticular tacking stitch using absorbable material (e.g. 4/0 Dexon). The skin edge is advanced slightly towards the centre of the defect as it is sewn. This management of the margin improves the chances of 'take' of the graft at the edges as there is no bare fat and the 'frame' is fixed so that shearing forces produce little movement. In addition, the otherwise punched-out appearance of a healed grafted defect is improved by a smoothing out of its edge contours.

7

The split skin graft used to resurface such defects is probably best not taken from the skin on the route of the lymphatic drainage from the primary tumour because of the increased risk of the development of in-transit metastases in the donor site.

The skin graft should be of intermediate thickness and can be applied in various ways. First, meticulous haemostasis of the graft bed must be obtained with accurately applied diathermy for all but venous and larger arterial bleeding points, which are ligated with fine absorbable material (e.g. 5/0 Dexon).

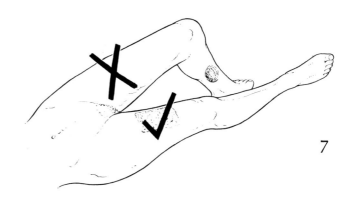

7

The graft can be fixed with marginal sutures, and if extra security is required these sutures are left long and tied over a bolus of polyurethane foam or of cotton wool impregnated with flavine and liquid paraffin.

A simpler, quicker and equally effective way of securing the graft is by means of an adhesive dressing, the least expensive of which is a single layer of cotton gauze applied after the outer surface of the graft and the skin surrounding the defect has been painted with mastic.

Alternatively, the same defect can be temporarily dressed with paraffin gauze and simple dressings while the split skin graft is stored in physiologically moist, sterile conditions at approximately 4°C. The graft can be applied to the defect in the ward 24–48 hours later when the patient is conscious and cooperative. An intelligent, self-disciplined patient will then take over responsibility for not knocking off the exposed graft. This exposed, delayed primary application of the graft is particularly successful in the healing of dorsal trunk tumour excision defects, where scapular movements will often shear off grafts held under dressings.

It is prudent to take up to twice as much skin graft as is necessary for a single application so that, should the first graft fail to take, stored skin can be applied without the need for a further operation.

When grafts are applied very near or over joints the 'take' is usually improved if the joint is splinted for the first week. Grafts on the leg benefit from firm support with a soft foam pad 1 cm thick and elasticated tubular bandage, which allows early ambulation without detriment to 'take'.

Dressed skin grafts are best examined at the fourth or fifth postoperative day so that any seroma beneath the graft can be released and haematoma evacuated by incising the graft and carefully removing the clot by swabbing and irrigation. At this time the replaced skin is usually still viable and can be vascularized satisfactorily.

Sites demanding special attention

8a, b & c

Digits

Subungual melanoma, although epidermal in origin, is intimately related to bone and the terminal interphalangeal joint. To achieve an adequate but not unduly mutilating clearance of the primary tumour only the distal one and a half phalanges should be amputated in the majority of cases. More radical complete digital ray amputation is of doubtful value unless the local tumour has already evidently spread more proximally than the distal joint.

Limbs

Primary malignant melanoma rarely penetrates deeply (except on the subungual site) and limb amputation for primary tumour has largely been abandoned. No advantage in terms of the length or quality of life follows such amputation as compared with less radical ablation.

Trunk

Nodular trunk melanoma in the male has a sinister prognosis and when a patient presents with satellite lesions a much wider area of excision of up to 100 mm in all directions is sometimes practised. Such a wide excision does not greatly increase disability and may reduce the chance of troublesome local recurrences.

Care after primary surgery

As in all cases of malignancy it is important that the patient should be reviewed regularly. Malignant melanoma is most likely to produce metastases in the first 2 or 3 years after excision of the primary. Although a grave prognostic sign, early recurrence is not always followed by a fatal outcome and demands early surgical treatment. In the early years after primary surgery the local area of the primary and any regional nodes to which it may drain should be examined every 4–8 weeks if recurrence is to be treated promptly and with some hope of success. Self-examination can be taught to patients to reduce the frequency of specialist follow-up.

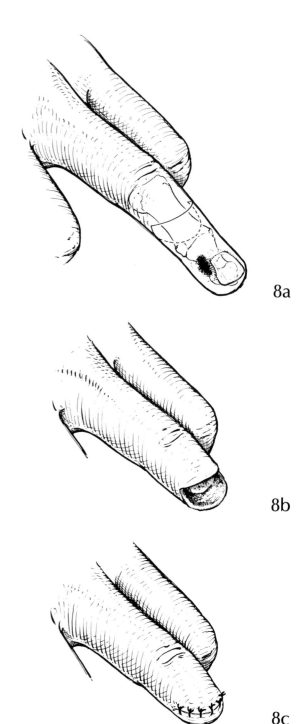

8a

8b

8c

SECONDARY TUMOUR

Local metastases

These are probably best treated as if they were primaries with further wide excision, but not all are controlled in this way. Secondaries limited to a limb can often be controlled by isolated limb perfusion with cytotoxic agents (*see* Volume on General Principles, Breast and Hernia, 'Isolated limb perfusion for chemotherapy of tumours', pp. 228–238).

Once the disease has spread systematically and declared itself clinically or has been revealed by simple radiology, computer assisted tomography or isotope scanning techniques cure is rare, but the natural progression of the local lesions may be very slow and the patient may survive for a long period. In these circumstances multiple small localized metastases can often be controlled by conservative excision, diathermy or cryosurgery or by the use of intralesional cytotoxic chemical injection, BCG or vaccinia. Dinitrochlorobenzene has been used to provoke a delayed hypersensitivity reaction at the site of any metastases, which destroys them. Although melanoma is relatively radioresistant, radiotherapy can be effective in the control of recurrences.

The more radical approach of integumentectomy for skin metastases which are limited to one limb but are extensive has been followed occasionally by good results and with far less disability than limb amputation. Amputation for secondary disease has largely been abandoned, just as for primary melanoma, because it produced a distressing disability in what was often a long terminal stage and with no more relief of symptoms than the more conservative measures.

Regional lymph node management

Controversy continues over the virtues of therapeutic versus prophylactic node excision and no overwhelming evidence yet exists to support one or condemn the other. Balch et al.[5] thought there was an advantage in prophylactic block dissection of nodes for tumours between 1.5 and 4.0 mm thick, but Veronesi et al. disagree.

There is significant morbidity following groin dissection, some 30 per cent of patients suffering from leg oedema if the operation has been carried out thoroughly. Many surgeons therefore adopt a 'watch-and-wait' policy, believing that lymph nodes play an immunologically defensive role and are best left to continue this until overwhelmed by tumour and clinically enlarged. Only then are they removed.

Axilliary nodes

Axilliary nodes should be cleared *en bloc* when clinically enlarged (*see* chapter on 'Axillary and inguinal node clearance', pp. 637–644). Complications are unusual, although seroma can persist for several weeks. Recurrence in the axilla after clearance is rare.

Inguinal nodes

There is controversy over whether to extend the inguinal node excision to include the iliac group. Many surgeons now take the view that if the disease has spread to involve the suprainguinal nodes it is beyond control and therefore only extend the dissection to remove these higher nodes when they are obviously enlarged and distressing to the patient. On the other hand some surgeons prefer always to carry out a full iliofemoral regional node clearance, believing that the number of patients returning with suprainguinal node enlargement after a purely superficial inguinofemoral clearance is significant both in number and in the severity of the problems which these higher metastases cause.

Inguinal node excisions are characterized by a high rate of delayed healing. The technique of the operation and measures to improve rates of healing are described in the chapter on 'Axillary and inguinal node clearance', pp. 637–644.

Distant systemic metastases

Apparently solitary deposits in the brain, lung, liver or gut are often worth resecting as removal of such secondary tumours has been followed by prolonged periods of freedom from symptoms and tumour progression.

Bony metastases are often very painful and relief usually follows radiotherapy even though the tumour is radiosensitive in less than 30 per cent of cases.

Widespread distant metastases are beyond surgical control. Contemporary systemic chemotherapy produces tumour regression in only some 25 per cent of cases and usually only for short periods. As such treatment is sometimes accompanied by unpleasant side effects it is usually reserved for patients who already have distressing symptoms due to their tumour. Newer drugs such as vindesine have fewer and less severe side effects and are being used with quite good effect in patients with symptom-free secondaries.

Patients with terminal debility, pain and nausea require sympathetic specialized nursing, appropriate and adequate analgesia and regular medical visitation. They also need ready access to relatives and friends and this and careful nursing are often best found at home or in a hospice.

Prevention?

Prevention of melanoma is not yet possible as our knowledge about its aetiology is very incomplete. Much has been written about the causative role of sunlight in melanoma, but it is clearly only one factor in its genesis. Nevertheless, the avoidance of overexposure to sunlight and other sources of ultraviolet light seems a prudent precaution. This is particularly applicable to western Europeans living or holidaying outside their native environment in sunnier climates.

Earlier diagnosis would appear to offer improved survival, particularly if the lesion can be caught when it is still thin according to Breslow's classification. Health teams and the public need to be better informed about the alarming increase in the incidence of this disease and the importance of early recognition and excision. In Britain the incidence has almost doubled in the past 15 years and in Australia it has risen at an even greater rate.

Earlier treatment is likely to improve survival figures, but whether or not it will improve real survival – that is, after discounting the time gained by the ealier diagnosis – remains to be seen (c.f. carcinoma of the breast).

References

1. Clark, W. H., Jr. A classification of malignant melanoma in man correlated with histogenesis and biologic behaviour. Advances in Biology of Skin 1966; 8: 621–647

2. Breslow, A. Thickness, cross-sectional areas and depth of invasion in the prognosis of cutaneous melanoma. Annals of Surgery 1970; 172: 902–908

3. Reed, R. J. Histopathology: microscopic anatomy and reaction patterns of the skin; controversies in dermatopathology. In: Reed, R. J. ed. New concepts in surgical pathology of the skin. pp. 27–60; 61–147. New York: Wiley, 1976

4. Olsen, G. The malignant melanoma of the skin. Copenhagen: Aarhuus Stiftsbogtrykkerie, 1966

5. Balch, C. M., Murad, T. M., Soong, S-J., Ingalls, A. L., Richards, P. C., Maddox, W. A. Tumour thickness as a guide to surgical management of clinical stage I melanoma patients. Cancer 1979; 43: 883–888

6. Veronesi, U., Adarius, J., Bandiera, D. C. et al. Delayed regional lymph node dissection in Stage I melanoma of skin and the lower extremity. Cancer 1982; 49: 2420–2430

Axillary and inguinal node clearance

Ronald W. Hiles FRCS, FRCS(Ed)
Consultant Plastic Surgeon, Frenchay Hospital, Bristol, Avon, UK

THE AXILLA

Surgical anatomy

The fibro-fatty tissue of the axilla contains many scattered lymph nodes. Division into pectoral, scapular, lateral, infraclavicular, central and apical groups indicates their distribution and all these groups are removed when the axilla is surgically cleared of metastatic tumour. The boundaries of the dissection are the axillary vein above and laterally; the posterior wall formed by the subscapularis, teres major and latissimus dorsi; the anterior wall formed by the pectoralis major, the subclavius and the clavipectoral fascia; and the medial wall formed by the serratus anterior and the chest wall. The apex is where the neurovascular contents of the axilla pass to the posterior triangle of the neck, at which conduit the clavicle is in front, the scapula behind and the outer border of the first rib medial.

The cords of the brachial plexus lie superior, lateral and posterior to the axillary artery and the overlying vein and will not be endangered if dissection in this area is confined to a line in front of the vein and inferior to it. The one nerve which crosses the vein near the apex which should be preserved is the lateral pectoral nerve to the pectoralis major muscle. The nerve to the serratus anterior emerges deep to the vein near the apex and runs down the medial wall, while the nerve to the latissimus dorsi emerges from below the vein slightly lower down and crosses the posterior wall. All three of these motor nerves should be preserved. The medial pectoral nerve to the pectoralis minor and to part of the pectoralis major beyond is usually sacrificed. Sensory nerves to the axillary and medial upper arm skin cross the axilla from the medial to the lateral side and have to be sacrificed to maintain the integrity of the *en bloc* excision and avoid seeding of the wound with tumour.

The axillary lymph nodes receive from the upper half of the trunk anteriorly and from the lateral half of the breast (pectoral group), from the upper half of the trunk posteriorly and from the axillary tail of the breast (scapular group), from the upper limb (lateral group), from the upper part of the breast and from the thumb (infraclavicular group) and from the floor of the axilla (central group). Lymph passes from all these groups via the apical group on to the right subclavian lymph trunk.

The operation

Positioning of the patient

The patient lies supine with the arm abducted to 90° and resting on an arm table in the plane of the trunk. Extension in abduction posterior to this plane should be avoided as it carries the risk of traction injury to the brachial plexus. If the arm is completely enveloped in sterile towels its position can be altered during surgery to give 90° of flexion and full adduction at the shoulder so as to relax the pectoral muscles and improve the access to the apex of the axilla. Slight head-up and arm-up lateral tilt of the table further improves exposure and access and reduces the tendency to venous congestion. The surgeon can be seated for comfort in the angle between the arm rest and the table.

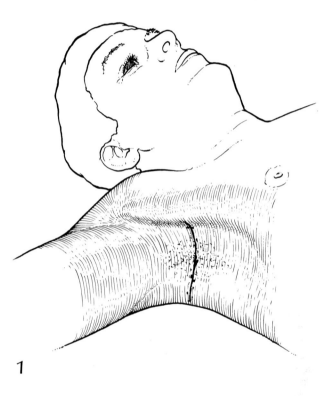

1

Skin incision

1

The transverse incision crossing the apex of the vault of the axillary skin gives adequate exposure, excellent healing and minimal problems with scar contracture. It can be extended anteromedially to improve the exposure to the clavipectoral area, but this is rarely necessary. A longitudinal incision running down the centre of the axilla from the arm is an alternative approach; healing is usually good, but the quality of the matured scar is not as good as with the transverse incision; it is occasionally complicated by a visible web of contracture but this is not sufficient to restrict movement.

The skin is dissected free from the underlying subcutaneous fat in all directions from the incision to the boundaries of the axilla. The raising of the skin must not interfere with the subdermal plexus of vessels but needs to be quite superficial.

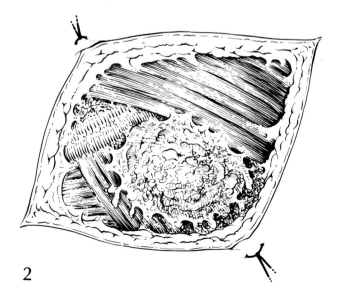

2

The node dissection

2

Clearance of the axilla is commenced by incising the deep fascia over the lateral margin of the pectoralis major. Passing medially, the deep surface of the muscle is cleaned until the lateral pectoral nerve arising from the lateral cord of the brachial plexus is seen and preserved as it pierces the clavipectoral fascia to supply the muscle.

3

The fully towelled arm is then adducted, in 90° of flexion, at the shoulder and held in this position by the assistant so as to relax the pectoralis major. This muscle can then be retracted to give excellent access to the pectoralis minor. To clear the infraclavicular group of lymph nodes the minor muscle is best divided close to its insertion at the coracoid process, ultimately to be removed with the specimen. The axillary vein can then be seen deep to the clavipectoral fascia. Commencing at the apex of the axilla and passing laterally along the line of the axillary vein, the fascia is divided and the fibro-fatty contents of the axilla cleared from it by sharp dissection. Tributaries passing to the main vein from the axilla are clipped, divided and ligated and the main specimen is drawn downwards to reveal the scapularis. Medially the long thoracic nerve supplying the serratus anterior and running deep to the loose areolar tissue, closely applied to the chest wall, is identified, preserved and dissected clear. Passing laterally again, any remaining branches of the axillary artery which cross the posterior wall of the axilla are ligated and divided. The long subscapular nerve running down from beneath the axillary vein across the posterior wall to supply the latissimus dorsi is preserved and cleared of its usually close association with the subscapular artery. If there is any prospect of a latissimus dorsi muscle flap being required the subscapular artery and vein are preserved intact.

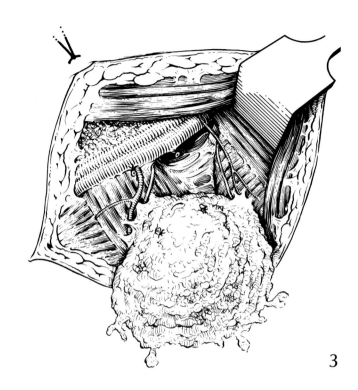

3

At this stage the arm is replaced on its support so as to straighten the axillary vein and make dissection of the lateral part of the specimen easier. Once the anterolateral border of the latissimus dorsi muscle is reached dissection reverts to the upper medial aspect of the specimen. The pectoralis minor is resected at its origin. As the specimen is withdrawn and the serratus anterior muscle and its nerve are cleaned, the whole of the medial wall of the axilla is revealed. The intercostobrachial nerve and several lower lateral cutaneous sensory branches of the upper intercostal nerves enter the specimen and have to be divided to complete the clearance of the medial wall. The anterior border of the latissimus dorsi is then cleaned, care being taken to preserve its nerve as it enters the muscle low on the posterior wall of the axilla, where it may be looped into the specimen and divided if this danger is not recognized.

Once the fat and nodal contents of the axilla have been delivered, complete haemostasis is checked, perforated suction tube drainage is inserted and the skin incision closed with subcuticular or small interrupted sutures. An airtight closure with suction applied to the drain will make bulky dressings and firm pressure unnecessary. This will facilitate shoulder movements, which should be encouraged early. The axilla is best dressed with a small gauze dressing held in place with one loose narrow strip of adhesive skin tape running from the mid-anterior to the mid-posterior axillary fold. The arm is nursed just short of complete adduction to allow ventilation and avoid maceration. Drainage may be necessary for up to 10 days to avoid seroma. As soon as suction drainage has dropped below 5 ml per day it is cut off and the drain covered with a dressing. It is withdrawn gradually over the next few days when the dressing is no longer moist.

In the case of malignant melanoma when the primary tumour presents with palpable axillary modes and is near to or in the axillary skin, the excision of skin and lymph nodes should be integrated *en bloc* and extensive split skin grafting may be necessary.

Postoperative complications

Seroma

If the suggested suction drainage routine is employed serous collections are rarely a problem, but the drain may need to be kept in the wound for quite a long time on occasion. If serous collections form after removal of the drain, needle aspirations repeated as necessary usually suffice.

Wound breakdown

If due regard is given to preservation of the subdermal vasculature of the skin, wound breakdown is extremely rare in the axilla. Small breakdowns can be safely left to heal spontaneously with appropriate simple dressings. Larger breakdowns which fail to heal within 2 weeks are best repaired with split skin grafts to reduce the risk of subsequent contractures.

Stiff shoulder

It is imperative that active movement of the shoulder joint is instituted from the first postoperative day as the longer the shoulder remains immobile the more difficult will it be to overcome the resultant stiffness. When the patient cooperates well a full range of movement at the shoulder should be regained by the 10th to 14th day.

Oedema of the arm

Slight oedema of the arm and hand following axillary clearance is not unusual but it is rarely severe, distressing or disabling. If it threatens to be progressive but is caught early it can often be controlled by the fitting of an elasticated glove and sleeve. Progressive postoperative oedema may indicate recurrence of axillary tumour and some degree of venous obstruction. It is a not uncommon sequel to axillary radiotherapy.

Extending the dissection above the line of the axillary vein, which is unnecessary for satisfactory clearance of the axilla and a danger to the cords of the brachial plexus, may also increase the risk of distal lymphoedema and should be avoided for these three reasons unless unusual extension of tumour demands it.

THE GROIN

Surgical anatomy

With the exception of a small area of skin over the heel, all the superficial tissues of the lower limb drain to the vertical chain of a superficial group of inguinal lymph nodes which lie alongside the termination of the long saphenous vein. The skin of the lateral side of the trunk and the back below the waist drains to a group lateral to the saphenous opening, while the skin of the anterior abdominal wall and perineum drains to a medial group.

The superficial nodes drain by efferent vessels through the cribriform fascia of the saphenous opening to deep nodes lying on the medial side of the femoral vein to join lymph from the deep tissues of the limb. The lymph drainage then passes through the femoral canal to the iliac nodes lying alongside the external and common iliac vessels.

Below the inguinal ligament the regional lymph nodes are contained within the femoral triangle bounded medially by the adductor longus and laterally by the sartorius. The floor of the triangle is formed mainly by the pectineus, psoas and iliacus from medial to lateral and the main neurovascular contents are the femoral vein, the femoral artery and femoral nerve from medial to lateral.

Above the inguinal ligament surgical access to the iliac nodes is via the three muscular lamini of the anterior-abdominal wall. The external iliac vein runs along the brim of the pelvis behind the artery, being joined by the internal iliac vein over the sacroiliac joint and becoming the common iliac vein. At this point artery and vein are crossed by the ureter and at a higher level by the presacral nerves. Anteriorly the vessels are covered loosely by peritoneum.

Also encountered in the dissection, working downwards from the common iliac vessels, is the obturator nerve running posteromedial to the external iliac vessels and turning forwards in the bifurcation between the internal and external iliac vessels on to the fascia over the obturator internus muscle. As it enters the pelvis the nerve is very close to the ovary, and near the obturator fossa it lies on the pubic bone. The femoral nerve lies deep to the iliac fascia in the groove between the iliacus and psoas and should not normally be disturbed or seen in the dissection above the inguinal ligament. Immediately above the inguinal ligament the inferior epigastric and deep circumflex iliac arteries arise from the external iliac artery.

In the femoral triangle superficial branches of the femoral nerve are given off to the skin of the upper thigh and some minor branches have to be sacrificed. In a similar way small vessels from the femoral artery supplying the skin over the triangle pass inextricably through the dissection and have to be sacrificed along with accompanying veins. Some of the larger main trunks of the named cutaneous arteries of the femoral triangle can usually be preserved without jeopardizing the integrity of the *en bloc* clearance. Certainly the superficial circumflex iliac artery, running superolaterally, is applied to the floor of the triangle and can usually be preserved. The superficial epigastric and superficial external pudendal arteries usually have to be sacrificed. The latter forms a landmark by passing immediately inferior to and in the angle between the junction of the long saphenous vein with the femoral vein at the saphenous opening. The deep external pudendal artery, as its name suggests, passes medially but relatively deeply and can often be preserved. Preserving two out of four of these vessels probably reduces the chance of skin necrosis alongside the incision without prejudicing the adequacy of the lymph node clearance. An added safeguard for primary wound healing is to excise a margin of 1–2 cm of skin on either side of the incision, which is the portion of skin most likely to be devascularized by the dissection. Provided that so much skin as to introduce undue tension is not excised this manoeuvre will usually prevent delay in healing and wound breakdown.

The operation

Positioning of the patient

The patient should be laid supine with the hip in full extension, some 20° abduction and externally rotated. Slight foot-up tilt reduces venous congestion.

4

Skin incision

The straight incision is preferred. The development of curved flaps or Z-plasties is likely to increase the risk of marginal skin necrosis. The incision commences 5 cm above the junction of the outer and middle thirds of the inguinal ligament and slopes downwards and medially to end at the inferior angle of the femoral triangle. The skin is dissected, leaving a thin layer of subcutaneous fat and the subdermal plexus of vessels intact. The dissection is carried to the lateral and medial borders of the femoral triangle below, to the anterosuperior iliac spine and the pubic tubercle above, and to clear the lower 6 cm of the anterior abdominal wall. A 1–2 cm margin of skin is excised on either side of the incision as discussed above.

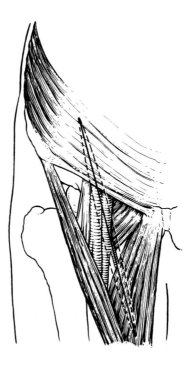

4

Radical or limited dissection?

Opinion differs as to whether it is always necessary to carry out the suprainguinal dissection or not. It is the policy of many surgeons to forego the iliac dissection in most cases unless there is an involved Cloquet's gland in the femoral canal, palpable secondary tumour above the inguinal ligament or radiographic (computer assisted tomography) evidence of enlarged iliac nodes. Others prefer always to carry out a radical clearance to include the regional nodes above and below the ligament, accepting the increased chance of troublesome lower limb oedema.

If radical ilio-inguinal clearance *en bloc* is to be carried out, as with most operations for cancer, it is probably best to work from above downwards, from iliac to inguinal, keeping the specimen as one and passing the iliac nodes beneath the inguinal ligament when both dissections are complete.

The inguinal dissection

5

The subcutaneous fat and deep fascia are incised at the margins of the superficial dissection to reveal the external oblique above, the sartorius laterally and the adductor longus medially. With dissection of the medial border completed and after ligation of the long saphenous vein and other smaller veins at the distal limit of this part of the dissection, the external oblique aponeurosis is then cleared, working from above downwards until the inguinal ligament is reached. Dissection proceeds cautiously below the medial end of the inguinal ligament until the femoral artery and vein are identified. The plane of dissection is carried downwards over the femoral vein to the junction of the saphenous vein with the femoral at the saphenous opening. The long saphenous vein is ligated and severed, with a flush tie of the stump at the junction. The superficial external pudendal artery is then usually encountered and ligated. Dissection of the femoral canal is completed and the specimen drawn downwards as it is cleared from the femoral vein distally. The specimen is drawn further laterally and downwards as it is cleared from the remainder of the floor of the femoral triangle. Lateral to the femoral artery several small perforating cutaneous branches of the femoral nerve are sacrificed above, while the larger branches to the lower thigh are preserved. The specimen becomes free as the lateral border of the femoral triangle is reached at the sartorius muscle. Haemostasis is then checked throughout the field of the dissection and the wound is ready for closure.

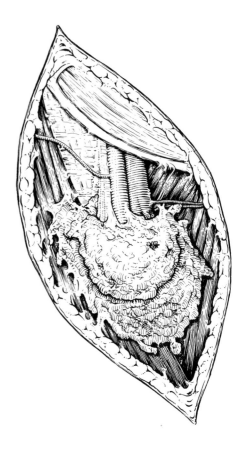

5

Only rarely are the femoral or external iliac veins intimately involved in adherent tumour. Usually tumour can be dissected free of the vessel wall, which is very rarely penetrated by tumour. If there is gross involvement of the vessel it is probably prudent to leave a narrow cuff of tumour to preserve the integrity of the vessel wall and to treat it with postoperative radiotherapy. If only a small portion of vessel wall is involved in tumour (and the expertise of the surgeon allows it) it can be excised after temporarily clamping or taping the vessel above and below. The defect is then patched with saphenous vein taken from the periphery of the field of dissection and the clamps removed.

6

The iliac dissection

The iliac group is approached by cleaning and splitting the external oblique aponeurosis parallel with the inguinal ligament and some 5 cm above it. The internal oblique and transversus abdominis muscle and fascia are then incised in the same line to reach the extraperitoneal 'space' over the main vessels. The peritoneum and the ureter are retracted as high as the bifurcation of the aorta and the pelvic viscera are retracted medially. It is helpful to have catheterized the urinary bladder to empty it before towelling the patient.

The iliac nodes are dissected clear of the common iliac vessels from above downwards, working from lateral to medial to leave clean vessels. The smaller group of obturator nodes are cleared by identifying and preserving the obturator nerve and then mobilizing the nodes, working from medial to lateral, to connect with the main dissection over the iliac vein. The dissected nodes are liberated to the femoral canal and ideally left to be cleared beneath the inguinal ligament in continuity with the femoral triangle dissection. If the iliac specimen is bulky it is reasonable to remove it separately after ligation at the upper limit of the femoral canal.

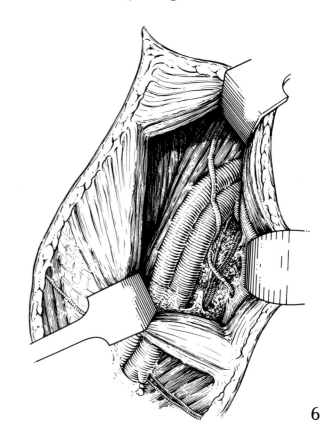

6

Closure

The iliac approach wound is closed in layers after checking absolute haemostasis in the pelvis. The pelvis can be drained by passing the suction tube drainage from the femoral triangle via the femoral canal into the pelvis. The femoral canal, if it has been enlarged by the dissection, is closed to its usual dimensions by a substantial suture between the inguinal and pectineal ligaments.

In the femoral triangle, if the femoral vessels have been involved and repaired or if there is doubt about viability of the skin cover, the vessels can be covered by transposition of the sartorius. The muscle is detached from its origin, its flimsy vascular pedicle is retained and the upper end of the muscle is reattached to the inguinal ligament above the femoral vessels with several interrupted sutures of 3/0 calibre. If skin viability is not in doubt and if the dissection has been uncomplicated there is no need to transpose the sartorius.

The wound margins having been excised, the fresh skin edges are approximated in two layers, using suture material which is not thicker than 4/0, care being taken to avoid undue tension and to distribute what tensions there are evenly. In this way the viability of the skin edge can be preserved and primary healing encouraged. The tubular suction drain is brought out 1 cm below the lower limit of the wound. With suction drainage there is no need for a compression dressing and the wound can be simply supported with adhesive translucent skin tapes which allow the colour of the wound edge to be observed after the operation.

The patient is nursed with the foot of the bed elevated and the whole leg is supported with an elastic stocking or evenly applied elastic bandage. Suction drainage usually needs to be maintained for at least 5 days and until serous aspirate drops to below 10 ml a day. Early ambulation with an elastic stocking is encouraged, but at rest the patient should always keep the foot elevated.

Postoperative complications

Wound breakdown

Failure of primary healing is not uncommon but is rarely a serious complication. Provided the skin adjacent to any area of breakdown is adherent the patient need not be retained in hospital but can be nursed at home with daily baths and dressings while the wound heals by second intention. Attempted secondary suture is rarely successful and best avoided. If an unusually large breakdown occurs the defect is best grafted with split skin.

Seroma

If wound suction is efficient and maintained for long enough, seroma is rare. Small collections slowly absorb spontaneously; larger collections demand occasional aspiration but sometimes require formal drainage and the insertion of a corrugated drain.

Lymphoedema

Some 30 per cent of patients suffer from lymphoedema of the leg after groin dissection, but in only a few is it severe and disabling. Primary uncomplicated healing and good elastic support to the leg mimimize the risk.

Flexion contracture

Scar contracture is rare and should not occur if primary healing is obtained. Where it does occur and is uncomfortable, which is exceedingly rare, it can warrant release and split skin graft.

Numbness

There is usually a relatively small area of numbness over the skin of the upper anterior thigh and patients should be warned of this before the operation.

Hernia

Abdominal wall, inguinal and femoral canal weakness should not occur if potential defects at this site are carefully repaired during closure. They are very uncommon complications.

Illustrated by Kevin Marks

Secondary surgery for burns

T. L. Barclay   ChM, FRCS(Ed), FRCS
Formerly Consultant Plastic Surgeon, Bradford Royal Infirmary and St Luke's Hospital, Bradford, UK

Introduction

The scars left after healing of burns or scalds which have damaged or destroyed the deeper part of the dermis will be associated with contracture across the flexor aspect of a joint if a significant area of the injury has had to heal by secondary intention. It is important to differentiate those scars which are associated with significant skin shortage from those whose appearance is lumpy and unsightly but which nevertheless do not restrict the full extension of a joint.

Scars not associated with contracture

Hypertrophic scars

Scars from recently healed burns should not be treated surgically. Split skin grafts are a poor substitute for skin which has been damaged but not destroyed, and good results can almost always be obtained by wearing of pressure garments, bandages or, best of all, rigid plastic splints moulded to the area to be treated, or quite often by the passage of time alone. If the scars are sufficiently bad to require treatment, pressure therapy continued for 9–12 months is well worth while. (For a full discussion of pressure bandaging and splintage, *see* Huang, Blackwell and Lewis[1].

Mature scars

Scars from which all hypertrophy has disappeared may be thin and papery, especially on extensor surfaces if the original injury was not treated by skin grafting. For these burnt-out, thin, shiny, easily injured scars, resurfacing with split skin graft is often worth while.

1

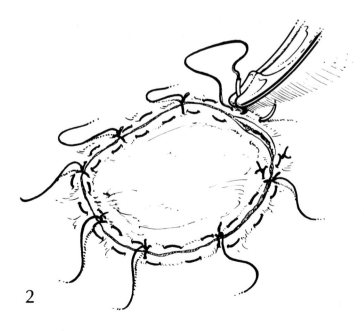

1

The thin epidermis is removed by sharp dissection, leaving the deeper part of the scar behind to act as a firm scaffold for the skin graft. Bleeding is usually scanty and easily controlled.

2

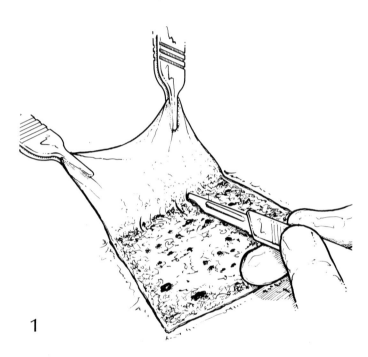

2

A skin graft of moderate thickness is cut from a suitable donor area and sutured into place, paying particular attention to accurate edge-to-edge apposition to avoid a step in the contour of the healed edge (which would detract from the appearance for weeks or months).

3

A good tie-over dressing completes the procedure.

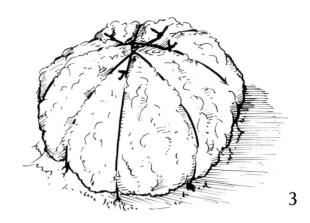

3

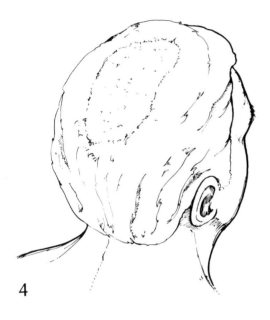

4

Scars of the scalp

If healed burns of the scalp are associated with significant hair loss, surgery should certainly be considered for children and for younger adults.

4 & 5

Excision and suture

Bald patches on the vertex can be substantially diminished in size or sometimes completely eliminated by excision and suture, repeated after an interval of some months if necessary. Only moderate tension on the scalp advancement flaps is permissible since, if the scalp is pulled very tight, the hair follicles in the edge may be sufficiently deprived of their blood supply to lose their hair-growing function, thus creating a further bald area at the sides of the scar.

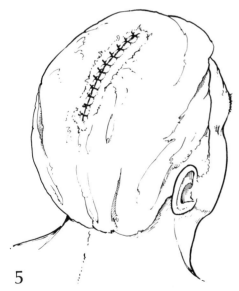

5

6

Hair transplants

An alternative is hair transplants, which do survive in thin scars although with a 'cobblestone' effect. It has been suggested that the first crop of grafts should be at the edge of the defect, gradually approaching the centre of the scar at later sessions.

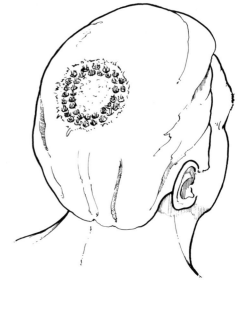

6

7

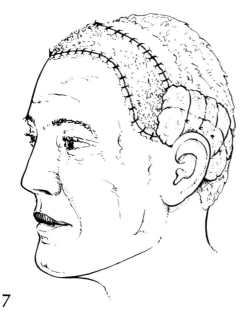

7

Hair-bearing flap

Significant disruption of the anterior hairline can sometimes be much improved by transposing a hair-bearing flap from an area where a secondary skin graft can easily be hidden. The procedure is often well worth while even though the growth of the hair in the transposed flap is in the wrong direction – hairstyling can be very effective.

The recently introduced method of tissue expansion by placing a silicone prosthesis beneath skin adjacent to a defect and expanding it by injection of fluid over a period of weeks enables quite large scalp defects to be closed with expanded hair-bearing scalp, and undoubtedly will have a place in secondary burns surgery. (*See* chapter on 'Tissue expansion in reconstructive surgery', p. 116, Illustration 4).

Scars associated with contracture

If the full range of extension of a joint is lost, because of shortage of the overlying integument in the long axis of a limb, full release must be obtained. Continued use of pressure garments which also stretch the affected flexure, especially the neck, is moderately effective but needs to be continued for at least a year. The alternative of surgery should be considered in every case, and especially for contractures where the operation to import skin across the divided scar is designed for a once and for all release.

The recent development of the fasciocutaneous flap has advanced surgical thinking and design, particularly for the surgery of burn contractures. It is now realized that scarred local skin can be used for the transfer, and that this is not only often possible but desirable. The secondary defect can be sited where closure by suture or by skin graft will produce a scar or graft whose subsequent contracture will *not* start again to impede the movement of the joint which has been released. The previous critisisms of surgical release of contracture, put forward by the proponents of splintage – that multiple operations are often required for release of even minor contractures and that surgical treatment takes as long as non-surgical splintage–are not now tenable in most cases.

Once a contracture across a flexure due to skin shortage is established additional skin in the long axis of the line is required for its release; improvement will not occur with the passage of time alone (in contrast to surface appearance). Scars on extensor surfaces seldom lead to loss of function except on the back of the hand or the dorsum of the foot. Extreme delay in healing over an extensor surface may produce an unstable scar which in the long term may undergo malignant change (Marjolin's ulcer). Treatment of such an ulcer is by simple wide excision and skin grafting, and calls for no special comment except that prognosis is good if the ulcer is still confined to the scarred area but very poor if the disease process has invaded normal skin.

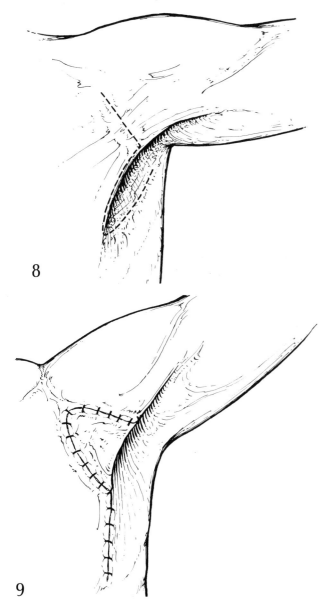

8

9

Z-plasty

Burns scars are seldom the result of linear skin loss (except sometimes those scars due to burns from direct contact with a hot object). Although there may be a web of scarred skin across a flexor surface, indicating longitudinal skin shortage, there is almost always lateral shortage as well. Therefore Z-plasty, which to be successful relies, on achieving extra length by importation of skin from the sides of the defect, has very limited use and is particularly disappointing in scars on the flexor surfaces of the fingers.

Fasciocutaneous transposed flap

A method of release far superior to Z-plasty of localized flexor surface contracture is provided by the transposition of small or medium-sized local fasciocutaneous flaps through 90°.

8 & 9

The main band of contracture is cut across two-thirds of its width, the incision continuing to one edge of the scar. A kite-shaped defect results. A flap large enough to fill the defect is raised in the remaining one-third through scar (or skin graft) and deep fascia. The integument is not disturbed from its attachment to the deep fascia. A length: breadth ratio of 3:1 is perfectly safe. It is important that the base of the flap is co-terminous with the remaining edge of the scar so that full release of the contracture is effected. In less severe contractures the secondary defect can usually be closed by suture. If this results in unacceptable tightness a skin graft may be applied. However, this should be avoided if possible as the graft may be unsightly because of the deep secondary defect and the graft's consequent adherence to muscle.

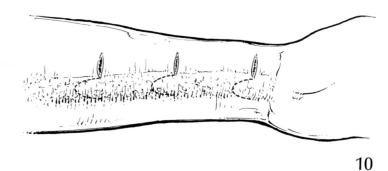

10

10, 11 & 12

For long tight bands on flexor surfaces which stand up slightly from the surrounding skin, multiple small fascio-cutaneous flaps are ideal. These can be based proximally or distally, provided the length:breadth ratio does not exceed 3:1.

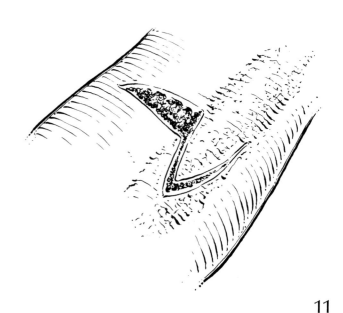

11

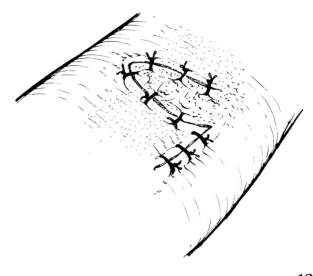

12

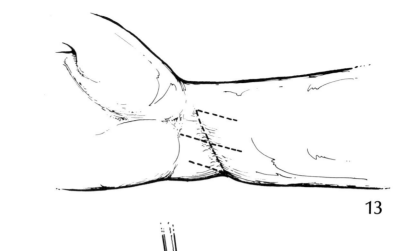

13

13, 14 & 15

Fasciocutaneous Z-plasty

This is very useful to eliminate grooves on extensor or lateral surfaces which are unsightly but not really restricting. The Z-plasty is designed at 60° in the usual way, but since scarred skin is being used the deep fascia must be included in the flap. The correct technique is to incise each side of the Z right through the fascia before lifting the tip with a skin hook, otherwise invariably the fascia is left behind and the scarred flap has insufficient vitality to survive transposition through 90°.

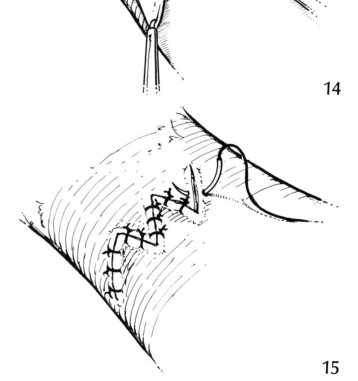

14

15

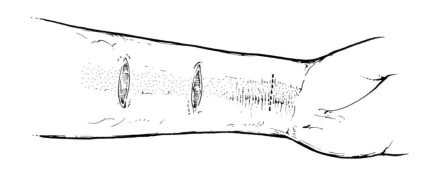

16

16 & 17

Cross-cut and skin graft

If the scar is judged unsuitable for fasciocutaneous flap repair or the surgeon is doubtful of his ability to raise viable flaps, simple cross-cut and skin graft may be acceptable. However, it should be remembered that the skin grafts will themselves contract and a further release may be required at a later date – the fasciocutaneous method provides material that will not shrink.

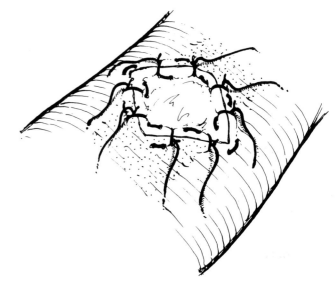

17

Burns of special areas

18a & b

Unstable scars behind the knee

This is a common problem, and can only be solved by adequate surgery. The scar must be excised, not cross-cut. The defect must be made to assume a diamond shape, if necessary by sacrifice of some normal skin at the midpoints of the edges, otherwise a further contracture of the junctional scars will require another (unnecessary) procedure. The skin graft should be as thick as is consistent with reasonable healing of the donor area in order to avoid secondary splintage for the knee, which would be necessary if the graft were thin and liable to shrinkage. (Splintage in extension for some weeks or months is usually quite acceptable for small children, especially in hand or finger burns, but less and less advisable with advancing years for fear of fibrosis in the capsule of the affected joint or joints.)

19 & 20

Cross-cut and conventional transposed skin flaps on the neck

Unscarred local skin may be chosen for resurfacing the cross-cut. In this case conventional skin flaps raised at the deep layer of the superficial fascia may be used so that the secondary defects on the lateral or extensor aspect of the limb can accept skin grafts which will not be adherent to muscle, and which will eventually have quite a good appearance. In practice, this time-consuming repair is seldom preferred to direct skin-grafting of the cross-cut. The exception is on the front of the neck, where even very thick skin grafts are notorious for shrinking to a miserable vestige of their former size.

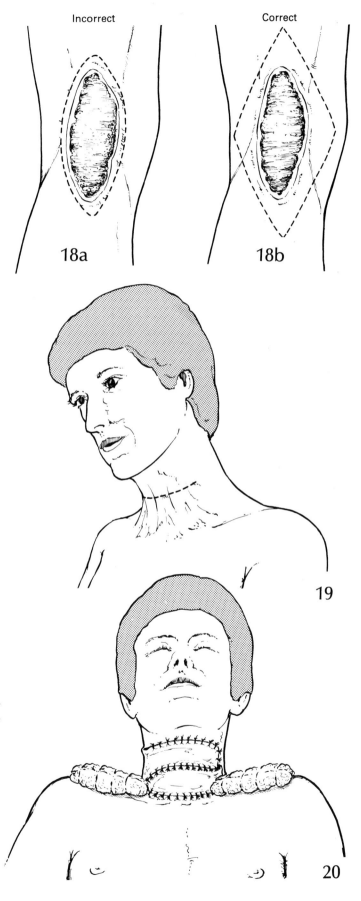

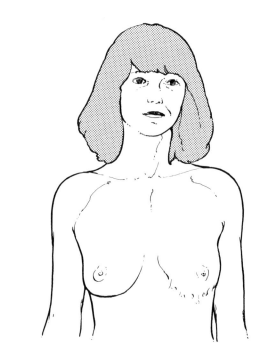

21

Contractures in the region of the breast

In contrast to the neck contracture, contracture under the breast in adolescent girls is best treated by free split skin grafts. The repair is not undertaken before breast development is reasonably well advanced for fear of inserting the graft too high up.

21, 22 & 23

A long curved incision is made across the scar, at the same level as the submammary crease on the opposite side. Then division of scar, fibrous tissue and, if necessary, fascia is continued until the nipple and areola maintain their normal position without tension. It is unusual for this operation to have to be repeated if the correction is undertaken at the right age, and if the release of the contracture has really been complete.

If the nipple and areola have been destroyed, it is seldom possible to produce a convincing substitute by plastic surgery, and in any case the extensive scarring will eliminate any desire on the part of the patient to expose it. A prosthetic nipple stuck on with glue may be helpful: alternatively the 'doughnut' operation may sometimes be worth while in that it does produce a small protuberance on an otherwise featureless mound.

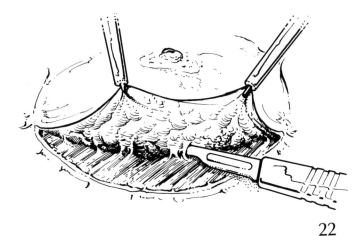

22

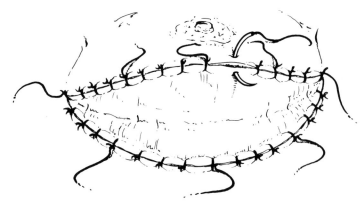

23

24

Two concentric circles are inscribed through the skin at the selected nipple site, the radius of these circles being 0.5 and 2 cm respectively. The wide circular defects so created between the plaques of skin are repaired either by advancement or skin graft. The edge of the skin or skin graft is turned well down the stalk of subcutaneous tissue underlying the skin plaques, and then epithelialization of the exposed fat by secondary intention with fibrosis perpetuates the prominence of the circles of skin, thus mimicking the nipple and areola respectively.

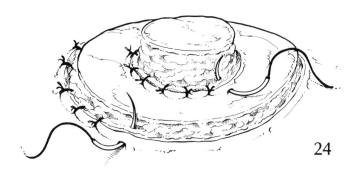

24

Pedicled skin replacement

Pedicled skin cover is required when only badly damaged skin is available locally or when free skin grafts will not be satisfactory – for example when the scar is adherent to bone or joint capsule, or when secondary contracture of the grafts will present a severe problem (e.g. the neck). This may be direct (e.g. cross-arm flap, cross-leg flap) or indirect (tube pedicle).

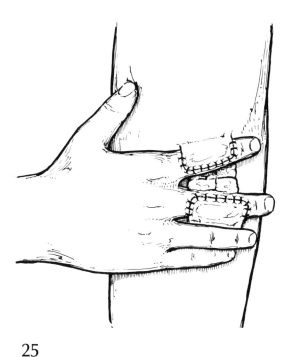

25

Cross-arm flaps

These repairs are particularly useful for resurfacing the extensor aspect of the fingers, when the damage has included destruction of part or all of the extensor tendon. Although there is usually little prospect of repairing or replacing the tendon itself, a good piece of resilient skin will often allow a surprising amount of extensor function to be regained provided the joint itself has not been damaged.

25

The scar is excised down to the mid-lateral line of the affected finger or fingers. Secondary fibrosis of the lateral slips of the extensor tendon is released by partial division of the collateral ligaments to allow the finger to be straightened and flexed at the interphalangeal joints. A pattern of the defect is made from jaconet or similar material and is carefully traced on the donor area on the outer side of the upper arm, allowing sufficient length for the flap to reach and cover the defect without tension. The flap is incised on three sides and raised at the level of the deep fascia. A skin graft is applied to the raw area on the arm and secured with a thin tie-over dressing. The skin flap is then radically thinned, applied to the finger(s) without tension or redundancy and sutured on three sides.

The hand is then secured to the elbow area with Elastoplast slings, leaving the opposite forearm and hand free. The pedicle of the flap is divided and inset at a second operation 2 weeks later.

Cross-leg flaps

Pedicled repairs around the ankle and foot are only occasionally required after burns. The same principles apply as with cross-arm flaps except that the cross-leg flap should not be thinned at the time of transfer because the blood supply of the skin of the leg is much less generous than that of the arm. In addition, an interval of 3 weeks is allowed before the pedicle is severed.

Tube pedicle repairs

26

The tube pedicle repair, although old-fashioned, still has a place in secondary burns surgery and should be considered for severe contractures of the neck, extensive damage to the hand and major tissue loss around the face. So often the patient who has recovered from an extensive severe burn is left with a defect which is not remediable with local tissue, because all surrounding damage, although less severe, has produced skin unacceptable for transfer. Tube pedicle repairs are very time-consuming, and if experienced microvascular expertise is available the same result may be achieved by using free flaps.

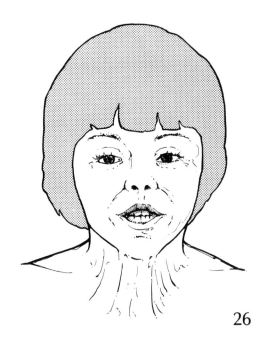

26

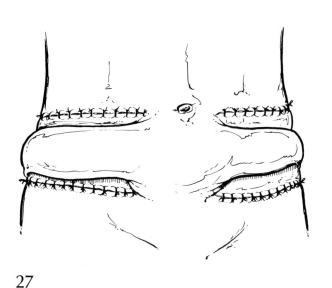

27

27 & 28

Tube pedicles may be constructed on any undamaged area of skin but commonly the lower abdomen is chosen. If the area has been used as a donor site for skin grafts, and a definite change in the appearance is visible, indicating dermal damage, an alternative site should be sought, because although a tube can be *constructed* in such an area, *transfer* will prove extremely hazardous and many 'delays' will be required.

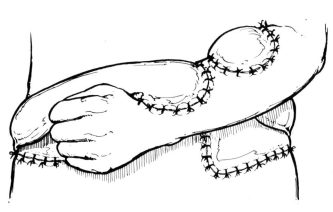

28

29–31

Three weeks are required between stages, but usually delays are unnecessary except for division of the second end on the abdomen. The whole repair should be planned so that end of the tube which is being worked on will *not* be in a dependent position for the first few days after its transfer. Once both ends have been transferred, considerable liberties can be taken to spread and thin the tissue to best advantage. Although the procedure is protracted and trying, the long-term result is almost always a sufficient reward for both the patient and the surgeon.

Reference

Huang, T. T., Blackwell, S. J., Lewis, S. R. Ten years of experience in managing patients with burn contractures of axilla, elbow, wrist and knee joints. Plastic and Reconstructive Surgery, 1978; 61: 70–76

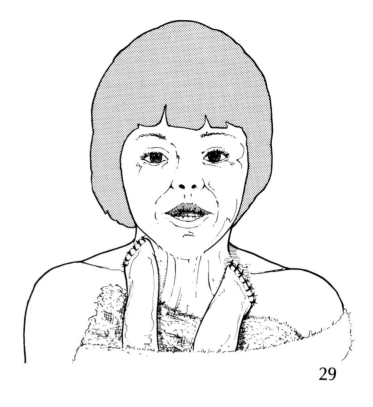

29

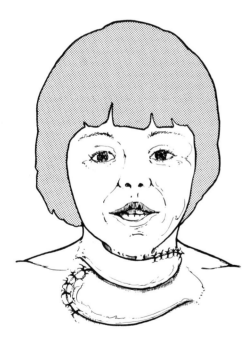

30

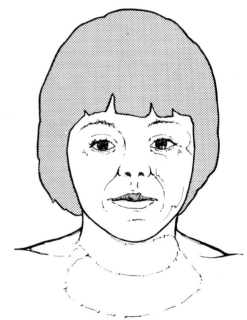

31

Illustrations by John W. Karapelou

Reduction mammoplasty

Norman E. Hugo MD
Professor of Surgery, College of Physicians and Surgeons, Columbia University
Chief, Plastic Surgery, Department of Surgery, Columbia–Presbyterian Medical Center, New York, USA

Indications

Mammary hypertrophy associated with back and neck pain, shoulder grooves from brassiere straps, slumped shoulders and kyphosis, intertrigo in the inframammary folds, dyspnoea, and nerve compression with arm and digital symptoms, as well as the generalized discomfort and poor self-image due to the exceptionally large size of the breasts are all indications for reduction mammoplasty.

Contraindications

Surgery is contraindicated when associated medical problems make the risk of operation unacceptably high.

Preoperative

Because of the difficulty of performing a satisfactory breast examination, a preoperative mammogram should be obtained, to be followed by a postoperative mammogram to document perioperative changes (fat necrosis) and to be used for comparison with future examinations.

All markings and measurements should be made the night before or on the morning of surgery with the patient standing erect (see below).

Anaesthesia

General endotracheal anaesthesia is necessary.

Position of patient

The patient lies supine, with the upper body flexed 20° and the arms abducted from the sides to 45°. Preoperative skin preparation and draping should be done widely, to include the clavicles, lateral chest walls just above the table and abdominal wall to the level of the umbilicus. Suturing or stapling the drapes to the skin is helpful.

Markings

1

Certain key lines are marked out on the erect patient to establish reference points. It is preferable to mark these lines with the patient standing. If sitting, the patient may list to one side and throw off the markings. The nipple line passes from the midclavicular point through the nipple. Using this line as the reference for superior elevation of the nipple–areolar complex enhances symmetry and maintains the nipple in proper position with the reconstructed mammary mound. The midsternal line extends from the sternal notch through the xiphoid to the umbilicus. The single most important step in breast reduction is the proper selection of the new nipple site.

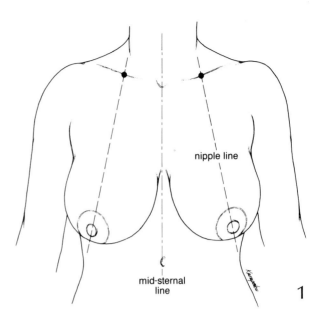

2

Regardless of the method employed to reduce the size of the breast, the initial step of determining where the nipple will be placed is critical and all other steps follow. The nipple should rest at the level of the inframammary fold. Its position is located by placing the fingers at the inframammary fold and the thumb opposite them on the nipple line.

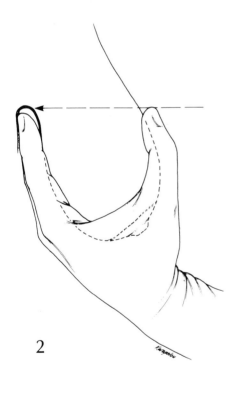

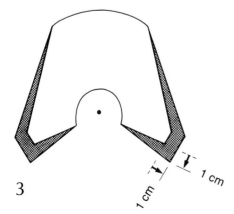

3

The Wise pattern or a modification is used to mark out the skin incisions. The modified pattern is 1 cm longer and each distal point 1 cm closer to the midline. This helps to reduce tension on the vertical closure, producing a more natural look. Before proceeding, the surgeon checks to see that vertical closure is possible simply by demonstrating that the vertical limbs will meet at the nipple line.

The operations

FREE GRAFT

4

The pattern is placed on the breast with its midpoints aligned on the nipple line. The nipple–areolar complex is marked out with a washer of 4.5 cm diameter.

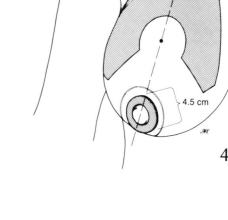

4

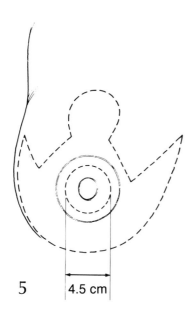

5 4.5 cm

5

The lines of incision are then drawn. The surgeon now decides how the nipple–areolar complex will be moved, by free graft (usually reserved for older patients with gigantomastia) or by pedicle. If a free graft is used, the nipple–areolar complex is amputated, making sure that it is of the correct size (4.5 cm in diameter).

6

The breast within the markings is amputated and the new nipple site de-epithelialized.

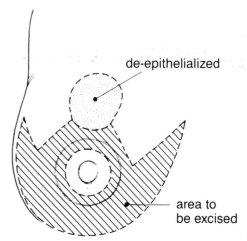

de-epithelialized

area to be excised

6

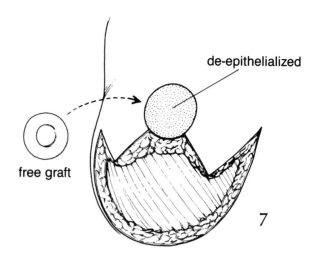

7 & 8

The nipple–areolar complex is sutured on to the de-epithelialized site and then secured by a tie-over bolus. The wound is closed in layers, using subcuticular sutures for the skin closure.

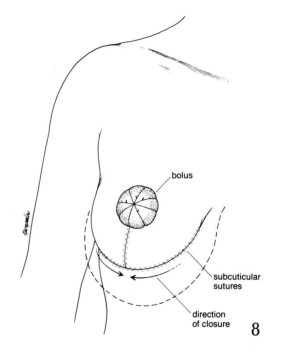

PEDICLE FLAPS

If the nipple–areolar complex is to be moved on a pedicle, this may be a bipedicle[1] or a single pedicle, based either superiorly[2] or inferiorly[3]. The vertical bipedicle technique is often used because of its dual blood supply. The disadvantages of this method are the prolonged operating time, the exposure of large raw areas during the operation, and a tendency postoperatively for the breast

to look bulky and square at its inferior aspect. The single superiorly based pedicle method is often used but the maximum length of this pedicle is limited to 18 cm, making it unsuitable for very large breasts. There is less tendency with this method to create a boxy look and the operating time is shorter. The inferiorly based pedicle retains vascular continuity with the chest wall through a substantial pedicle and this method is indicated when a massive reduction must be carried out.

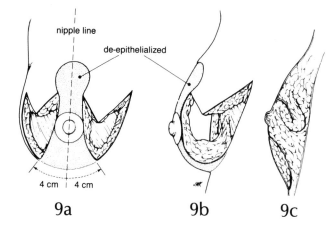

9a   9b   9c

Vertical bipedicle

9a–c

After the carrying pedicle for the nipple–areolar complex has been marked out for one of the three methods, the pedicle is de-epithelialized so that it can be moved and buried within the breast. In the vertical bipedicle method the inferior margin of the pedicle is 8 cm so as to incorporate as many vessels as possible. The breast is debulked by removing tissue medially and laterally, and by thinning of the pedicle. The inferior portion of the pedicle is thick to assure the blood supply.

The nipple–areolar complex is now advanced to its new location by folding the superior pedicle on itself.

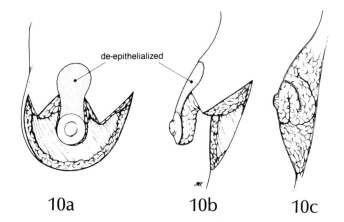

10a   10b   10c

Superiorly based pedicle

10a–c

In the superior pedicle method the pedicle is created in similar fashion to the inferior pedicle, except that the inferior pedicle is amputated. The superior pedicle can be as thin as one centimetre.

The nipple–areolar complex is relocated by folding the pedicle upon itself.

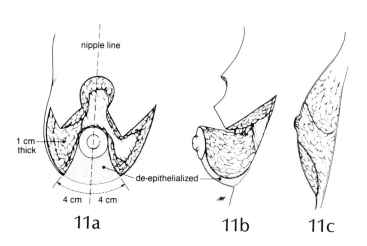

11a   11b   11c

Inferiorly based pedicle

11a–c

In the inferior pedicle method the pedicle is also created in similar fashion, except that the superior pedicle is amputated. The lateral portion of the breast is not removed to the depth of the pectoralis fascia but a layer of fat one centimetre thick is preserved lateral to the pedicle with the object of preserving sensation to the nipple. In addition, the inferior pedicle retains its entire attachment to the chest wall to retain as much vascularity as possible

The nipple–areolar complex is advanced to the new site without folding upon itself.

Wound closure

12

The wound is closed in layers, using absorbable sutures deep and subcuticular nylon sutures for the skin. The areolar is sutured·with continuous running sutures of fine nylon. Whatever the method chosen, the de-epithelialized pedicle is always buried. The horizontal closure progresses from the lateral and medial extremities to the midline in order to minimize 'dog-ears'. The use of drains is discretionary.

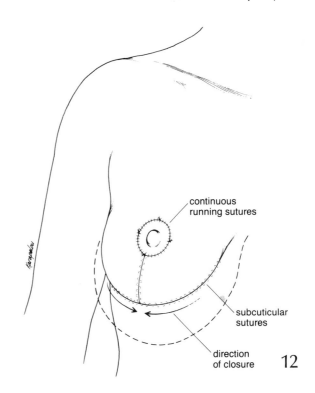

continuous
running sutures

subcuticular
sutures

direction
of closure   12

References

1. McKissock, P. K. Reduction mammoplasty with a vertical dermal flap. Plastic and Reconstructive Surgery 1972; 49: 245–252

2. Hugo, N. E., McClellan, R. M. Reduction mammoplasty with a single superiorly based pedicle. Plastic and Reconstructive Surgery 1979; 63: 230–234

3. Courtiss, E. H., Goldwyn, R. M. Reduction mammoplasty by the inferior pedicle technique: an alternative to free nipple and aveola grafting for severe macromastia or extreme ptosis. Plastic and Reconstructive Surgery 1977; 59: 400–407

Breast augmentation

Elethea H. Caldwell MD
Assistant Professor of Plastic Surgery, University of Rochester
School of Medicine and Dentistry, Rochester, New York, USA

Preoperative

Indications and patient selection

Breast augmentation is an appropriate procedure for patients with developmental mammary hypoplasia, atrophy of breast tissue following pregnancy, significant weight loss or mammary asymmetry. Careful patient selection is essential and must include an evaluation of both physical appearance and emotional stability. The patient's desire to improve her self-image is important in the evaluation of the latter.

Contraindications

Relative contraindications to breast augmentation are: recent breast abscess; diffuse cystic mastitis or breast tumour and true ptosis.

Anaesthesia

The procedure may be done under general or local anaesthesia. If local anaesthesia is used 30–50 ml of 0.5 per cent lignocaine (lidocaine) with adrenaline (epinephrine) 1:200 000 are injected into the retromammary space on each side.

Selection of prosthesis

Silicone elastomer mammary prostheses are used for most breast augmentation procedures. Various contours are available. A teardrop-shaped prosthesis is used where limited breast tissue is present and provides an accentuated profile. A round prosthesis offers a moderate profile and eliminates any concern about orientation of the prosthesis at the time of insertion. An inflatable prosthesis, which can be inserted through a very small incision, is particularly useful in mammary asymmetry because varying amounts of normal saline may be introduced into the filling valve to achieve the desired size. Contour and feel are similar to the gel-filled prosthesis.

Incisions

Mammary prostheses may be inserted through a submammary, periareolar or transaxillary incision. The submammary and periareolar incisions are most popular.

The operation

SUBMAMMARY APPROACH

1

The incision

A 5–6 cm incision is made in the submammary crease, placing one-third of the incision medial to a point dropped perpendicular from the nipple and two-thirds of the incision lateral to that point. If an inflatable prosthesis is used a 2 cm incision is required.

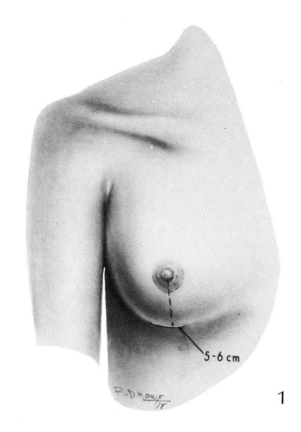

1

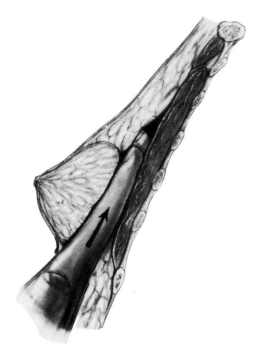

2

2

Development of the pocket

Following incision of skin, subcutaneous tissue and fat, haemostasis should be achieved. The correct plane of dissection is the retromammary space between the posterior capsule of the breast and the pectoralis major fascia. This plane appears as a fine areolar layer and is essentially a bloodless plane. The best method for developing the pocket is by blunt finger dissection.

3

The pocket position

The superior and lateral portion of the dissection to the anterior axillary line is achieved without difficulty. The medial portion of the dissection to the sternum is more difficult because of fibrous attachments between the skin and the costal cartilages. It is essential that the pocket be developed far enough medially or the breasts will appear too far apart. The pocket should be large enough so that there is no constriction of the prosthesis.

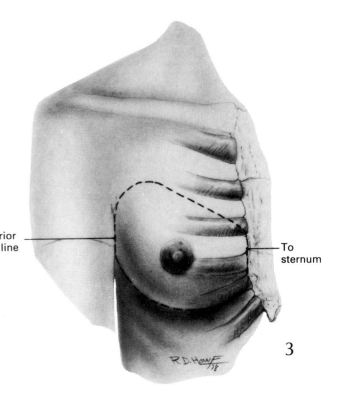

To anterior axillary line

To sternum

3

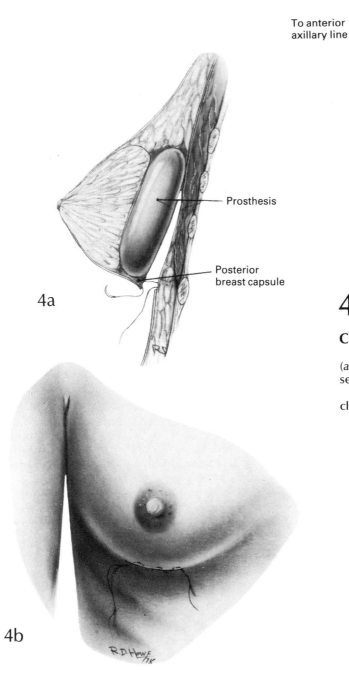

Prosthesis

Posterior breast capsule

4a

4b

4a & b

Closure of the incision

(a) The posterior capsule of the breast is sutured to the serratus anterior fascia using absorbable suture material.

(b) A continuous subcuticular suture is used for skin closure.

PERIAREOLAR APPROACH

If this approach is used an inflatable prosthesis should be employed.

5

The incision

A half-circle circumareolar incision is made.

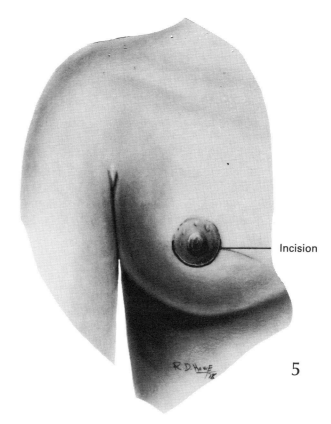

Incision

5

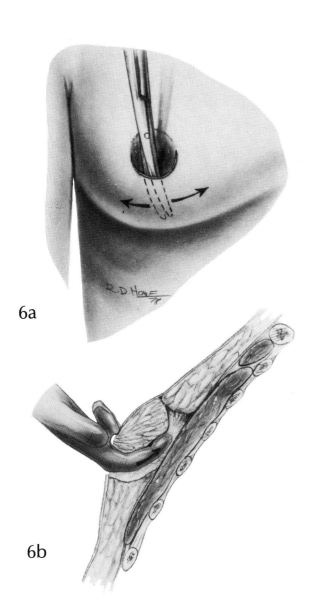

6a

6b

6a & b

Development of the pocket

The skin and subcutaneous tissue are undermined to the lower pole of the gland by blunt dissection using scissors. A pocket is created in the retromammary space using blunt finger dissection. This approach does not involve entering the gland.

7

Closure of the incision

A two-layer closure is carried out using a fine, absorbable suture in the subcutaneous layer and a continuous subcuticular suture of non-absorbable material in the cutaneous layer.

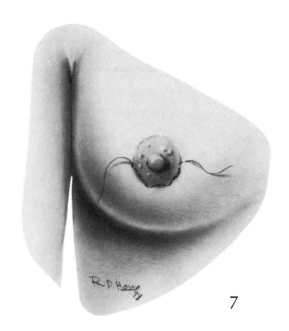

7

Postoperative care

No drains are required. A well-padded, secure dressing is constructed to provide support for the prostheses. This dressing is worn for 1 week and the patient then wears a soft bra night and day. The sutures remain for 2 weeks. Arm motion is restricted for 2 weeks after removal of the surgical dressing. At the end of the first week the patient is instructed on gentle massage of the mammary prostheses.

Complications

Early complications

Bleeding with haematoma formation and infection are the most common early complications. If meticulous haemostasis is achieved during the procedure and adequate sterile technique is observed, these complications should occur very infrequently.

Late complications

Capsular contracture is the most common late complication. In the body, the prosthesis is encapsulated by a fibrous envelope. If this envelope becomes thickened and develops progressive contracture, the breasts become hard to palpation and distorted in shape. The prosthesis migrates upwards with a downward migration of the nipple. Capsular contracture may be painful, requiring removal of the prosthesis or rupture of the capsule by external compression. A high rate of recurrence has been observed following rupture of the capsule.

Extrusion of the prosthesis is another late complication. It may be secondary to a haematoma or seroma which opens the incision spontaneously. Thin skin cover and scars may lead to extrusion of the prosthesis as the overlying skin may undergo avascular necrosis. Capsular contracture may also result in prosthetic extrusion. This is due to avascularity and inelasticity of the cutaneous incision as contracture occurs.

No association has been made between breast augmentation and the development of breast cancer. Breast augmentation does not alter the physiological function of the breast, and it is possible for the patient to breast-feed, although decrease in nipple sensation is sometimes experienced.

Further reading

Cronin, T. D., Greenberg, R. L. Our experiences with the Silastic gel breast prosthesis. Plastic and Reconstructive Surgery 1970; 46: 1–7

Gurdin, M., Carlin, G. A. Complications of breast implantations. Plastic and Reconstructive Surgery 1967; 40: 530–533

Regnault, P. Indications for breast augmentation. Plastic and Reconstructive Surgery 1967; 40: 524–529

Williams, J. E. Experiences with a large series of silastic breast implants. Plastic and Reconstructive Surgery 1972; 49: 253–258

Illustrated by Michael E. Leonard and Robert L. Margulies

Breast reconstruction

Gregory S. Georgiade MD
Assistant Professor, General and Plastic and Reconstructive Surgery,
Duke University Medical Centre, Durham, North Carolina 27710, USA

Nicholas G. Georgiade MD, FACS
Chairman and Professor, Division of Plastic and Reconstructive Surgery,
Duke University Medical Centre, Durham, North Carolina 27710, USA

Introduction

The following basic illustrations shows the techniques available to the surgeon attempting to reconstruct the breast mound and nipple and areola complex following a modified radical mastectomy for carcinoma of the breast.

The choice of technique depends on the severity of the deformity created by the mastectomy, the quality of the surrounding skin, and the muscles of the chest wall.

The operations

IMMEDIATE RECONSTRUCTION OF THE BREAST MOUND

Immediate reconstruction of the breast mound[1,2] at the time of the ablative procedure is the operation of choice in patients with small carcinomas requiring minimal skin resection who have a favourable prognosis for their primary breast cancer.

1

Immediately following the modified radical mastectomy, the serratus anterior muscle and the pectoralis major muscle are elevated from the underlying chest wall starting at the level of the seventh rib.

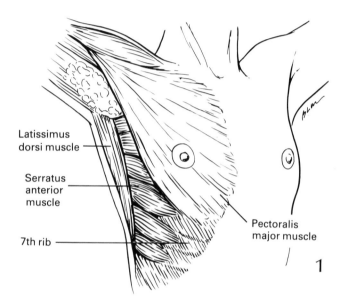

2

The completed elevation will include the inferior portion of the serratus anterior muscle to the level of the seventh rib, the pectoralis major muscle and medially a portion of the rectus abdominus fascia which will produce a large submuscular pocket suitable for prosthesis insertion.

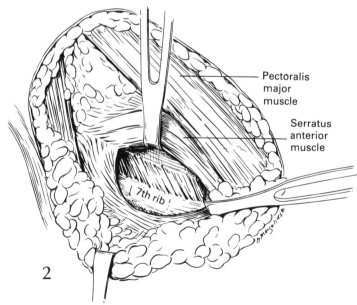

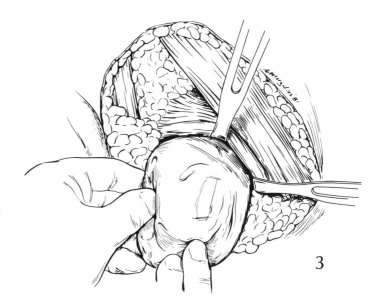

3

The prosthesis is inserted in the subserratus, subpectoral pocket, and the muscle defect is then closed after insertion of a suction drain in the lateral aspect of the muscular pocket. The skin closure is then accomplished in two layers after a drain has been placed in the area of the axillary dissection.

3

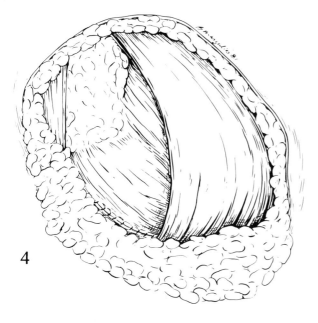

4

4

A sterile, bulky, compression dressing is then applied. The nipple areola complex can be reconstructed at the time of the immediate reconstruction, but in most patients it will be delayed until after the breast mound has gone through its natural process of settling and balancing with the opposite breast.

DELAYED BREAST MOUND RECONSTRUCTION OF POSTOPERATIVE DEFORMITY WITH PECTORAL MUSCLES AND SERRATUS MUSCLES INTACT

Correction of the postoperative deformity of the chest wall after a modified radical mastectomy will depend on the type of incision, presence or absence of pectoral muscle, and quality of skin coverage. This will vary widely from patient to patient. For this reason there are a number of different techniques which have been developed to facilitate reconstruction of the breast mound.

In the patient who has good quality skin coverage and intact innervated pectoral and serratus musculature, the breast mound can be reconstructed with a subserratus, subpectoral prosthesis in much the same manner just described in patients undergoing immediate reconstruction of the breast.

5

An incision is made at the level of either the sixth or seventh rib inferiorly through the skin of the anterior chest wall, approximately 1.5 cm below the contralateral inframammary skin crease level. After reconstruction of the breast mound, this incision will be situated in the inframammary crease region.

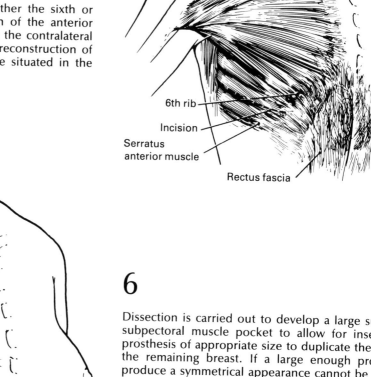

Pectoralis major muscle

6th rib

Incision

Serratus anterior muscle

Rectus fascia

5

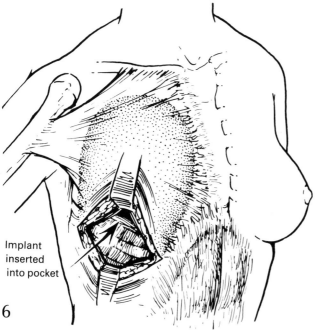

Implant inserted into pocket

6

6

Dissection is carried out to develop a large subserratus, subpectoral muscle pocket to allow for insertion of a prosthesis of appropriate size to duplicate the volume of the remaining breast. If a large enough prosthesis to produce a symmetrical appearance cannot be inserted at this time, then the breast mound can either be enlarged as a secondary procedure 4–6 months later or a tissue expander can be inserted.

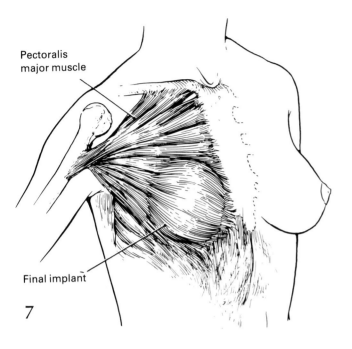

Pectoralis
major muscle

Final implant

7

7

The position of the prosthesis is shown in the subserratus, subpectoral pocket after suturing of the muscle edges prior to closure of the skin.

DELAYED BREAST MOUND RECONSTRUCTION OF POSTOPERATIVE DEFORMITY WITH DEFICIENCY OF SKIN AT OPERATIVE SITE

A postmastectomy patient who has a relative deficiency of skin in the area of the mastectomy but good quality skin in the surrounding loose abdominal tissues and upper chest tissues is a candidate for a procedure which requires wide undermining of these areas to affect reconstruction[3,4].

8

A new inframammary crease line must be created at the time of undermining. The wide area which is undermined is shown by the dotted region. This must be carefully planned to match the inframammary crease area of the contralateral breast.

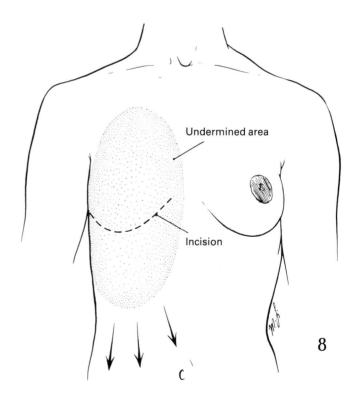

Undermined area

Incision

8

9

The abdominal tissue is advanced to the new infra-mammary line area and is sutured to the periosteum of the seventh rib.

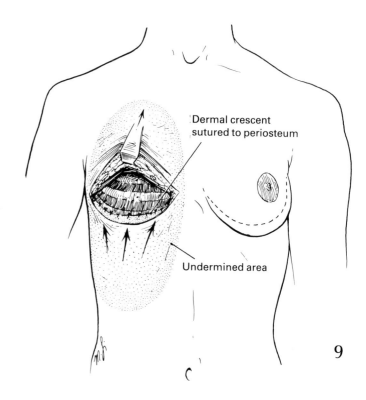

Dermal crescent sutured to periosteum

Undermined area

9

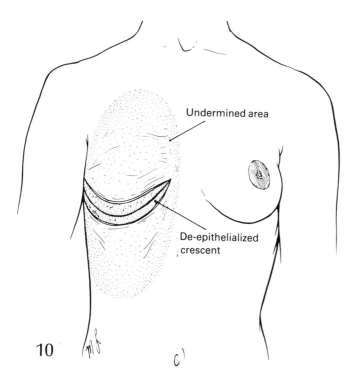

Undermined area

De-epithelialized crescent

10

10

The superior and inferior skin flaps are de-epithelialized and interpolated in order to buttress the newly created inframammary crease.

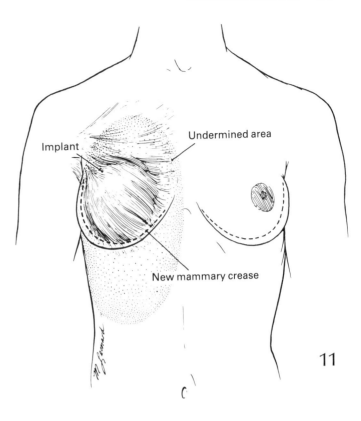

11

A suitably sized prosthesis is inserted in the subserratus subpectoral position, and the new inframammary crease is then closed with the overlapping of the superior and inferior de-epithelialized skin flaps.

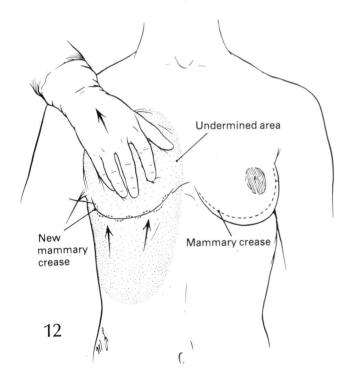

12

The final closure of the inframammary crease area is carried out with a subcuticular pull-out nylon suture.

PROGRESSIVE TISSUE EXPANSION WITH EXPANDABLE PROSTHESIS

Postoperative deformities with extensive scar contracture, which do not lend themselves well to the creation of a large submuscular pocket at the time of prosthesis insertion, may be managed by the gradual expansion of the skin pocket if there is adequate good quality skin and muscle within the region[5].

13

The initial incision can be made in the anterior axillary area or through the scar of the previous mastectomy incisions. A suitable area for the tissue expander can be undermined through these incisions as shown in the dotted areas.

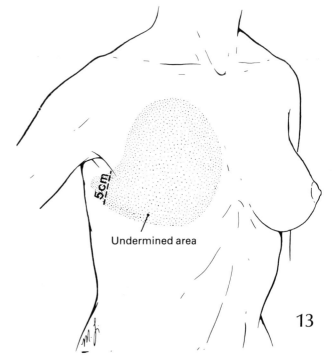

5 cm

Undermined area

13

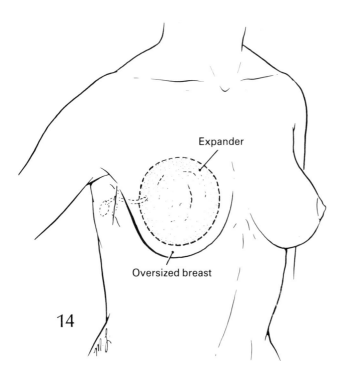

Expander

Oversized breast

14

14

The tissue expander of suitable size is then inserted and filled with saline to the point of creating tension on the overlying tissues, and the expanding valve is placed subcutaneously in the lateral axillary region.

15

Additional saline is added at monthly intervals in the axillary area. This addition can be carried out either blindly into the expanding valve or under direct vision, depending on the body habitus of the patient and the difficulty in identifying the valve.

The final breast prosthesis is inserted approximately 6 months later after adequate expansion of the chest wall tissue has been achieved. This can usually be carried out through the previous surgical approach to the area.

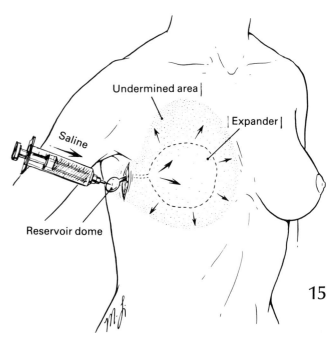

Undermined area

Expander

Saline

Reservoir dome

15

RECONSTRUCTION OF THE PATIENT WITH A LARGE SKIN OR MUSCLE DEFECT OF CHEST WALL

This procedure can be carried out with several different techniques which involve bringing tissue of adequate volume and texture into the area on its own vascular supply to provide for the necessary volume for reconstruction of the breast mound[6,7].

16

The latissimus dorsi muscle and its overlying skin can be used as a myocutaneous flap to provide a substitute for resected pectoral muscle, at the same time bringing in more skin to allow for adequate skin flaps to produce an appropriately sized breast mound. The skin island can be oriented in a number of directions, the most common of which is the oblique direction as shown.

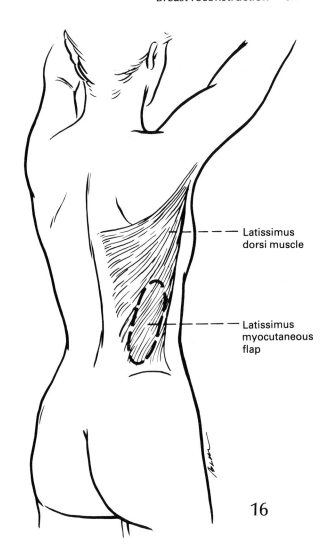

— Latissimus dorsi muscle

— Latissimus myocutaneous flap

16

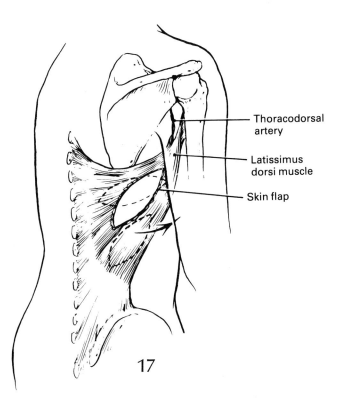

— Thoracodorsal artery

— Latissimus dorsi muscle

— Skin flap

17

17

The flap may also be oriented either transversely, or more horizontally as shown. Also note that blood supply to the muscle is through the thoracodorsal artery and vein which allows transposition of the myocutaneous unit on this vascular pedicle alone (*see Illustration 19*).

18

The previously designed skin and muscle flap is rotated to its new position on the chest wall where the latissimus muscle is fanned out and sutured in place with interrupted absorbable sutures. If possible this skin island is placed in a transverse position as shown. At the completion of the latissimus muscle transposition, a large submuscular pocket with sufficient overlying skin will have been created, allowing for prosthesis insertion to produce a breast mound of adequate size, shape and contour.

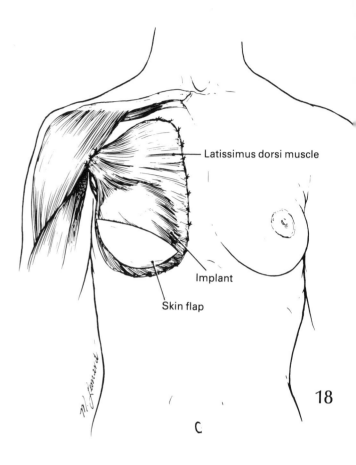

18

19

In some patients there will be adequate skin coverage but inadequate muscle coverage secondary to either denervation or resection of a portion of the pectoralis or serratus musclature. In this situation, a transposition of the latissimus muscle can be carried out to provide for adequate muscle coverage to allow for later prosthesis insertion. This is generally done through a small transverse incision on the back in the bra line to allow adequate exposure of the latissimus muscle at the point where it is freed from its insertion along the spine and spinal processes and transposed anteriorly, preserving the thoracodorsal blood supply.

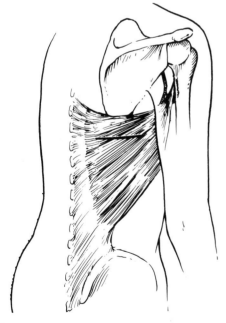

19

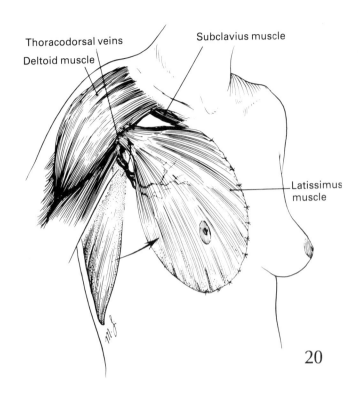

20

It is then fanned out and sutured into place in the same fashion as described for the myocutaneous flap and a prosthesis is again inserted behind it. Note the location of the thoracodorsal artery and vein.

20

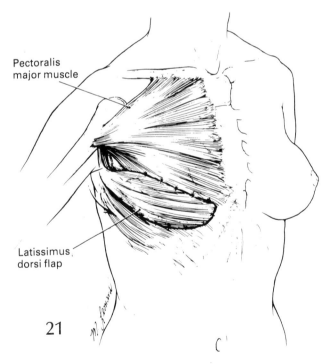

21

21

When only a portion of the pectoralis muscle has been removed during the ablative surgery a portion of the latissimus muscle can be transferred to recreate the necessary bulk to the pectoralis muscle.

ABSENCE OF PECTORALIS MUSCLE

In patients who have a post mastectomy deformity with absence of the pectoralis muscle, extensive scarring and denervation of the latissimus dorsi muscle, the rectus abdominus myocutaneous flap should be considered as the technique of choice for breast reconstruction. This flap, much like the latissimus dorsi myocutaneous flap, is a myocutaneous flap in which the carrier muscle provides the circulation to the overlying skin island, but unlike the latissimus flap the rectus abdominus flap has a much more extensive muscle pedicle[8, 9].

22

A large skin flap is developed on the lower abdominal area based on the blood supply to the rectus muscle on the side opposite the chest deformity to be reconstructed. This flap is supplied by the superior epigastric artery and vein from the internal mammary circulation.

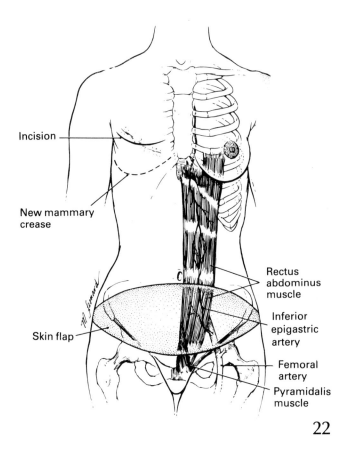

22

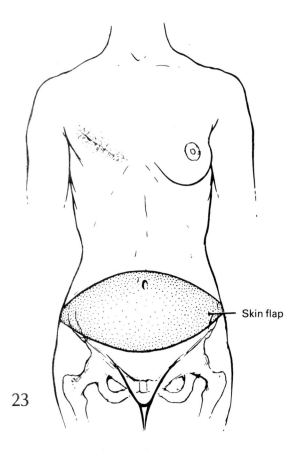

23

23

It is usually preferable if the myocutaneous unit designed on the abomen covers an area extending above the umbilicus. The ensures adequate circulation to the skin and reduces potential problems with postoperative hernia formation in the anterior abdominal wall. The skin of the anterior abdomen is elevated to the costochondral margins, and a large tunnel is created to contact with the elevated skin flaps from the prior mastectomy. A portion of the rectus fascia is incised medially and laterally, to be elevated later with the flap itself (*see Illustration 25*).

24

The abdominal skin flap is elevated until it reaches the area of the rectus fascia, with perforators through the fascia. These can be seen both medially and laterally. Either the rectus sheath is incised at this point, exposing the underlying rectus muscle, or a portion of the anterior rectus fascia is allowed to remain attached to the rectus muscle as shown. The latter option allows the rectus muscle to retain greater integrity and also saves operative time. The incision is carried to the skin flap and along the entire course of the rectus abdominus muscle. Note that a safer flap is created if the paraumbilical perforating vessels are included as shown in Illustration 23.

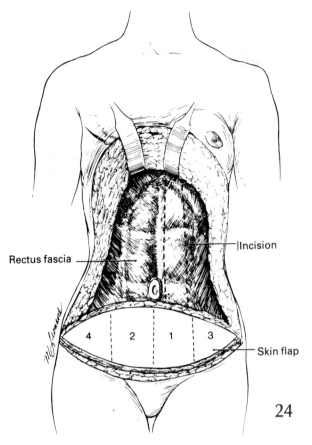

24

25

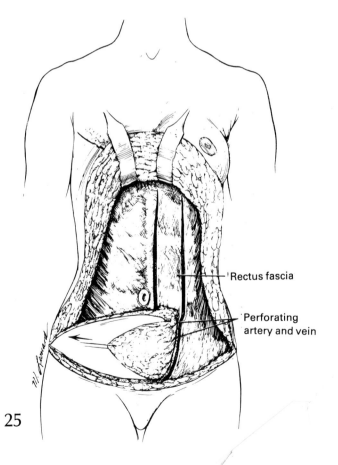

25

25

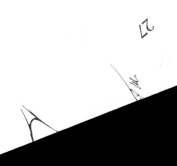

The inferior epigastric arte... inferior lateral portion ... ligated at the time th... the ches... wall are...

26

The rectus muscle is then freed from the underlying posterior rectus sheath, and the entire myocutaneous unit is transposed to the chest area.

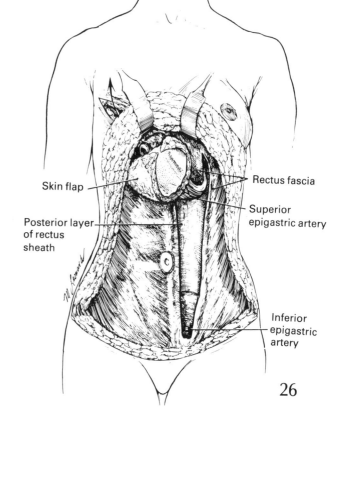

Skin flap

Posterior layer of rectus sheath

Rectus fascia

Superior epigastric artery

Inferior epigastric artery

26

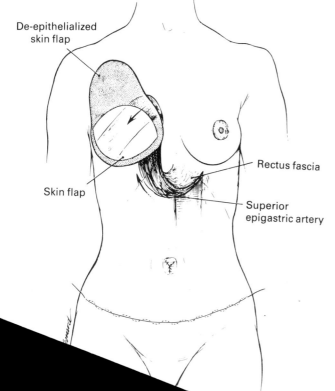

De-epithelialized skin flap

Skin flap

Rectus fascia

Superior epigastric artery

27

The skin of the chest wall has already been elevated. Next the rectus abdominus flap is brought into the area of the elevated skin flaps and is contoured in this position to match the opposite breast mound. Usually an area of the rectus skin flap will be de-epithelialized and inset under the skin flaps to provide for a suitable degree of ptosis and contouring of the breast mound to make it as symmetrical as possible to the opposite breast. The fascial defect in the lower abdomen is then closed with the addition of Marlex mesh if necessary and the abdominal skin is approximated with a new umbilicus created from the old umbilicus. Alternatively an umbilicus can be reconstructed if the umbilicus has remained part of the transposed flap.

RECONSTRUCTION OF THE NIPPLE AREOLA COMPLEX

The final step of breast reconstruction is the creation of the nipple areola complex. This can be carried out by a number of different techniques[10].

28

Creation of the nipple areola complex is most commonly carried out with the use of a combination of a full-thickness groin skin graft to create the areola, and nipple sharing from the opposite nipple. Prior to nipple areola reconstruction, the proposed site of the new complex is marked with the patient in a standing position and then a full-thickness skin graft is harvested from the groin area. This area is selected because the greater pigmentation of this region more closely matches the usual areolar colour.

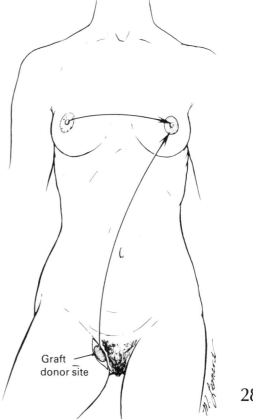

Graft donor site

28

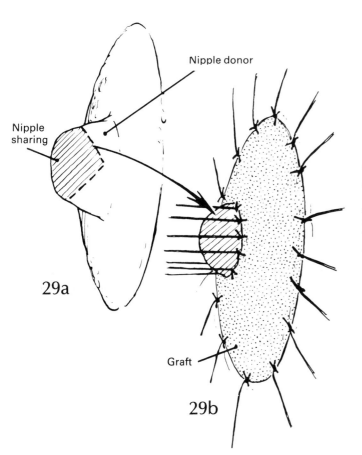

Nipple donor

Nipple sharing

29a

Graft

29b

29a & b

A wedge of the contralateral nipple is harvested and the nipple defect is closed. The groin skin graft is placed on the previously marked de-epithelialized area of the areola and sutured in place with interrupted sutures. The harvested nipple wedge is then placed in the central portion of the areola and sutured in place. A bolus tie-over dressing is used to fix the skin graft to its underlying bed.

CONSTRUCTION OF THE NIPPLE

30a–f

In this technique, the nipple is constructed using a central core of breast mound and wrap-around full-thickness skin graft to fill in the newly created defect and to yield a nipple-like projection. The use of an elevated plastic stent to maintain the newly created elevated nipple in position for approximately one week has also been found to be of advantage.

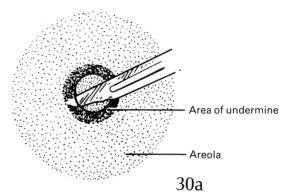

Area of undermine

Areola

30a

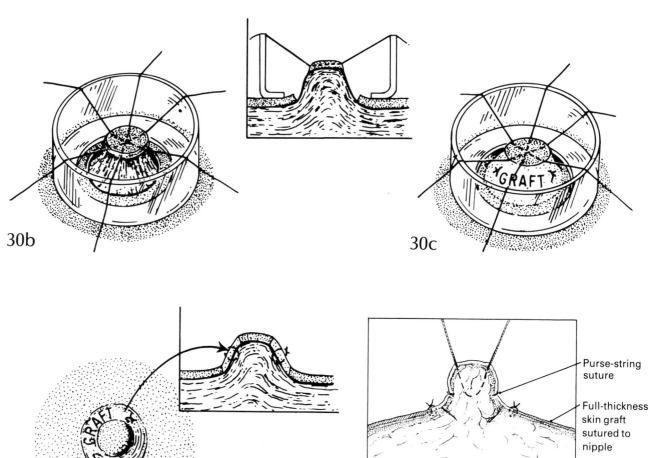

30b

GRAFT

30c

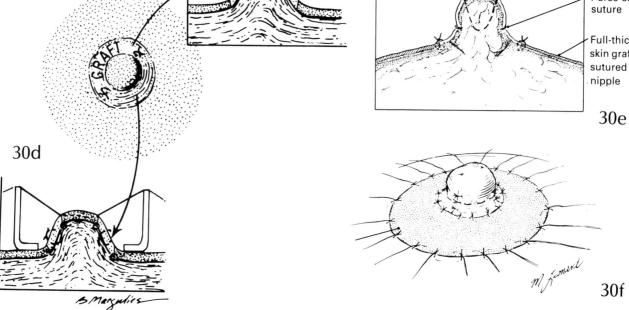

30d

GRAFT

Purse-string suture

Full-thickness skin graft sutured to nipple

30e

30f

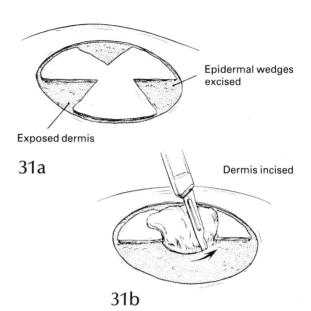

Epidermal wedges excised

Exposed dermis

31a

Dermis incised

31b

31a & b

This alternative technique involves creation of three large epithelial flaps sutured together to form a nipple projection.

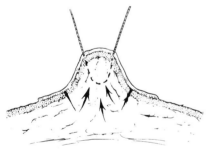

32a

Nipple raised
and remaining epidermis excised

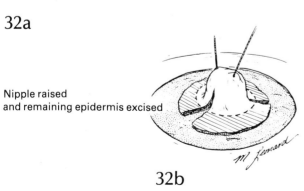

32b

32a & b

It is important to place a purse-string suture at the new nipple base. The remainder of unexcised skin is trimmed, and a full-thickness groin graft is used for the new areola.

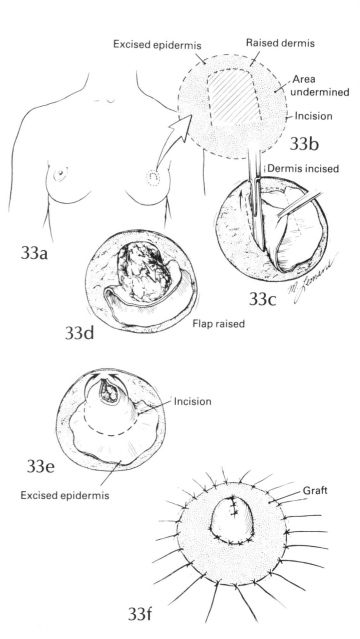

33a–f

Construction of the nipple can also be carried out utilizing either a superiorly or inferiorly based skin breast mound flap and underlying fat flap.

Note: The constructed nipple can be tattooed if increased pigmentation is needed. Undermined skin from the areola is used to wrap around the underlying elevated flap in order to create the nipple with projection (*see Illustrations 33d and 33e*). The excess is trimmed, and the areola is constructed using a groin full-thickness skin graft (*see Illustration 33f*).

References

1. Georgiade, N. G., ed. Breast reconstruction following mastectomy. St Louis: C. V. Mosby Co., 1979

2. Georgiade, G., Georgiade, N., McCarty, K. S. Jr., Seigler, H. F. Rationale for immediate reconstruction of the breast following modified radical mastectomy. Annals of Plastic Surgery 1982; 8: 20–28

3. Ryan, J. J. A lower thoracic advancement flap in breast reconstruction after mastectomy. Plastic and Reconstructive Surgery 1982; 70: 153–160

4. Lewis, J. R. Jr. Use of a sliding flap from the abdomen to provide cover in breast reconstruction. Plastic and Reconstructive Surgery 1979; 64: 491–497

5. Radovan, C. Breast reconstruction after mastectomy using the temporary expander. Plastic and Reconstructive Surgery 1982; 69: 195–208

6. Bostwick, J. III. Aesthetic and reconstructive breast surgery. St Louis: C. V. Mosby Co., 1983; 379

7. Bostwick, J. Vasconez, L., Jurkiewicz, M. J. Breast reconstruction after radical mastectomy. Plastic and Reconstructive Surgery 1978; 61: 682–693

8. Hartrampf, C. R., Scheflan, M., Black, P. W. Breast reconstruction with a transverse abdominal island flap. Plastic and Reconstructive Surgery 1982; 69: 216–225

9. Elliot, L. F., Hartrampf, C. R. Tailoring of the new breast using the transverse abdominal island flap. Plastic and Reconstructive Surgery 1983; 72: 887–893

10. Serafin, D., Georgiade, N. Nipple-areola reconstruction after mastectomy. Annals of Plastic Surgery 1982; 8: 29–34

Illustrations by Gillian Lee

Abdominal reduction

Paule C. L. Regnault MD, FRCS(C)
Former Professor Agrégé de Clinique, Montreal University, Montreal, Canada

The common deformities of the abdominal wall fall into three main categories, each requiring different surgical techniques for correction. Following a description of these procedures the possible complications and treatment thereof are dealt with as a whole.

THICK ADIPOSE ABDOMEN

Indications

The usual complaints requiring surgical relief are of excessive fat tissue, an adipose apron falling over the pubis, pain due to weight, and hernia. Difficulty is experienced in wearing normal clothing. In more severe, long-lasting cases eczema of the groins or varicose veins co-exists.

Contraindications

Poor-risk patients. These lipectomies may induce a state of shock from removal of massive portions of tissue with associated blood loss.

Preoperative

Preparation of patient

The patient is encouraged to lose as much weight as possible, but a fasting diet should be stopped about 3 weeks before surgery. Aspirin should not be taken for a period of 10 days before surgery.

If the patient is liable to constipation an enema is given the day before operation. The upper part of the pubic area is shaved. Blood should be available and cross-matched in patients undergoing large excisions.

Special instrumentation and apparatus

The operating table should be capable of placing the patient in a semi-Fowler (or jack-knife) position at the time of suturing. If this is not possible, pillows may be put under the knees before the operation. Strong retractors of Israel or Doyen type will be required.

Planning the excision

This is always estimated, either the day before or at the time of surgery, with the patient standing, using a dark felt pencil or silver nitrate. The markings are verified on the operating table, checking tissue elasticity and the symmetry of the markings.

Anaesthesia

General anaesthesia with endotracheal intubation is best and easiest for the surgeon. Spinal anaesthesia is excellent if the patient accepts this and if the local physical condition permits.

The operations

ADIPOSITY OF LOWER ABDOMEN AND MID-LINE

1

The technique indicated is the 'fleur-de-lis' type of resection. The lower incision is drawn like a high W, 2 cm above the inguinal folds and above the pubic hair line. The upper limit of the horizontal excision is traced by gently pulling the tissues downward to meet the lower limit of the excision. The lateral limits of the vertical portion are estimated by pulling the adipose layer medially from each side.

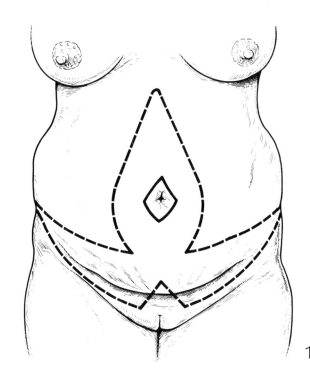

2

The operation is started from the lower incision line, working progressively upward. When both lower lateral portions of the 'fleur-de-lis' have been removed, the vertical incision is made on the right side and the fat dissected from the fascia to the left limit of the excision. The umbilicus is freed from the piece dissected, and this is more easily done by cutting from the umbilical site to one of the edges already detached. Before incising the left limit of the upper portion, a final estimation of the extent of the removal is made by pulling the tissues medially and downward in order to suture with moderate tension.

Large vessels are ligated while smaller ones are coagulated.

Divarication or hernia is repaired by plication with interrupted non-absorbable sutures. Occasionally a significant umbilical hernia is found. The umbilicus then has to be removed to avoid necrosis. When the divarication is too extensive to be repaired by plication, a synthetic mesh may be used. Some defatting is usually necessary in a small area at the upper limit of the vertical excision, and sometimes a small horizontal skin and fat excision is made to avoid a redundancy in this area.

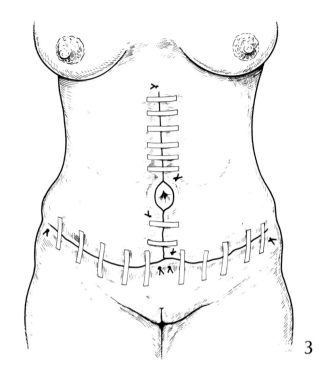

3

The vertical incision is sutured first, leaving a small space for the umbilicus by removing a piece of skin in the appropriate area. The subcutaneous layer is sutured with strong absorbable material. The superficial layer is closed with thin absorbable running suture. Adhesive strips maintain the suture line.

3

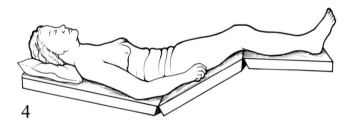

4

4

To facilitate closure of the horizontal incision the table may be placed in a moderate 'jack-knife' position. No drainage is usually necessary, as no undermined area has been left.

ADIPOSE LAYER THICKEST AT WAIST LINE AND PROTRUDING IN FRONT OF BODY

5

The T technique is indicated. The upper part of the abdominal fat, at the level of the waist line, is removed horizontally, while the lower part is removed vertically. Preoperative markings are made with the patient standing, and the extent of removal of skin and fat is roughly estimated at this time. The excision may be continued posteriorly, according to the degree of tissue redundancy there. The markings are finally adjusted on the operating table after skin disinfection and draping.

6

The incision is commenced on the vertical marking on the right side. The fat is detached from the fascia and the amount to be removed is judged by traction on the undermined skin and fat. This is followed by similar excision on the left side. The lower incisions of the horizontal portion of the T are then made and the fat is removed in the same way, working upwards. The umbilicus is incised as a triangular shape so that it can be located more easily in the final scar. The dissection of the umbilicus is made easier by dividing the flap. When both right and left arms of the horizontal excision have been detached, the amount to be removed is estimated and excised along the upper border of the T.

Careful haemostasis is necessary. Muscular divarication or hernia is repaired by plication of the fascia with non-absorbable sutures.

No undermining is done.

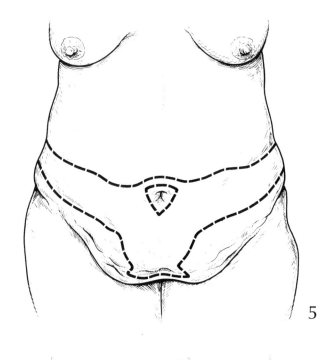

5

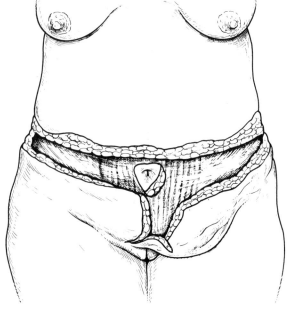

6

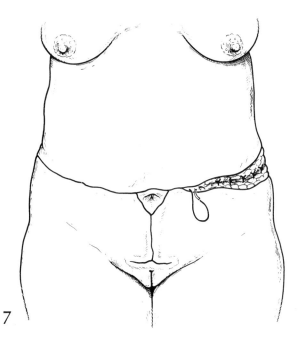

7

7

The edges of the wound are approximated in two layers, using heavy absorbable material on the fat and a subcuticular running suture on the skin. Drainage is usually unnecessary. The vertical incision is closed first; the operating table is then put in a jack-knife position to facilitate closure of the horiztontal incision.

CIRCULAR OPERATION

8, 9 & 10

The circular operation is indicated when the fat layer is located at the waist line and appears as a thick belt of fat and skin, which may be pendulous.

Usually the incisions respect the spinal area so that the excision is not quite circumferential. On the abdomen a vertical wedge may be removed medially and a small horizontal removal carried out above the pubic area, depending on the exact circumstances.

The operation is commenced posteriorly, with the patient lying on the abdomen. After suturing, the patient is turned over for the adbominal part of the excision. No undermining is usually necessary except laterally where the tissues are less elastic. Drainage is usually required.

Circular lipectomies are major operations and often require blood transfusion. They can be managed in two stages, the back first, leaving temporary huge 'dog ears' on each side, and the front one or more weeks later.

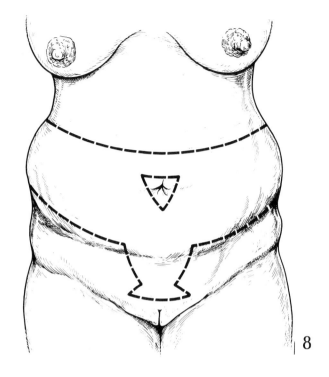

8

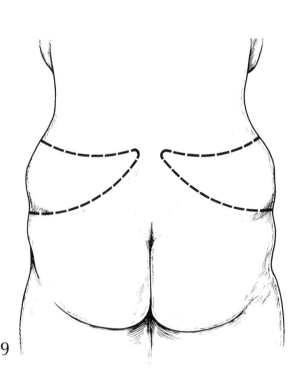

9

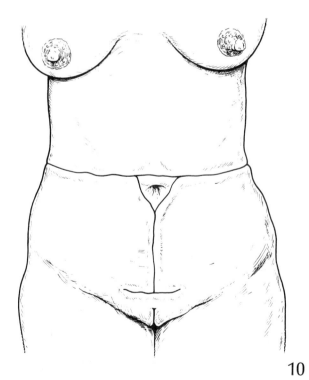

10

Postoperative care

The dressing is applied with moderate pressure, using elastic adhesive strapping. It is left for 48 hours while the patient is nursed in the same position as on the table. Mild sedatives are usually sufficient. Haemoglobin is checked but blood transfusion is rarely needed.

LOOSE STRETCHED SKIN – DERMOCHALASIS

Indications

Dermochalasis and striae in postpartum younger women, divarication of the recti and abdominal scars located below the umbilicus. Moderate excess fat, if present, is located predominantly below the umbilicus.

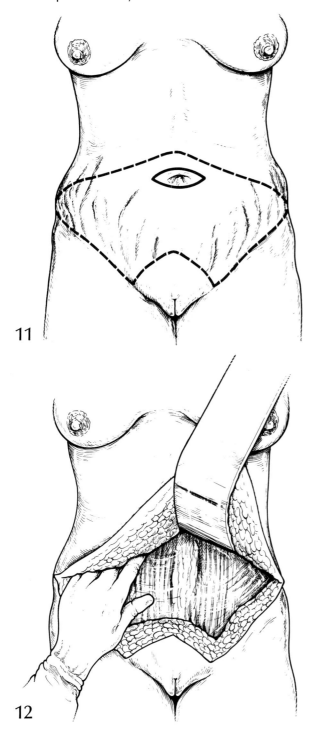

11

12

Contraindications

Scars located above the umbilicus, or a thick fat layer above the umbilicus.

Preoperative

Planning the excision

11

This is carried out preoperatively with the patient standing up. The W lines should follow the inguinal folds laterally so that the scar lies either in the folds or slightly above if the skin elasticity seems poor. The central portion of the W is within the pubic hair, at its upper limit or slightly above the hair line, depending on skin elasticity. Normally the lateral extensions of the W are longer than the medial ones. The upper limit of the excision is a straight line drawn from a point above the umbilicus to the lateral ends of the W. The length of the upper incision should be either equal to or shorter than the sum of the W branches. The umbilicus is circumscribed as a narrow ellipse or in a reverse W shape at the upper and a V at the lower incision.

The operation

After disinfection of the skin and draping the amount of tissue to be removed is verified by pinching the soft tissues, and the markings may be adjusted accordingly. The upper portion of the excision is scored with the scalpel, to be incised after undermining and checking the tissue elasticity.

12

The lower incision is made through the skin, but is carried obliquely upward through the fat so as to respect the inguinal lymph nodes. When reaching the fascia, the very fine cellular layer covering the fascia should be respected over the entire undermined area. This layer seems to play an important role in fluid resorption and in reducing postoperative pain. The undermining is carried out with blunt or sharp dissection, and very gently.

Haemostasis is achieved by clamping all perforating vessels. On reaching the umbilicus the flap is cut in the midline, the umbilicus is freed and the undermining continued upward to the xiphoid process and over the lower ribs.

Divarication of the recti muscles is repaired by plication of the aponeurosis with non-absorbable material. This shortens the umbilical stem, which will produce a nice dimpled umbilical effect.

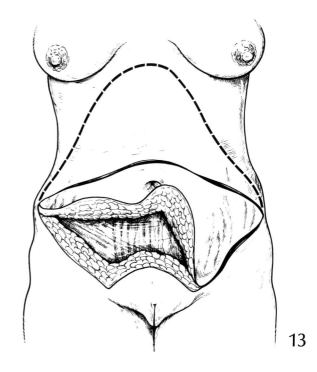

13

Resection of the flap usually follows the preoperative markings but it may be more extensive than planned if traction on the flap proves that a greater amount of tissue may safely be removed.

13

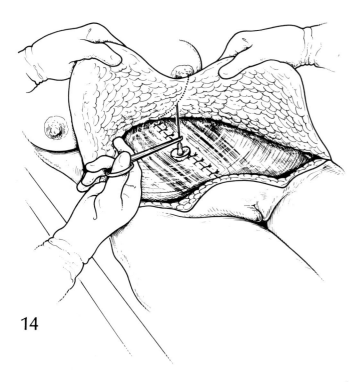

14

14

The new location of the umbilicus in the upper flap is determined before flap resection and before folding the operating table. A needle is held vertically (at 90°) on the navel while the flap is pulled with the estimated final pulling force. The needle should pierce the skin in the midline.

The operating table is put in a jack-knife position so that the wound edges come together easily. The angle of the table may be 90°–120°. This position is the key to easy closure without tension (see *Illustration 4*).

15a–c

Once the new location of the umbilicus has been determined, a straight horizontal incision is made in the midline, about 2 cm wide. When the reverse W umbilicus has been designed, another reverse W is incised at the location chosen.

A thread anchored to the umbilicus and passed through this wound allows easy suturing of the umbilicus after the lower incision has been closed.

Suturing is done in two layers, using heavy absorbable material for the fat and fascia and a subcuticular continuous fine suture for the skin. If the midportion at the pubis seems to form an unaesthetic sharp angle it may be rounded.

Adhesive strips are applied to all suture lines. Drains are retained for 48 hours.

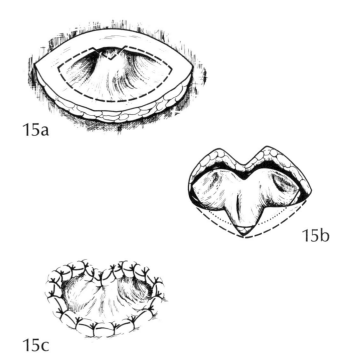

15a

15b

15c

Postoperative care

A moderate pressure dressing is applied with elastic adhesive bandages. The patient is transported to the bed in the same position and is left so for about 48 hours. Leg movements are encouraged. The bandage and drains are then removed, and the patient is allowed to get up. A soft elastic girdle is recommended for a few weeks.

INTERMEDIATE ABNORMALITY

Indications

The indications are excess fat or abdominal scars in the upper quadrants, dermochalasis limited to the periumbilical area, and minor dermochalasis of lower quadrants.

Planning

The proposed incisions are marked preoperatively, with the patient standing up. Tissue elasticity is estimated at the same time. The scars should be made horizontal if possible, if necessary with a compromise between the length of the final excision and its direction. Imagination is necessary for good planning. The problems most frequently encountered are dealt with as follows.

(1) Periumbilical folds are removed by a horizontal spindle-shaped excision.

(2) Cholecystectomy, splenectomy or other superiorly located scars are excised horizontally. Some limited undermining is done. The umbilicus is either transposed into the flap or remains in the suture line.

(3) Minor dermochalasis of the suprapubic area is removed by a low W excision with limited undermining. A small excision is often necessary at the upper border of the umbilicus.

Complications of abdominal lipectomies

Haematoma

Prevention

All coagulation abnormalities are corrected before operation. The operation should be performed after menstruation. Aspirin is stopped 10 days before operation. Perfect haemostasis must be achieved. Drainage is employed when necessary. Nausea is prevented. Ambulation is forbidden for 24 hours. A moderate pressure dressing or girdle is used.

Treatment

If haematoma should develop the area is evacuated as soon as possible, and repeatedly, until dry. A moderate pressure dressing or girdle is applied.

Infection

Systemic antibiotics are administered prophylactically when there is haematoma or necrosis, and to treat postoperative infection.

Necrosis

Prevention

Good planning and gentle surgery are essential, especially when using a W incision with extensive undermining. Tension should be maximal laterally rather than at the midline. The W operation should not be used in patients with transverse scars located too high to be removed. The patient should remain in the jack-knife position for at least 24 hours. Adhesive strips should be generously used to support the scars. Dressings should not be too tight and plaster casts or sandbags should be avoided on flaps. Umbilical sloughing is avoided by removing the umbilicus when a large umbilical hernia is repaired. The umbilicus should be left at least 2.5 cm wide when operating on the thick adipose abdomen.

Treatment

If any areas show vascular insufficiency it is best to wait until demarcation is obvious. All necrotic tissue is then removed and the area skin-grafted.

Hypertrophic and hypotrophic scars

Skin tension is relieved by generous subcutaneous suturing. Adhesive strips are maintained for several weeks. Wearing irritating clothes and the performance of exercises should be avoided for several weeks. After the strips have been removed scars should be massaged with body creams.

Hypertrophic scars are treated by injection of triamcinolone *in situ*, whereas hypotrophic scars are excised one or two years after surgery.

Redundant folds

Redundant folds are prevented by making sure that the margins of the wound are defatted in thick adipose cases and enough skin is removed. It is better to have longer scars than to leave excess tissue. Once the midline is closed, the horizontal incisions are sutured from their lateral extremities.

Persistent redundant folds are treated by excision and defatting a few months postoperatively.

Oedema of flaps

Early postoperative massage, exercises and soft girdles are used to prevent and treat flap oedema.

Unaesthetic location of the umbilicus

Incorrect placement of the umbilicus is avoided by carefully checking the location of the midline and the normal level of the umbilicus between waist and iliac crest at operation.

An incorrectly sited umbilicus must be excised and relocated.

Acute anaemia

Anaemia must be corrected before surgery and blood should be given if operative loss exceeds 500 ml.

Further reading

Castanares, S., Goethel, J. Abdominal lipectomy: a modification in technique. Plastic and Reconstructive Surgery 1967; 40: 378

Gonzolez-Ulloa, M. Belt lipectomy. British Journal of Plastic Surgery 1960; 13: 179

Regnault, P. Abdominal dermolipectomies. Clinics in Plastic Surgery 1975; 2: 411

Pressure sores

Bruce N. Bailey FRCS
Consultant Plastic Surgeon, Stoke Mandeville Hospital, Aylesbury, Buckinghamshire, UK

Christopher Khoo FRCS
Consultant Plastic Surgeon, Wexham Park Hospital, Slough, Berkshire, UK

Introduction

Pressure sores are lesions caused solely by pressure. Most develop when patients are confined to bed ('bedsores') or spend long periods in a sitting position. The skin and soft tissues overlying bony prominences are subjected to constant unrelieved compression or shearing between the bone and an external resistance.

Aetiology

The normal capillary blood pressure in skin is 32 mmHg. Prolonged exposure to pressures exceeding this causes tissue ischaemia. If pressure is unrelieved the initial inflammation is followed by irreversible changes which lead to tissue necrosis.

Pressure and shearing forces in the skin are the only cause of pressure sores, although anaemia, hypoproteinaemia, malnutrition, old age, debility and infection are often cited as predisposing factors. Additional features in neurological patients are paralysis and loss of protective sensation. Even if all these features are present, however, a patient will not develop a pressure sore unless the tissues are subjected to sufficient pressure long enough to cause ischaemia and tissue necrosis. Conversely, a full-blooded, well-muscled, healthy young individual may develop a pressure sore if subjected to immobilization and prolonged pressure (e.g. on an operating table). Proper wound management and total relief of pressure will heal all pressure sores, albeit slowly. Recovery may be delayed if the factors needed for normal healing are not present, but sores never start to heal unless pressure is totally relieved.

Gross appearances

The early visible changes include erythema of the skin, with oedema and then blistering. These appearances are suggestive of superficial damage which will heal quickly when pressure is relieved. Unrelieved ischaemia of the skin results in an eschar which then separates to reveal underlying ulceration. Infection is common and may be associated with further destruction of the soft tissues and the underlying bone. The sore cavity is often larger than suggested by the appearance of the area of skin necrosis over it.

Principles of wound management

1. There must be total relief of pressure

The patient is nursed in a position which allows the ulcerated area complete relief from pressure but which does not endanger other areas. In many cases (e.g. sacral, ischial, heel and trochanteric sores) this may be achieved by nursing the patient in a prone position. This position allows access for dressings and is tolerated, after some practice, by all patients, including those with ileostomies, colostomies, indwelling catheters and flexion deformities of the hip. However, quadriplegic patients may have difficulty in maintaining respiratory movements. Pillows should be placed in such a way that the anterior bony prominences of the knees and iliac spines are not themselves subjected to pressure. In the prone position pressure distribution may be facilitated by the use of moveable packs, a bed composed of inflated sacs (low air loss bed) or a fluidized bead bed, but these do not by themselves adequately relieve pressure and shearing forces on a sore. It is essential to have meticulous nursing care for healing to progress at its optimum rate. If the patient is nursed in a lateral position regular turnings must be carried out to prevent the development of pressure sores over the trochanters.

2. The wound must be properly cared for

Pressure sores may contain much infected and necrotic material and it is essential to remove this by scalpel or scissor dissection. This may be done at the bedside, and excision should be repeated at regular intervals until all obviously necrotic tissue is removed. A margin of skin may be incised or removed to allow access to a large underlying cavity. The wound should then be packed with ribbon gauze dampened with eusol and this dressing should be repeated three times a day. It is helpful to put the patient into the bath each day, using only mild soap in the bath water. The wound should be checked for bacterial growth by culturing from excised tissue and surface swabs taken from the granulations which come to line the cavity. Systemic antibiotic therapy is not indicated as there is poor antibiotic penetration into the lining of pressure ulcers. Topical antibiotics are also contra-indicated because of the likelihood of development of bacterial resistance.

Various topical agents have been used to treat pressure sores. These include absorbent dextran beads and enzymatic debriding agents such as streptokinase and streptodornase. These act at the surface of the wound and have little effect on the large amounts of necrotic material, for which mechanical removal is essential.

Superficial eschars such as those overlying heel sores may be softened by application of 0.2 per cent nitro-furazone cream and penetration may be increased by scoring the eschar. Once the eschar has separated the dressing should be changed to eusol-soaked gauze and the ulcer managed as a cavity.

With debridement and dressings infected ulcers are made ready for surgery over a period of 1 or 2 weeks. The healthy surface granulations which appear are dry, bright red and finely granular. There should be no odour, and a margin of purple secondary epithelium is seen growing in from the wound edge. When this stage has been reached the patient is in a healing phase and many pressure sores will progress to spontaneous healing (see Sacral Sores, below). Otherwise, these appearances may be taken to indicate a favourable time for surgical closure of the pressure sores.

The bacterial count will be greatly decreased and is reflected in a quantitative count of less than 10^5 organisms/g of tissue. Surface swabs are again taken and the results may be used as a guide to the selection of antibiotics for operative cover. The presence of bacteria is not in itself a contraindication to skin grafting or other surgery if the physical appearance of the wound is satisfactory.

3. The general management of the patient

In addition to the dressings, debridement, control of infection and avoidance of pressure, attention should be directed to the patient's nutritional status. Sphincter management is of importance in paraplegic patients.

Nutrition Many patients with long-standing pressure sores are grossly catabolic as a result of the original illness and from the effects of the open and infected sores themselves. Closure of a pressure sore with a skin graft may be indicated as a temporary expedient to control a hypercatabolic state and improve the patient's condition before definitive reconstruction with a flap.

The nitrogen balance should be calculated from an assessment of dietary intake and the 24-hour urinary urea excretion, and the serum albumin concentration measured. An individual diet rich in protein and calories should be given, and ideally the patient should be gaining weight at the time of surgery. Debilitated patients often have poor appetites, but the oral route is still preferred for nutrition. The ordinary diet should be supplemented with sip-feeds to provide an ideal intake. If the patient is unable or unwilling to take enough by mouth a fine-bore nasogastric tube should be inserted and nutrition provided by means of constant infusion over the entire 24-hour period with gravity infusion or, preferably, an infusion pump.

Patients who are chronically ill should receive additional vitamin C, zinc sulphate, trace elements and vitamins.

Anaemia The haemoglobin level should be at least 13g/dl before surgery and it should be maintained at this level afterwards. Blood transfusion may need to be repeated (especially at an early stage when frequent debridements are carried out) and any specific cause of anaemia apparent from the blood film (e.g. iron, vitamin B_{12} or folate deficiency) should be corrected.

Paraplegic patients These should be managed jointly with spinal physicians. Concurrent problems such as urinary tract infections should be treated. The bowels should be controlled and evacuations carried out as necessary. A low-residue diet is helpful during the period of surgery. Patients nursed prone will need either condom or catheter drainage. Spasms should be controlled if possible with diazepam, baclofen or dantrolene. Strong spasms make surgery difficult and general anaesthesia may be indicated for some patients even though the level of spinal injury means that there is no sensation at the site of the pressure sore.

Surgical management

Healing of pressure sores may be achieved by the following means:

1. Spontaneous healing by cicatrization or secondary epithelialization.
2. Closure with skin grafts, which may be split skin grafts applied as meshed grafts, postage stamp grafts or pinch grafts.
3. Direct closure after bone excision.
4. Flap closure after bone excision. Almost all pressure sores can be closed directly after adequate bony resection, and the use of flaps should be reserved for those instances in which a simpler method is not possible. Flaps may contain skin, muscle or both (cutaneous flaps, muscle flaps and musculocutaneous flaps). The use of a flap does not prevent subsequent development of a further pressure sore in the same area if pressure is not avoided.

Sacral sores

Sacral sores are the common 'acute sores' seen in patients confined to bed during medical and surgical emergencies such as pneumonia or fracture of the neck of the femur. Most severely ill patients are nursed in the supine position or in various degrees of hip flexion so that the sacrum is subjected to pressure and shearing forces and is always at risk.

Positioning of the patient

Sacral sores are triangular. The horizontal base runs between the posterior spines, and the apex points downwards towards the anus. The tissue damage may be superficial or deep. Superficial sores are characterized by erythema, vesiculation and coagulation of skin, and heal when pressure is removed. The nursing management of superficial sacral sores includes careful skin cleansing and positioning the patient so that further pressure on the sacrum is totally avoided. The patient should be nursed prone or turned from side to side. If continued supine nursing is unavoidable the patient should be lifted so that for 10 seconds every 20 minutes the tissues of the sacral area are perfused.

For patients in orthopaedic traction nursing on a low air loss bed will assist lifting and reduce pressure between lifts. Cut-away air sacs are available so that the sacrum may be free from pressure.

Deeper sacral sores may include full-thickness skin loss, fat necrosis and even destruction of the posterior sacral spines. These may also heal in response to proper management. A deep sacral sore should be cleaned with hydrogen peroxide and then packed lightly with surgical gauze wrung out in eusol. Dressings three times daily will keep the sore clean. The patient need not be confined to bed and may have a daily bath in warm soapy water. When in bed the patient must lie prone or on his sides, and never on the sore. He may sit in an upright chair so that weight is carried on the buttocks, and is allowed to walk. However, a semi-reclining position is absolutely forbidden as the combination of pressure and the shearing force on the coccyx or sacrum prolongs vascular damage and prevents healing.

Spontaneous healing

This follows one of two patterns, with predominant epithelialization or cicatrization.

1a & b

In the patient with loose buttock skin a granulating bed develops in the base of the sore. A thin purple fringe of secondary epithelium is present at the edge of the granulations, but as cicatrization is faster than epithelialization the wound edges are drawn to the centre (a). Closure occurs over a matter of weeks and the amount of secondary epithelium remaining in the centre of the healed wound is small.

If the buttock skin is tight closure is mainly by epithelialization (b). As long as the granulations remain healthy, healing will progress until the raw area is completely covered.

Cicatrization leaves a stable surface over the sacrum which can be subjected to normal trauma. However, a sore covered with secondary epithelium cannot withstand rough treatment and will break down again if the patient is put to bed in a supine position. It is nearly always to the patient's advantage to allow acute sores to heal spontaneously while exercise, physiotherapy and rehabilitation continue.

Excision and suture

Small sacral sores may be excised and the defect closed by direct suture of the edges. This method of closure is only possible if there is sufficient laxity of buttock skin to allow the edges to come together with light finger pressure on either side of the wound. Direct closure of large defects is only possible if the wound edges are sewn together under considerable tension with a significant risk of breakdown; such wounds should therefore not be closed directly.

Surgery is contraindicated if ambulation is desired because the patient should remain prone after surgery until the suture line is soundly healed. Closure is carried out in layers, using strong deep sutures (e.g. 0 Dexon), and it is advantageous to leave a subcutaneous nylon suture in place for 3–4 weeks to strengthen the suture line. After 3 weeks the patient may lie supine for brief periods. Frequent inspections are carried out to ensure that the area of the suture line is able to tolerate the pressure. Over the next week periods of weight-bearing may progress from 5 minutes each hour to constant pressure during the hour, and if there are no ill effects the patient is allowed to sleep supine thereafter.

Skin grafting

Skin grafting may be carried out as a temporary measure to achieve rapid closure in patients with large defects. In ambulant patients with normal sensation a skin graft alone may be an adequate means of managing the acute sacral sore. In paraplegic patients who are to live at home without constant supervision there is a risk that breakdown will occur if the graft is not protected and pressure avoided.

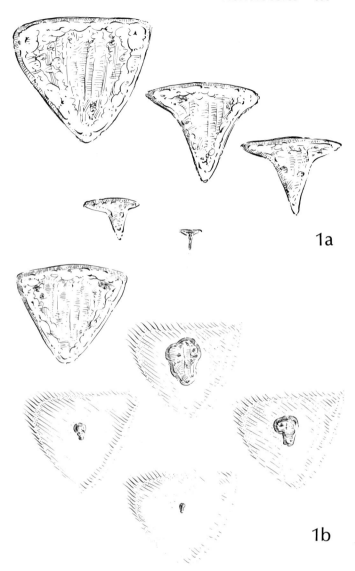

1a

1b

Skin grafts should be taken from non-weightbearing areas of the body (e.g. the medial aspects of the thighs or the lumbar hollows). They should be applied to a healthy granulating base and may be meshed to aid conformity with an irregularly contoured bed and to prevent the accumulation of seromata beneath the graft. Meshed split skin grafts applied to the defect are covered with a single layer of tulle gras, and warm saline-soaked gauze is applied over the tulle for 48 hours to prevent the exposed areas of granulation underneath the interstices of the mesh from drying out. The meshed graft should not be expanded. It is helpful to cover the moist gauze with a sheet of sterilized aluminium cooking foil to retain warmth and moisture. The graft should be inspected regularly to ensure that no displacement has occurred and the patient should remain prone until healing has occurred. The grafted area slowly consolidates and no weight should be borne until 3 weeks after the operation. Weight bearing commences with periods of a few minutes each hour and is allowed to progress until weight is taken on the graft for a period of an hour. Should any erythema of the graft or the adjacent tissues be seen weight bearing is reduced until further consolidation of the fresh graft has occurred.

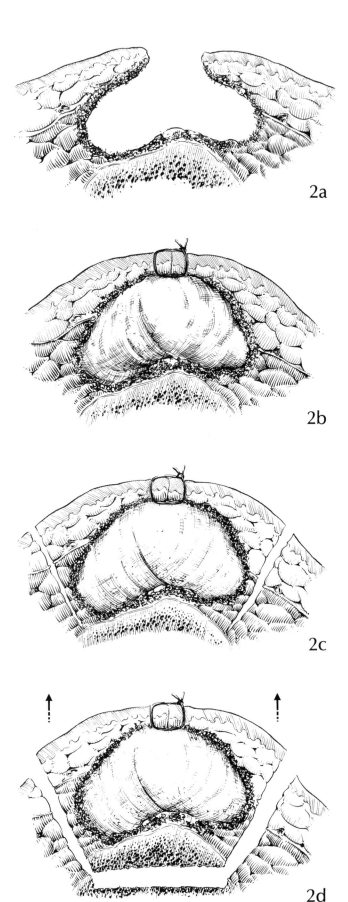

2a

Excision and flap closure

Excision of the sore

2a–d

Large sacral sores are often widely undermined and initial management should include frequent debridement and dressing until the patient is in a good healing phase (*a*).

Flap repair may also be carried out as a definitive procedure after previous skin grafting.

Excision of the wound margins and walls of an ulcer cavity is carried out with the 'pseudo-tumour' technique. Ribbon gauze soaked in iodine solution is packed into the cavity and sewn in (*b*) and the ulcer and surrounding tissues are then excised *in toto* around the gauze pack (*c*). The excision includes the underlying bony prominence of the posterior sacral spines (*d*), which are removed with a curved osteotome or a gouge. The bone surface is then rasped to produce a completely smooth surface. A powered reciprocating osteotome and bone rasp are helpful and allow precise degrees of bone excision.

The coccyx should then be disarticulated by scalpel excision and the bone end smoothed. Further bone excision is avoided because of the risk of damage to the sacral vascular plexus and the sacral nerves. Individual bleeding points may be tied off or coagulated, but the oozing cancellous bone surface should not be charred. The use of bone wax is not advised as the wax may act as a focus for subsequent infection. Haemostasis may be assisted by the application of bovine thrombin solution or the use of bovine collagen paste. It is absolutely essential that adequate drainage be provided, and one or two suction drains should be placed to ensure that haematoma is not allowed to collect. The initial drainage is often copious and the drains should remain in place until the drainage is serous and of small volume. Closure is carried out in layers.

2b

2c

2d

Gluteal skin rotation flap

3a & b

The sacral sore is excised to create a triangular defect. All areas of secondary epithelium and the underlying bony prominences are included in the excision. An inferiorly based gluteal rotation flap is designed by outlining the largest possible semicircle (*a*). The circumference of the flap should lie below the iliac crest so that the scar will not lie over a bony prominence. The margin of the flap passes over the trochanteric region, overlying any trochanteric sore, and downwards towards the ischium. The larger the semicircle, the less tension is developed in closure of the secondary defect.

The flap is raised down to the gluteal fascia and up to the diameter of the semicircle. Extensive undermining is necessary to ensure that the flap is able to move comfortably into position without shearing at its base, which may cause occlusion of the large gluteal vessels. After adequate mobilization the flap may be rotated comfortably with the flat of the hand to lie over the sore. The triangular primary defect is closed and the crescentic secondary defect may be closed either as an out-cut (*b*) or a back-cut (see below). Excision of a triangle from the outer line and closure under tension advances the outer portion of the flap and assists tension-free closure over the sore. The closure is begun with sutures of 0 Dexon, which are inverted so that the knot lies buried in the fat. The bite on each suture includes the full thickness of the fat and the dermis and several such interrupted sutures distribute tension. A second layer of 2/0 or 3/0 Dexon sutures includes the intervening subcutaneous fat and the dermis. Skin closure is performed with interrupted 4/0 nylon sutures which may be placed as half-mattress sutures. Large suction drains are inserted to drain the entire undersurface, and these remain until drainage is less than 10 ml/day. A sample of the drainage fluid is sent for bacterial culture before withdrawal of the drain.

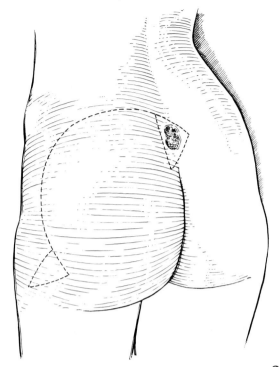

3a

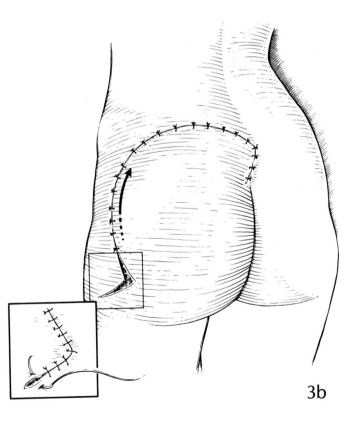

3b

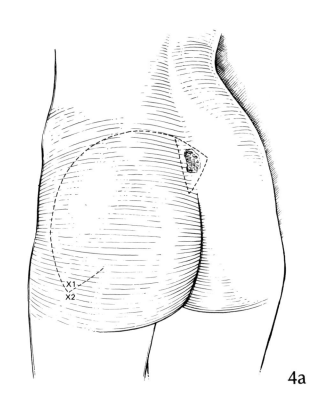

4a

4a & b

In younger patients with a good blood supply the flap may be rotated with a back-cut through the base of the flap (a). No tissue is discarded (as is the case with an out-cut), but closure produces tension across the base of the flap (b) and this procedure should be reserved for patients in whom a good vascular supply is assured. The back-cut is usually half the length of the triangular defect and as the cut is opened out into a triangle an increase in length of the flap margin sufficient for closure is obtained. It is necessary to undermine adequately on both sides of the back-cut so that skin from the surrounding area may be brought in to close the secondary defect. Closure is then carried out in the same manner as described for the out-cut.

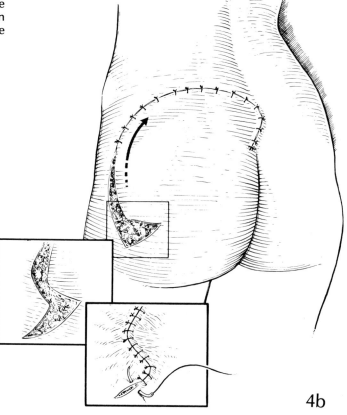

4b

Muscle flaps

5a & b

The gluteus maximus muscle is supplied by two separate vascular pedicles (*a*). The upper half of the muscle is supplied by the superior gluteal vessels while the lower half of the muscle is supplied by the inferior gluteal vessels, which emerge below the piriformis muscle to supply in addition the skin of the thigh.

The gluteus maximus muscle is exposed through a semicircular incision designed in the same way as a standard rotation flap. The flap may be based inferiorly or superiorly. With an inferiorly based flap dissection is performed in the normal manner at the level of the gluteal fascia. The plane between gluteus maximus and gluteus medius muscles is identified by finger dissection and the muscle is divided at its insertion into the iliotibial tract. The upper part of the muscle is split longitudinally along the line of its fibres and may now be swung backwards to cover the sacral defect. The vessels now lie on the superficial surface of the upturned muscle (*b*). The exposed muscle may be skin grafted or cutaneous flap cover may be provided by transposition of the skin flap medially with skin grafting of the secondary defect at the lateral margin of the flap. With this technique the inferior half of the gluteus maximus may be preserved in the lower buttock.

Alternatively, the entire gluteus maximus muscle may be raised together with the overlying skin as a musculocutaneous flap. The incision is made as for an inferiorly based cutaneous rotation flap and is extended deeply downwards through the origin of the muscle from the edge of the sacrum. The thick musculocutaneous unit is split from the underlying gluteus medius and piriformis muscles and rotated into the defect. Occasionally free movement of the flap is held back by the tightness of the superior gluteal vessels themselves; these may then be divided, as the entire skin and muscle unit will survive on the inferior gluteal pedicle.

The gluteus maximus muscle flap may also be approached through a skin incision as for a superolaterally based skin rotation flap. The margins of this flap extend in a semicircle from the sacrum, down across the ischium, and as far as the lateral margin of the buttock crease. The lower margin of the gluteus maximus is identified and the plane of dissection found by palpation of the sciatic nerve. The lower part of the muscle is detached from its insertion into the greater trochanter of the femur and dissection continues upwards until the upper portion of the muscle is located with its separate pedicle. The two halves of the muscle can then be used independently for coverage of ischial and sacral defects.

Other muscle and musculocutaneous flaps have been used for coverage of sacral defects and include the gracilis and tensor fasciae latae flaps. For most purposes, however, the straightforward cutaneous rotation flap is adequate and its use entails less extensive dissection.

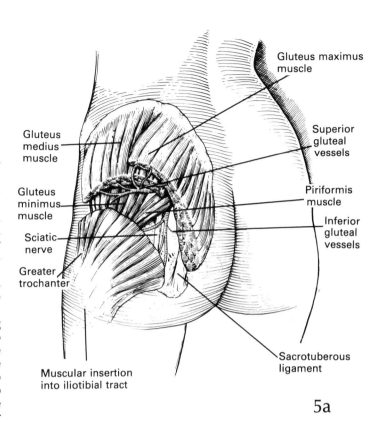

5a

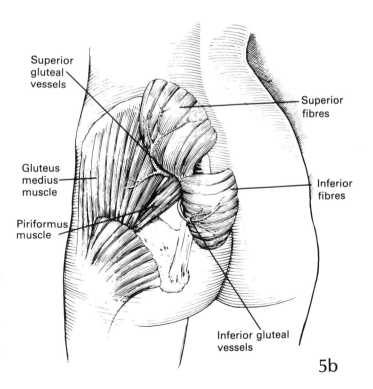

5b

6a & b

Muscle flaps provide thicker padding and their excellent vascularity increases the period of time that pressure may be suffered without permanent consequences. However, constant and unrelieved pressure over a muscle flap will still create pressure necrosis, and if this occurs through the skin and muscle of a musculocutaneous flap (a) the possibilities for further reconstruction using local tissue will be limited. When flaps are designed for sacral cover the largest possible flap should be designed, as a large flap will allow itself to be re-raised for rotation should breakdown occur and eventually for use as a transposition flap with skin grafting of the secondary defect (b).

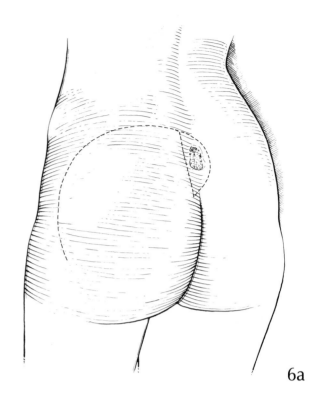

6a

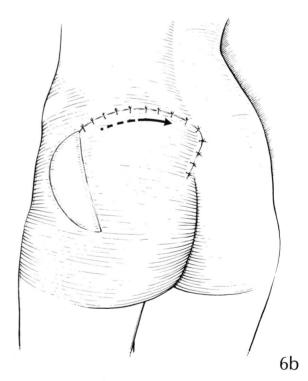

6b

Trochanteric sores

Excision and suture with retention of greater trochanter

Some trochanteric sores are suitable for excision and direct closure, which may eventually be possible after granulation and cicatrization in a healing sore have drawn the edges closer. When the patient is in a good healing state the shallow residual sore may be excised together with any secondary epithelium which has formed. Sores suitable for excision and direct closure are seldom more than 4 cm wide, though they may be longer. Aponeurotic structures may be exposed, but there should not be any evidence of osteomyelitis or of arthritis of the hip joint.

7a, b & c

Excision and suture with excision of greater trochanter

The sore is excised through skin and fat down to aponeurotic structures, and in the base of the wound the greater trochanter and any secondarily ossified tissues are exposed. The bone is removed by a chisel cut through the intertrochanteric notch to the lateral side of the femur (a). Further chisel cuts are made to ensure that the bone surface is smooth, and a coarse rasp may be used to smooth the surface. There is initial vigorous bleeding which then slows. The cancellous bone surface may be sealed with bovine collagen, but bone wax should be avoided as troublesome sepsis may occur in the presence of haematoma.

After skin excision the edges of the defect retract and it may seem that they cannot be apposed (b). After adequate bone excision, however, the retracted skin edges can be stretched back to close the cavity (c). A large-calibre suction drain is placed in the depths. The bone surface is covered with muscle or periosteum, if possible, and closure is commenced in layers, using 0 Dexon in the depths of the wound and proceeding to 3/0 Dexon, which is sufficient to appose the subcutaneous layer. The skin is closed with 4/0 nylon and the edges of the wound may be further protected against shearing forces with half-inch (1.25 cm) Steristrips. The patient is returned to bed and nursed off the repair. Drains are retained until only 1–2 ml of straw-coloured fluid is aspirated in any 6–hour period. Gentle external pressure may be applied to assist suction drainage and ensure that there is no internal pressure.

The sutures are removed after 2 weeks and it is about 6 weeks before weight may be fully borne on the suture line. Weight bearing may begin at 3 weeks with 5 minutes' pressure each hour and with the wound fully protected with Steristrips. If there are no signs of redness of the skin or suture line progressively longer periods are allowed until full weight bearing is achieved 6 weeks after surgery.

Flap closure

If it is not possible to achieve direct closure with deep 0 Dexon and subcutaneous 3/0 Dexon sutures a flap should be employed to avoid closure under tension. An inferiorly based gluteal rotation flap may be used, the direction of rotation being outwards, and the opposite of the direction of rotation for a sacral sore. Additional movement may be gained by transposing the flap outwards and skin grafting the secondary defect.

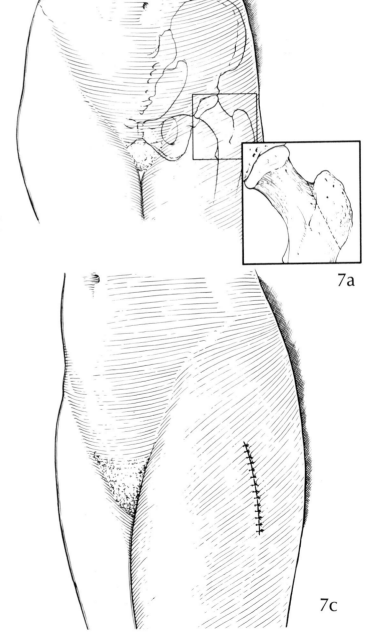

7a

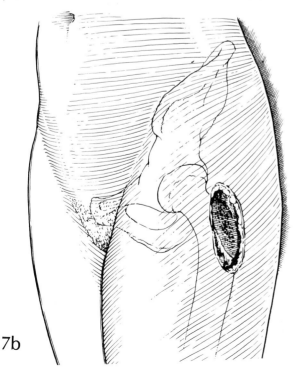

7b

7c

Superior transposition flap

8a & b

Alternatively, a local flap from the thigh may be used. An anterolateral, superiorly based flap may be transposed from a meaty part of the thigh, and although this donor site is weight bearing in the prone position, weight is taken on a flat muscular surface and there is no underlying bony prominence. A skin graft in this area is therefore not harmful. The flap is outlined generously (*a*) so that it can be swung into the defect without tension (*b*). A suction drain is inserted and with the vacuum the flap dips down into the defect and forms a concavity, obliterating the dead space.

Planning should provide for a flap that extends beyond the edge of the defect to be filled as the axis of movement of the flap is from the distant corner of the base to the proximal corner of the flap. The additional length of the flap should be at least the length of the base of the defect. As the secondary defect is to be skin-grafted there is no difficulty in closure as the skin graft may easily be cut to the necessary size. It is advantageous to mesh the skin graft and to apply it without expansion. This will avoid problems associated with the collection of haematoma under the graft.

The flap itself is undermined at the level of the deep fascia and must turn through 45–90° into the defect. Redundancy does not matter as the flap conforms exactly when suction is applied, sinking deeply into the defect. If it has not proved possible to close the raw bone surface with periosteal flaps the skin flap itself will closely appose to the bone for haemostasis. There is no tension and subcutaneous 3/0 Dexon sutures will hold the flap comfortably, while 4/0 nylon sutures are inserted to close the skin.

The suction drain is inserted away from the base of the flap, and the skin graft over the donor site is held with black silk sutures tied over a flavine wool dressing. While flap transposition and skin grafting of the flap donor site are being completed the skin graft donor site is covered with a damp gauze swab. At the end of the operation this is soaked off and oozing will have stopped. A single thickness of surgical gauze is applied to promote early coagulation and the donor site is then exposed.

Sutures are removed from the transposition flap margin after 2 weeks and Steristrips protect the edges thereafter. Weight may be borne at 4 weeks with the proviso that it is increased slowly, with close observation of the area. If the flap reddens the time of lateral lying must be decreased.

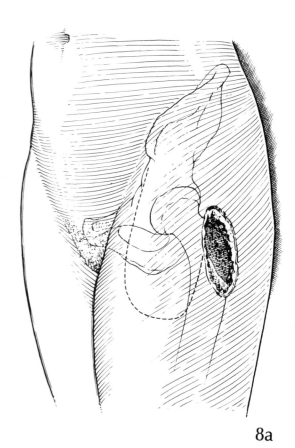

8a

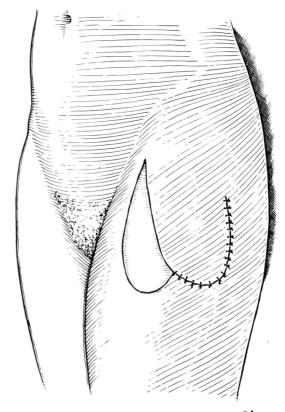

8b

Anterior bipedicled flaps

9a, b & c

An anterior bipedicled flap which is convex anteriorly may be used to close a trochanteric defect. The flap should be longer than the defect and wider than it (a). The flap is elevated down to the fascia lata and freed by finger dissection until it is able to swing backwards on its superior and inferior pedicles to cover the defect without tension. An elliptical secondary defect anteriorly is closed with a split skin graft (b).

This flap may also be designed as a musculocutaneous flap which includes the tensor fasciae latae muscle, which arises from the anterior superior iliac spine and inserts into the iliotibial tract (c), in its thickness. The skin markings are as for the cutaneous flap, but the level of undermining is deep to the tensor fasciae latae muscle. This flap is too tight at the muscle level to move backwards comfortably and it is necessary to divide the fascia lata transversely at the lower pedicle of the flap. The flap is then a cutaneous bipedicle but a proximally based muscle flap. The donor site and defect are then closed, the only difference being that an additional layer of sutures is used to hold the posterior edge of the fascia to the posterior margin of the defect.

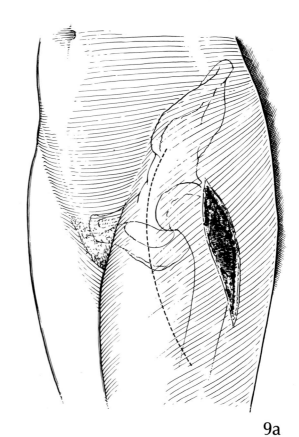

9a

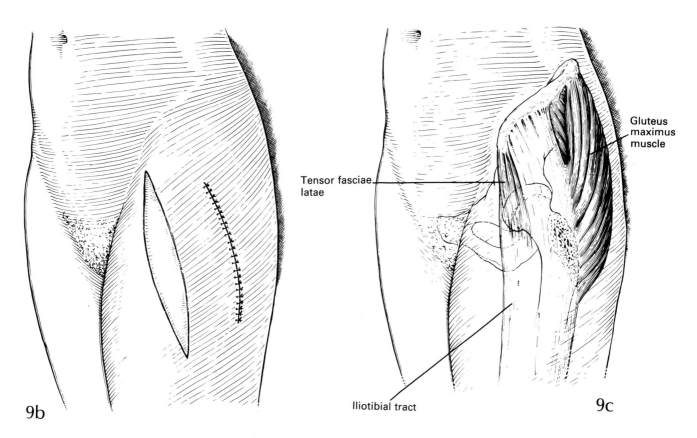

9b

Tensor fasciae latae

Gluteus maximus muscle

Iliotibial tract

9c

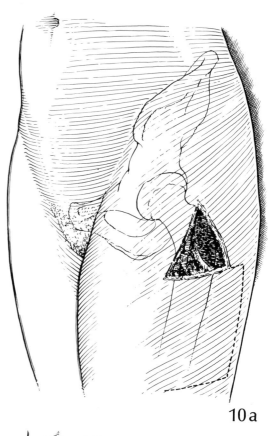

10a

10a & b

Anterior transposition flap

An anteriorly based flap may also be used, raised beneath the fascia and inferior to the defect (a). A back cut in the fascia is necessary to allow the flap to move upwards into the defect. A triangular secondary defect is created (b) and this is closed with a split skin graft. This technique leaves an area of skin graft on the outer aspect of the thigh, but the graft sits on muscle and there is no underlying bony prominence.

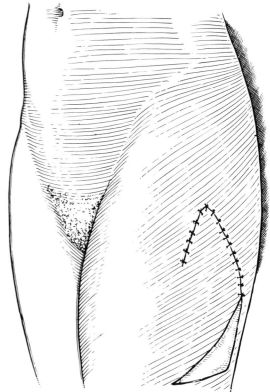

10b

Tensor fasciae latae musculocutaneous flap

11a, b & c

This flap may be designed up to 15 cm in width and is a superiorly based musculocutaneous flap whose anterior margin is delineated by a line passing from the anterior superior iliac spine down to the lateral femoral condyle (*a*). The posterior margin of the flap is parallel to this line and passes 15 cm behind it. This flap is based on the lateral femoral circumflex artery, which enters the tensor fasciae latae muscle 8 cm below the anterior superior spine, and the flap may be taken almost the whole length of the thigh. The thickness of the flap includes muscle and fascia lata and elevation is begun after ensuring that there is adequate length to reach and fill the defect. If the flap is transposed a large dog-ear is present; this may be avoided by designing the flap as an island, and it is safe to divide the skin proximally over the muscle pedicle of the flap. The donor site is closed with a split skin graft (*b*), though very small flap donor sites may be closed directly (*c*).

It should be noted that in the majority of cases excision of the bursa, ectopic bone and underlying greater trochanter will bring about enough relaxation of the skin to allow direct closure or closure with a small flap. The use of large musculocutaneous flaps is reserved for very large defects resulting from excision of the hip joint and upper femoral shaft. In these instances the flap provides a well-vascularized muscle to fill and heal the cavity and adequate skin for comfortable closure.

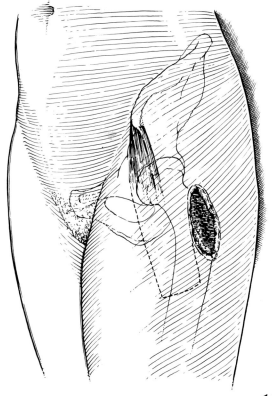

11a

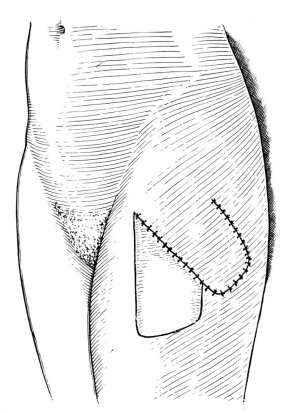

11b

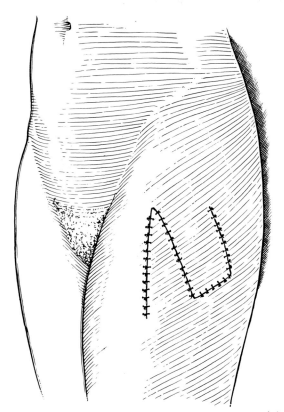

11c

Ischial sores

Spontaneous healing

There is no reason to skin-graft ischial sores. If a granulating surface develops cicatrization follows and forms a durable skin surface over the tuberosity. Closure will occur satisfactorily after adopting a prone position which provides skin laxity and pressure avoidance. Following cleansing and regular dressings the granulating wound is suitable for closure when the patient's general condition is satisfactory.

Excision of inferior pubic ramus and closure

The patient is positioned prone on the operating table with padding positioned to take the weight off the chest, rib margins, iliac crest, knees and the dorsum of the feet. In this position there is relaxation of tissue adjacent to the sore. The cavity is packed with ribbon gauze soaked in povidone iodine solution and the pack is retained with heavy silk sutures across the neck of the cavity. A mass or 'pseudotumour' is created and the sore can be excised. The iodine sterilizes the walls of the cavity and leakage of iodine during surgery indicates that the wall of the cavity has been breached.

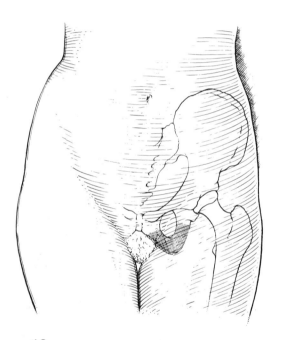

12

12

Adequate bone excision allows direct closure of almost all ischial sores. An incision is made into healthy skin around the rim of the sore and deepened down to the ischial tuberosity. When this is reached the aponeurosis and periosteum are incised around the base of the sore and these are excised in continuity with the sore. A Farabouef rougine is used to strip all soft tissue off the bone to the point where the obturator externus runs across the ilium laterally. Medially the periosteum, aponeurosis and muscle attachments are stripped up to the symphysis. A Gigli saw is passed through the obturator foramen and the inferior ramus is sawn through. Careful retraction by the assistant ensures that the skin edges are not injured. Laterally, the second cut passes through the ischial tuberosity and subacetabular ilium. The bone edges are nibbled back and smoothed.

13a & b

Large vessels are ligated and smaller vessels sealed with diathermy to ensure haemostasis. Closure is in layers over a suction drain left in the cavity. The skin is comfortably closed with 4/0 nylon. Direct excision and closure are always possible, except when there has been much previous surgery with extensive scarring. In this instance only, the inferior part of the gluteus maximus muscle may be turned over as a muscle flap to assist closure (a). Very large sores with ischial and trochanteric components in continuity may be closed with a single tensor fasciae latae musculocutaneous flap to fill both defects (b).

In the routine case, however, it is unnecessary to advance the gluteus maximus muscle or to turn over the hamstring muscles. It is unphysiological to pinch muscle between the ischial tuberosity and a seat, as in the normal subject the gluteus maximus slides out of the way when the sitting position is assumed. It is of greatest importance to remove the underlying bony prominence, and when this is done there is enough relaxation of adjacent tissues to allow direct closure. For this reason the biceps and other hamstring muscle flaps are not needed.

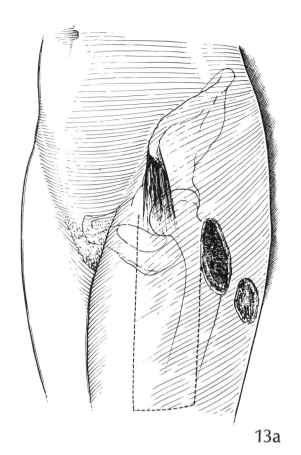

13a

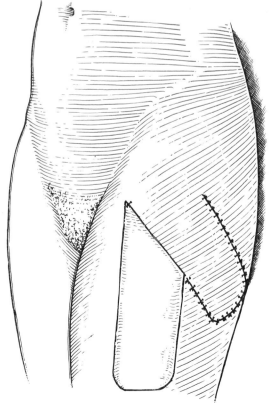

13b

OTHER PRESSURE SORES

The heel

Cutaneous skin flaps around the heel are dangerous and should be avoided. The vascular supply of tissue in this area is not dependable, especially in patients with peripheral vascular disease, or in elderly patients. Loss of skin flap creates a defect larger than the original pressure sore.

Vascularized flaps based on the plantar vessels have been described, but simple pinch grafts applied when the ulcer has responded to cleansing and dressings constitute a durable repair without the creation of a secondary defect. The secondary defect which is grafted after transposition of a vascularized flap is not in a weight bearing area but is still undesirable because the junction of the flap and skin graft often forms a mass of keratin which may give rise to secondary pressure sores.

Other sites

Pressure sores occur on many other areas of the body: the occiput, scapular spines, posterosuperior iliac spines, olecranon processes, costal margins, anterior superior iliac spines, medial sides of the knees, medial malleoli and the dorsum of the feet.

Sores in these areas should all be managed by removal of pressure and regular dressings. Bone removal is usually unnecessary and healing by cicatrization occurs rapidly once the first breakdown is heeded. If healing is slow pinch grafts may be used to speed the process and occasionally local flaps may be designed to fill unusually large defects.

Treatment of skin defects of the leg and foot

John R. Cobbett FRCS
Consultant Plastic Surgeon, The Queen Victoria Hospital, East Grinstead, and Lewisham Hospital, UK

Introduction

Acute soft tissue injuries of the lower limb, with or without bony involvement, are not usually seen in the first instance by the plastic surgeon. They are managed along standard lines, i.e. by adequate debridement, primary closure of clean wounds, and delayed primary closure of seriously contaminated or gunshot wounds.

If there is skin loss a free split skin graft may be applied initially or taken at the time of wound debridement, stored at 4°C and applied 48 hours later.

Rarely there may be exposed bone, tendon (see later), ligament or joint, in which case a pedicle graft of some sort will be required, as a split skin graft will not take on such a bed.

A common injury worthy of special mention is a V-shaped laceration on the front of the calf, usually the result of tripping upstairs, and particularly common in elderly females. The major portion of the 'V' flap is usually not viable, and time can often be saved by excising most of the flap and using a free split skin graft to fill the resulting defect as a primary repair. Suturing the flap back into place in its entirety usually leads to necrosis of its tip and often the need for a secondary graft.

Major degloving injuries of the limb usually occur in the plane just superficial to the deep fascia. Split skin grafts can be cut from the avulsed skin and applied directly to the deep fascia, discarding all subcutaneous tissue. Attempted replacement of all partially avulsed flaps *in toto* is liable to be followed by considerable areas of necrosis due to the trauma sustained by the tissues at the time of the injury.

An ulcer on the lower limb, if kept reasonably at rest, will heal unless prevented by:

1. vascular insufficiency;
2. local acute or chronic infection;
3. the presence of a foreign body;
4. certain systemic diseases (anaemia, diabetes mellitus);
5. local malignancy;
6. exposure of bare bone, ligament, tendon or metal; or
7. deliberate action of the patient.

Large uncomplicated ulcers will heal more rapidly if covered with a simple split skin graft, but healing will occur even without this. The commonest cause of chronicity is probably local ischaemia secondary to varicose veins or, more rarely, arterial insufficiency. The treatment of these conditions is outside the scope of this chapter but it must be noted that in the presence of such disease no plastic surgical techniques are likely to produce stable healing. Repeated applications of reconstituted lyophilized skin changed every 2–3 days will accelerate cleaning of such a vascular ulcer and help to prepare it for grafting with autogenous skin. Application of specially prepared amnion has been shown to increase the vascularity of the base of such an ulcer, thus facilitating the take of a free split skin graft[1].

Acute local infection will be obvious and is normally easily controlled. Specific chronic infections are now rare but their presence, and that of systemic disease, can be excluded by appropriate laboratory investigations.

A foreign body may be suspected from the history and can often be confirmed by radiography.

Malignant ulceration is uncommon. In plastic surgical practice malignant melanoma is probably the commonest cause. The usual history is of an enlarging, bleeding, ulcerating, pigmented lesion. If the diagnosis is in doubt, excision biopsy under a tourniquet, with immediate frozen sections, is probably a justifiable alternative to immediate undiagnosed wide excision, which in any case, should be done if the frozen sections are positive or indeterminate. There is no place for the removal of part of such a lesion for histological examination, as this will almost certainly cause further dissemination of the tumour. The other cutaneous malignancy causing leg ulceration is a Marjolin ulcer, a squamous cell carcinoma occurring in an old burn or ulcer scar. Local biopsy is permissible in this case.

The author has never knowingly seen dermatitis artefacta appearing in the leg, but the possibility of interference by the patient should always be borne in mind.

The majority of patients with unhealed leg ulcers presenting to the plastic surgeon have bare tendon, bone or metal plate exposed in the base of the ulcer. In those with exposed bone there is usually an associated fracture.

Tendon exposure

If there is paratenon covering the tendon a free split skin graft will suffice to heal the wound. If the tendon is unimportant, such as a toe extensor, and dessicated or necrotic, the easiest course is often to excise it through the length of the wound and use a free graft to cover the resultant defect. The loss of such a tendon is usually not a total disaster, as the fibrous tissue underlying a successful graft takes on the function of a tendon, often to a surprising degree. Large tendons – or those that are definitely viable – require early cover as for bare bone.

Metal exposure

Although there may be exceptions, metal that has become exposed by skin necrosis is usually best removed. If the associated fracture is unstable, a plaster cast with suitable windows may be used for immobilization, although such a cast tends to get in the way of whatever repair is required. Some form of external/internal fixation, rigid but allowing access to all aspects of the limb, is chosen.

Bare tibial cortex will sequestrate after some months, leaving a bed of granulation tissue which may be covered with a free graft, but the resulting scar is often unstable. Exposed bone or tendon, or an open joint, usually require a pedicle flap for cover. As elsewhere, pedicle flaps may be local or distant. Local flaps commonly used on the leg may be cutaneous, fasciocutaneous or myocutaneous, or they may be simple muscle flaps covered in turn by a free skin graft. Distant flaps include free revascularized flaps, cross-leg flaps and, on very rare occasions, open jump or tube pedicle flaps. In addition, in special circumstances local axial pattern flaps containing a known artery may be used. The skin over the pedicle of such flaps may be retained or it can be removed, creating an 'island' pedicle flap. The advent of fasciocutaneous and myocutaneous flaps has greatly reduced the difficulties previously found in closing lower limb defects. The de-epithelialized 'turnover' flap described by Thatte[2] would appear to be an acceptable alternative to fasciocutaneous flaps, but in the majority of cases the latter repair is simpler and at least as safe.

Choice of repair

The precise choice of cover for a lower limb defect is a matter of experience, but some guidelines can be given here. It is best discussed by dividing the limb into six zones.

1–4

THE THIGH

It is rare to need a pedicle flap for coverage in the thigh since a bare portion of femur is extremely uncommon. However, exposure of the main vessels is occasionally an indication for such a procedure. Laterally the tensor fascia lata flap has a wide radius of application; medially the gracilis myocutaneous flap has similar properties. Both flaps can be safely raised distally to within 7.5 cm (3 inches) of the knee joint. Laterally the skin and deep fascia are raised together deep to the fascia from inferiorly upwards until the blood vessel supplying the tensor muscle is found under the superior end of the rectus femoris. Medially the gracilis usually has two vascular pedicles. Division of the lower one, if necessary, is usually safe. Although the overlying skin receives its blood supply from vessels associated with the underlying muscle or fascia, it is surprisingly (and disastrously) easy to separate the two in the plane superficial to the deep fascia. It is strongly recommended that the skin and deep fascia (or muscle) be sutured together at their edges as the flaps are raised in order to prevent this mishap. This advice is equally true for similar flaps raised elsewhere on the lower limb, or indeed the rest of the body. The secondary defect resulting from the raising of such a flap may be capable of direct closure, or may require a free split skin graft.

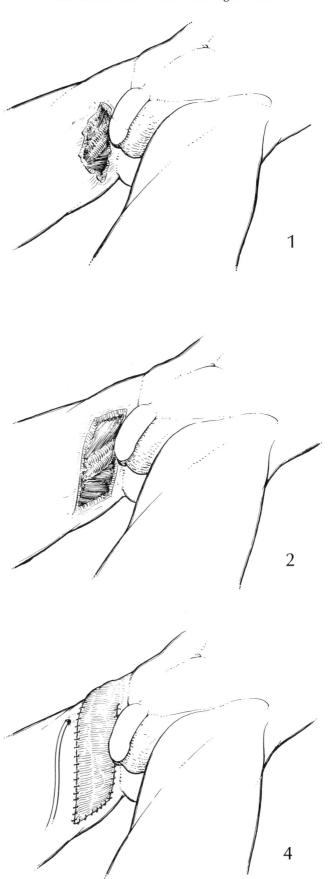

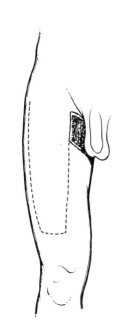

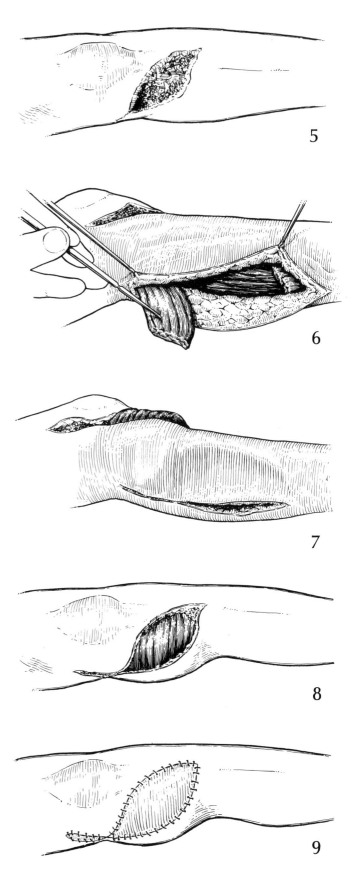

5–9

THE KNEE JOINT

An open knee joint requires urgent closure with viable tissue. Because fasciocutaneous flaps are difficult to raise in this area without exposing bone or joint capsule, muscle flaps from the calf are usually chosen and are extremely reliable. Either the lateral or medial belly of the gastrocnemius muscle can be separated from its fellow, and from the underlying soleus, and mobilized sufficiently to cover any aspect of the knee joint while retaining its superior blood supply. A free skin graft over the mobilized and sutured muscle completes the repair, thus leaving the integument over the soleus muscle intact.

10–12

UPPER TWO-THIRDS OF TIBIA

Exposed bone in this area is best covered with a
fasciocutaneous flap taken from either side of the wound
and transposed across the bare area of bone. A split skin
graft will be required to fill the secondary defect. Such
fasciocutaneous flaps can be cut to proportions of at least
three to one (length to breadth of base), thanks to the rich
blood supply on the the surface of the deep fascia, the
anatomy of which was described by Haertsch[3].

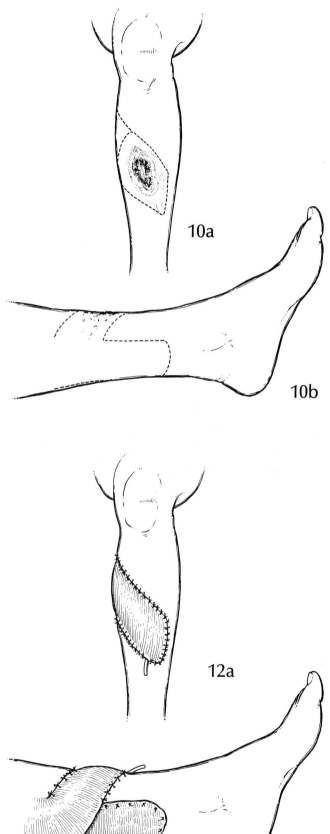

10a

10b

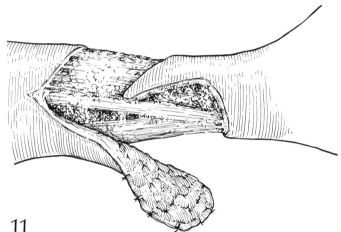

11

Skin cover in the three zones defined above is not
difficult to achieve and may confidently be undertaken by
any surgeon without extensive training in plastic surgery.
Skin cover in the remaining lower part of the limb is very
much more difficult, and without the availability of special
skills and experience the surgeon may do well to consider
most seriously the quick and easy solution of amputation.
Amputation should also be considered when there is
massive chronic infection of the bone, with the likelihood
of recurrent long-term problems.

12a

12b

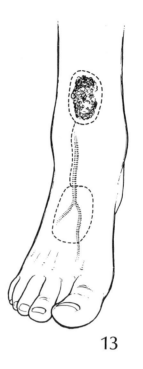

13

LOWER THIRD OF TIBIA AND ANKLE JOINT

Here there is a paucity of fasciocutaneous and myo-cutaneous flaps, although small examples of the former may be possible. A knowledge of the remaining vascular anatomy in the individual patient may become very important, and angiograms may be required before a decision can be taken on the best means of repair.

13–15

A small defect in the lower third of the tibia can be closed most easily by an island dorsal foot flap. The skin on the dorsum of the foot, extending if necessary to include the skin of the first interdigital web, is taken as an island based on the dissected-out dorsalis pedis vessels and tunnelled under any intervening skin to fill the defect. The lower part of the extensor retinaculum may be divided to increase the range of the island flap. The dissection requires care. The first dorsal metatarsal artery should be included if the web skin is taken, and considerable care should be taken to ensure that adequate soft tissue is left over the tendon of the extensor hallucis longus, as exposure of this structure by a failed skin graft can lead to very prolonged healing in the donor site.

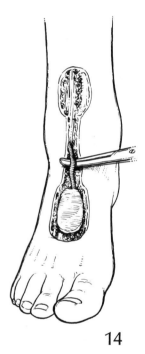

14

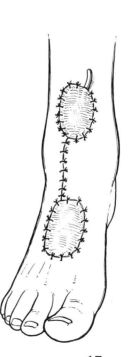

15

16–19

A large defect will require either a free flap, perhaps from groin or scapular areas, with direct microvascular anastomoses of donor and recipient vessels, or a cross-leg flap. The use of a free flap in these circumstances is often complicated by previous vascular damage and by spasm in the recipient vessels. The procedure should only be undertaken by a surgeon with considerable microvascular experience, and an arteriogram is virtually essential.

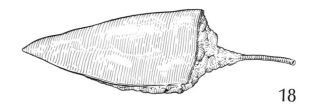

18

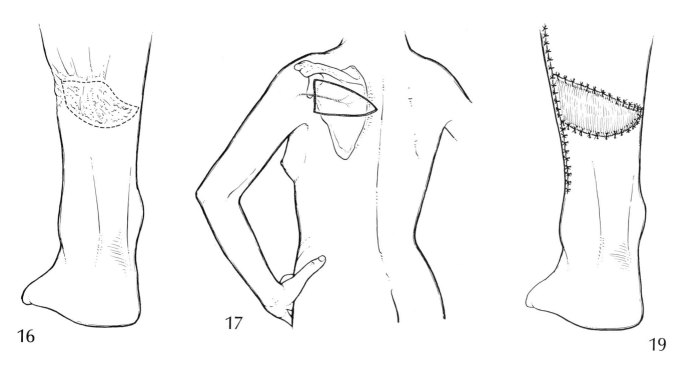

16

17

19

20

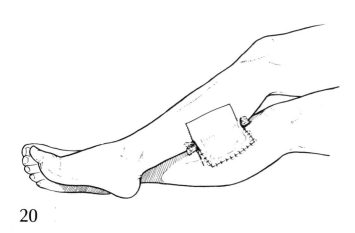

20

A cross-leg flap may thus be the only solution for a surgeon without extensive reconstructive surgery experience. The flap is normally taken – after careful preoperative planning using appropriate patterns of suitable material – from the posterior surface of the opposite calf. The flap should include the deep fascia and, if based on the medial aspect of the calf, as is usual, the long saphenous vein should be spared so as to ensure adequate venous drainage for the flap. The length of the flap from base to end should not be greater than the width of the flap at its base. If the defect on the recipient leg is such that a suitably tailored flap would be longer than its base, then the defect itself should be enlarged so that a 'square' shaped flap will fill it. The defect should be made to fit the flap, not the other way round.

While the flap is still attached to both limbs care must be taken to avoid pressure from one leg on to the other. Windowed plaster casts on both legs, although necessitating longer flaps because of their sheer thickness, may in the long run be worth while by ensuring immobility and, if correctly applied, absence of pressure sores.

THE HEEL

21–23

This is another very difficult area. On the weight bearing area a medial plantar flap of skin and soft tissue and containing the medial plantar vessels will solve most problems. More posteriorly, an island dorsal foot flap may be possible. Failing this a cross-leg flap may be required. A distally based muscle flap of the soleus has been used, but this is probably unreliable unless the posterior tibial artery is included, when the flow therein will be retrograde, feeding the muscle from the dorsalis pedis, through the foot anastomoses. Preoperative angiograms are essential for this, and the procedure is not recommended for the occasional reconstructor. Pressure sores on the posterior aspect of the heel are best treated conservatively with appropriate surgical debridement followed by a period of wet dressings until adequate granulations for a skin graft are present.

THE SOLE

This is another problem area. Pedicle graft cover can be obtained by a cross-limb flap from calf or thigh, or, in a thin individual, even from the back of the ipsilateral thigh, with the knee in full flexion. However, any such repair will leave skin that, while of good quality, is anaesthetic and hence prone to ulceration on weight bearing. Various free flaps possessing a nerve supply which can be linked to the local sensory nerves at the recipient site are available, but these techniques are beyond the scope of this chapter.

References

1. Bennett, J. P., Matthews, R., Faulk, W. P. Treatment of chronic ulceration of the legs with human amnion. Lancet 1980; 1: 1153–1156

2. Thatte, R. L. One-stage random-pattern de-epithelialised 'turn over' flaps in the leg. British Journal of Plastic Surgery 1982; 35: 287–292

3. Haertsch, P. A. The blood supply to the skin of the leg: a post-mortem investigation. British Journal of Plastic Surgery 1981; 34: 470–477

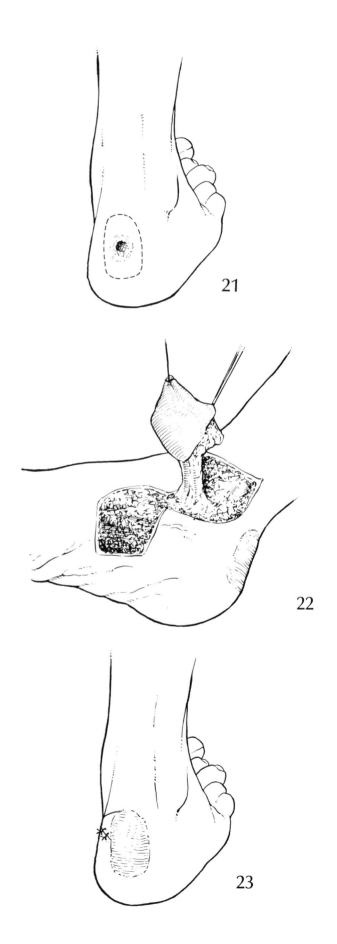

21

22

23

Illustrations by Patrick Elliott and Gwynne Gloege

Surgical management of lymphoedema of the extremity

Timothy A. Miller MD, FACS
Professor of Surgery, UCLA School of Medicine;
Chief of Plastic Surgery, Wadsworth Veterans Administration Medical Center, Los Angeles, California, USA

Introduction

In spite of the large number of different operative procedures described in the literature, lymphoedema of the lower extremity remains one of the more resistant and as yet incurable clinical problems. The aetiology of this condition is obscure. It is likely that an inborn error in the lymphatic system (resulting in fewer collecting channels than are normally present) is responsible in many patients but clinical lymphoedema of an extremity can occur in the presence of normal lymphangiographic appearances. Conversely, individuals with abnormal lymphangiographic findings may have no clinical evidence of lymphoedema.

It is likely that the familiar anatomical explanation of lymphoedema may offer some, but not all, of the answers regarding this challenging and poorly understood condition.

Some functional abnormality within the lymphatics may also in part account for the symptoms of oedema. For example, patients who go on to develop lymphoedema following axillary node dissection or irradiation consistently do not develop symptoms for at least one year. If the oedema were the result of a decrease in lymphatic drainage channels, why is there no clinical swelling for the intervening year?

Because of the uncertainties regarding the aetiology of lymphoedema and our imperfect understanding of the pathophysiology of the accumulation of large amounts of protein-rich fluid within the intercellular space, a large number of operative procedures have been described for its management. Unfortunately, because of our inability to cure this condition and produce an extremity of normal dimensions, postoperative results tend to be evaluated subjectively. In addition, few long-term follow-up studies have been carried out.

While acknowledging that no operative procedure can cure this problem, it is my firm belief that staged skin and subcutaneous excision beneath skin flaps provides the most reliable and consistent postoperative improvement. In general, the greater the amount of skin and subcutaneous tissue removed the better the postoperative result.

The operations

SKIN AND SUBCUTANEOUS EXCISION FOR LYMPHOEDEMA OF THE LEG

Stage I

1

The procedure is performed with a pneumatic tourniquet placed on the proximal thigh. The initial incision courses along the mid-portion of the medial thigh and calf, curving posterior to the medial malleolus. In almost all cases a substantial ellipse of skin, to be excised later in the procedure, is outlined at the time when the skin flaps are developed. Additional skin is usually excised on completion of the operative procedure.

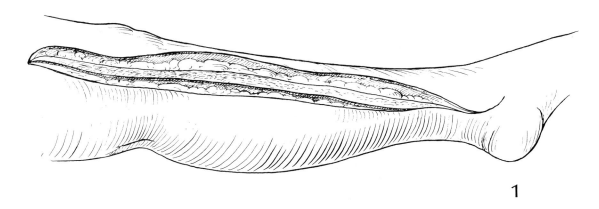

1

2

A large skin flap is developed anteriorly to expose the entire medial surface of the tibia, and posteriorly to the mid-sagittal plane of the extremity. These flaps are approximately 1–2 cm thick. In order to maintain their vascularity, undermining in the superior and inferior poles of the dissection (particularly in the region of the ankle) is limited to approximately 4–5 cm. When the flaps have been completely developed, a transverse incision is made across the mid-calf, extending down through the subcutaneous tissue and deep muscle fascia investing the gastrocnemius and soleus muscles.

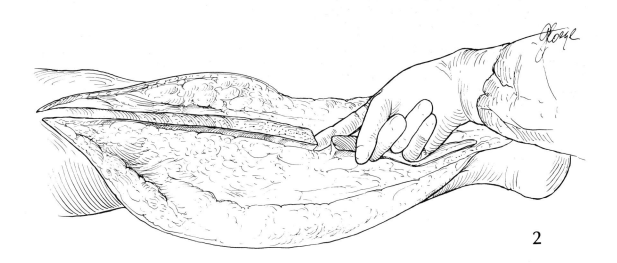

2

3

Once the muscle compartment has been opened, the sural nerve is identified adjacent to the deep muscle fascia and preserved. The dissection then proceeds superiorly towards the knee, excising all the fatty tissue overlying the periosteum of the tibia, the deep fascia of the calf muscles and the overlying subcutaneous tissue.

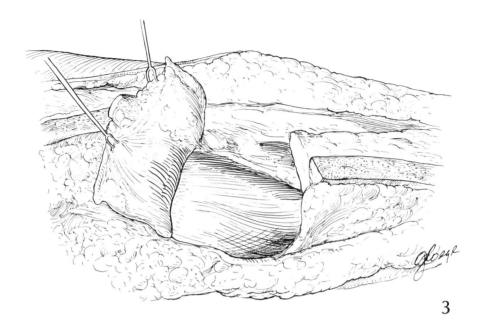

3

4

As the proximal gastrocnemius muscle tapers towards its origin, the level of dissection continues above the thick ligamentous tissues of the medial knee joint capsule. All of the subcutaneous tissue overlying the knee joint capsule and medial thigh adductor muscles is removed.

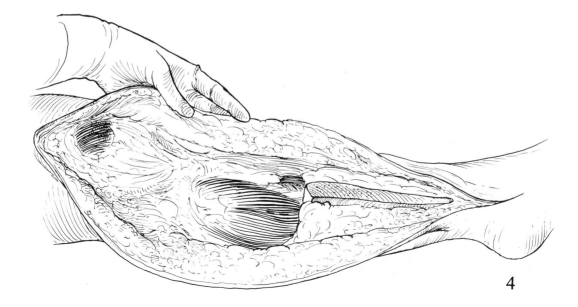

4

5

The dissection then proceeds inferiorly to completely expose the muscle bellies of the gastrocnemius and soleus by removing the overlying fascia. In the ankle region the level of dissection lies just above the deep fascia that joins the medial malleolus to the tendo calcaneus. This limits potential damage to the posterior tibial artery, which lies deep to these fascial structures. At the conclusion of this stage of the procedure the pneumatic tourniquet is decompressed and haemostasis established before final trimming of the skin flaps.

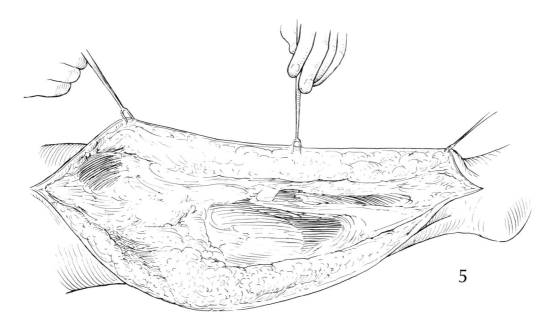

5

6

Following excision of the subcutaneous fatty tissues and deep fascia there is considerable skin redundancy. As much of this excess skin as possible is removed.

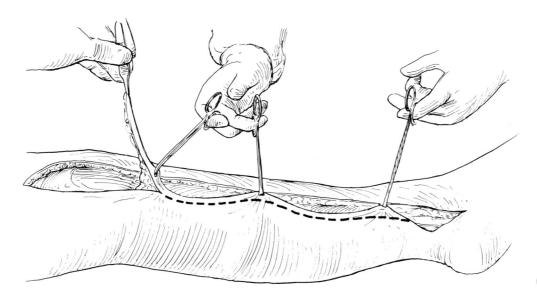

6

Wound closure

7

Subcutaneous or dermal suturing has not been found to be effective. Sutures through the skin and including some of the deep muscle or fascial structures ensure adherence of the skin flaps and allow contouring in the areas of the ankle and knee regions. It is absolutely essential that a large suction catheter is placed in the dependent portion of the posterior skin flap and kept on constant suction.

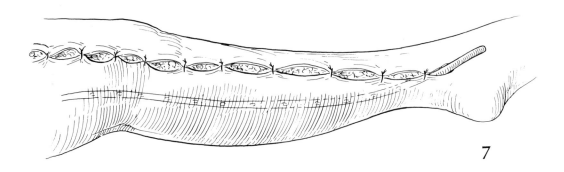

7

Postoperative care

The entire extremity is immobilized in a well-padded posterior plaster splint and elevated for at least 8 days postoperatively. Sutures are removed on the 8th postoperative day and replaced by benzoin and tape closure.

The extremity is dangled on the 9th day and the patient can walk on the 10th day postoperatively. Allowing the leg to become dependent sooner than this results in the accumulation of serous fluid and the risk of haematoma.

Stage II

8

The second stage of the skin and subcutaneous excision for lymphoedema is performed on the lateral aspect of the extremity at least 3 months later. The extent of excision varies with each patient. The principal objective is to remove skin and subcutaneous tissue from the lower two-thirds of the lateral calf, the ankle and the dorsum of the foot. The incision is positioned along the mid-lateral aspect, and again skin flaps are dissected anteriorly and posteriorly. Much less fatty tissue is excised on the lateral aspect of the extremity than on the medial aspect. The skin flaps can be somewhat thinner – often 1 cm or less in thickness.

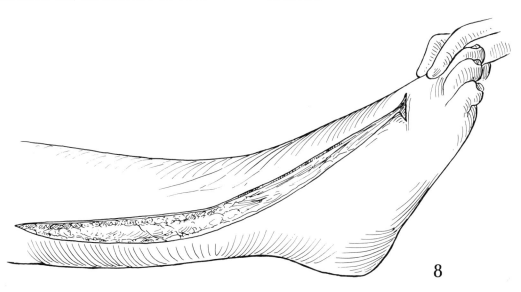

8

9

During this part of the dissection the superficial branch of the peroneal nerve is identified as it exits from the extensor retinaculum of the ankle. This nerve is preserved for later reinnervation of the skin flap, providing sensation to the dorsum of the foot. Considerable contouring can be achieved by using curved Mayo scissors on the undersurface of the pedicle flap to excise excess fatty tissue. Again, at the conclusion of the excision, large amounts of redundant skin can be excised.

Wound closure and postoperative management are the same as for the medial aspect.

Long-continued use of a supporting elastic bandage is essential after this procedure if ulceration and scar breakdown between the grafts are to be kept to a minimum. Provided this is done, troublesome intermittent inflammatory attacks can be largely prevented for many years.

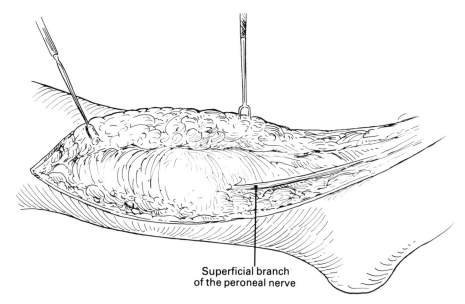

Superficial branch
of the peroneal nerve

9

ABLATIVE SURGERY FOR LYMPHOEDEMA OF THE LOWER LEG

Long-standing lymphoedema of the lower limb occasionally leads to gross and disabling enlargement of the limb which does not decrease in size when the limb is elevated. The thickened hard skin and subcutaneous tissue of the limb are of such an unyielding nature as to offer little chance of achieving a satisfactory result by simply reducing the bulk of the limb by the raising, thinning and re-suture of flaps. In these cases a stage has been reached where consideration might reasonably be given to amputation.

As an alternative, radical excision of the whole of the skin and subcutaneous tissue of the lower leg can be carried out. The raw area is then resurfaced with a split or full thickness skin graft taken from the excised tissue. If the skin on the tissue removed is unsuitable for use as a graft, split skin may be taken from elsewhere in the body.

The result, particularly when split skin grafting is performed, is often less than ideal. Cosmetically the contrast between the thin lower leg and bulky thigh is unattractive. Split skin grafts can be unstable and sometimes leak fluid, leading to intertrigo and fungal infections between the toes and an eczematous appearance of the skin grafts. The use of full thickness skin grafts would therefore seem preferable when this is possible.

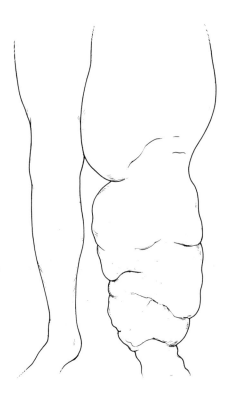

10

Chronic, long-standing and irreversible lymphoedema is best treated by the Charles procedure. It is preferable to admit the patient to hospital a few days before surgery to have the limb elevated and as much oedema drained from the leg as possible.

10

11

'Ice tong' calipers are used to elevate the limb to a vertical position, as this makes excision of the skin and subcutaneous tissue much easier. A pneumatic tourniquet is placed around the thigh and inflated to provide a bloodless field. A 'stocking seam' incision is marked along the posterior midline of the calf. Above, a circumferential incision is marked just below the tibial tubercle; below, the circumferential incision passes just above the malleoli and then extends downwards to the base of the toes to include all the skin on the dorsum of the foot.

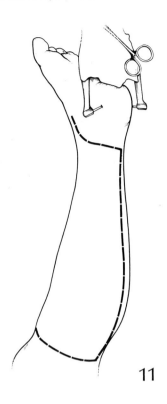

11

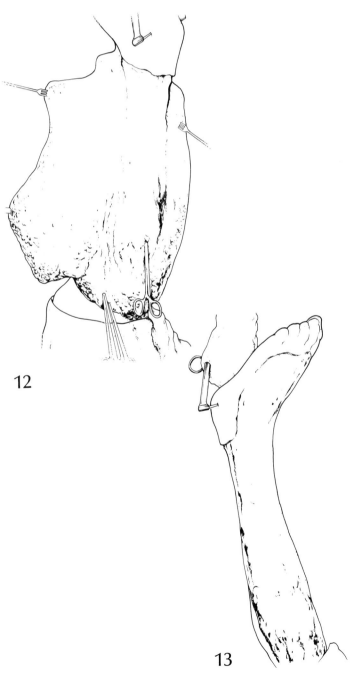

12

13

12 & 13

The incisions are made and, working progressively from posterior to anterior, the skin and subcutaneous tissue are separated from the underlying fascia. Some tissue must be left over the Achilles tendon to provide a vascularized bed for the skin graft.

The wound can be pressure-wrapped with an elastic bandage at this stage and the tourniquet released while the skin graft is cut from the specimen.

14

The skin grafts can be cut from the specimen with a Brown electric dermatome or a Reese dermatome. Both have the disadvantage of requiring multiple strips of graft. Gibson and Ross have developed a special dermatome (shown here) to remove all the required skin in a single sheet.

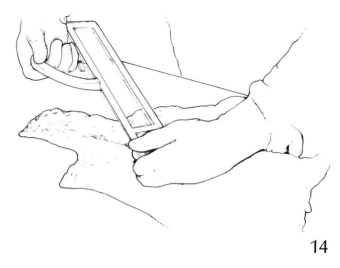

14

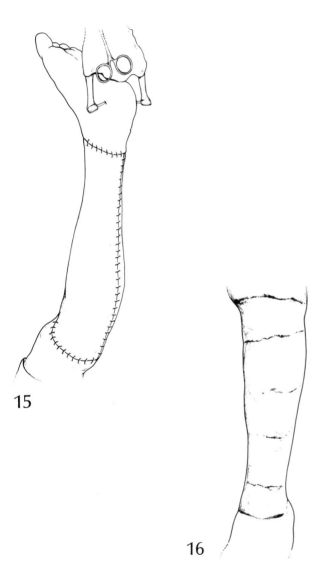

15

15

After complete haemostasis has been secured, the skin graft is applied to the wound and sutured to itself and to the wound margins as shown. If necessary, several strips of graft may be used. A pressure dressing is applied over the graft and the leg is immobilized in a cast. The leg should be kept elevated postoperatively until the graft is adequately vascularized.

16

At the first graft dressing the junctions between the skin grafts are still visible.

16

17

The final result shows that, while bulk is reduced, the aesthetic result is less than pleasing. Also, the skin grafts tend to thicken and, particularly on the dorsum of the foot, to weep, and intertrigo between the toes is a frequent problem.

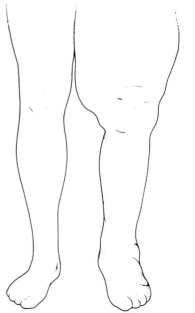

17

SKIN AND SUBCUTANEOUS EXCISION FOR POST-MASTECTOMY OEDEMA OF THE ARM

18

Preoperatively, the patient is confined to bed, with the arm elevated for at least 48 hours. This results in considerable resolution of the oedema, allowing the amount of excess skin to be estimated. The operative procedure is the same as for the lower extremity except that in the forearm much more skin than subcutaneous tissue is excised.

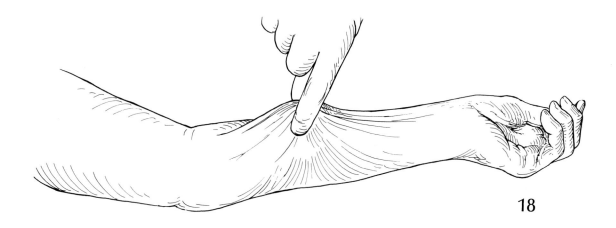

18

19

A large ellipse of skin and subcutaneous tissue is excised along the ulnar aspect of the forearm and upper arm. This part of the procedure is performed with a pneumatic tourniquet on the upper arm. The tourniquet is then removed and the excision continued along the medial aspect of the proximal upper arm and extending to the posterior axillary fold. It is in this area that considerable amounts of skin and subcutaneous tissue are excised.

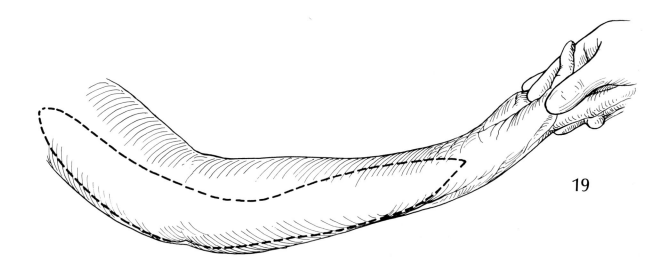

19

20

The ulnar nerve is identified to prevent inadvertent injury to it. It is most vulnerable just above the medial epicondyle.

Wound closure is accomplished as described for the lower extremity. Suction catheters are placed in the posterior portion of the wound along the dependent skin flap.

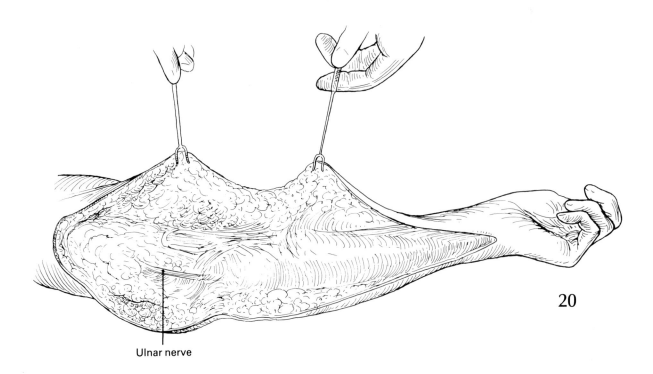

Ulnar nerve

20

Hypospadias

John D. Noonan MD, FACS
Associate Professor, Division of Plastic Surgery, Albany Medical College, Albany, New York, USA

Charles E. Horton MD
Professor and Chairman, Department of Plastic Surgery, Eastern Virginia Medical School, Norfolk, Virginia, USA

Charles J. Devine, Jr MD
Professor and Chairman, Department of Urology, Eastern Virginia Medical School, Norfolk, Virginia, USA

Introduction

1a–g

Hypospadias, derived from the Greek (hypo, meaning under, plus spadon, meaning a tear or a rent), is a common developmental anomaly which affects approximately 1 per 300 live male births[1]. In this condition the urethral meatus is situated on the undersurface of the penis proximal to its normal location in the glans. It may be located in a variety of places extending from the perineum to the base of the glans, leading to a practical classification based on each variant anatomical location. These are listed from proximal to distal as: (a) perineal; (b) scrotal; (c) penile-scrotal junction; (d) penile; (e) distal penile; and (f) glanular.

Extending around the abnormal urethral meatus distally there appears a fan-like projection of abnormal congenital fibrous tissue, the apex of which originates from the aberrant meatus and extends to the base of the glans, inserting there along a broad cuff. This anomaly, known as chordee (Latin, meaning string), produces a curvature and tends to buckle or bow-string the distal portion of the penis. Since the fibrous band lacks elasticity, the ventral curvature becomes more prominent during erection and may prevent or at least hinder normal sexual activity. Chordee is not seen in all hypospadias cases (g). It is usually more severe in the perineal or scrotal varieties.

History

This affliction has occurred in men (and women) from the earliest recorded times. Usually it is not necessary to treat hypospadias in the female. Many methods of management for male hypospadias have been mentioned in ancient manuscripts. Early Greek surgeons amputated the penis distal to the meatus and remoulded the tip with a glowing cautery.

Modern-day surgical treatment began with the first successful repair, which was reported by John Peter Mettauer of Virginia in 1842[2]. At the end of the nineteenth and beginning of the twentieth century, Duplay[3], Thiersch[4], Anger[5], Nove'Josserand[6], Ombredanne[7] and many other authors presented theses on the surgical repair of hypospadias. To date, there have been over 250 procedures described for the correction of this condition. Modification of older procedures have been reworded and reworked with minor variations to produce both functionally and cosmetically better technical repairs. When the literature on techniques of repair contains so many alternatives and discrepancies in beneficial results, the surgeon may wonder about the efficacy of such repairs. In order to understand the variety of approaches it is first necessary to understand the developmental embryology and surgical anatomy.

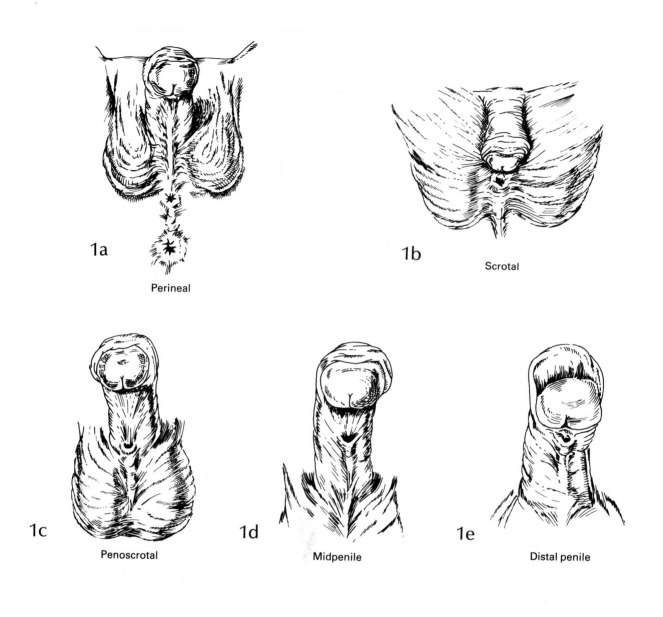

1a   Perineal

1b   Scrotal

1c   Penoscrotal

1d   Midpenile

1e   Distal penile

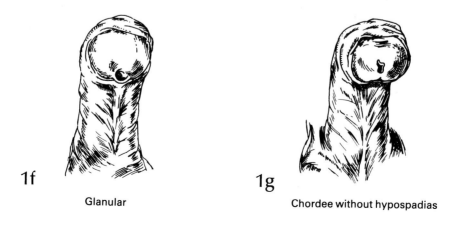

1f   Glanular

1g   Chordee without hypospadias

Embryology

2a, b & c

Although sex is determined at conception, the first 6 weeks of gestation have been named the 'indifferent period' because the sex of the embryo cannot be determined accurately either grossly or by gonadal sectioning. It is during this time that the genital system makes its appearance. At the end of the fifth week embryos develop a conical genital tubercle projection with a medially positioned urogenital groove covered by a thin urogenital membrane and lateral side walls which are known as the urogenital folds. During the seventh week the genital tubercle elongates into a somewhat cylindrical phallus with its tip moulding into an eventual glans. Lateral to the base of the phallus a rounded ridge also makes its appearance on each side; they are genital swellings which eventually differentiate into labial or scrotal landmarks. Rupture of the urogenital membrane in the region near the base of the phallus provides an external opening for the urogenital sinus at about the end of the second month. Proceeding from this basic framework the external genital organs of the male and female develop acording to their predestined design. In the male the formation of an external penis with a penile urethra continues steadily towards completion during the ensuing gestation. At 12 weeks the progressive modelling of the male genitalia has resulted in characteristics that are recognizable as distinctly masculine. The scrotal swellings have shifted posteriorly and are separated by the median raphe; the phallus has become the penis, while the urogenital groove has elongated along the ventral aspect of the phallus to form the potential urethra. The lateral urethral folds gradually unite from proximal to distal to incorporate the urethra completely within the shaft of the penis. By the 14th week the urethra has closed as far as the glans and ultimately the urethra takes its normal anatomical position in the glans.

In the patient afflicted with hypospadias there is failure to complete this embryological progression. Instead of the normal growth and differentiation, this process is arrested in the early stages of development and ventrally located urethral meatus is thus formed. The aetiology of this error is not clear. Several hypotheses have been advanced which suggest decreased or abnormal hormonal stimulation but solidarity of proof remains questionable.

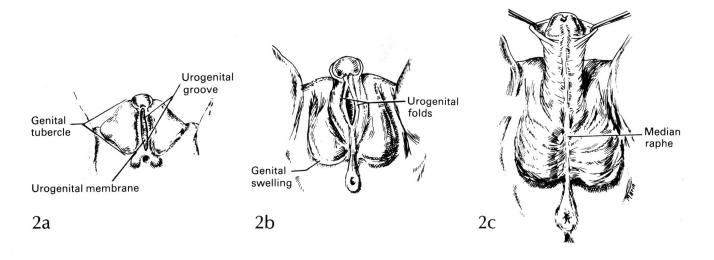

2a

2b

2c

3

Diagnosis of hypospadias is made by physical examination. Minimal degrees are often overlooked and it is not surprising that parents may be the first to recognize the problem. It is important to make sure that the meatal opening is large enought to allow free voiding. A child with severe hypospadias should have a complete urological investigation including intravenous pyelogram and cystoscopy. The finding of this congenital anomaly should alert the physician to search for the possibilities of other anomalies. There are several major points to be considered following the diagnosis of hypospadias: (1) A child should *not* be circumcised. This is of the utmost importance, since the surgical repair may depend on the availability of preputial skin. (2) Where the meatus is too deficient to allow adequate free voiding, a meatotomy should be fashioned along the *distal rim* of the meatus in order to avoid injury to the proximal urethra. The patient should be followed up at approximately 3-monthly intervals until the penis is of adequate size to facilitate surgery. This is usually between the ages of 1 and 2 years. At this time the growth of the penis slows but the fascial layers of the penis gradually become thicker and more adherent after the age of 2 years, thus making the dissection more difficult in the older child. It is important to note that chromosomal studies may be necessary, especially in the presence of ambiguous genitalia. Chromosomal studies, however, of themselves have shown no abnormality associated with hypospadias.

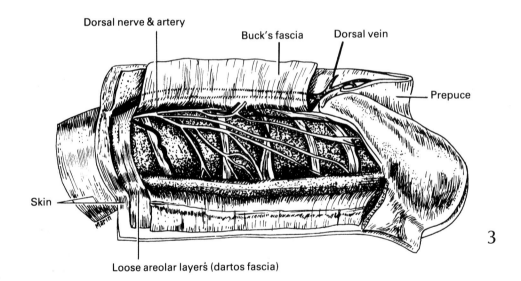

Dorsal nerve & artery

Buck's fascia

Dorsal vein

Prepuce

Skin

Loose areolar layers (dartos fascia)

3

The surgical management of hypospadias

Surgery requires a twofold approach; first, the correction of the abnormally curved penis and, second, construction of the distal urethra. The end-result must be aesthetic and the child should be subjected to the minimum amount of hospitalization. It should likewise be kept in mind that the correction should be completed prior to school age to avoid social harassment and embarrassment with lasting psychological problems. The utmost care must be taken to preserve the dorsally located neurovascular network necessary for viability and tactile sensation.

Originally, a multistage approach was advocated due to the inability to attain and/or verify adequate chordee release. The conservative approach therefore was initially to excise the tissues causing the chordee and then wait at least 6 months to determine that no chordee persisted. However, more surgeons are finding that adequate extirpation of the tissues causing chordee can be achieved and a concomitant urethroplasty can be performed at the same operation.

4a, b & c

Complete chordee release can be facilitated by creating an artificial erection during the operation to ensure that no residual fibrotic bands have been left behind. In order to accomplish this a tourniquet fashioned with a soft red rubber catheter is placed at the base of the phallus and held there with a clamp. A simulated erection can be produced by injecting normal saline through a small gauge needle into the corpus cavernosum[8].

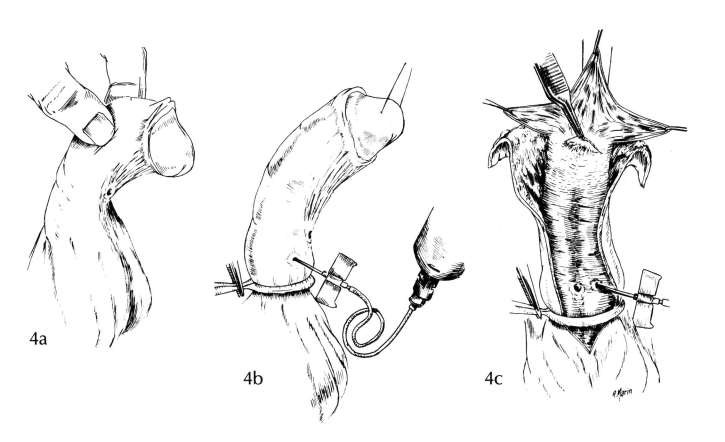

4a

4b

4c

Operative technique

5a–e

The Horton-Devine operation was designed to obviate multistage procedures and at the same time incorporate the basic concept of obtaining a successful urethral repair to the tip of the glans[9]. A traction suture of 4/0 silk is placed in the dorsal anterior portion of the glans to aid in manipulation and exposure during the operative procedure. It has also proved beneficial to infiltrate 0.25–0.5 ml of 1:100 000 epinephrine solution along the anticipated incision line. This substantially decreases haemorrhage during dissection through the vascular tissue of the phallus. Bleeding is likewise minimized by continued deep general anaesthesia which inhibits venous engorgement of the corpus cavernosum. A circumferential coronal incision is extended along the ventral shaft of the penis and eventually encircles the abnormal meatus. The tissue causing chordee is excised totally. Aided by the simulated erection, it can be determined with certainty that the penis will be straight on erection. A V-flap meatal reconstruction of the glans assures an adequate neomeatal orifice at the normal anatomical site. Lateral glans flaps cover the ventral surface of the new urethral meatus[10].

The type of construction of the distal urethra is related to anatomical location. If the meatal opening is distal, the circumferential incision around the urethral orifice is made to incorporate an elliptical area of ventral skin that can be based at the urethra and turned forward into a tubed local flap (flip-flap). Ventral skin coverage is obtained from the redundant prepuce.

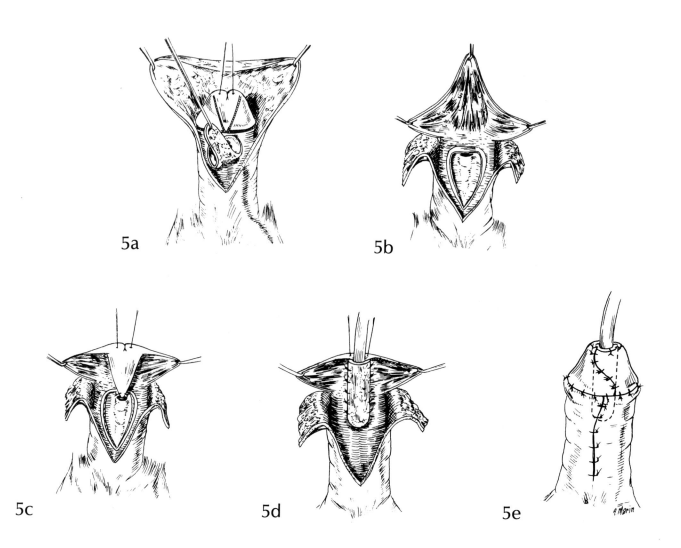

5a

5b

5c

5d

5e

6a–d

If the hypospadiac meatus is more proximal, a circular incision made around the orifice is used and a full-thickness preputial skin graft is then designed for the construction of the distal neourethra. The graft is tubed with the raw surface out and sutured into place over a catheter brought out through the neomeatus in the glans penis.

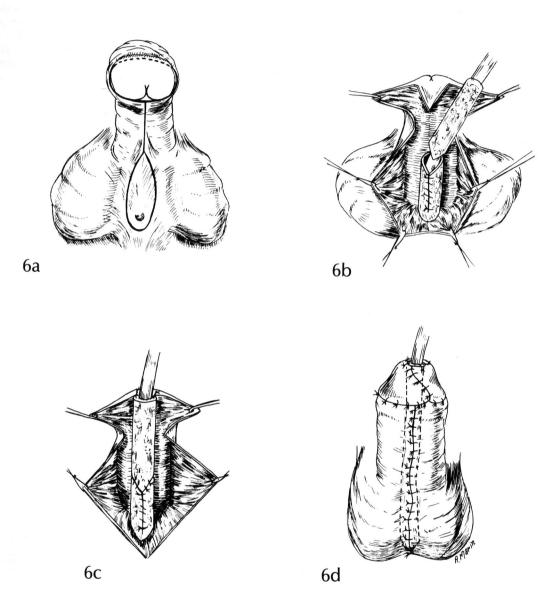

6a

6b

6c

6d

7a–g

For a perineal hypospadias repair again the same basic technique is used; however, the proximal local *hairless* scrotal skin can be tubed and the remainder of the distal urethra is constructed with a preputial graft. The authors prefer 6/0 chromic catgut sutures throughout the repair as they will absorb and do not have to be removed. The tube graft should have a large tongue and groove anastomosis proximally and distally to avoid anastomotic stenosis. A small catheter is placed through the flip-flap type of repair for approximately 3 days for urinary drainage. In more proximal hypospadias both a stent and perineal urinary diversion is preferred. This catheter is left in place 3–4 days following removal of the neourethral stent.

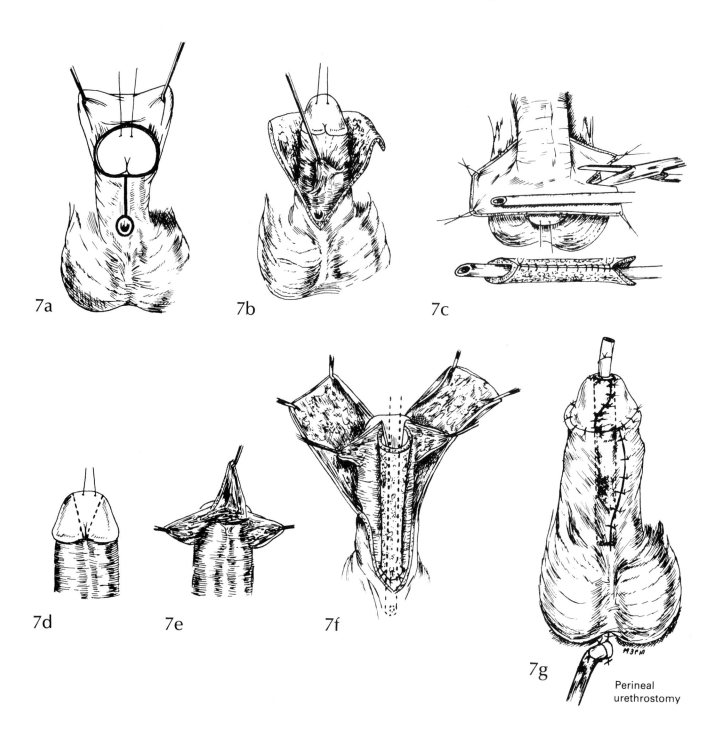

7a

7b

7c

7d

7e

7f

7g

Perineal
urethrostomy

8 & 9

Several other one-stage procedures have been devised which offer an alternative to the Horton-Devine approach. Broadbent[11] uses a spiral flap of preputial skin to create the neo-urethra. Hodgson[12] takes advantage of the redundant dorsal coronal skin fold by passing the penis through the base of the preputial skin and reflecting a tubed graft from its underside. Toksu[13] utilizes this same principle with a glanular modification.

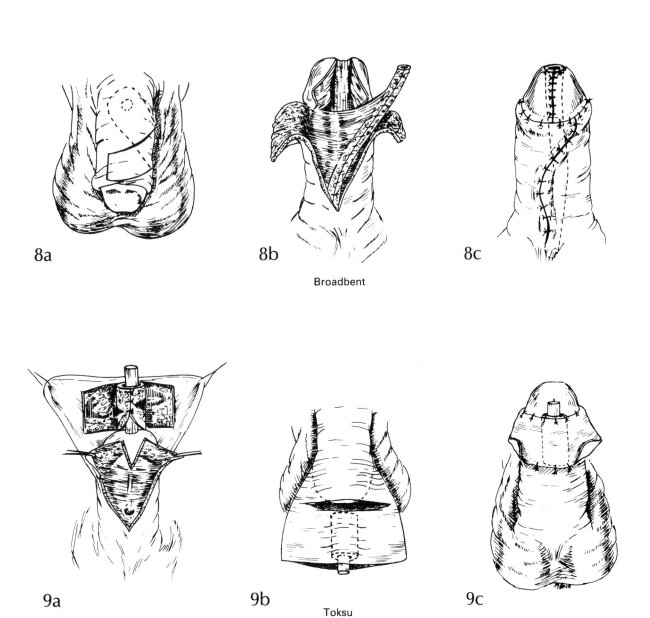

8a   8b   8c

Broadbent

9a   9b   9c

Toksu

10a–f

There are other important techniques that must be available to the hypospadias team, in the event of a problem case necessitating a diversified approach. The Byars' (Thiersch-Duplay) is an excellent multistaged procedure[14, 15]. At the first operation the chordee is released closure being achieved with the redundant preputial skin. This is accomplished by using a circumcoronal incision with a dorsal slit, thereby elevating paired skin flaps or preputial skin. These are then used to resurface the ventral defect. The second stage is performed at approximately 4–5 years of age which is adequate time for maturation and softening of the previous first-stage scars. At the second stage of the Byars' procedure an elliptical incision is made from the anticipated glanular meatus back to and circumferentially around the hypospadiac meatus. This ventral flap of skin is then tubed on itself for the neourethra and the skin is closed above it.

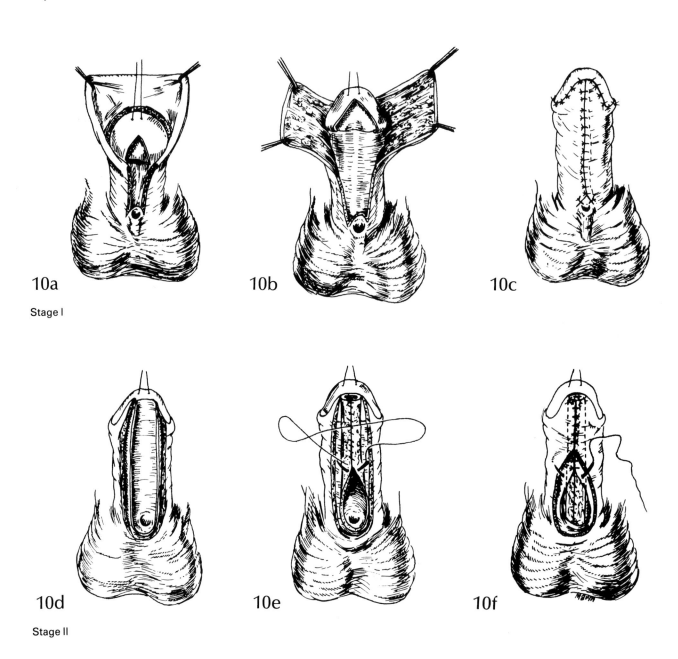

10a

Stage I

10b

10c

10d

Stage II

10e

10f

11a, b & c

A second type of multistaged procedure described by Sir Denis Browne[16] is a modification of the previous method initially suggested by Duplay in 1874. His procedure takes advantage of the fact that a buried strip of skin will form into a tube. This operation has many advocates and was popular in recent years, with satisfactory results being obtained by those surgeons specifically trained in this technique. The first stage is similar to Byars' operation. The second procedure is performed at the age of 4 or 5 years, at which time a paired incision along the ventral aspect of the penile shaft is made and tapered both distally onto the glans and proximally behind the hypospadiac meatus. This creates a longitudinal skin strip. The lateral skin is elevated in a superficial plane and a dorsal relaxing incision is made to release tension. The ventral skin edges are approximated over the buried strip of skin. In time, the buried island will tube itself and form the distal portion of the urethra.

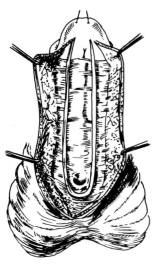

11a

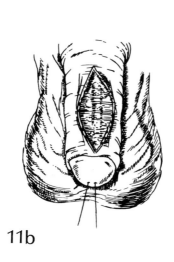

11b

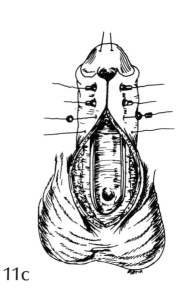

11c

12, 13 & 14

For penile hypospadias the Cecil-Culp operation with several modifications is another alternative[17,18]. The first-stage operation is the same as the Byars or Browne operation. The chordee is released and the incision closed without tension along the ventral aspect of the penile shaft. At the second stage, a skin island is developed along the ventral aspect of the penile shaft and tapered at the glans. The incision is carried back behind the hypospadiac urethral meatus and the skin is then tubed on itself. An extension of the incision posteriorly along the scrotal raphe allows scrotal-skin undermining and the penis is folded downward so that the corporal bodies can be sewn to the superficial dartos fascia of the scrotum with fine catgut sutures. The incision is then closed using fine subcuticular sutures to approximate the scrotal skin to the penile shaft skin. This gives ample coverage to the neourethra and the ventral aspect of the penile shaft. At a third stage of this operation the penis is released from the scrotum, taking a generous portion of scrotal skin bilaterally in order to cover the ventral aspect of the penis. Thus the ventral surface of the penis is covered partly by scrotal skin. The scrotal defect is closed primarily.

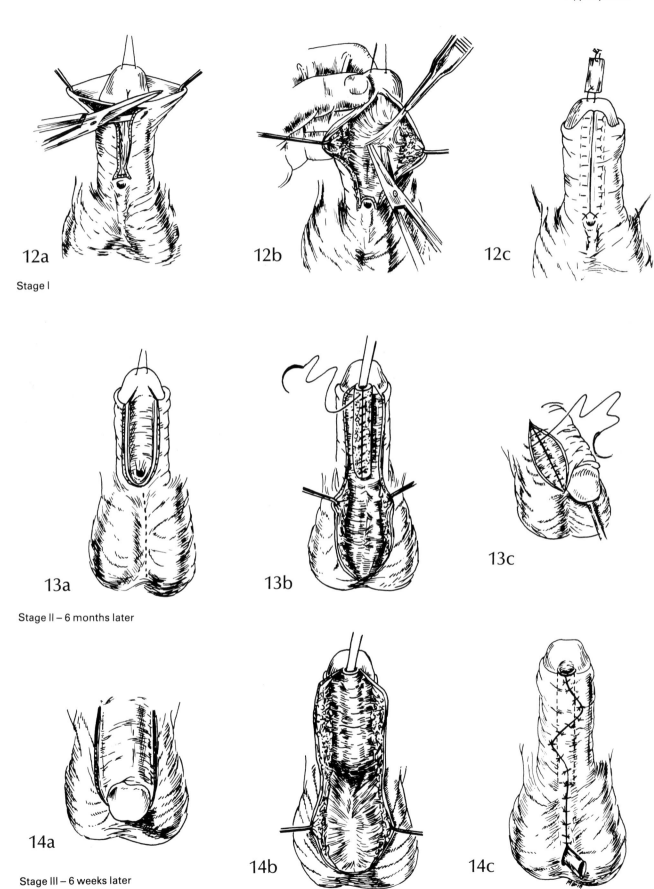

12a

12b

12c

Stage I

13a

13b

13c

Stage II – 6 months later

14a

14b

14c

Stage III – 6 weeks later

15a–d

A recent procedure described by Van der Meulen[19] again utilizes the principle of Duplay's skin strip. Using a circumpreputial incision, retaining the meatus distally, and by a dorsal preputial backcut, adequate ventral coverage can be obtained if there is no significant chordee.

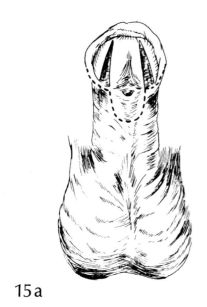

15a

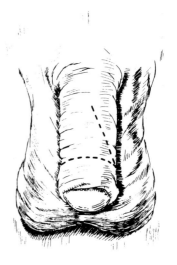

15b

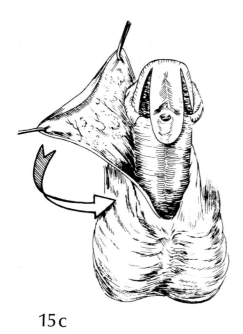

15c

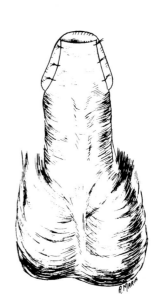

15d

16 & 17

When the tissues causing chordee must be transected and/or the meatus is more proximal the procedure is performed in two stages. First the release is accomplished and ventral coverage is procured by rotation and cutback of the preputial skin. At a subsequent stage the neourethra is formed by covering a ventral skin island by the previously banked excess preputial skin.

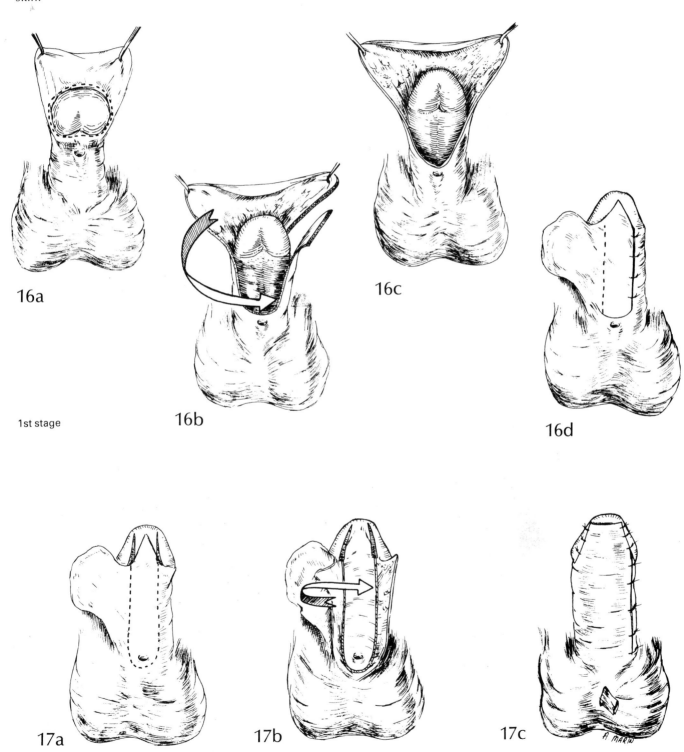

16a

1st stage

16b

16c

16d

17a

2nd stage

17b

17c

Complications

The major early complications in hypospadias repair are (*1*) haematoma formation and (*2*) infection. Acute bleeding can occur immediately postoperatively or within the first 24–48 hours. The extravasation of blood under flaps or grafts not only produces a physical barrier to new ingrowth of nutrient vessels but also carries with it the potential of a nidus for infection. If infection does not occur, the mere fact that haematoma is present may produce eventual fibrosis and scarring resulting in the formation of new chordee. Thus great attention should be directed to haemostasis and to the immediate postoperative course.

Infection may cause wound dehiscence, graft or flap necrosis and severe cicatrization. In order to minimize this complication the patient is placed on a prophylactic antimicrobial agent. If infection does occur with dehiscence of the wound, it is advisable to await secondary healing with the institution of sterile sitz baths and continued appropriate antimicrobial coverage in order to minimize the destruction. After an adequate time interval, usually 3–6 months, a secondary repair can be made.

The most common late secondary complications include: (*1*) fistula, (*2*) stricture, (*3*) diverticulum and (*4*) occasional urethral hair growth with calculi formation. Should a fistula occur, immediate re-repair is *not* recommended. A common site of breakdown is at the proximal anastomosis. This may be due to many factors, including multiple suture lines, the calibre of the lumen and the local quality of the graft or flaps. Small fistulae have been known to close spontaneously when adequate drainage has been established by the insertion of a drainage catheter. Most fistulae, however, require surgical closure[20].

Stricture formation may occur early or late in the convalescent period. The neourethra and suture lines should be given adequate time to resolve any initial oedematous or inflammatory stricture. The graft also must be given time to soften and adapt to an adequate size. Instrumentation at this point may cause deleterious effects. When possible, most patients are watched for approximately 4–6 months in order to obtain an adequate softening of the tissues. If the stricture does not abate within this time span surgical intervention should be carried out. The repair is performed by opening the urethra to a normal calibre and using a patch of penile or preputial skin to rebuild the circumference of the urethra to normal. Hairless skin grafts can be used with excellent results.

A diverticulum when initially diagnosed should be approached surgically through an incision directly over it. The neck of the diverticulum should be identified and divided flush with the neourethra. The urethral opening is best closed with individual chromic catgut sutures.

A urethral beard arises from using hair-bearing skin to form the neourethra. This should never be a problem if careful attention to the source of the urethral reconstructive material has been given. If hair within the urethra is a problem the hair-bearing skin must be excised and a new urethra constructed. Electrolysis of abundant hairgrowth has not produced adequate results in the authors' experience.

References

1. Backus, L. H., DeFelice, C. A. Hypospadias, then and now. Plastic and Reconstructive Surgery 1960; 25: 146–160

2. Mettauer, J. P. Practical observation on those malformations of the male urethra and penis, termed hypospadias and epispadias with an anomalus case. American Journal of the Medical Sciences 1842; 4: 43–57

3. Duplay, S. De l'hypospadias perineo-scrotal et de son traitement chirurgical. Archives Générales de Médecine 1874; 23: 513–530; 657–690

4. Thiersch, C. Ueber die Entstehungsweise und operative Behandlung der Epispadie. Archiv Heilkunde 1869; 10: 20

5. Anger, M. Th. A recemment présente à la société de chirurgie (séance du 21 janvier, 1874). Reported by M. F. Guyon in Bull. Soc. Nat. Chir. 1915; 1: 188

6. Nove'Josserand, G. Traitment de Chypospadias; nouvelle méthode. Lyon méd. 1897; 85: 198–200

7. Ombredanne, L. Précis Clinique et Médical Operative de Chirurgie Infantile 1932, 3rd edn. Paris: Masson et Cie; 851

8. Horton, C. E., Devine, C. J., Jr. Simulated erection of the penis with saline injection: a diagnostic maneuver. Plastic and Reconstructive Surgry 1977; 59: 138–139

9. Horton, C. E., Devine, C. J. Jr., Crawford, H. H., Adamson, J. E., Devine, T. C., Devine, C. J. Sr. A one-stage hypospadias repair. In: Transaction of the 3rd International Congress of Plastic Surgery: 1963, 900–903. Washington, D.C, Excepta Medica, 1964

10. Bialas, R. F., Horton, C. E., Devine, C. J. The adaptability of the glans flap in hypospadias repair. Plastic and Reconstructive Surgery. 1977; 60: 416–420

11. Broadbent, T. R., Woolf, R. M., Toksu, E. Hypospadias: one stage repair. Plastic and Reconstructive Surgery 1961; 27: 154–159

12. Hodgson, N. B. A one stage hypospadias repair. Journal of Urology 1970; 104: 281–283

13. Toksu, E. Hypospadias, one stage repair. Plastic and Reconstructive Surgery 1970; 45: 365–369

14. Byars, L. T. A technique for consistently satisfactory repairs of hypospadias. Surgery Gynecology and Obstetrics 1955; 100: 184–190

15. Wray, R. C., Ribaude, J. M., Weeks, P. M. The Byars hypospadias repair. A review of 253 consecutive patients. Plastic and Reconstructive Surgery 1976; 58: 329–331

16. Brown, D. Hypospadias. Postgraduate Medical Journal 1949; 25: 367–372

17. Cecil, A. B. Modern treatment of hypospadias. Journal of Urology 1952; 67: 1006–1011

18. Culp, O. S. Experience with 200 hypospadias, evolution of a therapeutic plan. Surgical Clinics of North America 1959; 39: 1007–1023

19. Van der Meulen, J. C. The correction of hypospadias. Plastic and Reconstructive Surgery 1977; 59: 206–215

20. Mustardé, J. C. One stage correction of distal hypospadias and other penile fistulae. British Journal of Plastic Surgery 1965; 18: 413–422

21. Nove'Josserand, G. Resultats éloignes de l'urethroplastie par la tunnellisation et la greffe dermo-epidermique dans les formes graves de l'hypospadias et de l'epispadias. Journal d'Urologie Médicale et Chirurgicale 1914; 5: 393–406

Further reading

Blair, V., Brown, J. B. The correction of scrotal hypospadias and epispadias. Surgery, Gynecology and Obstetrics. 1933; 57: 646–653

Bucknall, R. T. H. A new operation for penile hypospadias. Lancet 1907; 2: 887–890

Horton, C. E. (Ed.) Plastic and Reconstructive Surgery of the Genital Area. Boston: Little, Brown & Co., 1973

Horton, C. E., Devine, C. J. Jr., Crawford, H. H., Adamson, J. E. One hundred one-stage hypospadias repairs. In: Transactions of the 4th International Congress of Plastic and Reconstructive Surgery 1967; 962–964. Amsterdam; Excepta Medica. 1969

Horton, C. E., Devine, C. J., Jr. Hypospadias. In: Plastic Surgery in Infancy and Childhood, Ed. Mastardé, J. C. Philadelphia: W. B. Saunders, 1971: 396–426

Horton, C. E., Devine, C. J., Jr. Hypospadias and epispadias. CIBA Clinical Symposia 1972; 24: (3)

Horton, C. E., Devine, C. J., Jr. Urethral fistulas. In: Plastic and Reconstructive Surgery of the Genital Area, Ed. Horton, C. E. Boston: Little, Brown & Co., 1973: 397–403

Horton, C. E. et al. Hypospadias, epispadias, and exstrophy of the bladder. In: Plastic Surgery, Eds. Grabb, W. C., Smith, J. W. Boston: Little, Brown & Co., 1973

Mayo, C. H. Hypospadias. Journal of the American Medical Association 1901; 36: 1157. Quoted by C. D. Creevy. The correction of hypospadias: A review. Urological Survey 1958; 8: 2–47

McCormack, R. M. Simultaneous chordee repair and urethral reconstruction for hypospadias; experimental and clinical studies. Plastic and Reconstructive Surgery 1954; 13: 257

Congenital absence of the vagina

Percy Jayes FRCS
Formerly Consultant Plastic Surgeon, St Bartholomew's Hospital, London and
Queen Victoria Hospital, East Grinstead, Sussex, UK

Introduction

Congenital absence of the vagina is an uncommon condition for which many widely different types of operation have been devised. Isolated loops of bowel have been used to make a vagina but this method is unpopular in view of the complexity of the operation and the troublesome mucus discharge from the cavity. Williams[1] has described a simple operation which is essentially a high perineorrhaphy that is particularly suitable for minor cases of shortening of the vagina.

The standard method of vaginal reconstruction is to dissect a space between the bladder and rectum and to insert therein a mould carrying a split-skin graft as described by McIndoe and Read[2].

In most cases the external genitalia are normal, the vagina is completely absent and the uterus is represented by a nubbin of fibrous tissue. Occasionally a functioning uterus is present.

The operation

1

With the patient in the lithotomy position, the labia are retracted and a vertical incision is made in the vulval dimple. The space between the bladder and rectum is opened up, mainly by blunt dissection with fingers and blunt scissors. A sound in the urethra identifies that structure but particular care must be exercised not to damage the rectal wall posteriorly. It is sometimes helpful to introduce a finger into the rectum. In the event of perforation of the rectal wall the operation should be abandoned and a further attempt made after an interval of about 3 months.

The dissection continues until a cavity is created which is approximately the size of the normal vagina. Every effort is made to ensure complete haemostasis and a temporary pack is introduced into the cavity.

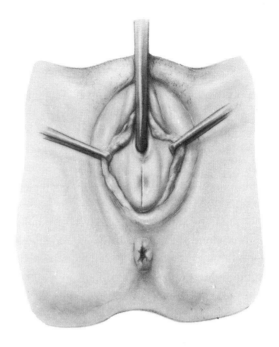

1

2, 3 & 4

The patient is taken down from the lithotomy position while a medium-thickness split-skin graft, measuring at least 24 × 10 cm, is cut from the inner aspect of the thigh, The graft must be in one piece and not too thin, otherwise it may tear while being stitched or inserted.

The graft is folded in half with the raw surface outwards and the lateral edges are sewn together with fine plain catgut on an atraumatic needle in order to produce a skin-lined sack. A large Fergusson speculum is introduced into the skin sack and a cylinder of polyurethane foam is pushed inside the speculum slightly projecting from its distal end. The donor area on the thigh is dressed with tulle gras, dry gauze, cottonwool and a crêpe bandage.

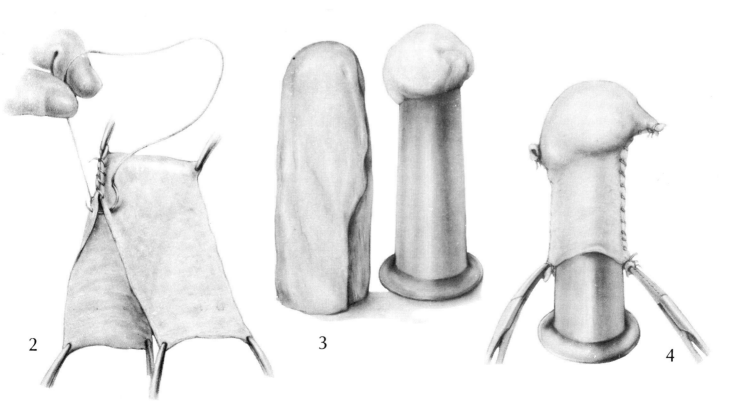

2   3   4

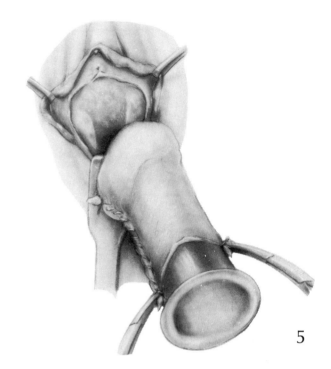

5

5 & 6

The patient is put back in the lithotomy position and the speculum carrying the skin graft is gently introduced into the vaginal cavity. The polyurethane foam is then pushed on into the skin sack and the speculum is withdrawn.

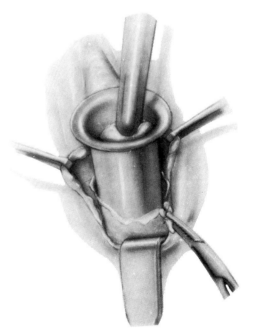

6

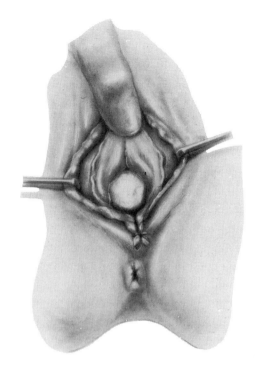

7

7 & 8

The operation is completed by suturing the labia together over the foam. A self-retaining catheter is introduced into the bladder and a pad and T-bandage applied over the vulva. The patient is put on a systemic antibiotic and kept in bed at rest.

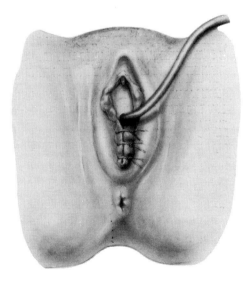

8

9

Ten to 14 days later the patient is again anaesthetized and put in the lithotomy position. The stitches in the labia are removed and the foam gently taken out of the cavity which is then irrigated with normal saline solution. After carefully trimming away any loose excess skin, an acrylic mould is inserted. The labia are split longitudinally and sutured together to form a strong barrier in the perineum. This keeps the mould in place for 3 or 4 months until the contractile phase of the graft is over. The perineum is then opened up and the mould removed.

The advantages of using polyurethane foam initially[3] rather than the acrylic mould are:

1. greater comfort for the patient in the immediate postoperative period;
2. the risk of serious complications, especially rectovaginal fistula and occasionally urethrovaginal fistula due to pressure necrosis from the rigid mould, is completely avoided;
3. the cylinder of foam is about a third larger in all dimensions than the normal vagina and soft, even pressure is maintained over the whole of the cavity;
4. the graft is kept in close contact with the walls of the vagina and this ensures a complete take of the graft and minimal risk of postoperative haemorrhage.

In rare cases with a functioning uterus the same technique is used initially, but after removal of the foam a plastic dilator is fitted with a central lumen to allow free exit of menstrual blood.

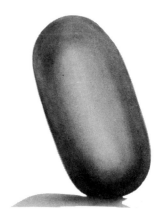

9

After completion of the reconstruction no special care is necessary but in the absence of regular sexual intercourse patients are advised to insert the acrylic mould occasionally to make sure that no contraction of the vaginal cavity is occurring.

References

1. Williams, E. A. Congenital absence of the vagina: a simple operation for its relief. Journal of Obstetrics and Gynaecology of the British Commonwealth. 1964; 71: 511–512

2. McIndoe, A. Treatment of congenital absence and obliterative conditions of the vagina. British Journal of Plastic Surgery 1950; 2: 254–267

3. Jayes, P. H. The establishment of the speciality of plastic surgery and its contributions to other specialities. Annals of the Royal College of Surgeons of England. 1966; 38: 210–218

Index